Rare Liver and Biliary Tract Diseases

Thilo Hackert • Aiste Gulla
Editors

Rare Liver and Biliary Tract Diseases

Surgical Management

Springer

Editors
Thilo Hackert, MD
General, Visceral, Thoracic Surgery
University Hospital Hamburg-Eppendorf
Hamburg, Hamburg, Germany

Aiste Gulla, MD, PhD, FACS
Clinic of Surgery
Gastroenterology and Nephrourology,
Institute of Clinical Medicine,
Faculty of Medicine
Vilnius, Lithuania

Department of Surgery
George Washington University,
School of Medicine and Health Sciences
Washington, DC, USA

ISBN 978-3-032-15075-2 ISBN 978-3-032-15076-9 (eBook)
https://doi.org/10.1007/978-3-032-15076-9

This Springer imprint is published by the registered company Springer Nature Switzerland AG
The registered company address is: Gewerbestrasse 11, 6330 Cham, Switzerland

Preface

The liver and biliary tract, though often overshadowed by more commonly discussed organ systems, play a central role in human physiology. Within this complex and vital domain lies a subset of conditions that are not only rare but also diagnostically and therapeutically challenging. *Rare Liver and Biliary Tract Diseases* is a timely and essential contribution to surgical practice, offering a comprehensive exploration of these often-overlooked disorders.

This textbook brings together the collective expertise of leading hepatologists, gastroenterologists, pathologists, and researchers from around the world. It serves as both a clinical guide and a scientific reference, bridging the gap between cutting-edge research and bedside care. From genetic cholestatic syndromes to rare hepatic tumors, from autoimmune biliary disorders to metabolic liver diseases, the chapters within provide clarity, depth, and practical insight.

What sets this work apart is its commitment to precision and accessibility. Each chapter is meticulously crafted to support clinicians in making accurate diagnoses, understanding pathophysiological mechanisms, and navigating the complexities of treatment in the context of limited evidence and evolving guidelines.

As rare diseases often demand a multidisciplinary approach and a high index of suspicion, this textbook will be an invaluable resource not only for hepatology specialists but also for internists, pediatricians, radiologists, and surgeons who may encounter these conditions in their practice.

In an era where personalized medicine and rare disease research are gaining unprecedented momentum, this book stands as a testament to the importance of knowledge, collaboration, and compassion in the care of patients with rare liver and biliary tract diseases.

Hamburg, Germany — Thilo Hackert
Washington, DC, USA — Aiste Gulla

Acknowledgement

Prof. T. Hackert and Prof. A. Gulla extend their sincere appreciation to their colleagues, friends, and fellow surgeons worldwide—Europe, Japan, and across the United States—whose dedication to advancing the understanding of rare liver and biliary tract diseases made this textbook possible. This truly international collaboration, grounded in exceptional expertise, rigorous scholarship, and a common commitment to hepatobiliary surgery, has shaped every chapter of this work.

Contents

1 Alagille Syndrome

Alberto Ferrarese, Lara Biribin, and Patrizia Burra

Abbreviations

ALGS	Alagille syndrome
BA	Biliary atresia
LT	Liver transplantation
PEBD	Partial external biliary diversion
QoL	Quality of life

1.1 Introduction

Alagille syndrome (ALGS) is a rare multisystemic disorder with autosomal dominant inheritance and a wide variability in clinical features, usually diagnosed during neonatal or paediatric age. First described in 1969 by Daniel Alagille [1], this syndrome typically involves the liver, heart, eyes, skeleton, face, vasculature, and kidneys [2]. The estimated incidence is between 1:30.000 and 1:50.000 live births, many cases perhaps being still undiagnosed because several patients with genetic mutations may only have mild clinical features [3].

1.2 Pathogenesis

JAG1 gene mutation has been found in 94–96% of ALGS patients, whereas a minority is affected by NOTCH2 mutations. Most mutations are acquired de novo and cause the disease through a haploinsufficiency mechanism (i.e. the loss of a single allele determines a reduced production of a protein, which is insufficient to support downstream function).

The Notch pathway is involved in intercellular signalling and becomes essential for promoting cell differentiation in many organs (e.g. liver, heart, and skeleton) during foetal age. Mammalian Notch signal transduction requires transmembrane receptors that, after interaction with Notch-specific ligands (such as the JAGGED protein), send transcriptional signals to the nucleus.

In the liver of mammalian embryos, cholangiocyte differentiation from multipotential hepatoblasts activates the expression of specific keratins (such as CK-19) and transcription factors (such as SOX9) that distinguish cholangiocytes from hepatocytes. Cholangiocytes then acquire a polarization and a spatial positioning, forming simple ductules (namely, intrahepatic biliary ducts) [4]. Notch signalling plays a key role in cholangiocyte differentiation, their spatial localization near the portal vein, and the formation of intrahepatic biliary ducts [5]. Therefore, mutations of the JAG1 gene,

A. Ferrarese · L. Biribin · P. Burra (✉)
Multivisceral Transplant Unit, Gastroenterology, Padua University Hospital, Padua, Italy
e-mail: alberto.ferrarese@unipd.it; lara.biribin@aopd.veneto.it; burra@unipd.it

T. Hackert, A. Gulla (eds.), *Rare Liver and Biliary Tract Diseases*,
https://doi.org/10.1007/978-3-032-15076-9_1

impairing Notch-mediated activation of intercellular signalling during embryogenesis, affect this process.

The pathophysiology of such a disease is even more complex, however. Indeed, experimental mouse models demonstrate that, post-natally, cholangiocytes may be able to alleviate cholestasis through the formation of de novo intrahepatic biliary ducts despite the persistent Notch inactivation [6], suggesting that more pathways are involved. Additionally, abnormalities on vascular architecture, close to intrahepatic biliary ducts, have been observed in such a disease [7]. Histological studies showed that the loss of function of Notch signalling also influences repair mechanisms. Indeed, ALGS livers are characterized by few reactive ductular cells and low-degree fibrosis (especially if compared with livers affected by biliary atresia (BA)). This point may be of help to understand the relatively mild progression to end-stage liver disease and portal hypertension, if compared with other neonatal cholangiopathies [8].

Considering extrahepatic organs, the multisystemic involvement of ALGS relies on the landmark role played by Notch-mediated signalling during embryogenesis. It stimulates the vascular smooth muscle differentiation of undifferentiated mesenchyme; regulates cardiac specification and ventricular and valvular morphogenesis; promotes segmentation of the axial skeleton, regulates osteoblast and osteoclast differentiation and function; and mediates nephron segmentation [9, 10].

1.3 Clinical Manifestations

ALGS portends a highly variable expressivity. Individuals with the same mutations, including members of the same family, may show discordance in both the overall phenotype and/or severity of the phenotype; therefore, other modifiers (epigenetic or environmental factors) can be implied [11–14].

1.4 Hepatic Manifestations

Hepatic involvement is a common feature, although not invariably observed. *Cholestasis* can vary from mild to severe and cause many complications, the most debilitating of which are jaundice and *pruritus*. The latter usually develops at around 3–6 months of life and may persist despite the resolution of jaundice [2, 15, 16]. Biochemical liver profile mirrors cholestasis (serum bilirubin, bile acids, γ-glutamyl transferase, and alkaline phosphatase), whereas serum aminotransferases are only mildly elevated, and markers of synthetic function are usually normal at presentation. An additional clinical feature related to chronic cholestasis is the development of *xanthomas* as a result of severe hypercholesterolemia. These typically painless lesions appear on the extensor surfaces of the hands and knees, improve with the resolution of cholestasis during childhood, and invariably disappear after liver transplantation (LT) [17]. *Hepatomegaly* is evident in 70–100% of ALGS patients, while splenomegaly is quite uncommon in the early phase but can occur in 70% of patients reaching adulthood, as a result of fibrosis and portal hypertension [12]. Features of *portal hypertension*, such as ascites or GI bleeding, often occur in early adulthood: recent data showed that ascites develops in 22.3–36% of young adult AGLS patients, whereas high-risk varices and GI bleeding develop in 12–16% of ALGS patients, respectively [15, 18].

1.5 Extrahepatic Manifestations

Congenital heart diseases are commonly observed in ALGS patients, occurring in up to 94% [19]. Abnormalities of the pulmonary artery tree, tetralogy of Fallot, pulmonary valve stenosis, and pulmonary atresia are frequently diagnosed during the neonatal age, significantly impairing survival when compared with children without cardiac involvement (6-year survival: 40% vs. 95%) [12, 20, 21]. Notably, survival remains significantly worse even after correction of the cardiac defect if compared with that of patients without cardiovascular defects [22].

A broad range of *vascular abnormalities* has been described in ALGS, the majority involving the cerebrovascular district (cerebral aneurysms, moyamoya syndrome [a progressive intracranial arterial occlusive disease], and dolichoectasia of the internal carotid arteries). Therefore, ALGS patients carry a high risk of ischaemic or haemorrhagic stroke, with a significant impact on mortality [21, 23]. Systemic abnormalities are also found in the abdominal vasculature and should be carefully investigated before abdominal surgery or liver transplantation (LT).

Characteristic *facial and vertebral anomalies* are described in up to 90% and 66% of cases, respectively [12, 24, 25]. The common facial features are a prominent forehead, with a pointed chin, which together create a triangular appearance; protrusion of orbital bones; and hypertelorism. Among skeletal anomalies, the common butterfly vertebrae originate from vertebral bodies, whose anterior arches fail to fuse.

Ocular abnormalities do not typically affect vision but can be helpful for diagnostic purposes. There is a wide range of ocular findings, such as peripheral chorioretinal changes or posterior embryotoxon. The latter has been widely described in ALGS, with variable prevalence across studies, but it is not disease-specific, being detected in healthy children too [26].

Despite not being included in classic diagnostic criteria, recent studies showed that *renal disease* can be found in a large percentage of patients (39–85%) [27, 28]. The most common manifestations are tubular acidosis and chronic kidney disease, which must be carefully investigated at the time of LT or after surgery.

Growth failure has been observed in up to 50–90% of patients affected by ALGS. Its aetiology is multifactorial, related to fat malabsorption, poor caloric and nutrient intake, and repeated hospitalizations. Recent data showed a correlation between growth retardation and the degree of cholestasis, providing useful information about subgroups of children who should be carefully screened for growth retardation and intensively managed [18, 29, 30].

Table 1.1 Common extrahepatic manifestations in Alagille syndrome

Extrahepatic organ(s)	Prevalence	Common manifestations
Heart and lung	Up to 94% of patients have at least one cardiac malformation	Pulmonary artery stenosis Tetralogy of Fallot Pulmonary valve stenosis Pulmonary atresia
Vessels	30%	Cerebral aneurysms Moyamoya syndrome Aorta aneurysm or coarctation
Skeleton	60%	Butterfly vertebrae Square-shaped proximal part of fingers Ulna shortening
Eye	50–90%	Posterior embryotoxon Chorioretinal diseases
Kidney	39–85%	Renal dysplasia Tubular acidosis Chronic kidney disease
Whole body	50–90%	Growth failure Malnutrition

Table 1.1 summarizes the most common extrahepatic manifestations of ALGS.

1.6 Diagnosis

According to the above-mentioned characteristics of ALGS, diagnosis is not always achieved in a timely fashion, especially in patients with mild presentation or low-degree cholestasis. The classic diagnostic criteria of ALGS included biopsy-proven intrahepatic bile duct paucity, in addition to the presence of three out of the following five features: chronic cholestasis, cardiac disease, skeletal anomalies, ocular abnormalities, and characteristic facial features. Nevertheless, with advances in genetic testing, ALGS can be diagnosed in patients who do not fulfil these criteria, especially in the presence of a positive family history. Moreover, *liver biopsy* is no longer required for diagnosis, also given the potential pitfalls (see below), although it remains a useful tool in clinical practice, especially where molecular testing is not available in a timely fashion, in doubtful cases mirroring other cholangiopathies, and for disease staging. The hallmark of liver biopsy in ALGS is bile duct paucity, which is defined when the ratio of interlobular bile ducts to portal tracts is ≤0.5. Bile duct paucity is not always present, especially in biopsies performed at the neonatal age, and is not pathognomonic of ALGS since it can be found in other conditions, such as infections, metabolic diseases, immunological diseases, or drug-related liver injury [31, 32]. Other findings in ALGS liver biopsies may include cholestasis, portal inflammation, and giant cell transformation. As discussed above, fibrosis may be present but in a milder fashion than in livers affected by biliary atresia (BA). Moreover, the latter condition is characterized by ductular proliferation, which is mostly absent in ALGS [12, 33].

Genetic diagnosis confirms clinical suspicion (or clinical diagnosis) in up to 96% of patients. Since most ALGS-associated mutations are found in JAG1 (chromosome 20), sequencing of this gene occurs first, enabling the identification of approximately 90% of mutations. In the absence of an identified mutation in JAG1, sequencing of the NOTCH2 gene (chromosome 1) should be performed since it can identify another 2–3% of mutations. For practical reasons and cost-effectiveness, simultaneous testing of both genes is now carried out by commercially available next-generation sequencing panels [34].

Given the heterogeneous presentation, the unavailability of worldwide gene sequencing, and the above-mentioned pitfalls given by liver biopsy, other techniques have been proposed, not only to diagnose ALGS but also to differentiate this disease from other cholangiopathies, especially BA. Ultrasound and magnetic resonance cholangiopancreatography may highlight a small gall bladder, abnormalities of the gall bladder wall, and common bile duct non-visualization. However, these conditions are not specific and are seen in a variable percentage of cases, thereby carrying low diagnostic accuracy. Intraoperative cholangiography, usually performed before Kasai portoenterostomy, is useful to evaluate the common bile duct, which is commonly not visualized in BA. This point is of interest since a misdiagnosed ALGS patient undergoing Kasai portoenterostomy may be associated with a poorer prognosis [35].

In view of the multiple extrahepatic manifestations, a patient with clinically diagnosed or genetically proven ALGS should undergo several evaluations after diagnosis, including cardiac ultrasound, antero-posterior and lateral chest Rx, renal function tests and renal ultrasound, ophthalmologic evaluation, nutritional assessment, and measurement of growth parameters. Finally, genetic counselling for family screening is advised [36].

1.7 Disease Course and Quality of Life

The natural history of ALGS is not easily predictable at the time of diagnosis, especially regarding the liver-related outcome. However, data coming from multicentre studies gave basic prognostic information that can help in identifying those patients at the highest (or lowest) risk of progression. Indeed, we have learnt that children with mild liver disease in early childhood rarely have disease progression in later life and that there is no late onset of cholestasis (e.g. beyond childhood). According to a multicentre study, simple biochemical parameters (bilirubin, transaminases, and platelets) showed a linear relationship with the risk of death or liver transplantation. As an example, children having lower bilirubin levels within 12 months of age showed a significantly better overall and transplant-free survival. Conversely, high bilirubin levels (≥10.0 mg/dl) predicted the likelihood of developing clinically significant portal hypertension and its manifestations (ascites and variceal bleeding) [15]. Recent data have demonstrated a possible prognostic role of liver stiffness measurements in paediatric cholangiopathies, including ALGS: further (and larger) data are awaited [37]. Considering the natural history and long-term follow-up, the leading causes of death are liver-related (22%), followed by heart-related and non-cardiovascular complications [15].

Given the multisystemic involvement, ALGS patients have a significantly impaired QoL. In a study by Elisofon et al., poor QoL has been associated with repeated cardiac invasive procedures and depression. Factors that could contribute to the psychological burden include short stature, delayed pubertal maturation, pruritus, and other physical disabilities [38]. Indeed, another study showed that QoL was significantly reduced when compared with that of patients with alpha1-antitrypsin deficiency, especially in physical domain scores, growth failure being a major determinant [39].

1.8 Preliminary Considerations Regarding the Management of ALGS

Like other multisystemic diseases, ALGS is a complex condition that requires a multidimensional and multidisciplinary management, involving many healthcare professionals, such as (transplant) hepatologists, (transplant) surgeons, anaesthesiologists, cardiologists, paediatricians, and psychologists. Therefore, referral to tertiary centres appears to be of utmost importance to achieve the most appropriate management.

Unlike other conditions, the phenotype is protean, and several complications can occur at different ages. Therefore, patients and families require a longitudinal—as smooth as possible—follow-up, including psychological counselling whenever needed and medical counselling tailored to issues arising throughout life stages (e.g. schooling, sexuality, pregnancy, and transition from child to adult healthcare services), such as for other chronic liver diseases or after LT [40–43]. Finally, the complexity of care for ALGS patients is associated with significant healthcare resource utilization, as well as an economic burden for families. According to recently published data, healthcare resource utilization has been estimated to be up to 70 times the average annual healthcare expenditure for healthy children, being higher than patients with chronic liver diseases, such as BA [44]. This issue should be highlighted, especially to policymakers.

1.9 Medical Treatment of Hepatic Manifestations in ALGS

The first point to consider is that no effective medical treatment for ALGS has yet been developed. Therefore, the management of cholestasis-related complications is the backbone in symptomatic patients, together with the treatment of portal hypertension in those with advanced liver disease. Until recent years, *pruritus* treatment shared commonalities with other cholestatic diseases, including the use of ursodeoxycholic acid [45], antihistamines, cholestyramine, rifampin, or a combination of two or more drugs. Recently, the landscape has changed after the publication of interesting data from preliminary trials on apical sodium-dependent bile acid transporter inhibitors (odevixibat and maralixibat) [46–48]. Robust data came from a study published in *The Lancet* that showed a significant reduction of serum bile acids in patients treated with maralixibat when compared with a placebo, with a concurrent reduction of pruritus and an improvement in QoL [49]. Results were consistent after the extension of follow-up [50]. It is not currently known, however, if these new drugs represent game changers in the natural history of the disease or if they may be used only for pruritus relief.

As in other cholestatic diseases, hypercholesterolemia does not carry a significant risk of atherosclerosis and should be treated only in the presence of other cardiovascular risk factors, which are often uncommon at a young age [51].

Correction of fat-soluble vitamin deficiency typically starts by mouth, but parenteral formulations can be considered if serum levels remain inadequate. Prothrombin time should be reassessed in patients with advanced cholestatic disease after vitamin K supplementation in order to rule out prolongations due to vitamin K malabsorption. Regarding *growth retardation and malnutrition*, parents and children should be counselled about food, especially in those with profound cholestasis. Since medium-chain triglycerides do not require micellar formation for absorption, they should be added to the everyday diet. Supplemental caloric intake by nasogastric tube (or by percutaneous gastrostomy) can be considered in the sickest patients. Low *bone mineral density*, usually associated with cholestasis and growth retardation, should be diagnosed and treated whenever possible [52].

Regarding *portal hypertension*, ALGS patients require management and surveillance through the same algorithms as patients with other chronic, advanced liver diseases [53]. Hepatocellular carcinoma is a rare complication, and anecdotal cases have been reported. It may arise both in underlying cirrhotic livers and in patients without cirrhosis. It should not be confused with the commonly seen regenerative liver nodules, which do not possess malignant potential [54, 55]. Anyway, surveillance for hepatocellular carcinoma through ultrasound is advised, at least in patients with advanced disease, even if specific guidelines have not been developed to date.

Finally, the management of patients with ALGS should aim at improving their global health, including QoL. Notably, pruritus, severity of liver disease, and extrahepatic comorbidities have been associated with worse QoL, and this is expected. However, other important features (xanthomas and low height) may reflect a stigma that should be remembered and faced by healthcare professionals.

According to the data coming from large registries, more than 40% of ALGS patients will reach 18 years of age without transplantation. Therefore, genetic counselling for fertility and pregnancy should be available, as well as close follow-up during childbearing and early after delivery [43]. Although guidelines for the management of pregnancy in ALGS have not been established to date—due to its rarity—chorionic villus sampling may represent a useful tool to screen for the presence of the classical JAGGED1 gene mutation in the foetus of an affected mother if the associated liver dysfunction does not represent a contraindication. Non-invasive prenatal screening tests can have a promising role too. They can be applied not only in cases with a positive family history but also when the foetal ultrasound shows abnormalities [56]. Pregnancy outcome has rarely been described in women with ALGS. Of the 31 pregnancies reported in a recently published series, only 11 were successful. Foetal growth restriction was present in seven pregnancies, pre-eclampsia in two, and postpartum maternal pulmonary oedema in one [57]. Possible causative factors for foetal growth restriction in women with ALGS include toxicity from bile acids, maternal vascular disease resulting in placental dysfunction, and alteration in placental growth factors. Considering mothers' health, the severity of liver disease, the presence of portal hypertension, and cardiac dysfunction and pulmonary hypertension should be carefully evaluated before conception and managed during pregnancy and delivery.

Available therapeutic options, according to the common signs and symptoms, are summarized in Table 1.2.

Table 1.2 Medical and surgical options for Alagille syndrome, according to signs/symptoms

Sign/symptom	Type of treatment	Therapy
Pruritus	Medical	Ursodeoxycholic acid Antihistamines Cholestyramine Rifampin Apical sodium-dependent bile acid transporter inhibitors
	Surgical	PEBD Ileal exclusion Liver transplantation
Fat-soluble vitamin deficit	Medical	Oral (and/or parenteral) vitamin D and K supplementation
Growth retardation	Medical	Enteral (or, in rare cases, parenteral) supplemental nutrition
	Surgical	Liver transplantation
Features of portal hypertension	Medical	Management as the standard of care for patients with cirrhosis
End-stage liver disease	Medical	Management as the standard of care for patients with cirrhosis
	Surgical	Liver transplantation

1.10 Surgical Treatment of Hepatic Manifestations in ALGS

There are three main surgical options that commonly involve patients with ALGS: Kasai portoenterostomy, biliary diversions, and liver transplantation (LT).

Kasai portoenterostomy represents the treatment of choice in patients with BA, which is the most common inherited cholangiopathy. Differential diagnosis between BA and ALGS is often difficult, especially at the neonatal age, even after the performance of liver biopsy or cholangiograms; therefore, several ALGS patients misdiagnosed with BA still undergo portoenterostomy. The surgical technique consists of the excision of extrahepatic bile duct remnants and the gall bladder and the end-to-side anastomosis between the portal plate and jejunum mobilized in a Roux-en-Y loop. The prognostic role of Kasai portoenterostomy in ALGS has been debated, with doubts of a potentially detrimental outcome being raised from small cohorts [58]. Recently published data from a large multicentre registry showed that 102 out of 1184 (9%) ALGS patients underwent Kasai portoenterostomy: these patients seemed to have a threefold higher risk of death/LT than patients who did not undergo surgery [15].

The primary aim of *biliary diversions* is to improve the quality of life and children's symptoms (especially pruritus) through a reduction of total bile acids. This can be achieved both by diverting bile acids and reducing the enterohepatic cycle. Nevertheless, biliary diversions do not halt the pathophysiology of ALGS; therefore, they should be reserved for patients having (mild-to-severe) cholestasis causing pruritus but no liver failure. Moreover, improvements in pruritus persist for a limited period of life. As an example, ileal exclusion may elicit a counterregulatory mechanism of increased bile acid reabsorption in the remaining ileum [59].

Among biliary diversions, the most common is partial external biliary diversion (PEBD), which has been proposed since 1988 as an effective surgical option for pruritus relief [59–61]. In this procedure, the gall bladder content is externally drained through a jejunal conduit, providing an improvement in pruritus. Several technical modifications have been proposed, such as the laparoscopic approach, the use of a gastrostomy tube to divert the gall bladder content, and cholecysto-appendicostomy [62–64]. Partial internal biliary diversion has the same aim as PEBD, without the presence of the external stoma. Usually, through a jejunal conduit, the gall bladder content flows into the colon, bypassing enterohepatic circulation [65, 66]. The potential oncogenic role of bile flow into colic mucosa has not yet been extensively studied; therefore, routine surveillance colonoscopies have been advocated. There are a few contraindications to PEBD, the most important being a previous cholecystectomy. Moreover, the site of stoma placement should be chosen carefully in order to avoid displacements or dysfunctions during the child's growth. The main complications reported after PEBD are high-volume stoma output (which often leads to conversion to ileal exclusion or LT), bleeding from anastomosis or from stomal varices, stoma dysfunction, and cholangitis.

Ileal exclusion creates an entero-colic anastomosis between the ileum and—usually—the ascending colon, aiming at "excluding" the terminal ileum, where bile salts are usually absorbed. According to the above-mentioned retrospective study [15], only 5% of patients underwent biliary diversion during their life, usually at 2 years of age.

Liver transplantation (LT) has become an effective treatment option for ALGS patients, even if it remains a minor indication among cholestatic diseases. According to the European Database, from 1968 to 2017, only 334 out of 14,515 children (2%) underwent LT for ALGS [67]. According to the Italian National Transplant Center Registry, 53 paediatric LTs have been performed for ALGS in Italy between 2002 and 2020, accounting for 3.6% of all paediatric LTs in Italy during the same period. Forty-eight were deceased-donor LTs, whereas five were living-donor LTs (3.6% and 3.8% of deceased-donor and living-donor transplants performed during the above-mentioned period, respectively).

Primary *indications* for LT in ALGS children are complications of cholestasis (debilitating pruritus, growth failure, and metabolic bone disease), liver failure, and severe portal hypertension.

The peculiar multisystemic presentation, as well as the disease stage at the time of transplant evaluation; possible abnormalities; and prior surgery require careful consideration and thorough preoperative planning. Similarly, these unique features should be taken into account for a tailored post-transplant management, with immunosuppression schedules without steroids at least in osteopenic patients and non-teratogenic drugs (Fig. 1.1).

Before transplant, a thorough evaluation of *cardiac* function should be carefully performed at trained centres through invasive investigation, focusing on right ventricular function and pulmonary arterial pressure. Indeed, acute heart failure and fluid overload can commonly be seen intraoperatively, especially in patients with right ven-

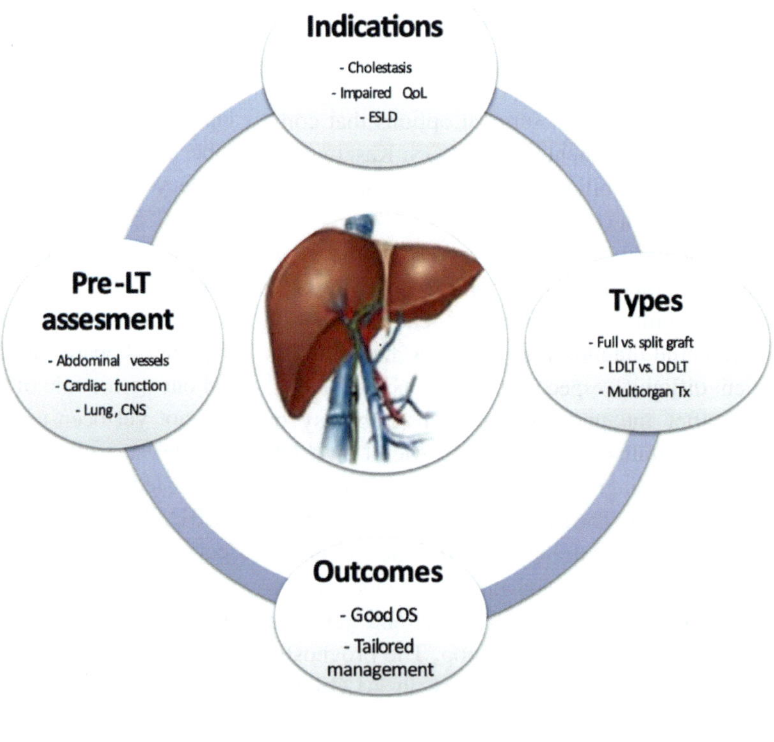

Fig. 1.1 Liver transplantation in Alagille syndrome: indication, pre-transplant assessment, type of transplant, and outcomes. Abbreviations: ESLD: end-stage liver disease, LDLT: living-donor liver transplantation, DDLT: deceased-donor liver transplantation, OS: overall survival, and CNS: central nervous system

tricular hypertrophy, who are not able to cope with fluid overload [68–70].

Cerebral vessel abnormalities, pulmonary vasculature disease, and kidney dysfunction should be carefully investigated and, when diagnosed, corrected prior to transplant whenever possible [71, 72]. To date, few cases of combined liver–kidney transplants have been described [73]. Angiography may be of help as a preliminary study in cases of small-calibre hepatic artery, median arcuate ligament, or other vascular abnormalities. When standard vascular anastomoses (e.g. termino-terminal donor to recipient hepatic artery anastomosis) are precluded, pre-surgical planning involving experienced surgeons should be attempted [74, 75]. Previous abdominal surgeries, such as PEBD or Kasai portoenterostomy, may make LT much harder, even if they do not influence post-LT survival [76].

Regarding the type of transplant, a few cases of living-donor LT from parents have been collected and published. Given the autosomal dominant transmission of the disease, as well as the protean disease phenotype, a careful evaluation of the donor—including genetic testing and liver biopsy—is warranted [77, 78]. The recipient's age and size (given the risk of growth retardation) are essential information for considering full-size vs. split LT. Notably, most ALGS patients usually undergo LT at a paediatric age, but transplantations in adulthood, allocating full-size grafts, have been described [79].

Even if congenital biliary diseases have the best post-LT outcome among paediatric indications, ALGS patient survival seems worse than that of matched patients with BA, probably due to extrahepatic comorbidities that impair early post-operative outcomes [80]. More recently, Black et al. analysed the outcomes of ALGS patients transplanted before reaching 21 years of age and compared those with matched patients transplanted for biliary atresia between 2002 and 2018. The cumulative 1-, 3-, and 5-year patient survival rates were 95.2%, 94.2%, and 94.2% in ALGS, without a significant difference if compared with patients with BA (97.9%, 97.5%, and 97.5%, respectively), even if ALGS patients more commonly had a diagnosis of heart disease and a history of cardiac interventions [81]. In Italy, the largest case series published to date on LT for ALGS (21 patients) confirmed a good post-operative outcome (1- and 5-year patient and graft survival: 90% and 85% and 80% and 75%, respectively) [82]. Composite goals going beyond survival must be pursued in ALGS LT patients. For instance, growth, improvement of QoL, metabolic diseases, and mental health are other significant end points [83–85]. According to a preliminary study by Elisofon et al. [38], there was no difference in QoL between children with ALGS who underwent transplantation and those who did not, but this topic certainly requires further investigation [38]. A careful management of immunosuppression must be pursued too, taking into account recipients' age, schooling, and chronic kidney disease, in order to provide the simplest, safest scheme possible, balancing the risk of rejection and adherence [86].

Acknowledgement We are grateful to Dr. Silvia Trapani (Italian National Transplant Center, National Institute of Health) for providing data about paediatric liver transplantation for Alagille syndrome in Italy.

References

1. Alagille D, Odièvre M, Gautier M, Dommergues JP. Hepatic ductular hypoplasia associated with characteristic facies, vertebral malformations, retarded physical, mental, and sexual development, and cardiac murmur. J Pediatr. 1975;86(1):63–71.
2. Mitchell E, Gilbert M, Loomes KM. Alagille Syndrome. Clin Liver Dis. 2018;22(4):625–41.
3. Leonard LD, Chao G, Baker A, Loomes K, Spinner NB. Clinical utility gene card for: Alagille Syndrome (ALGS). Eur J Hum Genet. 2014;22(3):435.
4. Takashima Y, Terada M, Kawabata M, Suzuki A. Dynamic three-dimensional morphogenesis of intrahepatic bile ducts in mouse liver development. Hepatology. 2015;61(3):1003–11.
5. Kodama Y, Hijikata M, Kageyama R, Shimotohno K, Chiba T. The role of notch signaling in the development of intrahepatic bile ducts. Gastroenterology. 2004;127(6):1775–86.
6. Thakurdas SM, Lopez MF, Kakuda S, Fernandez-Valdivia R, Zarrin-Khameh N, Haltiwanger RS, et al. Jagged1 heterozygosity in mice results in a congenital cholangiopathy which is reversed by concomitant deletion of one copy of Poglut1 (Rumi). Hepatology. 2016;63(2):550–65.

7. Strazzabosco M, Fabris L. Development of the bile ducts: essentials for the clinical hepatologist. J Hepatol. 2012;56(5):1159–70.
8. Fabris L, Fiorotto R, Spirli C, Cadamuro M, Mariotti V, Perugorria MJ, et al. Pathobiology of inherited biliary diseases: a roadmap to understand acquired liver diseases. Nat Rev Gastroenterol Hepatol. 2019;16(8):497–511.
9. MacGrogan D, Münch J, de la Pompa JL. Notch and interacting signalling pathways in cardiac development, disease, and regeneration. Nat Rev Cardiol. 2018;15(11):685–704.
10. Zanotti S, Canalis E. Notch signaling in skeletal health and disease. Eur J Endocrinol. 2013;168(6):R95–103.
11. Kamath BM, Bason L, Piccoli DA, Krantz ID, Spinner NB. Consequences of JAG1 mutations. J Med Genet. 2003;40(12):891–5.
12. Emerick KM, Rand EB, Goldmuntz E, Krantz ID, Spinner NB, Piccoli DA. Features of Alagille syndrome in 92 patients: frequency and relation to prognosis. Hepatology. 1999;29(3):822–9.
13. Elmslie FV, Vivian AJ, Gardiner H, Hall C, Mowat AP, Winter RM. Alagille syndrome: family studies. J Med Genet. 1995;32(4):264–8.
14. Izumi K, Hayashi D, Grochowski CM, Kubota N, Nishi E, Arakawa M, et al. Discordant clinical phenotype in monozygotic twins with Alagille syndrome: possible influence of non-genetic factors. Am J Med Genet A. 2016;170A(2):471–5.
15. Vandriel SM, Li LT, She H, Wang JS, Gilbert MA, Jankowska I, et al. Natural history of liver disease in a large international cohort of children with Alagille syndrome: results from the GALA study. Hepatology. 2023;77(2):512–29.
16. Subramaniam P, Knisely A, Portmann B, Qureshi SA, Aclimandos WA, Karani JB, et al. Diagnosis of Alagille syndrome-25 years of experience at King's College Hospital. J Pediatr Gastroenterol Nutr. 2011;52(1):84–9.
17. Garcia MA, Ramonet M, Ciocca M, Cabrera H, Lapunzina P, Alvarez E, et al. Alagille syndrome: cutaneous manifestations in 38 children. Pediatr Dermatol. 2005;22(1):11–4.
18. Kamath BM, Ye W, Goodrich NP, Loomes KM, Romero R, Heubi JE, et al. Outcomes of childhood cholestasis in Alagille syndrome: results of a multicenter observational study. Hepatol Commun. 2020;4(3):387–98.
19. McElhinney DB, Krantz ID, Bason L, Piccoli DA, Emerick KM, Spinner NB, et al. Analysis of cardiovascular phenotype and genotype-phenotype correlation in individuals with a JAG1 mutation and/or Alagille syndrome. Circulation. 2002;106(20):2567–74.
20. Fattouh AM, Mogahed EA, Abdel Hamid N, Sobhy R, Saber N, El-Karaksy H. The prevalence of congenital heart defects in infants with cholestatic disorders of infancy: a single-centre study. Arch Dis Child. 2016;101(9):803–7.
21. Kamath BM, Spinner NB, Emerick KM, Chudley AE, Booth C, Piccoli DA, et al. Vascular anomalies in Alagille syndrome: a significant cause of morbidity and mortality. Circulation. 2004;109(11):1354–8.
22. Bauser-Heaton H, Borquez A, Han B, Ladd M, Asija R, Downey L, et al. Programmatic approach to management of tetralogy of fallot with major aortopulmonary collateral arteries: a 15-year experience with 458 patients. Circ Cardiovasc Interv. 2017;10(4):e004952.
23. Emerick KM, Krantz ID, Kamath BM, Darling C, Burrowes DM, Spinner NB, et al. Intracranial vascular abnormalities in patients with Alagille syndrome. J Pediatr Gastroenterol Nutr. 2005;41(1):99–107.
24. Sanderson E, Newman V, Haigh SF, Baker A, Sidhu PS. Vertebral anomalies in children with Alagille syndrome: an analysis of 50 consecutive patients. Pediatr Radiol. 2002;32(2):114–9.
25. Sokol RJ, Heubi JE, Balistreri WF. Intrahepatic "cholestasis facies": is it specific for Alagille syndrome? J Pediatr. 1983;103(2):205–8.
26. da Palma MM, Igelman AD, Ku C, Burr A, You JY, Place EM, et al. Characterization of the spectrum of ophthalmic changes in patients with Alagille syndrome. Invest Ophthalmol Vis Sci. 2021;62(7):27.
27. Di Pinto D, Adragna M. Renal manifestations in children with Alagille syndrome. Arch Argent Pediatr. 2018;116(2):149–53.
28. Kamath BM, Podkameni G, Hutchinson AL, Leonard LD, Gerfen J, Krantz ID, et al. Renal anomalies in Alagille syndrome: a disease-defining feature. Am J Med Genet A. 2012;158A(1):85–9.
29. Rovner AJ, Schall JI, Jawad AF, Piccoli DA, Stallings VA, Mulberg AE, et al. Rethinking growth failure in Alagille syndrome: the role of dietary intake and steatorrhea. J Pediatr Gastroenterol Nutr. 2002;35(4):495–502.
30. Arvay JL, Zemel BS, Gallagher PR, Rovner AJ, Mulberg AE, Stallings VA, et al. Body composition of children aged 1 to 12 years with biliary atresia or Alagille syndrome. J Pediatr Gastroenterol Nutr. 2005;40(2):146–50.
31. Hoffenberg EJ, Narkewicz MR, Sondheimer JM, Smith DJ, Silverman A, Sokol RJ. Outcome of syndromic paucity of interlobular bile ducts (Alagille syndrome) with onset of cholestasis in infancy. J Pediatr. 1995;127(2):220–4.
32. Deprettere A, Portmann B, Mowat AP. Syndromic paucity of the intrahepatic bile ducts: diagnostic difficulty; severe morbidity throughout early childhood. J Pediatr Gastroenterol Nutr. 1987;6(6):865–71.
33. Russo P, Magee JC, Anders RA, Bove KE, Chung C, Cummings OW, et al. Key histopathologic features of liver biopsies that distinguish biliary atresia from other causes of infantile cholestasis and their correlation with outcome: a multicenter study. Am J Surg Pathol. 2016;40(12):1601–15.
34. Gilbert MA, Bauer RC, Rajagopalan R, Grochowski CM, Chao G, McEldrew D, et al. Alagille syndrome mutation update: comprehensive overview of JAG1 and NOTCH2 mutation frequencies and insight into missense variant classification. Hum Mutat. 2019;40(12):2197–220.

35. Han S, Jeon TY, Hwang SM, Yoo SY, Choe YH, Lee SK, et al. Imaging findings of Alagille syndrome in young infants: differentiation from biliary atresia. Br J Radiol. 2017;90(1077):20170406.
36. Turnpenny PD, Ellard S. Alagille syndrome: pathogenesis, diagnosis and management. Eur J Hum Genet. 2012;20(3):251–7.
37. Shneider BL, Goodrich NP, Ye W, Sawyers C, Molleston JP, Merion RM, et al. Nonfasted liver stiffness correlates with liver disease parameters and portal hypertension in pediatric cholestatic liver disease. Hepatol Commun. 2020;4(11):1694–707.
38. Elisofon SA, Emerick KM, Sinacore JM, Alonso EM. Health status of patients with Alagille syndrome. J Pediatr Gastroenterol Nutr. 2010;51(6):759–65.
39. Kamath BM, Chen Z, Romero R, Fredericks EM, Alonso EM, Arnon R, et al. Quality of life and its determinants in a multicenter cohort of children with Alagille syndrome. J Pediatr. 2015;167(2):390–6.e3.
40. Ferrarese A, Germani G, Lazzaro S, Cananzi M, Russo FP, Senzolo M, et al. Short-term outcomes of paediatric liver transplant recipients after transition to Adult Healthcare Service. Liver Int. 2018;38(7):1316–21.
41. Vajro P, Fischler B, Burra P, Debray D, Dezsofi A, Guercio Nuzio S, et al. The health care transition of youth with liver disease into the adult health system: position paper from ESPGHAN and EASL. J Pediatr Gastroenterol Nutr. 2018;66(6):976–90.
42. Burra P. The adolescent and liver transplantation. J Hepatol. 2012;56(3):714–22.
43. Ferrarese A, Senzolo M, Burra P. Successful pregnancy in Alagille Syndrome. Dig Liver Dis. 2015;47(1):86–7.
44. Ebel NH, Goldstein A, Howard R, Mogul DB, Marden JR, Anderson A, et al. Health care resource utilization by patients with Alagille syndrome. J Pediatr. 2023;253:144–51.e1.
45. Narkewicz MR, Smith D, Gregory C, Lear JL, Osberg I, Sokol RJ. Effect of ursodeoxycholic acid therapy on hepatic function in children with intrahepatic cholestatic liver disease. J Pediatr Gastroenterol Nutr. 1998;26(1):49–55.
46. Shneider BL, Spino C, Kamath BM, Magee JC, Bass LM, Setchell KD, et al. Placebo-controlled randomized trial of an intestinal bile salt transport inhibitor for pruritus in Alagille syndrome. Hepatol Commun. 2018;2(10):1184–98.
47. Gonzales E, Hardikar W, Stormon M, Baker A, Hierro L, Gliwicz D, et al. Efficacy and safety of maralixibat treatment in patients with Alagille syndrome and cholestatic pruritus (ICONIC): a randomised phase 2 study. Lancet. 2021;398(10311):1581–92.
48. Baumann U, Sturm E, Lacaille F, Gonzalès E, Arnell H, Fischler B, et al. Effects of odevixibat on pruritus and bile acids in children with cholestatic liver disease: phase 2 study. Clin Res Hepatol Gastroenterol. 2021;45(5):101751.
49. Kamath BM, Goldstein A, Howard R, Garner W, Vig P, Marden JR, et al. Maralixibat treatment response in Alagille syndrome is associated with improved health-related quality of life. J Pediatr. 2023;252:68–75.e5.
50. Shneider BL, Spino CA, Kamath BM, Magee JC, Ignacio RV, Huang S, et al. Impact of long-term administration of maralixibat on children with cholestasis secondary to Alagille syndrome. Hepatol Commun. 2022;6(8):1922–33.
51. Sorokin A, Brown JL, Thompson PD. Primary biliary cirrhosis, hyperlipidemia, and atherosclerotic risk: a systematic review. Atherosclerosis. 2007;194(2):293–9.
52. Loomes KM, Spino C, Goodrich NP, Hangartner TN, Marker AE, Heubi JE, et al. Bone density in children with chronic liver disease correlates with growth and cholestasis. Hepatology. 2019;69(1):245–57.
53. de Franchis R, Bosch J, Garcia-Tsao G, Reiberger T, Ripoll C, Faculty BV. Baveno VII – renewing consensus in portal hypertension. J Hepatol. 2022;76(4):959–74.
54. Schindler EA, Gilbert MA, Piccoli DA, Spinner NB, Krantz ID, Loomes KM. Alagille syndrome and risk for hepatocellular carcinoma: need for increased surveillance in adults with mild liver phenotypes. Am J Med Genet A. 2021;185(3):719–31.
55. Tsai S, Gurakar A, Anders R, Lam-Himlin D, Boitnott J, Pawlik TM. Management of large hepatocellular carcinoma in adult patients with Alagille syndrome: a case report and review of literature. Dig Dis Sci. 2010;55(11):3052–8.
56. Mohan P, Lemoine J, Trotter C, Rakova I, Billings P, Peacock S, et al. Clinical experience with non-invasive prenatal screening for single-gene disorders. Ultrasound Obstet Gynecol. 2022;59(1):33–9.
57. Morton A, Kumar S. Alagille syndrome and pregnancy. Obstet Med. 2021;14(1):39–41.
58. Kaye AJ, Rand EB, Munoz PS, Spinner NB, Flake AW, Kamath BM. Effect of Kasai procedure on hepatic outcome in Alagille syndrome. J Pediatr Gastroenterol Nutr. 2010;51(3):319–21.
59. Wang KS, Tiao G, Bass LM, Hertel PM, Mogul D, Kerkar N, et al. Analysis of surgical interruption of the enterohepatic circulation as a treatment for pediatric cholestasis. Hepatology. 2017;65(5):1645–54.
60. Whitington PF, Whitington GL. Partial external diversion of bile for the treatment of intractable pruritus associated with intrahepatic cholestasis. Gastroenterology. 1988;95(1):130–6.
61. Lemoine C, Superina R. Surgical diversion of enterohepatic circulation in pediatric cholestasis. Semin Pediatr Surg. 2020;29(4):150946.
62. Metzelder ML, Bottländer M, Melter M, Petersen C, Ure BM. Laparoscopic partial external biliary diversion procedure in progressive familial intrahepatic cholestasis: a new approach. Surg Endosc. 2005;19(12):1641–3.
63. Clifton MS, Romero R, Ricketts RR. Button cholecystostomy for management of progressive familial intrahepatic cholestasis syndromes. J Pediatr Surg. 2011;46(2):304–7.

64. Rebhandl W, Felberbauer FX, Turnbull J, Paya K, Barcik U, Huber WD, et al. Biliary diversion by use of the appendix (cholecystoappendicostomy) in progressive familial intrahepatic cholestasis. J Pediatr Gastroenterol Nutr. 1999;28(2):217–9.
65. Bustorff-Silva J, Sbraggia Neto L, Olímpio H, de Alcantara RV, Matsushima E, De Tommaso AM, et al. Partial internal biliary diversion through a cholecysto-jejunocolonic anastomosis--a novel surgical approach for patients with progressive familial intrahepatic cholestasis: a preliminary report. J Pediatr Surg. 2007;42(8):1337–40.
66. Flores CD, Yu YR, Miloh TA, Goss J, Brandt ML. Surgical outcomes in Alagille syndrome and PFIC: a single institution's 20-year experience. J Pediatr Surg. 2018;53(5):976–9.
67. Baumann U, Karam V, Adam R, Fondevila C, Dhawan A, Sokal E, et al. Prognosis of children undergoing liver transplantation: a 30-year European Study. Pediatrics. 2022;150(4):e2022057424.
68. Kamath BM, Schwarz KB, Hadzić N. Alagille syndrome and liver transplantation. J Pediatr Gastroenterol Nutr. 2010;50(1):11–5.
69. Razavi RS, Baker A, Qureshi SA, Rosenthal E, Marsh MJ, Leech SC, et al. Hemodynamic response to continuous infusion of dobutamine in Alagille's syndrome. Transplantation. 2001;72(5):823–8.
70. Ovaert C, Germeau C, Barrea C, Moniotte S, Van Obbergh L, Sokal E, et al. Elevated right ventricular pressures are not a contraindication to liver transplantation in Alagille syndrome. Transplantation. 2001;72(2):345–7.
71. Gandhi SK, Reyes J, Webber SA, Siewers RD, Pigula FA. Case report of combined pediatric heart-lung-liver transplantation. Transplantation. 2002;73(12):1968–9.
72. Madan N, Arnon R. Evaluation of cardiac manifestations in pediatric liver transplant candidates. Pediatr Transplant. 2012;16(4):318–28.
73. McGahan RK, Tang JE, Iyer MH, Flores AS, Gorelik LA. Combined liver kidney transplant in adult patient with Alagille syndrome and pulmonary hypertension. Semin Cardiothorac Vasc Anesth. 2021;25(3):191–5.
74. Shehata MR, Yagi S, Ogura Y, Ogawa K, Iida T, Mori A, et al. Use of recipient's left colic artery for arterial reconstruction during liver transplantation in Alagille syndrome with vasculopathy: a case report. Transplantation. 2012;93(6):e20–1.
75. Sanada Y, Naya I, Katano T, Hirata Y, Yamada N, Okada N, et al. Visceral artery anomalies in patients with Alagille syndrome. Pediatr Transplant. 2019;23(2):e13352.
76. Gunadi, Kaneshiro M, Okamoto T, Sonoda M, Ogawa E, Okajima H, et al. Outcomes of liver transplantation for Alagille syndrome after Kasai portoenterostomy: Alagille syndrome with agenesis of extrahepatic bile ducts at porta hepatis. J Pediatr Surg. 2019;54(11):2387–91.
77. Valamparampil JJ, Reddy MS, Shanmugam N, Vij M, Kanagavelu RG, Rela M. Living donor liver transplantation in Alagille syndrome-single center experience from South Asia. Pediatr Transplant. 2019;23(8):e13579.
78. Hori T, Egawa H, Takada Y, Oike F, Kasahara M, Ogura Y, et al. Long-term outcomes after living-donor liver transplantation for Alagille syndrome: a single center 20-year experience in Japan. Am J Transplant. 2010;10(8):1951–2.
79. Arnon R, Annunziato R, Schiano T, Miloh T, Baisley M, Sogawa H, et al. Orthotopic liver transplantation for adults with Alagille syndrome. Clin Transpl. 2012;26(2):E94–E100.
80. Kamath BM, Yin W, Miller H, Anand R, Rand EB, Alonso E, et al. Outcomes of liver transplantation for patients with Alagille syndrome: the studies of pediatric liver transplantation experience. Liver Transpl. 2012;18(8):940–8.
81. Black K, Ziogas IA, Thurm C, Hall M, Hafberg E, Alexopoulos SP, et al. Pediatric liver transplant survival in Alagille syndrome is comparable to biliary atresia-a linked database analysis. J Pediatr Gastroenterol Nutr. 2022;75(3):257–63.
82. Maldini G, Torri E, Lucianetti A, Guizzetti M, Pinelli D, Bertani A, et al. Orthotopic liver transplantation for Alagille syndrome. Transplant Proc. 2005;37(2):1174–6.
83. D'Antiga L, Ballan D, Luisetto G, Cillo U, Guariso G, Zancan L. Long-term outcome of bone mineral density in children who underwent a successful liver transplantation. Transplantation. 2004;78(6):899–903.
84. Loeb N, Owens JS, Strom M, Farassati F, Van Roestel K, Chambers K, et al. Long-term follow-up after pediatric liver transplantation: predictors of growth. J Pediatr Gastroenterol Nutr. 2018;66(4):670–5.
85. Lund LK, Grabhorn EF, Rüther D, Buchholz A, Lang M, Herden U, et al. Long-term outcome of pediatric liver transplant recipients who have reached adulthood: a single-center experience. Transplantation. 2023;107:1756.
86. Burra P, Ferrarese A, Feltrin G. Quality of life and adherence in liver transplant recipients. Minerva Gastroenterol Dietol. 2018;64(2):180–6.

2 Bile Duct Injury

Daniel Ansari, Jenny Rystedt, and Roland Andersson

2.1 Introduction

Most bile duct injuries (BDIs) are iatrogenic in nature. They are usually sustained during cholecystectomy (emergency and elective). BDIs may also occur during other abdominal procedures, during endoscopic and percutaneous interventions on the bile ducts, or in the setting of hepatobiliary trauma. Cholecystectomy is the primary treatment for symptomatic gallstone disease and one of the most common general surgical procedures worldwide, with over 1.2 million procedures performed annually in the United States alone [1]. The surgeon Carl Langenbuch developed the technique of cholecystectomy through cadaveric dissection and, in the year 1882, performed the first successful open cholecystectomy in a patient who had been suffering from biliary colic for many years [2]. In 1985, the surgeon Erich Mühe performed the first laparoscopic cholecystectomy [3], which has now become the gold standard. More than 90% of cholecystectomies are nowadays performed laparoscopically in the United States [4]. The benefits of the laparoscopic approach have been well-established, including decreased postoperative pain, faster functional recovery, and better cosmesis [5]. However, a major concern with laparoscopic cholecystectomy has been the reported higher frequency of BDIs compared to open surgery [6]. Early recognition of BDI is essential for a good clinical outcome, as undiagnosed injuries may lead to biliary peritonitis, sepsis, multiple organ failure, and mortality. The late clinical course of BDIs includes strictures and recurrent cholangitis, resulting in secondary biliary cirrhosis and portal hypertension, ultimately necessitating liver transplantation.

The patient perspective of a BDI is tragically depicted by the famous case of Sir Anthony Eden, a British Prime Minister, who suffered a BDI during cholecystectomy, which resulted in a lifetime of complications and reoperations [7]. Experienced surgeons may also cause BDIs, which is exemplified by the Eden case, in which the primary operation was performed by a senior surgeon. The repeated occurrence of BDIs, even in experienced hands, has led to intense research into the predisposing factors for BDIs during cholecystectomy and the methods of prevention [8]. Following BDIs, medical malpractice claims are common, especially if there is a delay in diagnosis or if the management is incorrect [9].

This chapter focuses on the diagnosis and treatment of BDIs. Considering the rarity of BDIs, most of the evidence for the management of these injuries has been derived from BDIs after cholecystectomy.

D. Ansari · J. Rystedt · R. Andersson (✉)
Department of Surgery, Clinical Sciences Lund, Lund University, Skåne University Hospital, Lund, Sweden
e-mail: daniel.ansari@med.lu.se; jenny.lundmark_rystedt@med.lu.se; roland.andersson@med.lu.se

T. Hackert, A. Gulla (eds.), *Rare Liver and Biliary Tract Diseases*,
https://doi.org/10.1007/978-3-032-15076-9_2

2.2 Postcholecystectomy Bile Duct Injury

2.2.1 Incidence

The incidence of BDIs after laparoscopic cholecystectomy ranges from 0.25% to 0.74% for major lesions, involving the common bile duct, the common hepatic duct, or the right hepatic duct. For minor lesions, including bile leaks from the cystic duct or small Luschka ducts, rates from 0.28% to 1.70% are reported, while traditional open surgery historically reported BDI rates of 0.1–0.3% [10]. These early findings likely reflected the initial learning curve. In the modern era, BDI rates for laparoscopic cholecystectomy have decreased to levels seen in open surgery [5, 11, 12].

2.2.2 Diagnosis

BDI may be suspected during cholecystectomy when there is unexpected bile staining. If routine intraoperative cholangiography (IOC) is used, rates of intraoperative detection of BDIs of 90% and higher are reported [13–16]. During IOC, a clip is placed on the cystic duct–infundibular junction, and a small incision is made on the anterior surface of the cystic duct. A catheter is advanced through a cystic ductotomy, and a cholangiogram is obtained that can visualize the biliary anatomy, the flow into the duodenum, and the presence or absence of bile duct stones (Fig. 2.1). A normal IOC does not exclude the occurrence of BDI, but the positioning of the catheter in the operative field and its relation to the cholangiogram may help reduce anatomical misinterpretation and, hence, reduce the risk of aggravating the injury by proceeding to dissect any wrong anatomical structures [18]. Routine IOC has been found to reduce BDIs and is preferred over its selective use [14, 19]. An alternative approach is ICG fluorescence cholangiography [20], which combines the intravenous injection of ICG, a fluorescent dye, and near-infrared (NIR) light to provide real-time imaging of the biliary anatomy.

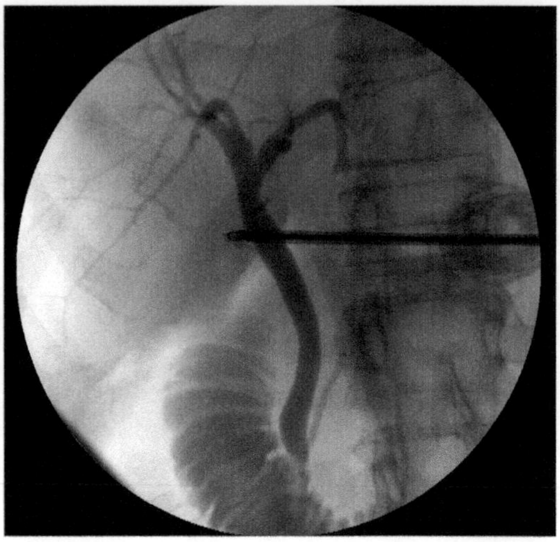

Fig. 2.1 Normal intraoperative cholangiography [17]. (With permission)

Bile duct anatomy can also be clarified with IOUS, which uses an ultrasound probe that is inserted into the peritoneal cavity [21–23].

However, many BDIs go unnoticed during the index operation and manifest postoperatively as bile leakage, with abdominal pain and sepsis, or biliary obstruction, with or without cholangitis, usually within the first postoperative week. If a drain is in place from the index operation, biliary discharge may be noted, and the patient may have milder symptoms due to the clearance of bile. Some laboratory tests may be indicative of BDI, such as increases in liver function tests, including aspartate transaminase (AST), alanine transaminase (ALT), alkaline phosphatase (ALP), and bilirubin. For patients presenting postoperatively, any available imaging method can be used to identify fluid collections in the gallbladder fossa and ductal dilation. Fluid collections should be drained expeditiously to avoid pain, biliary peritonitis, and sepsis. A triphasic computed tomography (CT) is needed to detect any concomitant vascular injury, and a contrast-enhanced magnetic resonance cholangiopancreatography (MRCP) may be used as an adjunct to map the bile ducts and any bile leakage and aid in treatment planning. Late biliary strictures may manifest clinically for up to 10 years after the injury and often need surgical treatment for the definitive release of symptoms, such as recurrent cholangitis [24].

It is important to detect BDIs early. Patients with BDIs detected intraoperatively have a better prognosis than patients whose injuries are detected postoperatively [25]. IOC can aid in the early detection of injuries and thereby reduce mortality.

2.2.3 Differential Diagnosis

The term "postcholecystectomy syndrome" (PCS) comprises a heterogeneous group of symptoms, such as abdominal pain, dyspepsia, and jaundice, with a high incidence of up to 40% [26]. These symptoms may be attributed to biliary causes, including BDIs, biliary strictures, retained bile duct stones, and sphincter of Oddi dysfunction. Bile leakage by the unrecognized transection of aberrant bile ducts in the liver bed (i.e., segment 6 ducts) is an important differential diagnosis for major BDIs. Patients may also have PCS due to extrabiliary causes, such as peptic ulcer disease, pancreatitis, and irritable bowel syndrome.

2.2.4 Classification

A proper diagnosis and classification of BDIs is of utmost importance for the choice of treatment. How to best classify BDIs is a matter of much debate, as illustrated by the multitude of classifications that are available, such as Bismuth [27, 28], Strasberg [29], Stewart-Way [30], Hannover [31], and ATOM classifications [32]. The Hannover classification was developed with a specific focus on laparoscopic injury patterns (Fig. 2.2). The benefit of the Hannover classification is the high association between the discrimination of classifiable injuries and the type of treatment [31]. The ATOM classification proposed by the European Association for Endoscopic Surgery (EAES) includes Anatomic characteristics, Time Of detection, and Mechanism of injury [32]. Despite its comprehensive nature, the ATOM classification is often regarded as too elaborate to be used in everyday clinical practice.

2.2.5 Risk Factors

Aberrant biliary anatomy, severe inflammation and fibrosis in the triangle of Calot, obesity, male sex, inappropriate exposure and bleeding, and other technical difficulties are known risk factors for BDIs [33]. However, most BDIs have been reported to be due to visual perceptual illusion and misidentification of ductal anatomy [15, 34]. No single measure to prevent BDIs during cholecystectomy has been reported to be successful. A combination of awareness of the known risk factors for BDI and intraoperative visualization of the bile ducts to fit to the operative field is the best available strategy, together with good assistance to prevent confirmation bias.

2.2.6 Preventive Surgical Strategies

The critical view of safety (CVS) is a strategy applied during laparoscopic cholecystectomy to reduce BDIs (Fig. 2.3) [29]. For the CVS to be complete, the hepatocystic triangle and the lower part of the cystic plate need to be dissected clear from tissue to expose the cystic duct and cystic artery. The CVS should be obtained during laparoscopic cholecystectomy before clipping or transecting any tubular structures. Technical challenges may arise in the setting of severe inflammation, anatomical variations, and Mirizzi's syndrome, when an impacted stone in the cystic duct compresses the common bile or common hepatic duct. If the CVS cannot be obtained, conversion to open surgery or a bailout procedure such as subtotal cholecystectomy may be necessary. When converting to open surgery, a fundus-first approach is often used, but caution must be exercised when there is severe inflammation because of the risk of damage to the right portal pedicle [36]. Subtotal cholecystectomy is a method in which the gallbladder is opened above the infundibulum and all stones are removed. The

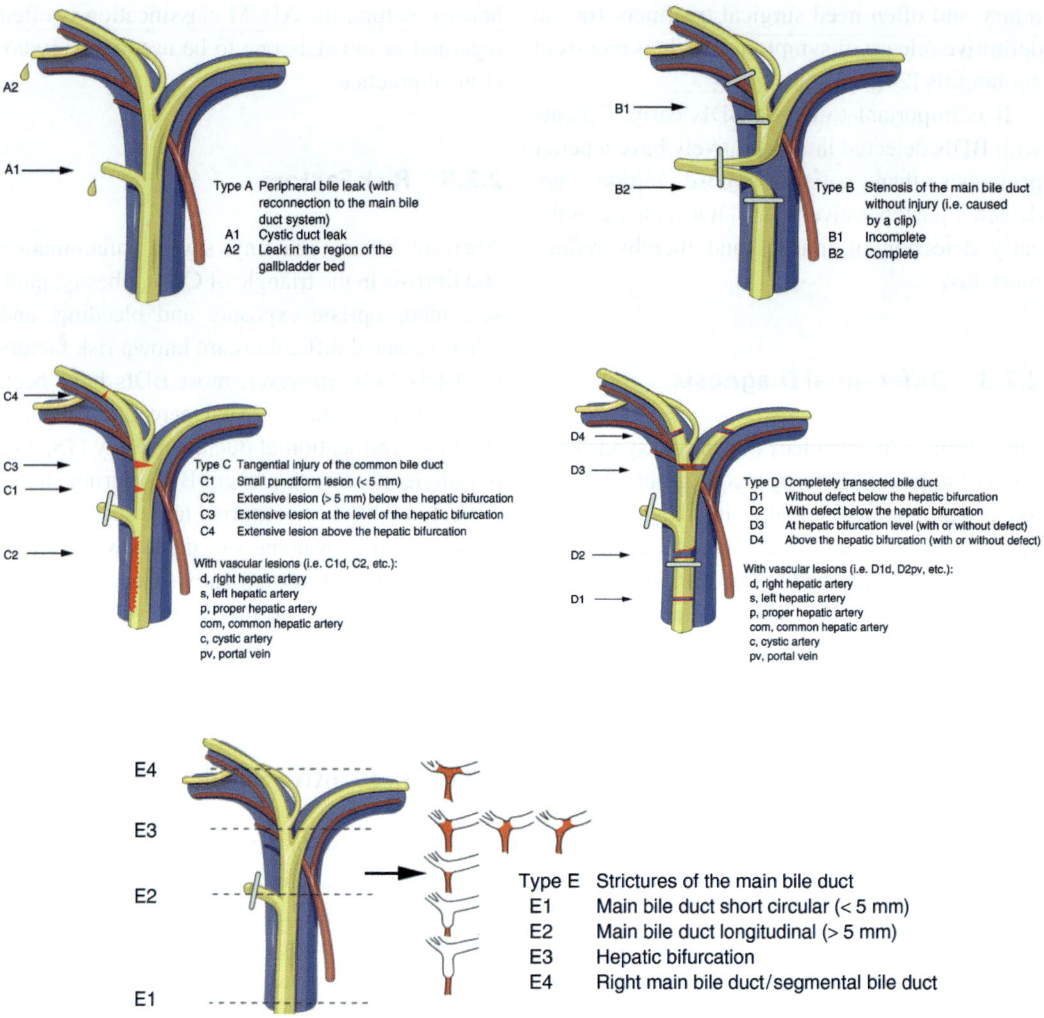

Fig. 2.2 Hannover classification of iatrogenic bile duct injuries [31]. (With permission. Copyright Oxford University Press)

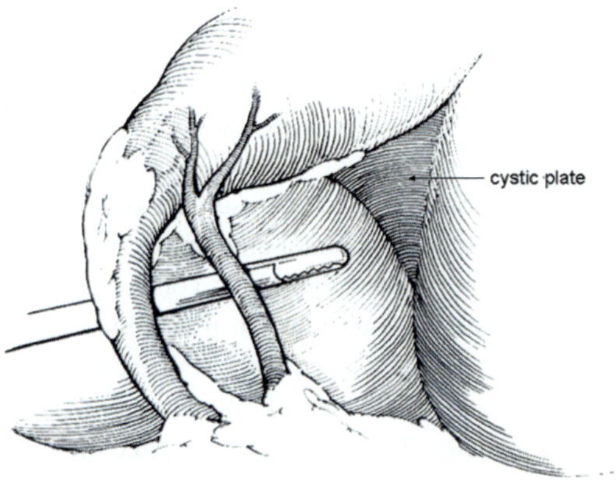

Fig. 2.3 Critical view of safety [35]. (With permission. Copyright Wolters Kluwer Health, Inc.)

"fenestrating" subtype leaves the remnant gallbladder open (cystic duct may be sutured internally), while the "reconstituting" subtype closes the remnant gallbladder [37]. IOC, ICG, and IOUS are all different modalities for the intraoperative visualization of the bile ducts and to detect anatomical variations, aberrant ducts, and iatrogenic injuries. Routine use of IOC has been reported to be superior to on-demand use, and this can probably be extrapolated to the other methods. In the event of technical difficulties and a suspected BDI, a well-established method for detecting and diagnosing BDI is optimal.

2.2.7 Treatment

2.2.7.1 Intraoperative Repair

Minor BDIs are minor lesions, typically caused by electrocautery or sharp dissection. When detected intraoperatively, treatment for these lesions is suture repair, potentially over T-tube drainage or internal stent, if no or limited thermal damage is present (Fig. 2.4). Intraoperative detection of a minor BDI and its immediate repair result in long-term quality of life comparable to an uneventful cholecystectomy [38].

2.2.7.2 Endoscopic or Percutaneous Biliary Drainage

Endoscopic retrograde cholangiopancreatography (ERCP) and percutaneous transhepatic biliary drainage (PTBD) are cornerstones in BDI management, as they allow for the mapping of the site of injury and a reduction of the transpapillary pressure gradient through stent/catheter placement (Fig. 2.5). For minor BDIs in general and cystic duct leakage specifically, endoscopic/percutaneous treatment is successful for over 95% of the patients.

2.2.7.3 Biliary Reconstruction

Major BDIs are associated with tissue loss and often require reconstruction with a Roux-en-Y hepaticojejunostomy (Fig. 2.6). Referral to an HPB center is recommended if surgical expertise is not available at the local hospital. The timing of BDI repair has shown an impact on the patency (stricture rate) and long-term quality of life, but immediate and early repair are only possible when the BDI is diagnosed intraoperatively. Excellent clinical outcomes have been reported after BDI repair, with an outreach service from a tertiary referral HPB center for enabling early

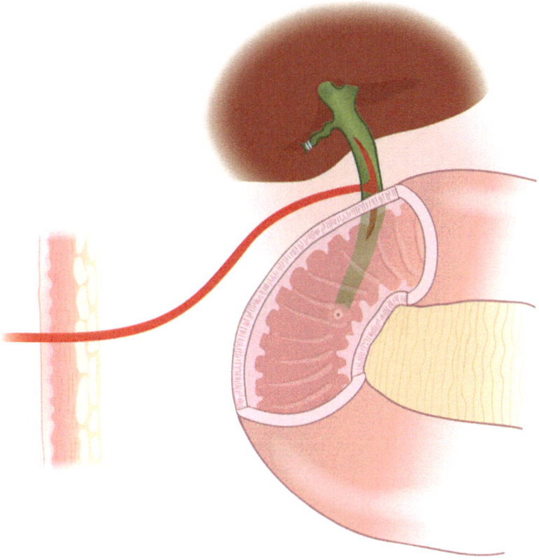

Fig. 2.4 T-tube [17]. (With permission)

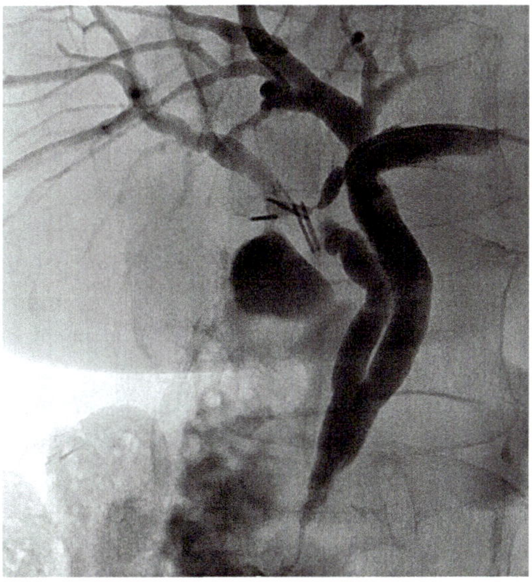

Fig. 2.5 PTBD with clips on the right hepatic duct (and the cystic duct) with proximal contrast leakage. (With permission (Jenny Rystedt))

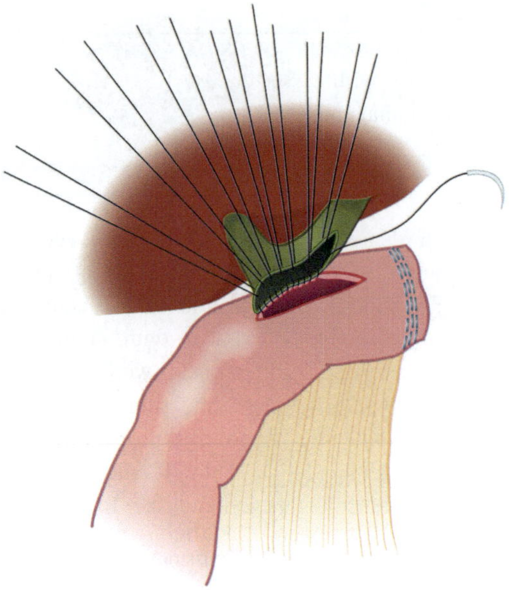

Fig. 2.6 Hepaticojejunostomy [17]. (With permission)

repair of major injuries as well [39]. The optimal timing for reconstructive surgery has been evaluated in a multicenter setting, and no differences were reported between early and late repair [40]. For concomitant vascular injuries (hepatic artery or portal vein), the consensus is to delay repair to enable revascularization via the hilar plate, imaging, and precise planning [41]. Partial hepatectomy and, to some extent, liver transplantation are reserved for the select few patients in whom reconstructive surgery is unsuccessful or not possible due to liver failure [42].

2.3 Traumatic Bile Duct Injuries

Non-iatrogenic traumatic injury to the biliary tree is infrequent and represents less than 5% of all BDIs [43]. Traumatic BDIs have an incidence of 0.1% among hospital admissions for blunt and penetrating trauma, and the treatment is often staged due to concomitant vascular injury [44]. Most traumatic BDIs are associated with hepatic trauma and present as contusions, partial tears, or complete transections of the biliary tree. Because intrahepatic BDIs are often associated with liver parenchymal damage, the American Association for the Surgery of Trauma (AAST) liver injury scale is recommended (Table 2.1), while extrahepatic BDIs have a separate classification, as shown in Table 2.2. For patients in shock, damage control principles should be used. Hemorrhage control is the first priority of management when there is associated vascular injury. Once hemorrhage is controlled, minor BDI injuries can be primarily repaired, possibly over a T-tube or an internal stent, but for major BDI injuries, drainage and delayed repair with biliary reconstruction is preferred when the patient's physiology has improved. Severe distal bile duct

Table 2.1 AAST liver injury scale [45]

Grade	Description of injury
I	Subcapsular hematoma <10% surface area
	Parenchymal laceration <1 cm depth
II	Subcapsular hematoma 10–50% surface area; intraparenchymal hematoma <10 cm in diameter
	Laceration 1–3 cm in depth and ≤10 cm length
III	Subcapsular hematoma >50% surface area; ruptured subcapsular or parenchymal hematoma
	Intraparenchymal laceration >10 cm
	Laceration >3 cm depth
	Any injury in the presence of a liver vascular injury or active bleeding contained within the liver parenchyma
IV	Parenchymal disruption involving 25–75% of a hepatic lobe
	Active bleeding extending beyond the liver parenchyma into the peritoneum
V	Parenchymal disruption >75% of the hepatic lobe
	Juxtahepatic venous injury to include the retrohepatic vena cava and the major central hepatic veins

AAST American Association for the Surgery of Trauma

Table 2.2 AAST extrahepatic biliary injury tree scale [46]

Grade	Description of injury
I	Gallbladder contusion/hematoma
	Portal triad contusion
II	Partial gallbladder avulsion from the liver bed; cystic duct intact
	Laceration or perforation of the gallbladder
III	Complete gallbladder avulsion from the liver bed
	Cystic duct laceration
IV	Partial or complete right hepatic duct laceration
	Partial or complete left hepatic duct laceration
	Partial common hepatic duct laceration (<50%)
	Partial common bile duct laceration (<50%)
V	>50% transection of the common hepatic duct
	>50% transection of the common bile duct
	Combined right and left hepatic duct injuries
	Intraduodenal or intrapancreatic bile duct injuries

AAST American Association for the Surgery of Trauma

injuries with simultaneous damage to the pancreatic head may require complex reconstruction with a pancreatoduodenectomy.

2.4 Recommendations

BDI may occur as an iatrogenic complication during surgical procedures, primarily cholecystectomy, or, less frequently, following hepatobiliary trauma. Visual misperception during laparoscopy and a misunderstanding of the biliary anatomy are the most common causes of postcholecystectomy BDIs. The implications of BDIs can be profound due to the increased morbidity and mortality, decreased quality of life, increased costs, and potential for litigation [9, 41, 47, 48]. Methods to enable safer laparoscopic cholecystectomy include a knowledge of the risk factors for BDI, obtaining the CVS, the use of intraoperative imaging (e.g., IOC, ICG, or IOUS), the recognition of aberrant biliary anatomy, conversion to open surgery, and the application of bailout procedures. In the event of a BDI, early detection and diagnosis, including referral to an HPB center with associated interventional radiologic and endoscopic facilities, is recommended, as patients with BDIs benefit from multidisciplinary management.

References

1. Jones MW, Guay E, Deppen JG. Open cholecystectomy. In: StatPearls. Treasure Island: StatPearls Publishing; 2022.
2. Langenbuch C. Ein fall von exstirpation der gallenblase wegen chronischer cholelithiasis. Heilung. Berl Klin Wochenschr. 1882;19:725–7.
3. Mühe E. 296. Die erste Cholecystektomie durch das Laparoskop. Langenbecks Arch Chir. 1986;369(1):804.
4. Csikesz NG, Singla A, Murphy MM, Tseng JF, Shah SA. Surgeon volume metrics in laparoscopic cholecystectomy. Dig Dis Sci. 2010;55(8):2398–405.
5. Keus F, de Jong JA, Gooszen HG, van Laarhoven CJ. Laparoscopic versus open cholecystectomy for patients with symptomatic cholecystolithiasis. Cochrane Database Syst Rev. 2006;(4):CD006231.
6. Brunt LM, Deziel DJ, Telem DA, Strasberg SM, Aggarwal R, Asbun H, et al. Safe cholecystectomy multi-society practice guideline and state of the art consensus conference on prevention of bile duct injury during cholecystectomy. Ann Surg. 2020;272(1):3–23.
7. Braasch JW. Anthony Eden's (Lord Avon) biliary tract saga. Ann Surg. 2003;238(5):772–5.
8. Eikermann M, Siegel R, Broeders I, Dziri C, Fingerhut A, Gutt C, et al. Prevention and treatment of bile duct injuries during laparoscopic cholecystectomy: the clinical practice guidelines of the European Association for Endoscopic Surgery (EAES). Surg Endosc. 2012;26(11):3003–39.
9. Kapoor VK. Medico-legal aspects of bile duct injury. J Minim Access Surg. 2016;12(1):1–3.
10. Christou N, Roux-David A, Naumann DN, Bouvier S, Rivaille T, Derbal S, et al. Bile duct injury during cholecystectomy: necessity to learn how to do and interpret intraoperative cholangiography. Front Med (Lausanne). 2021;8:637987.
11. Halbert C, Pagkratis S, Yang J, Meng Z, Altieri MS, Parikh P, et al. Beyond the learning curve: incidence of bile duct injuries following laparoscopic cholecystectomy normalize to open in the modern era. Surg Endosc. 2016;30(6):2239–43.
12. Mangieri CW, Hendren BP, Strode MA, Bandera BC, Faler BJ. Bile duct injuries (BDI) in the advanced laparoscopic cholecystectomy era. Surg Endosc. 2019;33(3):724–30.

13. Alvarez FA, de Santibanes M, Palavecino M, Sanchez Claria R, Mazza O, Arbues G, et al. Impact of routine intraoperative cholangiography during laparoscopic cholecystectomy on bile duct injury. Br J Surg. 2014;101(6):677–84.
14. Rystedt JML, Tingstedt B, Montgomery F, Montgomery AK. Routine intraoperative cholangiography during cholecystectomy is a cost-effective approach when analysing the cost of iatrogenic bile duct injuries. HPB (Oxford). 2017;19(10):881–8.
15. Way LW, Stewart L, Gantert W, Liu K, Lee CM, Whang K, et al. Causes and prevention of laparoscopic bile duct injuries: analysis of 252 cases from a human factors and cognitive psychology perspective. Ann Surg. 2003;237(4):460–9.
16. Rystedt J, Lindell G, Montgomery A. Bile duct injuries associated with 55,134 cholecystectomies: treatment and outcome from a national perspective. World J Surg. 2016;40(1):73–80.
17. Rystedt J. Bile duct injury – the importance of intraoperative detection. Doctoral thesis, Lund University, Faculty of Medicine. 2017.
18. Rystedt JML, Montgomery AK. Author response to: routine versus selective intraoperative cholangiography during cholecystectomy: a systematic review, meta-analysis, and health economic model analysis of iatrogenic bile duct injury. BJS Open. 2022;6(2):zrac054.
19. Rystedt JML, Wiss J, Adolfsson J, Enochsson L, Hallerback B, Johansson P, et al. Routine versus selective intraoperative cholangiography during cholecystectomy: systematic review, meta-analysis and health economic model analysis of iatrogenic bile duct injury. BJS Open. 2021;5(2):zraa032.
20. Boogerd LSF, Handgraaf HJM, Huurman VAL, Lam HD, Mieog JSD, van der Made WJ, et al. The best approach for laparoscopic fluorescence cholangiography: overview of the literature and optimization of dose and dosing time. Surg Innov. 2017;24(4):386–96.
21. Biffl WL, Moore EE, Offner PJ, Franciose RJ, Burch JM. Routine intraoperative laparoscopic ultrasonography with selective cholangiography reduces bile duct complications during laparoscopic cholecystectomy. J Am Coll Surg. 2001;193(3):272–80.
22. Hublet A, Dili A, Lemaire J, Mansvelt B, Molle G, Bertrand C. Laparoscopic ultrasonography as a good alternative to intraoperative cholangiography (IOC) during laparoscopic cholecystectomy: results of prospective study. Acta Chir Belg. 2009;109(3):312–6.
23. Pfluke JM, Bowers SP Jr. Laparoscopic intraoperative biliary ultrasonography: findings during laparoscopic cholecystectomy for acute disease. J Laparoendosc Adv Surg Tech A. 2011;21(6):505–9.
24. Halle-Smith JM, Marudanayagam R, Mirza DF, Roberts KJ. Long-term outcomes of delayed biliary strictures following cholecystectomy. HPB (Oxford). 2022;24(2):209–16.
25. Tornqvist B, Stromberg C, Persson G, Nilsson M. Effect of intended intraoperative cholangiography and early detection of bile duct injury on survival after cholecystectomy: population based cohort study. BMJ. 2012;345:e6457.
26. Jaunoo SS, Mohandas S, Almond LM. Postcholecystectomy syndrome (PCS). Int J Surg. 2010;8(1):15–7.
27. Bismuth H, Majno PE. Biliary strictures: classification based on the principles of surgical treatment. World J Surg. 2001;25(10):1241–4.
28. Bismuth H. Postoperative strictures of the bile duct. In: Blumbart LH, editor. The biliary tract. Clinical surgery international. Edinburgh: Churchill Livingstone; 1982. p. 209–18.
29. Strasberg SM, Hertl M, Soper NJ. An analysis of the problem of biliary injury during laparoscopic cholecystectomy. J Am Coll Surg. 1995;180(1):101–25.
30. Stewart L, Robinson TN, Lee CM, Liu K, Whang K, Way LW. Right hepatic artery injury associated with laparoscopic bile duct injury: incidence, mechanism, and consequences. J Gastrointest Surg. 2004;8(5):523–30; discussion 30–1.
31. Bektas H, Schrem H, Winny M, Klempnauer J. Surgical treatment and outcome of iatrogenic bile duct lesions after cholecystectomy and the impact of different clinical classification systems. Br J Surg. 2007;94(9):1119–27.
32. Fingerhut A, Dziri C, Garden OJ, Gouma D, Millat B, Neugebauer E, et al. ATOM, the all-inclusive, nominal EAES classification of bile duct injuries during cholecystectomy. Surg Endosc. 2013;27(12):4608–19.
33. Shallaly G, Cuschieri A. Nature, aetiology and outcome of bile duct injuries after laparoscopic cholecystectomy. HPB (Oxford). 2000;2(1):3–12.
34. Dekker SW, Hugh TB. Laparoscopic bile duct injury: understanding the psychology and heuristics of the error. ANZ J Surg. 2008;78(12):1109–14.
35. Strasberg SM, Brunt LM. Rationale and use of the critical view of safety in laparoscopic cholecystectomy. J Am Coll Surg. 2010;211(1):132–8.
36. Strasberg SM, Gouma DJ. "Extreme" vasculobiliary injuries: association with fundus-down cholecystectomy in severely inflamed gallbladders. HPB (Oxford). 2012;14(1):1–8.
37. Strasberg SM, Pucci MJ, Brunt LM, Deziel DJ. Subtotal cholecystectomy-"fenestrating" vs "reconstituting" subtypes and the prevention of bile duct injury: definition of the optimal procedure in difficult operative conditions. J Am Coll Surg. 2016;222(1):89–96.
38. Rystedt JM, Montgomery AK. Quality-of-life after bile duct injury: intraoperative detection is crucial. A national case-control study. HPB (Oxford). 2016;18(12):1010–6.
39. Perera MT, Silva MA, Hegab B, Muralidharan V, Bramhall SR, Mayer AD, et al. Specialist early and

immediate repair of post-laparoscopic cholecystectomy bile duct injuries is associated with an improved long-term outcome. Ann Surg. 2011;253(3):553–60.
40. Rystedt JML, Kleeff J, Salvia R, Besselink MG, Prasad R, Lesurtel M, et al. Post cholecystectomy bile duct injury: early, intermediate or late repair with hepaticojejunostomy – an E-AHPBA multi-center study1. HPB (Oxford). 2019;21(12):1641–7.
41. de'Angelis N, Catena F, Memeo R, Coccolini F, Martinez-Perez A, Romeo OM, et al. 2020 WSES guidelines for the detection and management of bile duct injury during cholecystectomy. World J Emerg Surg. 2021;16(1):30.
42. Renz BW, Bosch F, Angele MK. Bile duct injury after cholecystectomy: surgical therapy. Visc Med. 2017;33(3):184–90.
43. Michele M. Chapter 8: Traumatic bile duct injuries. In: Garbuzenko DV, editor. Actual problems of emergency abdominal surgery. Rijeka: IntechOpen; 2016.
44. Thomson BN, Nardino B, Gumm K, Robertson AJ, Knowles BP, Collier NA, et al. Management of blunt and penetrating biliary tract trauma. J Trauma Acute Care Surg. 2012;72(6):1620–5.
45. Kozar RA, Crandall M, Shanmuganathan K, Zarzaur BL, Coburn M, Cribari C, et al. Organ injury scaling 2018 update: spleen, liver, and kidney. J Trauma Acute Care Surg. 2018;85(6):1119–22.
46. Moore EE, Jurkovich GJ, Knudson MM, Cogbill TH, Malangoni MA, Champion HR, et al. Organ injury scaling. VI: Extrahepatic biliary, esophagus, stomach, vulva, vagina, uterus (nonpregnant), uterus (pregnant), fallopian tube, and ovary. J Trauma. 1995;39(6):1069–70.
47. Sturesson C, Hemmingsson O, Mansson C, Sandstrom P, Stromberg C, Taflin H, et al. Quality-of-life after bile duct injury repaired by hepaticojejunostomy: a national cohort study. Scand J Gastroenterol. 2020;55(9):1087–92.
48. Andersson R, Eriksson K, Blind PJ, Tingstedt B. Iatrogenic bile duct injury--a cost analysis. HPB (Oxford). 2008;10(6):416–9.

3 Hepatic Epithelioid Hemangioendothelioma

Ali Ramouz, Uta Merle, and Arianeb Mehrabi

3.1 Incidence

Epithelioid hemangioendotheliomas (EHs) are rare vascular tumors that invade visceral organs and soft tissue, including the liver, lungs, and mediastinum [1]. The term EH was first introduced by Weiss and Enzinger in 1982 and was classified as a lesion with metastatic potential by the World Health Organization in 2002 [2, 3]. These tumors are characterized by epithelioid and histiocytoid vascular endothelial cells and range from benign hemangiomas to aggressive angiosarcomas [4]. Generally, EHs are considered to have a low-to-medium grade of malignancy.

EH tumors most commonly affect the liver, and these tumors are called primary hepatic EHs (HEHs) [4]. The overall estimated incidence of HEH is 1–2 cases in 1,000,000, and HEH is mainly reported in the white population [5, 6]. HEH usually appears between 30 and 50 years of age and affects more females than males (3:2) [7]. These tumors can present as single, multiple, diffuse, and multifocal lesions [8] and increase in size and complexity as the disease progresses. During the early phases of the disease, tumors are mainly nodular, and they become more diffuse in the later stages. Histologically, HEH is composed of dendritic-like cells and epithelioid tumor cells, which infiltrate the hepatic sinuses [9] and then the hepatic vessels and the portal vein [1]. Distant metastases can also occur in the advanced stages of HEH [10].

3.2 Etiology

The etiopathogenic factors correlated with HEH development are still unclear. Unlike other primary liver tumors, chronic liver disease does not predispose to HEH, and HEH has been diagnosed in the absence of hepatic insult or systemic disease. No clear causal relationship between the development of HEH and several putative risk factors has been demonstrated to date. These potential risk factors include oral contraceptives, vinyl chloride, asbestos, thorotrast, Crohn's disease, major liver trauma, viral hepatitis, primary biliary cirrhosis, and alcohol consumption [10, 11].

The molecular mechanisms of HEH pathology have not been well-studied but are thought to involve genes associated with cell cycle control, cell signaling, and epigenetic modification. The

A. Ramouz · A. Mehrabi (✉)
Department of General, Visceral, and Transplantation Surgery, University of Heidelberg, Heidelberg, Germany
e-mail: Ali.ramouz@med.uni-heidelberg.de; Arianeb.mehrabi@med.uni-heidelberg.de

U. Merle
University Hospital Heidelberg, Department of Gastroenterology, Hepatology and Infectious Diseases, Heidelberg, Germany
e-mail: Uta.merle@med.uni-heidelberg.de

T. Hackert, A. Gulla (eds.), *Rare Liver and Biliary Tract Diseases*,
https://doi.org/10.1007/978-3-032-15076-9_3

vascular endothelial growth factor (VEGF) signaling pathway was recently shown to be activated in patients with HEH [12]. Moreover, a special translocation t (1/3) (P36/25) has also been named as a specific mutation for HEH, although the correlation between the fusion transcripts and tumorigenesis remains unclear [13]. Recurrent WWTR1-CAMTA1 gene fusion has also been detected in patients with HEH [14–16]. These mutations retain WWTR1 in the nucleus, which is thought to result in oncogenesis.

3.3 Clinical Presentation

The clinical manifestations of HEH remain unclear because it is usually detected incidentally by ultrasonography or computed tomography (CT) scans carried out for other reasons [17]. According to the literature, 25% of patients with HEH are asymptomatic at the time of diagnosis [7, 18]. HEH also presents a heterogeneous clinical manifestation with a wide spectrum, from unspecific abdominal complaints to portal hypertension and liver failure (Table 3.1) [7, 19]. These variable and atypical clinical manifestations result in misdiagnosis in up to 80% of patients, and HEH is first detected by histopathological examination [7, 20, 21].

Table 3.1 Frequency of signs and symptoms of hepatic epithelioid hemangioendothelioma in patients

Signs and symptoms	%
Right upper quadrant pain	39–48
Hepatosplenomegaly	15–20
Weight loss	10–15
Weakness	8–10
Anorexia	8–13
Abdominal fullness/discomfort	5–10
Epigastric mass	1–8
Ascites	7–8
Jaundice	6–9
Nausea/emesis	4–7
Fever	4–5
Chest pain/shoulder pain/costal arch pain	2–8
Others	3–10
Asymptomatic	24–27

The main symptoms of HEH are abdominal pain (particularly in the right upper quadrant), hepatomegaly or abdominal mass, anorexia, and weight loss. If the diagnosis is late, more advanced symptoms can be observed, such as ascites, jaundice, portal hypertension, liver failure, and spontaneous rupture of the tumor [5, 7, 22–24]. If the major hepatic veins are affected, Budd–Chiari syndrome can also be observed [11, 25]. Most HEH cases (80%) have a multifocal presentation [7, 26] and most commonly affect the right lobes [7, 27]. In addition, in one-third of the patients, extrahepatic manifestations are observed at the time of diagnosis [7, 10]. The most common sites of extrahepatic invasion are the lungs, regional lymph nodes, peritoneum, bone, spleen, and diaphragm [1, 10, 20], but other sites can also be affected, such as the pleura, mediastinum, myocardium, pericardium, brain, common bile duct, pancreas, and uterus.

3.4 Diagnostic Workups

3.4.1 Laboratory Tests

There are no definitive laboratory findings for HEH, and laboratory parameters show no pathological abnormality in 15% of HEH patients [7]. The main laboratory finding that might indicate HEH is the elevation of alkaline phosphatase; however, levels of other liver enzymes can also increase, such as γ-glutamyl transpeptidase, aspartate aminotransferase, and alanine aminotransferase [28–30]. Elevated bilirubin levels have also been reported in 20% of patients [7], but levels of other common markers for liver malignancies are not altered in HEH, so they are useful for ruling out other cancers.

3.4.2 Imaging and Diagnostic Tools

Different imaging modalities have been used to detect HEH, including ultrasonography, CT scans, magnetic resonance imaging (MRI), and positron emission tomography (PET). Other modalities (including plain abdomen radiography and endoscopic retrograde cholangiopancreatography) have also provided useful data on the lesions, but the diagnostic efficacy of these other techniques has not been established. A HEH diagnosis should be confirmed via pathological examination, but radiological features play an important role in limiting differential diagnoses [17, 31].

Different presentations have been reported for HEH, ranging from avascular and calcified small nodules to large tumors that coalesce over the whole liver parenchyma. HEH can also occur peripherally and extend to the liver's capsule. This may result in flattening or retraction of the liver capsule due to fibrosis, as well as compensatory hypertrophy of the unaffected segments. These features may also provide diagnostic clues [32]. As mentioned earlier, the type of HEH can also indicate the stage of the disease. However, while imaging results can suggest HEH, they cannot give a definite diagnosis. For example, a nodular HEH tumor identified by radiology has a similar form to a hepatic metastasis, so a biopsy is needed to make a specific diagnosis. In another example, diffuse lesions indicate hepatic vascular invasion and advanced-stage disease. However, these diffuse lesions are difficult to differentiate from cholangiocarcinoma, hepatocellular carcinoma, and veno-occlusive hepatic disease.

3.4.2.1 Ultrasonography

Ultrasonography is usually the first technique used to assess abdominal complaints, and it is rare that HEH is not detected by ultrasonography (although the results are operator-dependent). HEH typically appears as a peripheral hypoechoic lesion on an ultrasound, but other patterns are possible. The echogenicity of HEH does not depend on the lesion size but on the lesion type, and discrete nodules or diffuse regions can both be seen on the ultrasound. Doppler ultrasonography can also evaluate the vascularity of the HEH tumor, whereas ultrasonography can evaluate portal hypertension and hepatomegaly. Recently, contrast-enhanced ultrasound (CEUS) has been used to enhance the detection of multifocal HEH lesions. These appear as a peripheral nodular enhancement with centripetal fill-in and washout in the portal venous and late venous phase (PVLP), as a rim-like arterial enhancement with washout in the PVLP, and as an inverted target sign with or without washout in the PVLP [33–35]. These features, particularly washout in the PVLP, can help determine the malignancy of HEH in some patients, although some might also be detected in patients with more common focal liver lesions, such as hemangioma and cholangiocarcinoma.

3.4.2.2 CT Scan

Most HEH lesions have a low-density pattern in CT scans [19, 36] and can also present as calcifications, capsular retraction, and compensatory hypertrophy. Lesion-induced fibrosis seems to be the main cause of capsular retraction of the adjacent liver, but this can be caused by other pathologies, such as metastatic lesions and cholangiocarcinomas [7]. The type of HEH lesion influences how it manifests in a CT scan [37]. Nodular lesions appear as nonspecific, multinodular lesions, whereas diffuse lesions appear as a large mass that may represent the coalescence of smaller nodules. The following criteria on a CT scan may indicate a diffuse HEH lesion [20, 38–40]: (1) large peripheral tumors with gradual growth and no liver capsule protrusion due to fibrotic changes; (2) peripheral enhancement of contrast agent and central lesions with peripheral hypervascularization and nodular merging, with no traceable venous structure; and (3) portal hypertension with compensatory hypertrophy of the unaffected liver segments, as well as splenomegaly and local calcifications.

On a non-contrast CT scan, tumor nodules usually have a hypodense appearance, and subcapsular lesions may show associated capsular retraction [18, 20]. Therefore, unenhanced CT images may better estimate the extent of the lesion [28]. On a contrast CT scan, HEH appears as both peripheral and central enhancements. Smaller nodules (<2 cm) tend to show homogeneous enhancement [20], whereas 2–3-cm tumors show a ring-like enhancement during the arterial phase and central filling on the delayed and portal phases (the "halo sign") [12, 37]. Larger lesions may show heterogeneous enhancement, including a "lollipop sign" (an enhancing vein terminating at the periphery of a hypodense mass); this is the most characteristic feature of HEH on a CT scan, as it is rarely observed in other hepatic lesions [38, 41]. Infiltration of the sinusoids, venules, and veins via HEH narrows or occludes these pathways, which taper or terminate the portal and hepatic veins adjacent to the lesion. As a result, the contrast agent is tapered and terminated. Considering these features, the "lollipop sign" in CT-scan is a rare finding in other hepatic lesions and can serve as the most characteristic finding of the HEH.

3.4.2.3 MRI

MRI is a common technique for diagnosing HEH since it can detect small subcapsular lesions. HEH tumors show a low signal in T1-weighted imaging and a high signal in T2-weighted imaging [38, 42, 43]. On non-contrast enhanced MRI, a HEH lesion typically appears as a "halo sign," with three varying signals at different phases [44]. In T1-weighted imaging, HEH presents as a hypointense core with a hyperintense rim [1, 38] whereas in T2-weighted imaging, HEH shows a hyperintense core and a hypointense rim. The presence of a central sclerotic zone and a peripheral region of cellular proliferation is the main clarification for the target appearance of the tumor [45, 46]. The central low-signal areas represent hemorrhage, coagulation necrosis, and calcification, whereas the peripheral high-signal areas represent edematous connective tissue and viable tumor tissue. With diffusion-weighted imaging, more than half of the lesions also show a hyperintense external rim and core.

Contrast administration in MRI affects the appearance of HEH tumors in a similar way to a contrast-enhanced CT scan. In the arterial phase, HEH presents as a mild homogeneous enhancement, a ring-like enhancement, or a heterogeneous pattern, which correlates with the size of the tumor [33]. After administration of gadopentetate dimeglumine, an avascular zone appears between the liver parenchyma and the tumor, which shows as a peripheral enhancement, with a thin and unenhanced rim exposing the margin [46, 47]. Ferumoxide-enhanced T1-weighted imaging is the best technique for evaluating tumor extension [48]. Similar to the CT scan, enhanced imaging of the clear tumor mass and the blocking of adjacent veins contribute to the characteristic lollipop sign in MRI (Fig. 3.1).

3.4.2.4 PET-CT Scan

In an 18F-labeled fluoro-2-deoxyglucose (FDG) PET-CT scan, FDG is taken up more homogenously by healthy hepatocytes than by abnormal hepatocytes. This makes the uptake and excretion of FDG by HEH cells unpredictable, and up to one-third of HEHs have an FDG uptake similar to healthy cells. To address this problem, double-time 18F-FDG PET-CT has been used to detect and evaluate the progression of HEH. Lesions

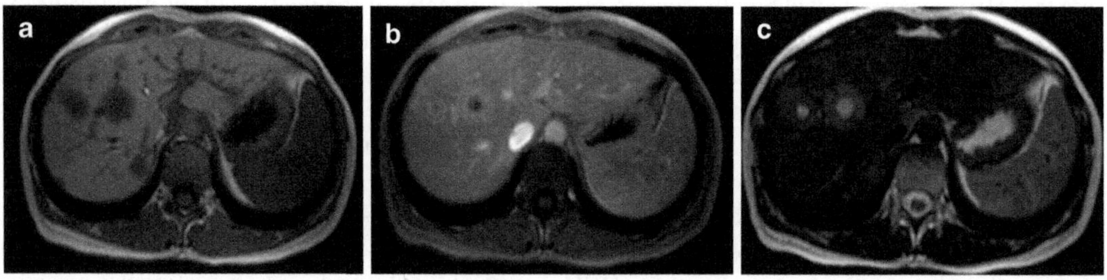

Fig. 3.1 Magnetic resonance images (MRIs) of hepatic epithelioid hemangioendothelioma (HEH). (**a**) Multiple hypointense lesions with necrosis in T1-weighted MRI (lollipop sign). (**b**) Reduced enhancement of the lesions and central necrosis in contrast-enhanced, T1-weighted MRI. (**c**) Hyperintense lesions and central necrosis with a target appearance in T2-weighted MRI (target sign). (Figure from Mehrabi et al. [7]. Copyright 2006 by John Wiley and Sons. Adapted with permission (License number: 5484870879424, Date: 09.02.2023))

that were not detected during the early phases of the disease can be detected by this delayed scanning [49]. 18F-FDG PET-CT has also been used to detect metastases [1, 50] and can distinguish between HEH lesions (with low FDG uptake) and cholangiocarcinomas (with high FDG uptake) [51]. However, diagnosing HEH with 18F-FDG PET-CT scanning is in its early stages and requires further assessment.

3.4.3 Histopathological Aspects

Histopathological examination is key to the diagnosis of HEH. Most specimens are collected surgically for diagnosis and, rarely, through fine-needle aspiration cytology. If precisely extracted and studied by an experienced pathologist, core biopsies can help diagnose HEH, although the histology might be confused with sclerosing hemangioma and sclerosing adenocarcinoma in some cases [52–54]. Because the histology results can be inconclusive, immunohistochemistry should also be performed to confirm endothelial cell differentiation [54]. Epithelial-like cells, dendritic-like cells, and intermediate cells are all present in HEH lesions [55–57], and the known biomarkers for HEH in these cells are factor VIII [24, 58], CD34, and CD31 [57, 59, 60]. Other less specific biomarkers are factor XIIIa, vimentin, type IV collagen, cytokeratin, and smooth muscle actin. Although histology is key to diagnosing HEH, no correlation has been reported between histological findings and the clinical course of the disease.

3.5 Differential Diagnosis

HEH might be misdiagnosed in up to 80% of cases because of variable tumor patterns. HEH lesions are mainly confused with angiosarcoma, cholangiocarcinoma, hepatocellular carcinoma, metastatic carcinoma, and sclerosing hemangioma (Table 3.2). Other less common misdiagnoses include mixed hamartoma, spindle cell neoplasm, inflammatory pseudotumors, bile duct adenoma, cirrhosis, carcinoma with chondromyxoid change, veno-oclusive disease, fibrolamellar carcinoma, postnecrotic fibrosis, and Budd–Chiari syndrome [7, 32, 60]. The main reasons for these misdiagnoses are similar results from immunohistochemistry profiling and hematoxylin–eosin staining. However, there are distinguishing features of HEH, including the infiltrative growth pattern with the preservation of the hepatic acinar landmarks (portal areas) and vascular invasion with the tufting of portal vein branches and terminal hepatic venules [7]. HEH can also be distinguished by epithelioid and dendritic tumor cells, especially if intracytoplasmic lumina are present, or by delayed expression of epithelial differentiation markers, including cytokeratins [1, 60].

Table 3.2 Differential diagnosis between hepatic epithelioid hemangioendothelioma and other primary and secondary hepatic lesions

Tumor type	Imaging characteristics	Immunohistochemical staining markers					Molecular biology	
		CD31	CD34	Vimentin	Factor VIII antigen	Pancytokeratin	Fusion gene	WWTR1-CAMTA1
HEH	Halo sign, target sign, lollipop sign, capsular retraction	+	+	+	+	–	+	+
Angiosarcoma	Heterogeneous centripetal enhancement	+	+	–	+	–	–	–
Hepatic hemangioma	Hypoattenuating, bright dot sign, irregular fill-in	–	–	–	–	–	–	–
Cholangiocarcinoma	Capsular retraction, gradual centripetal enhancement, central fibrosis	–	–	–	–	+	–	–
Hepatocellular carcinoma	Hypo- and hyperechoic enhancement	–	–	–	–	+	–	–
Metastatic carcinoma	Bull's-eye sign	–	–	–	–	+	–	–

3.6 Treatment

There are no standardized guidelines for HEH treatment, and therapeutic decisions are typically based on the liver lobes involved, the number and size of hepatic lesions, and the presence of extrahepatic disease [61]. Possible interventions include wait and watch, chemotherapy, radiotherapy, percutaneous ablative techniques, transarterial chemoembolization, liver resection, and liver transplantation (LT). However, HEH is a rare disease, so no randomized controlled trials have compared the efficacy of these treatments. Surgical treatment, within the frame of liver resection and liver transplantation, seems to be the only curative option for HEH that can increase long-term survival (Table 3.3). These treatment options are discussed below.

3.6.1 Watch and Wait

The "watch and wait" strategy involves allowing the disease to progress naturally without treatment [7]. In a few cases, spontaneous regression of the HEH tumor was reported, but in other cases, the patients died within weeks of their diagnosis because no treatment was initiated [62, 63]. The unpredictable nature of HEH makes it impossible to tell whether a tumor is aggressive or not and whether a "wait and watch" approach is suitable. This approach can be considered together with regular follow-ups (3-month intervals) in patients who have known regressive HEH lesions.

Table 3.3 5-Year overall survival of patients with hepatic epithelioid hemangioendothelioma after different therapeutic modalities

Therapy	5-Year survival rate (%)
Overall	55–70
Liver transplantation	64–95
Liver resection	75–88
Radiochemotherapy	30–43
None	<5

3.6.2 Systemic Therapy

The treatment of HEH with chemotherapy has unknown efficacy, with some studies reporting lower survival with chemotherapy than without. Systemic therapy has also been used to manage HEH, particularly in patients with extrahepatic disease [64]. Because HEH has a vascular origin and because VEGF receptors are expressed in HEH lesions [65, 66], VEGF inhibitors such as sorafenib, pazopanib, and bevacizumab have been used to treat HEH and have been shown to increase survival by 6 months [67–69]. A combination of VEGF inhibitors with cell cycle inhibitors (such as capecitabine) might improve survival outcomes even more.

3.6.3 Interventional Therapies

The most common interventional therapies for HEH are selective internal radiotherapy, transarterial chemoembolization, and radiofrequency ablation. Transarterial chemoembolization has shown the most promising outcomes, with a 3-year survival of >80% [7, 12]. Radiofrequency ablation has also been considered a safe intervention and has negligible morbidities in patients with HEH tumors <3 cm [70, 71]. Selective internal radiotherapy has led to significant remission of HEH lesions [72]. However, these modalities are not well-reported in the literature, so their efficacy remains to be clarified.

3.7 Surgical Management

3.7.1 Liver Resection

The most common surgical treatments for HEH are liver transplantation and liver resection, both of which have acceptable 5-year survival rates. HEH is rare, so treatments cannot be compared in a randomized controlled trial, and the choice between liver resection and liver transplantation remains debatable. Liver resection is reserved for single, intrahepatic, and monolobar lesions. The reported postoperative mortality rate following liver resection for HEH is 0–3%, and the 5-year survival rate is 75%. Anatomical liver resection is thought to be the best surgical approach because it preserves most of the liver parenchyma, but the appropriate curative surgical resection margin has not been determined. Some reports have suggested a surgical margin of 1 cm from the principal lesion, but there is currently no correlation between this resection margin and local HEH recurrence [73]. Others have shown that a negative surgical margin is sufficient in all liver sarcomas, including HEH [74, 75], suggesting that a resection margin of >1 cm is not necessary in patients with HEH [75]. However, underlying liver diseases, such as cirrhosis, are rare in patients with HEH, which permits complex liver resections. In a retrospective study from Mayo Clinic comprising 30 patients with HEH, the criteria for liver resection in patients with HEH were defined as <10 lesions, a tumor diameter of <10 cm, and lesions in ≤4 liver segments [76]. However, most cases have extensive liver involvement at the time of first diagnosis, and radical liver resection may cause posthepatectomy liver failure in these patients. On the other hand, conservative resection may not completely eradicate the tumor, leading to local recurrence or distant metastases. Portal vein embolization can be used to increase the remnant liver volume before radical resection of extensive tumors. Another possible approach for increasing the remnant liver volume is associating liver partition with portal vein ligation for staged hepatectomy (ALPPS). However, the recurrence rate is higher after liver resection than after liver transplantation [61].

The role of minimally invasive (MI) liver resection in HEH treatment has not been well-investigated. However, most HEH lesions are subcapsular, making them good candidates for MI resection. MI liver resection reduces intraoperative blood loss, hospital stay, and the rate of postoperative morbidity. These positive outcomes may be further improved by robotic liver surgery, which has shown promising outcomes for the management of benign and malignant liver lesions. MI liver surgery would also make repeated liver resection of recurring HEH tumors possible, either MI or open, since MI eliminates the disadvantages of the open resection, such as adhesion.

3.7.2 Liver Transplantation

Liver transplantation represents the best therapeutic option for unresectable HEH since liver resection might not be possible among patients with multinodular or bilobar involvement of the liver. In the literature, fewer than 300 cases have been reported. Three leading series have been reported from multicenter Western surveys, with the highest population of 149 patients with HEH from Europe [54]. Although no strong patient selection criteria and no algorithm have been introduced for the optimal management of HEH, liver transplantation has been recommended due to a better prognosis, with 5-year survival rates of up to 95% in some studies. A more detailed American study with 110 HEH cases reported a 5-year survival of 64% [77]. A more recent European study reported 5- and 10-year survival rates of 83% and 74%, respectively. The presence of extrahepatic metastases was not considered an absolute contraindication for liver transplantation in these surveys. To determine the risk of HEH recurrence after liver transplantation, Lai et al. proposed an HEHE-LT score to define the risk factors [78]. Independent predictors of HEH recurrence, and therefore relative contraindications to liver transplantation, include macrovascular involvement, a waiting time of less than four months before transplantation, and the presence of hilar nodal metastases. Patients without the risk factors had a 5-year disease-free survival of >90%, and this reduced to 40% in patients fulfilling these criteria. However, two out of the three criteria mentioned above can only be evaluated after hepatectomy, so they cannot be used for preoperative decision-making. Other risk factors for HEH recurrence after transplantation include tumor growth under immunosuppressive therapy and a lack of effective postoperative oncologic anticancer therapy. Therefore, the role of anticancer therapy after liver transplantation needs further investigation.

Surgical management by means of liver transplantation and liver resection is the best curative strategy for improving long-term survival in patients with HEH. Unresectable HEH without extrahepatic metastases is an excellent indication for liver transplantation, and HEH with extrahepatic disease should not be an absolute contraindication for liver transplantation in patients with severe liver dysfunction. Even HEH patients with extrahepatic invasion or multiple bilobar hepatic lesions are suitable candidates for liver transplantation. Furthermore, successful liver transplantation promotes long-term survival even in patients with distal metastases and should be considered a treatment to avoid liver failure in complicated intrahepatic disease and in cases where the tumor is difficult to resect. However, liver transplantation is associated with higher rates of morbidity and mortality than liver resection. Particularly, hepatic artery thrombosis (HAT) is more common in patients with HEH, leading to graft failure in 4.5% of patients after liver transplantation, which is more common compared to 0.5% of HAT for non-HEH patients [79].

3.8 Recommendations and Follow-Up

The diagnosis of HEH during the early stages of the disease remains challenging because of the low incidence and nonspecific signs and symptoms. As a result, most patients are diagnosed at advanced stages when bilobar liver involvement or distant metastases have occurred. Surgery is

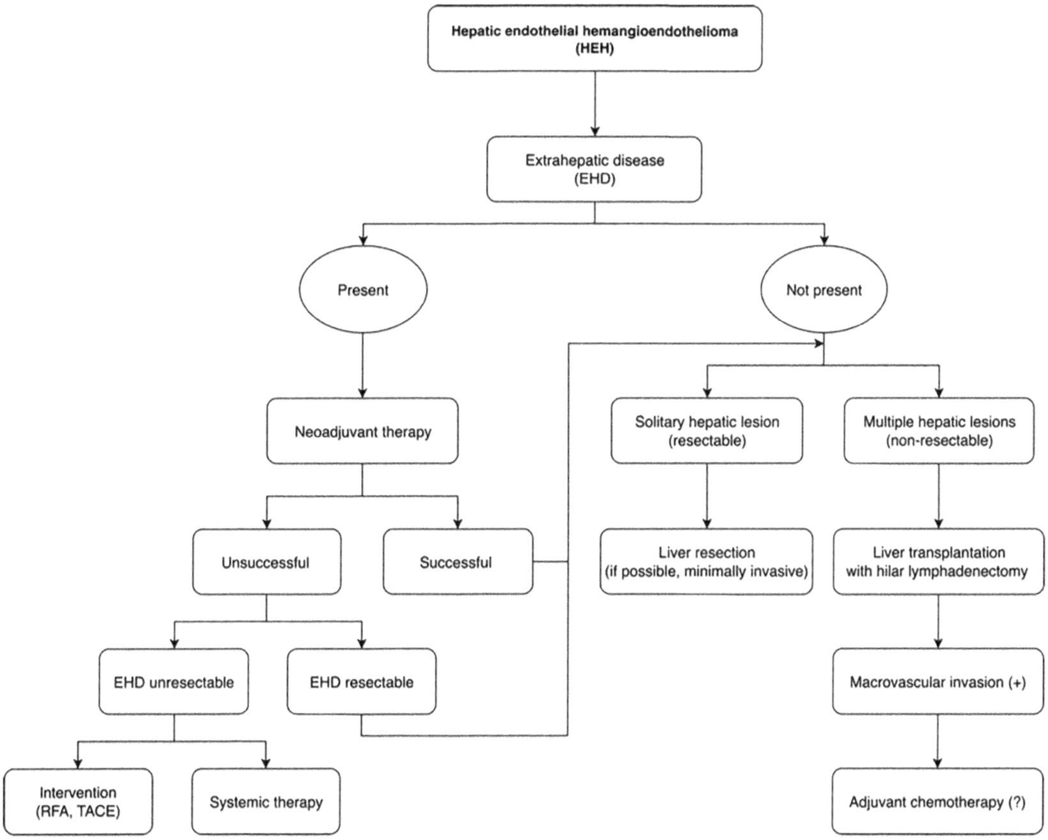

Fig. 3.2 Schematic tree of therapeutic strategies for patients with hepatic epithelioid hemangioendothelioma (HEH) based on the current literature

the only curative treatment for HEH, but the suitability of surgery in patients with advanced disease remains controversial. Recent data suggest that there should be no principal reluctance to perform liver resection or transplantation in patients with systemic disease. Based on these findings, we suggest a therapeutic schema for HEH (Fig. 3.2), in which surgical treatment is an option for all patients with HEH, except those with unresectable or diffuse extrahepatic disease. In these patients, neoadjuvant chemotherapy is recommended before surgery, but the efficacy and success rates of this approach are not clear. Liver transplantation should be considered the last resort for curative treatment, although systemic disease may prevent some patients from being eligible for transplantation. Because HEH is rare, randomized trials to compare treatments are likely not possible despite the need for this evidence.

The reported rate of HEH recurrence is 27%, regardless of the treatment modality. Disease-free survival has ranged between 11% and 94% in HEH patients after liver transplantation, and most studies have reported a 5-year disease-free survival rate of more than 60%. The recurrence of HEH is higher after liver resection than after liver transplantation, but recent reports have revealed a 5-year disease-free survival of more than 50% after resection. The HEHE-LT score might be a good way to identify those patients at a higher risk of HEH recurrence after liver transplantation, although the validity of this score has not been confirmed. The role of adjuvant chemotherapy after surgical treatment, particularly liver resection, is not well-established. Till a clarification of these pitfalls and questions is received, a structured and regular follow-up with imaging diagnostics should be carried out after surgical treatment (resection or transplantation) to detect HEH recurrence as quickly as possible.

References

1. Kou K, Chen YG, Zhou JP, Sun XD, Sun DW, Li SX, et al. Hepatic epithelioid hemangioendothelioma: update on diagnosis and therapy. World J Clin Cases. 2020;8(18):3978–87.
2. Weiss SW, Ishak KG, Dail DH, Sweet DE, Enzinger FM. Epithelioid hemangioendothelioma and related lesions. Semin Diagn Pathol. 1986;3(4):259–87.
3. Fletcher CD, Unni K, Mertens F. World Health Organization classification of tumours. Pathology and genetics of tumours of soft tissue and bone. IARC Press; 2002.
4. Ishak KG, Sesterhenn IA, Goodman MZD, Rabin L, Stromeyer FW. Epithelioid hemangioendothelioma of the liver: a clinicopathologic and follow-up study of 32 cases. Hum Pathol. 1984;15(9):839–52.
5. Elleuch N, Dahmani W, Aida Ben S, Jaziri H, Aya H, Ksiaa M, et al. Hepatic epithelioid hemangioendothelioma: a misdiagnosed rare liver tumor. Presse Med. 2018;47(2):182–5.
6. Hertl M, Cosimi AB. Liver transplantation for malignancy. Oncologist. 2005;10(4):269–81.
7. Mehrabi A, Kashfi A, Fonouni H, Schemmer P, Schmied BM, Hallscheidt P, et al. Primary malignant hepatic epithelioid hemangioendothelioma: a comprehensive review of the literature with emphasis on the surgical therapy. Cancer. 2006;107(9):2108–21.
8. Langrehr J, Petersen I, Pfitzmann R, Lopez-Hänninen E. Malign epithelioid hemangioendothelioma of the liver. Results of surgical treatment strategies: Ergebnisse der chirurgischen Behandlung. Chirurg. 2005;76:1161–7.
9. Bruegel M, Muenzel D, Waldt S, Specht K, Rummeny EJ. Hepatic epithelioid hemangioendothelioma: findings at CT and MRI including preliminary observations at diffusion-weighted echo-planar imaging. Abdom Imaging. 2011;36(4):415–24.
10. Gurung S, Fu H, Zhang WW, Gu YH. Hepatic epithelioid hemangioendothelioma metastasized to the peritoneum, omentum and mesentery: a case report. Int J Clin Exp Pathol. 2015;8(5):5883–9.
11. Shah PM, Dhakre VW, Nagral A. Primary hepatic hemangioendothelioma in a patient with Budd-Chiari syndrome. BMJ Case Rep. 2017;2017:bcr-2017-221103.
12. Lazăr DC, Avram MF, Romoşan I, Văcariu V, Goldiş A, Cornianu M. Malignant hepatic vascular tumors in adults: characteristics, diagnostic difficulties and current management. World J Clin Oncol. 2019;10(3):110–35.
13. Neofytou K, Chrysochos A, Charalambous N, Dietis M, Petridis C, Andreou C, et al. Hepatic epithelioid hemangioendothelioma and the danger of misdiagnosis: report of a case. Case Rep Oncol Med. 2013;2013:243939.
14. Errani C, Zhang L, Sung YS, Hajdu M, Singer S, Maki RG, et al. A novel WWTR1-CAMTA1 gene fusion is a consistent abnormality in epithelioid hemangioendothelioma of different anatomic sites. Genes Chromosomes Cancer. 2011;50(8):644–53.
15. Mendlick MR, Nelson M, Pickering D, Johansson SL, Seemayer TA, Neff JR, et al. Translocation t(1;3)(p36.3;q25) is a nonrandom aberration in epithelioid hemangioendothelioma. Am J Surg Pathol. 2001;25(5):684–7.

16. Flucke U, Vogels RJ, de Saint Aubain Somerhausen N, Creytens DH, Riedl RG, van Gorp JM, et al. Epithelioid hemangioendothelioma: clinicopathologic, immunhistochemical, and molecular genetic analysis of 39 cases. Diagn Pathol. 2014;9:131.
17. Liu X, Yu H, Zhang Z, Si S, Huang J, Tan H, et al. MRI appearances of hepatic epithelioid hemangioendothelioma: a retrospective study of 57 patients. Insights Imaging. 2022;13(1):65.
18. Studer LL, Selby DM. Hepatic epithelioid hemangioendothelioma. Arch Pathol Lab Med. 2018;142(2):263–7.
19. Mistry AM, Gorden DL, Busler JF, Coogan AC, Kelly BS. Diagnostic and therapeutic challenges in hepatic epithelioid hemangioendothelioma. J Gastrointest Cancer. 2012;43(4):521–5.
20. Zhou L, Cui MY, Xiong J, Dong Z, Luo Y, Xiao H, et al. Spectrum of appearances on CT and MRI of hepatic epithelioid hemangioendothelioma. BMC Gastroenterol. 2015;15:69.
21. Zis P, Assi A, Kravaritis D, Sevastianos VA. Ischemic stroke as the first manifestation of hepatic epithelioid hemangioendothelioma. J Stroke Cerebrovasc Dis. 2014;23(3):e237–40.
22. Yang JW, Li Y, Xie K, Dong W, Cao XT, Xiao WD. Spontaneous rupture of hepatic epithelioid hemangioendothelioma: a case report. World J Gastroenterol. 2017;23(1):185–90.
23. Kim K-H, Kim S-J, Lee S-H. Living-donor liver transplantation for hepatic epithelioid hemangioendothelioma with early recurrence in an adult: a case report. Transplantation. 2018;102:S905.
24. Afrit M, Nasri M, Labidi S, Mejri N, El Benna H, Boussen H. Aggressive primary hepatic epithelioid hemangioendothelioma: a case report and literature review. Cancer Biol Med. 2017;14(2):187–90.
25. Din NU, Rahim S, Asghari T, Abdul-Ghafar J, Ahmad Z. Hepatic epithelioid hemangioendothelioma: case series of a rare vascular tumor mimicking metastases. Diagn Pathol. 2020;15(1):120.
26. Mulazzani L, Alvisi M. Imaging findings of hepatic epithelioid hemangioendothelioma and fibrolamellar hepatocellular carcinoma: a critical appraisal of current literature about imaging features of two rare liver cancers. Transl Cancer Res. 2019;8:S297–310.
27. Choi KH, Moon WS. Epithelioid hemangioendothelioma of the liver. Clin Mol Hepatol. 2013;19(3):315–9.
28. Hu HJ, Jin YW, Jing QY, Shrestha A, Cheng NS, Li FY. Hepatic epithelioid hemangioendothelioma: dilemma and challenges in the preoperative diagnosis. World J Gastroenterol. 2016;22(41):9247–50.
29. Wu X, Li B, Zheng C, Hong T, He X. Clinical characteristics of epithelioid hemangioendothelioma: a single-center retrospective study. Eur J Med Res. 2019;24(1):16.
30. Kim SJ, Kim YC. Unusual extrahepatic metastasis to the soft tissue of the left cervical neck area from hepatic epithelioid hemangioendothelioma. Hepatology. 2011;54(4):1480–1.
31. Schwab M. Encyclopedia of cancer. Springer; 2017.
32. Mehrabi A, Kashfi A, Schemmer P, Sauer P, Encke J, Fonouni H, et al. Surgical treatment of primary hepatic epithelioid hemangioendothelioma. Transplantation. 2005;80(1S):S109–S12.
33. Dong Y, Wang WP, Cantisani V, D'Onofrio M, Ignee A, Mulazzani L, et al. Contrast-enhanced ultrasound of histologically proven hepatic epithelioid hemangioendothelioma. World J Gastroenterol. 2016;22(19):4741–9.
34. Treska V, Daum O, Svajdler M, Liska V, Ferda J, Baxa J. Hepatic epithelioid hemangioendothelioma – a rare tumor and diagnostic dilemma. In Vivo. 2017;31(4):763–7.
35. Wang L, Lv K, Chang XY, Xia Y, Yang ZY, Jiang YX, et al. Contrast-enhanced ultrasound study of primary hepatic angiosarcoma: a pitfall of non-enhancement. Eur J Radiol. 2012;81(9):2054–9.
36. Zhao M, Yin F. Hepatic epithelioid hemangioendothelioma: clinical characteristics, diagnosis, treatment, and prognosis. World J Clin Cases. 2022;10(17):5606–19.
37. Woodall CE, Scoggins CR, Lewis AM, McMasters KM, Martin RC. Hepatic malignant epithelioid hemangioendothelioma: a case report and review of the literature. Am Surg. 2008;74(1):64–8.
38. Gan LU, Chang R, Jin H, Yang LI. Typical CT and MRI signs of hepatic epithelioid hemangioendothelioma. Oncol Lett. 2016;11(3):1699–706.
39. Fulcher AS, Sterling RK. Hepatic neoplasms: computed tomography and magnetic resonance features. J Clin Gastroenterol. 2002;34(4):463–71.
40. Beers BV, Roche A, Mathieu D, Menu Y, Delos M, Otte J-B, et al. Epithelioid hemangioendothelioma of the liver: MR and CT findings. J Comput Assist Tomogr. 1992;16(3):420–4.
41. Miller WJ, Dodd GD 3rd, Federle MP, Baron RL. Epithelioid hemangioendothelioma of the liver: imaging findings with pathologic correlation. AJR Am J Roentgenol. 1992;159(1):53–7.
42. Paolantonio P, Laghi A, Vanzulli A, Grazioli L, Morana G, Ragozzino A, et al. MRI of hepatic epithelioid hemangioendothelioma (HEH). J Magn Reson Imaging. 2014;40(3):552–8.
43. Larochelle O, Périgny M, Lagacé R, Dion N, Giguère C. Best cases from the AFIP: epithelioid hemangioendothelioma of bone. Radiographics. 2006;26(1):265–70.
44. Mamone G, Miraglia R. The "Target sign" and the "Lollipop sign" in hepatic epithelioid hemangioendothelioma. Abdom Radiol (NY). 2019;44(4):1617–20.
45. Lyburn ID, Torreggiani WC, Harris AC, Zwirewich CV, Buckley AR, Davis JE, et al. Hepatic epithelioid hemangioendothelioma: sonographic, CT, and MR imaging appearances. Am J Roentgenol. 2003;180(5):1359–64.
46. Ros LH, Fernández L, Villacampa VM, Ros PR. Epithelioid hemangioendothelioma of the liver-

-characteristics on magnetic resonance imaging: case report. Can Assoc Radiol J. 1999;50(6):387–9.
47. Alomari AI. The lollipop sign: a new cross-sectional sign of hepatic epithelioid hemangioendothelioma. Eur J Radiol. 2006;59(3):460–4.
48. Kehagias D, Moulopoulos L, Antoniou A, Psychogios V, Vourtsi A, Vlahos L. Hepatic epithelioid hemangioendothelioma: MR imaging findings. Hepato-Gastroenterology. 2000;47(36):1711–3.
49. Kitapci MT, Akkaş BE, Gullu I, Sokmensuer C. FDG-PET/CT in the evaluation of epithelioid hemangioendothelioma of the liver: the role of dual-time-point imaging. A case presentation and review of the literature. Ann Nucl Med. 2010;24(7):549–53.
50. Maeda T, Tateishi U, Hasegawa T, Ojima H, Arai Y, Sugimura K. Primary hepatic angiosarcoma on coregistered FDG PET and CT images. AJR Am J Roentgenol. 2007;188(6):1615–7.
51. Kim YJ, Yun M, Lee WJ, Kim KS, Lee JD. Usefulness of 18F-FDG PET in intrahepatic cholangiocarcinoma. Eur J Nucl Med Mol Imaging. 2003;30(11):1467–72.
52. Chaudhary P, Bhadana U, Singh RA, Ahuja A. Primary hepatic angiosarcoma. Eur J Surg Oncol. 2015;41(9):1137–43.
53. Wong JW, Bedard YC. Fine-needle aspiration biopsy of hepatic angiosarcoma: report of a case with immunocytochemical findings. Diagn Cytopathol. 1992;8(4):380–3.
54. Lerut JP, Orlando G, Adam R, Schiavo M, Klempnauer J, Mirza D, et al. The place of liver transplantation in the treatment of hepatic epitheloid hemangioendothelioma: report of the European liver transplant registry. Ann Surg. 2007;246(6):949–57; discussion 57.
55. Makhlouf HR, Ishak KG, Goodman ZD. Epithelioid hemangioendothelioma of the liver: a clinicopathologic study of 137 cases. Cancer. 1999;85(3):562–82.
56. Earnest F, Johnson CD. Case 96: hepatic epithelioid hemangioendothelioma. Radiology. 2006;240(1):295–8.
57. Campione S, Cozzolino I, Mainenti P, D'Alessandro V, Vetrani A, D'Armiento M. Hepatic epithelioid hemangioendothelioma: pitfalls in the diagnosis on fine needle cytology and "small biopsy" and review of the literature. Pathol Res Pract. 2015;211(9):702–5.
58. Naqvi J, Ordonez NG, Luna MA, Williams MD, Weber RS, El-Naggar AK. Epithelioid hemangioendothelioma of the head and neck: role of podoplanin in the differential diagnosis. Head Neck Pathol. 2008;2(1):25–30.
59. Wang ZB, Wei LX. Primary hepatic angiosarcoma: a clinical and pathological analysis. Zhonghua Bing Li Xue Za Zhi. 2013;42(6):376–80.
60. Virarkar M, Saleh M, Diab R, Taggart M, Bhargava P, Bhosale P. Hepatic hemangioendothelioma: an update. World J Gastrointest Oncol. 2020;12(3):248–66.
61. Cao L, Hong J, Zhou L, Ye Y, Liu Y, Yu J, et al. Selection of treatment for hepatic epithelioid hemangioendothelioma: a single-center experience. World J Surg Oncol. 2019;17(1):183.
62. Otrock ZK, Al-Kutoubi A, Kattar MM, Zaatari G, Soweid A. Spontaneous complete regression of hepatic epithelioid haemangioendothelioma. Lancet Oncol. 2006;7(5):439–41.
63. Makhlouf HR, Ishak KG, Goodman ZD. Epithelioid hemangioendothelioma of the liver. Cancer. 1999;85(3):562–82.
64. Lau A, Malangone S, Green M, Badari A, Clarke K, Elquza E. Combination capecitabine and bevacizumab in the treatment of metastatic hepatic epithelioid hemangioendothelioma. Ther Adv Med Oncol. 2015;7(4):229–36.
65. Young RJ, Woll PJ. Anti-angiogenic therapies for the treatment of angiosarcoma: a clinical update. Memo. 2017;10(4):190–3.
66. Agulnik M, Yarber JL, Okuno SH, von Mehren M, Jovanovic BD, Brockstein BE, et al. An open-label, multicenter, phase II study of bevacizumab for the treatment of angiosarcoma and epithelioid hemangioendotheliomas. Ann Oncol. 2013;24(1):257–63.
67. Läuffer JM, Zimmermann A, Krähenbühl L, Triller J, Baer HU. Epithelioid hemangioendothelioma of the liver. A rare hepatic tumor. Cancer. 1996;78(11):2318–27.
68. Chevreau C, Le Cesne A, Ray-Coquard I, Italiano A, Cioffi A, Isambert N, et al. Sorafenib in patients with progressive epithelioid hemangioendothelioma: a phase 2 study by the French Sarcoma Group (GSF/GETO). Cancer. 2013;119(14):2639–44.
69. Kobayashi N, Shimamura T, Tokuhisa M, Goto A, Ichikawa Y. Sorafenib monotherapy in a patient with unresectable hepatic epithelioid hemangioendothelioma. Case Rep Oncol. 2016;9(1):134–7.
70. Kamarajah SK, Robinson D, Littler P, White SA. Small, incidental hepatic epithelioid haemangioendothelioma the role of ablative therapy in borderline patients. J Surg Case Rep. 2018;2018(8):rjy223.
71. Shiina S, Tateishi R, Arano T, Uchino K, Enooku K, Nakagawa H, et al. Radiofrequency ablation for hepatocellular carcinoma: 10-year outcome and prognostic factors. Am J Gastroenterol. 2012;107(4):569–77; quiz 78.
72. Bostancı EB, Karaman K, Turhan N, Dalgıç T, Özer İ, Soydal C, et al. Selective internal radiotherapy for hepatic epithelioid hemangioendothelioma. Turk J Gastroenterol. 2014;25(Suppl 1):252–3.
73. Agostini-Vulaj D, Pehlivanoglu B, Weiss SW, Krasinskas A, Feely MM, Hornick JL, et al. Intrasinusoidal spread of hepatic epithelioid hemangioendothelioma: implications for the diagnosis in minimal samples. Am J Surg Pathol. 2019;43(4):573–9.
74. Konstantinidis IT, Nota C, Jutric Z, Ituarte P, Chow W, Chu P, et al. Primary liver sarcomas in the modern era: resection or transplantation? J Surg Oncol. 2018;117(5):886–91.
75. Giovanardi F, Larghi Laureiro Z, Meo GA, Hassan R, Lai Q. The challenging surgical management of hepatic epithelioid hemangioendothelioma: a narrative review. Chin Clin Oncol. 2022;11(4):27.

76. Grotz TE, Nagorney D, Donohue J, Que F, Kendrick M, Farnell M, et al. Hepatic epithelioid haemangioendothelioma: is transplantation the only treatment option? HPB. 2010;12(8):546–53.
77. Rodriguez JA, Becker NS, O'Mahony CA, Goss JA, Aloia TA. Long-term outcomes following liver transplantation for hepatic hemangioendothelioma: the UNOS experience from 1987 to 2005. J Gastrointest Surg. 2008;12(1):110–6.
78. Lai Q, Feys E, Karam V, Adam R, Klempnauer J, Oliverius M, et al. Hepatic epithelioid hemangioendothelioma and adult liver transplantation: proposal for a prognostic score based on the analysis of the ELTR-ELITA registry. Transplantation. 2017;101(3):555–64.
79. Brahmbhatt M, Prenner S, Bittermann T. Liver transplantation for hepatic epithelioid hemangioendothelioma is facilitated by exception points with acceptable long-term outcomes. Transplantation. 2020;104(6):1187–92.

Surgical Management of Liver Flukes

4

Aya Maekawa, Hiromichi Ito, Yosuke Inoue, and Yu Takahashi

4.1 Introduction

Fluke, or Trematoda, is a class within a group of parasitic flatworms. Liver flukes infect various mammals, including humans, and reside in their intestines, bile duct, and liver. Among digenean parasites affecting the human liver, three trematode families are involved: Opisthorchiidae, Fasciolodae, and Dicrocoeliidae [7]. Despite many preventative efforts against flukes by local public health authorities, their prevalence remains high in some areas of East and Southeastern Asia and sub-Saharan Africa [23]. While the symptoms caused by liver flukes are mild to minimal in general, chronic infection can cause severe consequences of carcinogenesis if it is left untreated [1, 2, 20].

In this chapter, we focus on common liver flukes and describe the association between fluke infection and the risk of hepatobiliary cancer.

4.2 Epidemiology

Liver flukes have three distinct hosts in their life cycles [5] (Fig. 4.1). The eggs are excreted into the definitive hosts' stool, embryonated, and hatch when reaching freshwater, ingested by intermediate snail hosts. The parasites grow as cercariae in the snails and then swim in the water, transmitting to various freshwater fishes, where they become infectious metacercariae. Humans and other mammals are infected as definitive hosts by ingesting raw or undercooked fish and contaminated vegetables containing metacercariae. After entering the human body, immature flukes migrate through the intestinal wall and the peritoneal cavity and specifically enter the liver and biliary ducts, where they mature into adults in 3–4 months. Adult flukes feed on the bile duct epithelia, live in the bile duct system, and continue to spawn in the bile for 20–30 years.

Liver fluke infection remains a major public health problem, with approximately 50 million people infected and over 700 million at risk [5, 12]. The geographic distribution of liver flukes differs between the species. *Clonorchis sinensis*, the so-called Chinese liver fluke, is found in China, Eastern Russia, South Korea, and Vietnam, infecting over 35 million people [21]. *Opisthorchis viverrini*, the so-called Southeast liver fluke, is endemic in northeast Thailand and Laos. Cholangiocarcinoma (CCA) is the leading cause of cancer-associated mortality, whereas

A. Maekawa · H. Ito (✉) · Y. Inoue · Y. Takahashi
Division of Hepatobiliary and Pancreatic Surgery, Cancer Institute Hospital, Japanese Foundation for Cancer Research, Tokyo, Japan
e-mail: aya.maekawa@jfcr.or.jp; hiromichi.ito@jfcr.or.jp; yosuke.inoue@jfcr.or.jp; yu.takahashi@jfcr.or.jp

T. Hackert, A. Gulla (eds.), *Rare Liver and Biliary Tract Diseases*,
https://doi.org/10.1007/978-3-032-15076-9_4

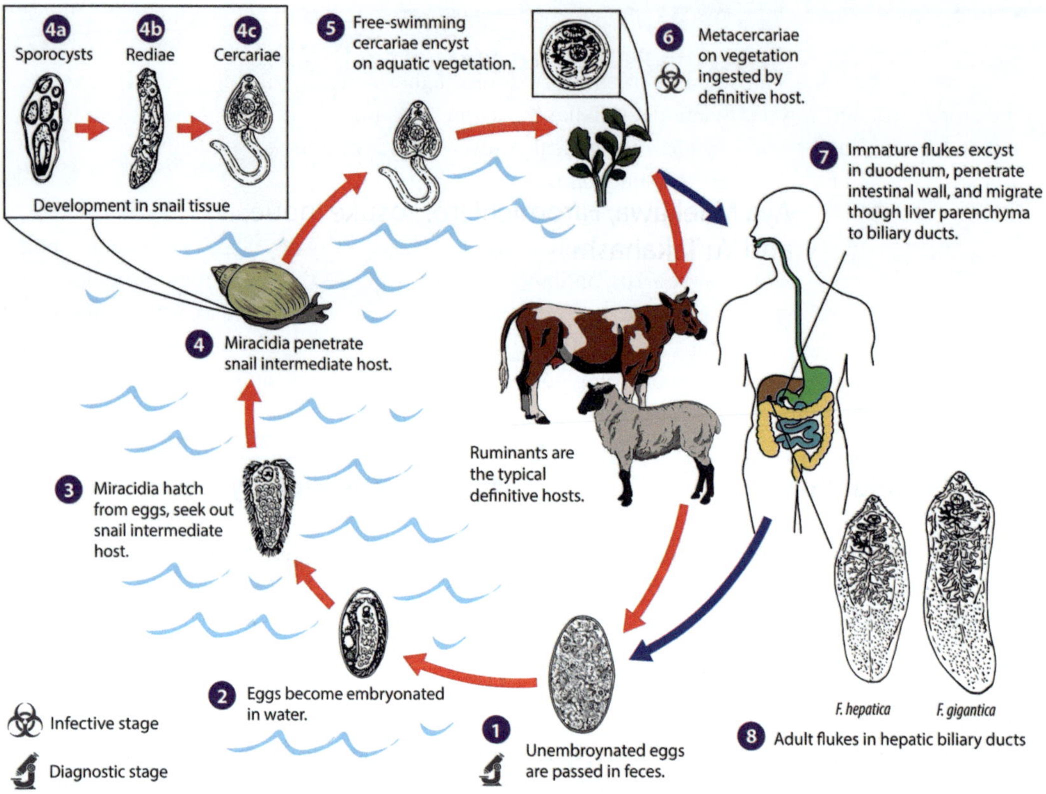

Fig. 4.1 Life cycle of liver flukes. (From Life cycle developed by Centers for Disease Control and Prevention (https://www.cdc.gov/parasites/fasciola/biology.html). The image is otherwise available on the agency website for no charge)

hepatocellular carcinoma is the most common type of primary liver cancer worldwide [15]. *Opisthorchis felineus* is one of the few zoonoses found in Southern Europe, with eight outbreaks reported in Italy [16]. Despite sanitation and hygiene promotion, liver fluke prevalence has not decreased as expected. This may be likely because of the increased awareness of this neglected disease and the expanding endemic geographical range due to globalization.

4.3 Clinical Presentation

The disease process for liver fluke infection can be classified into acute and chronic phases. Although most patients are asymptomatic in the acute phase, some can develop nonspecific symptoms, including intermittent fever, abdominal pain, malaise, nausea, hives, and weight loss, when it causes acute liver damage. Without adequate treatment to eradicate the disease, benign hepatobiliary complications such as cholangitis, cholecystitis, hepatomegaly, splenomegaly, and bile duct stone formation can occur subsequently. In particular, the ova, fluke worms, and mucin can cause chronic mechanical obstruction in the biliary flow, resulting in an increased risk of choledocholithiasis and cholangitis. In the chronic phase, liver cirrhosis can develop because of microvasculature obstruction due to granuloma caused by local reaction or the residing eggs. Additionally, persistent inflammation in the biliary system over decades can lead to cancer development. While CCA occurring secondary to fluke infection can anatomically arise anywhere within the biliary tract, depending on the site of infection, predilection sites have been known to differ among species; *Clonorchis* and *Opisthorchis* species are commonly found in the intrahepatic biliary tree, whereas *Fasciola* species prefer the extrahepatic bile ducts [17].

Several potential mechanisms by which CCA is developed through chronic fluke infection have been speculated, and they include mechanical damage to the biliary epithelia, immunopathology due to infection-related inflammation, and toxic effects of parasite secretion. Genetic and epigenetic aberrations have been reported, comparing fluke-related and non-fluke-related CCA. Despite its different etiology and biological background, the clinical presentation for patients with fluke-related CCA is not different from those with non-fluke-related CCA. They remain asymptomatic, and their diagnosis is often delayed until the tumor causes biliary obstruction and cholangitis.

4.4 Workup Investigation

4.4.1 Microscopic Inspection of Stool

A fecal examination is the most commonly used approach for diagnosing liver fluke infection because of the simplicity of sample collection and its low cost. Fecal samples are evaluated microscopically for the presence of eggs by various methods, including the formalin–ether technique or the spontaneous sedimentation technique using Lugol's staining solution, Kato-Katz method using methylene blue-stained cellophane, or direct smear microscopy [3, 10]. Although the fecal examination is highly specific, the test result depends on the burden of flukes and the prepatent period of infection before eggs are produced; thus, this method is inefficient for patients with chronic infection when egg production is sporadic. Repeated examinations are needed to improve diagnostic sensitivity. Also, parasitic infections can be superimposed, making microscopic differentiation between the eggs of liver flukes and other trematodes difficult. In this way, both the sensitivity and specificity of parasite identification rely on the technician's experience. Eggs from ingested food containing infected animal livers can be detected in the stool, leading to misdiagnosis. Thus, patients should be asked to avoid such a liver diet containing animal liver for several days prior to the stool test.

4.4.2 Blood Tests

Serum antibodies to the flukes become detectable 2–4 weeks after infection. This immunological test is useful for detection in the early stages of infection before eggs are produced and in chronic stages where egg production is sporadic or low. Enzyme-linked immunosorbent assay has a high sensitivity and specificity rate of over approximately 98% for fascioliasis [9]. Also, it can discriminate *Fasciola*-infected individuals from those with other concurrent parasitic infections.

Complete blood counts and serum testing may show anemia, eosinophilia, elevated erythrocyte sedimentation rate, liver enzymes, and gamma globulin. However, these results are nonspecific to liver fluke infection.

4.4.3 Imaging Diagnosis

Ultrasonography, computed tomography (CT), magnetic resonance imaging (MRI), and endoscopic retrograde cholangiopancreatography (ERCP) are commonly performed to evaluate the liver and biliary tracts. In acute phases, ultrasound and CT imaging may detect hypodense masses, hepatomegaly, and cysts due to infection. ERCP is utilized for both the diagnosis and treatment of liver flukes [24]. By direct visualization, ova or adult worms can be removed when they cause obstruction of the bile duct. Also, definitive histological or cytological diagnosis can be obtained during ERCP through bile duct biopsy and/or bile cytology. In general, it is challenging to determine whether liver fluke infection is the underlying cause of abnormal hepatobiliary conditions through radiological evaluations alone.

4.5 Differential Diagnosis

Symptoms of liver fluke infection are generally nonspecific, making early and accurate diagnosis challenging. Differential diagnoses include other parasitic infections, rheumatic diseases causing fever of unknown origin, digestive disorders such as gastroesophageal reflux, and non-fluke-related hepatobiliary disorders, such as viral hepatitis, cholangitis, cholecystitis, bile duct stones, and liver malignancies [22].

For most physicians in non-endemic regions, making the diagnosis of liver flukes is quite difficult because of the low index of suspicion or a lack of medical knowledge of this disease.

4.6 Treatments

4.6.1 Anthelmintics

Praziquantel is an anthelmintic agent used predominantly in treating liver flukes, schistosomiasis, and cysticercosis [18]. The World Health Organization (WHO)–recommended dose of praziquantel is 25 mg/kg orally three times a day for 2–3 days, resulting in an egg reduction rate of over 98% for both *O. viverrini* and *C. sinensis* infection. A single-dose 40 mg/kg oral praziquantel has been used for an opisthorchiasis control program in Thailand, given the high efficacy and safety of the drug [14]. Adverse events include fatigue, abdominal discomfort, dizziness, headache, and nausea, although these symptoms may come from the primary fluke infection.

An albendazole dose of 10 mg/kg once a day for 5–7 days is an alternative regimen recommended by the US Centers for Disease Control and Prevention. However, a longer treatment duration is required compared to praziquantel.

Tribendimidine is a relatively new anthelmintic agent from China, also effective for ancylostomiasis, ascariasis, and enterobiasis [19]. The egg reduction rate of a single-dose 400 mg tribendimidine treatment for *O. viverrini* and *C. sinensis* was reported to be as high as 98–99%, comparable to the praziquantel treatment, with fewer adverse effects. Patients in endemic areas with a coinfection of liver flukes and roundworms would benefit from the broad-spectrum coverage of tribendimidine.

Triclabendazole is a narrow-spectrum anthelminthic with high efficacy in treating fascioliasis. The WHO administered a donation program for triclabendazole for fascioliasis treatment in endemic countries in the 1990s, and this anthelminthic remains the only treatment recommended.

Drug resistance has become a major problem for both human and livestock infections [4, 8]. New drugs have been developed; however, the appropriate usage of conventional treatment is critical to prevent the unnecessary spread of resistance. Re-treatment may be necessary for patients with severe parasitic infections or those resistant to the primary treatment. Genomic and transcriptomic studies have been investigated; however, no effective vaccines have been developed to date [4].

4.6.2 Endoscopic Biliary Treatment

ERCP is clinically beneficial for biliary complications at various phases of the disease [24]. Crescent-shaped or linear filling defects on cholangiography suggest the presence of adult worms in the biliary tract. Endoscopic clearance and decompression of the biliary tract improve cholangitis or jaundice caused by parasitic obstruction and fluke infection–related biliary stones. Dilatation or stent placement is performed for biliary strictures caused by chronic inflammation. This procedure is not only utilized in active infection but may also be necessary in cases where the obstruction occurs from dead flukes after medical treatment.

4.6.3 Surgical Planning/Management

The earliest surgical intervention for liver flukes was choledocholithotomy with cholecystectomy, reported in 1941 by Manson-Bahr and Walton [11]. Nowadays, most patients with early and mild infections can be successfully treated with anthelmintics and/or endoscopic intervention for biliary obstruction as needed, and the need for surgical intervention is less common. The type of surgical intervention will depend on the stage of infection and hepatobiliary pathological changes.

For acute/chronic cholecystitis, open or laparoscopic cholecystectomy should be performed. When ERCP is unsuccessful in retrieving large bile duct stones, choledocholithotomy or hepaticojejunostomy is necessary. Pathologic evaluation for these stones may reveal parasite ova.

Surgical resection is the only curative treatment for CCA, and as mentioned above, the management of fluke-induced CCA is not different from that in non-fluke-related patients. Abnormal liver malfunction and liver fibrosis from chronic inflammation can increase the risk of perioperative complications. It is important to note that mid-to-long-term follow-up is crucial for patients diagnosed with liver fluke to monitor the chronic course of the disease, including carcinogenesis.

4.7 Follow-Up/Recommendations

Fluke infection remains a clinically important disease for public health in East Asia and Africa, as it increases the incidence of hepatobiliary cancer and the associated mortality in endemic areas. The parasites can survive for decades within their hosts, and many have recently developed multidrug resistance to frontline medications. Therapeutic intervention at an early stage of infection is desirable, though many patients take a long time to be diagnosed because of a lack of symptoms. Although fluke infections are a rare cause of biliary tract disease in industrialized countries, climate change, expanded international travel, and immigration from endemic regions have increased the incidence of these infrequent parasitic infections [13]. Thorough travel and exposure history taking are essential to reach a correct diagnosis for patients with atypical presentations of hepatobiliary disorders.

The treatment strategy for infected patients alone is insufficient for successful liver fluke control. Health education is vital to prevent both primary infection and reinfection after initial treatment [6]. To control this foodborne infection effectively, measures for recognition and education for the general public need to be implemented by the public health department and the food industry. Consumption of raw or undercooked aquatic plants, vegetables, liver, and freshwater fish from endemic areas must be avoided. The flukes remain alive in lightly salted, smoked, fermented, or pickled fish; the Food and Drug Administration recommends cooking fish to an internal temperature of at least 63 °C and storing by freezing at ≤ -20 °C for at least 7 days or ≤ -35 °C until solid.

Recent research advances have allowed us to better understand the neglected parasite's biology and pathogenesis. Early treatment and prevention of the disease spread can reduce the incidence of hepatobiliary disorders and deadly cancers.

References

1. Bouvard V, Baan R, Straif K, Grosse Y, Secretan B, El Ghissassi F, Benbrahim-Tallaa L, Guha N, Freeman C, Galichet L, Cogliano V, WHO International Agency for Research on Cancer Monograph Working Group. A review of human carcinogens--part B: biological agents. Lancet Oncol. 2009;10:321–2.
2. Brindley PJ, Bachini M, Ilyas SI, Khan SA, Loukas A, Sirica AE, Teh BT, Wongkham S, Gores GJ. Cholangiocarcinoma. Nat Rev Dis Primers. 2021;7:65.
3. Calvopina M, Romero-Alvarez D, Diaz F, Cevallos W, Sugiyama H. A comparison of Kato-Katz technique to three other methods for diagnosis of Amphimerus spp. liver fluke infection and the prevalence of infection in Chachi Amerindians of Ecuador. PLoS One. 2018;13:e0203811.
4. Canevari J, Ceballos L, Sanabria R, Romero J, Olaechea F, Ortiz P, Cabrera M, Gayo V, Fairweather I, Lanusse C, Alvarez L. Testing albendazole resistance in Fasciola hepatica: validation of an egg hatch test with isolates from South America and the United Kingdom. J Helminthol. 2014;88:286–92.
5. Chai JY, Darwin Murrell K, Lymbery AJ. Fish-borne parasitic zoonoses: status and issues. Int J Parasitol. 2005;35:1233–54.
6. Chavengkun W, Kompor P, Norkaew J, Kujapun J, Pothipim M, Ponphimai S, Kaewpitoon SJ, Padchasuwan N, Kaewpitoon N. Raw fish consuming behavior related to liver fluke infection among populations at risk of cholangiocarcinoma in Nakhon

Ratchasima province, Thailand. Asian Pac J Cancer Prev. 2016;17:2761–5.
7. Coma SM, Bargues MD. Human liver flukes: a review. Res Rev Parasitol. 1997;57:145–218.
8. Fairweather I, Brennan GP, Hanna REB, Robinson MW, Skuce PJ. Drug resistance in liver flukes. Int J Parasitol Drugs Drug Resist. 2020;12:39–59.
9. Gonzales Santana B, Dalton JP, Vasquez Camargo F, Parkinson M, Ndao M. The diagnosis of human fascioliasis by enzyme-linked immunosorbent assay (ELISA) using recombinant cathepsin L protease. PLoS Negl Trop Dis. 2013;7:e2414.
10. Katz N, Chaves A, Pellegrino J. A simple device for quantitative stool thick-smear technique in Schistosomiasis mansoni. Rev Inst Med Trop Sao Paulo. 1972;14:397–400.
11. Manson-Bahr P, Walton J. The surgical removal of fasciola hepatica from the common bile-duct with a commentary upon this infection in man. Br J Surg. 1941;28:380–3.
12. Mas-Coma S. Epidemiology of fascioliasis in human endemic areas. J Helminthol. 2005;79:207–16.
13. Mas-Coma S. Human fascioliasis emergence risks in developed countries: from individual patients and small epidemics to climate and global change impacts. Enferm Infecc Microbiol Clin (Engl Ed). 2020;38:253–6.
14. Olliaro PL, Coulibaly JT, Garba A, Halleux C, Keiser J, King CH, Mutapi F, N'Goran EK, Raso G, Scherrer AU, Sousa-Figueiredo JC, Stete K, Utzinger J, Vaillant MT. Efficacy and safety of single-dose 40 mg/kg oral praziquantel in the treatment of schistosomiasis in preschool-age versus school-age children: an individual participant data meta-analysis. PLoS Negl Trop Dis. 2020;14:e0008277.
15. Perakanya P, Ungcharoen R, Worrabannakorn S, Ongarj P, Artchayasawat A, Boonmars T, Boueroy P. Prevalence and risk factors of Opisthorchis viverrini infection in Sakon Nakhon province, Thailand. Trop Med Infect Dis. 2022;7:313.
16. Pozio E, Armignacco O, Ferri F, Gomez Morales MA. Opisthorchis felineus, an emerging infection in Italy and its implication for the European Union. Acta Trop. 2013;126:54–62.
17. Prueksapanich P, Piyachaturawat P, Aumpansub P, Ridtitid W, Chaiteerakij R, Rerknimitr R. Liver fluke-associated biliary tract cancer. Gut Liver. 2018;12:236–45.
18. Qian MB, Patel C, Palmeirim MS, Wang X, Schindler C, Utzinger J, Zhou XN, Keiser J. Efficacy of drugs against clonorchiasis and opisthorchiasis: a systematic review and network meta-analysis. Lancet Microbe. 2022;3:e616–24.
19. Sripa B, Hong ST. Tribendimidine: an alternative anthelmintic for liver flukes? Lancet Infect Dis. 2011;11:77–8.
20. Sripa B, Brindley PJ, Mulvenna J, Laha T, Smout MJ, Mairiang E, Bethony JM, Loukas A. The tumorigenic liver fluke Opisthorchis viverrini--multiple pathways to cancer. Trends Parasitol. 2012;28:395–407.
21. Sripa B, Suwannatrai AT, Sayasone S, Do DT, Khieu V, Yang Y. Current status of human liver fluke infections in the Greater Mekong Subregion. Acta Trop. 2021;224:106133.
22. Vg B, Ng P, En G. Early differential diagnosis of icteric variants of viral hepatitis, acute opisthorchiasis and sporadic pseudotuberculosis. Klin Med. 1981;59:73.
23. Wang T, Mitchell PD. Liver fluke infection throughout human evolution. Gastro Hep Adv. 2022;1:500–7.
24. Yilmaz S, Akici M, Simsek M, Okur N, Ersen O, Tuncer AA. Endoscopic retrograde cholangiopancreatography for biliary system parasites. Turk J Surg. 2018;34:306–10.

5 Mucinous Cystic Neoplasms of the Liver

Samantha M. Ruff and Timothy M. Pawlik

5.1 Introduction

Liver cysts occur in approximately 5–10% of the population. In 2010, the World Health Organization (WHO) reclassified cystic neoplasms of the liver into mucinous cystic neoplasms (MCNs) and intraductal papillary mucinous neoplasm of the bile duct (IPMN-BD). MCNs consist of lesions previously designated as biliary cystadenomas (BCAs) and biliary cystadenocarcinomas (BCACs). The WHO defines MCN as a neoplasm composed of cuboidal-to-columnar, mucin-producing epithelium that can be associated with ovarian-type stroma. These tumors are extremely rare and slow-growing. As a result, most of the literature is derived from small case series and case reports [1, 2].

5.2 Incidence and Origin

MCNs constitute less than 5% of all cystic liver lesions [3]. The incidence of BCA is 1 in 20,000–100,000. Historically, the risk of malignant transformation to BCAC was reported to be as high as 20–23% [4, 5]. However, some data suggest that malignant transformation may be closer to 3–6% with the discrepancy attributed to the inclusion of IPMN-BD prior to the diagnostic/nomenclature clarification [6]. It can be difficult to characterize the incidence of BCACs, given that these lesions are even more rare than BCAs. While the origin of MCNs remains unclear, there are multiple theories. One theory is that MCNs arise from a congenital event during development. In recent years, due to the consistent presence of ovarian-type stroma in MCNs, there has been a shift toward believing that MCNs arise from ectopic primordial germ cells that eventually develop into the embryonic gonads. During migration from the upper abdomen to the pelvis, these cells pass through the dorsal mesentery that gives rise to the body and tail of the pancreas. This process is thought to be a potential origin of pancreatic MCNs. While the primordial germ cells do not migrate through the liver, these cells are in close proximity and may enter the ventral mesentery, where the liver is developing. In addition, the peritoneal surface of the gonads is lined with bulging cells as opposed to flattened epithelium. As such, epithelial cells covering the gonads may be activated and may be able to detach and migrate to nearby organs with a peritoneal surface [5, 7]. The aberrant detachment and transfer of these cells to the liver may account for the development of liver MCNs. The transcription factor GATA4 that is responsible for

S. M. Ruff · T. M. Pawlik (✉)
Department of Surgery, Division of Surgical Oncology, The Ohio State University Wexner Medical Center and James Comprehensive Cancer Center, Columbus, OH, USA
e-mail: samantha.ruff@osumc.edu; tim.pawlik@osumc.edu

T. Hackert, A. Gulla (eds.), *Rare Liver and Biliary Tract Diseases*,
https://doi.org/10.1007/978-3-032-15076-9_5

gonadal development also drives the growth of the liver and pancreas [8]. This theory is supported by immunohistochemical studies that demonstrate that MCNs express estrogen and progesterone receptors and can experience rapid growth with oral estrogen contraceptive therapy [5, 9]. This theory may similarly apply to mucinous neoplasms of the pancreas and peritoneal cavity.

Not all MCNs contain ovarian-type stroma; however, MCNs may arise from more than one type of cell. Other theories include that MCNs originate from ectopic embryonic bile duct cells or intrahepatic peribiliary glands [2, 5, 10]. On final pathology, over 90% of BCACs have components of benign BCAs. Based on this finding, some BCACs may arise from the malignant transformation of BCAs [2, 11, 12]. BCACs that arise sporadically without a preexisting BCA may do so due to changes in the biliary ducts secondary to ischemia or carcinogens [2].

5.3 Clinical Presentation

Traditionally, MCNs were thought to occur predominantly in young women. While recent case series have demonstrated that approximately 90% of BCAs occur in women with an average age at presentation of 45 years old, BCACs tend to be more evenly distributed between men and women and have a later age of presentation [2]. MCNs more commonly occur in the left lobe of the liver [6, 13, 14].

Most MCNs are found incidentally, but patients can also present with vague, nonspecific symptoms like abdominal distention, pain, nausea, or vomiting. In rare circumstances, patients can present with obstructive jaundice, cholangitis, intra-cystic hemorrhage, or cyst rupture [15]. Presenting with these symptoms does not necessarily correlate with malignant disease; instead, these symptoms are typically due to the extrahepatic location of the MCN. Approximately 20% of patients will present with elevated liver function tests and/or hyperbilirubinemia [2, 10]. Rarely, in the presence of invasive MCNs (BCACs), patients can also present with metastatic (bone, lung, intra-abdominal peritoneum, and omentum) or regional/extrahepatic lymph node disease [12].

5.4 Differential Diagnosis and Workup

5.4.1 Imaging

The list of potential diagnoses is long and includes simple cysts (with or without hemorrhagic component), infections (e.g., hydatid cysts due to *Echinococcus granulosus*), biliary duct cysts (e.g., Caroli disease and bile duct duplication cysts), polycystic liver disease, and neoplasms (e.g., cholangiocarcinoma with cystic component, MCN, and IPMN-BD) (Table 5.1) [1, 2]. Imaging is the most valuable way to differentiate between different cystic lesions, but imaging must be used in conjunction with the

Table 5.1 Differential diagnosis of hepatic cystic neoplasms

Hepatic cystic neoplasms	Diagnosis
Developmental	Simple benign cyst Adult polycystic liver disease Caroli disease

Inflammatory	Pyogenic
	Parasitic
	  Entamoeba histolytica
	  Hydatid (echinococcal)
	Abscess
	  Fungal
	  Bacterial

Neoplastic	Primary
	  Undifferentiated embryonal carcinoma
	  Biliary cystadenoma or cystadenocarcinoma
	  Embryonal sarcoma
	  Cavernous hemangioma
	  Intraductal papillary neoplasms
	Secondary
	  Cystic metastasis

Traumatic	Hemorrhagic or hematoma Seroma Biloma Pseudocyst

Used with permission [5]

patient's clinical picture to narrow the diagnosis. On ultrasound (US), MCNs are hypoechoic, with thickened, irregular walls and mural nodules, internal debris, and thickened septa (Fig. 5.1a) [1]. Mural or septum nodules increase the suspicion of a malignancy such as BCAC [16–18]. While simple cysts do not have any septations or papillary projections, these findings can appear in complicated cysts, hydatid cysts, or simple cysts with hemorrhagic contents. Echinococcal cysts are often associated with calcifications, debris within the cyst, or daughter cysts that help differentiate these lesions on imaging. Positive serology can help confirm the diagnosis of hydatid cysts, while serum will be negative among patients with MCNs [1].

While ultrasound is more sensitive to detect the details of cystic lesions, CT provides a more accurate size depiction, as well as a better definition of the anatomic location/extent of the lesion (Fig. 5.1b). On CT scan, MCNs appear as a low-attenuation mass (less than 30 Hounsfield units) with enhanced loculations, septations, and/or a thickened/irregular wall. Abscesses will also have septations and will be multiloculate yet will often have a thicker wall than MCNs [1, 2]. In addition, patients with a liver abscess will usually present with systemic signs of an infection (e.g., leukocytosis, fever, tachycardia, and hypotension) and a potentially identifiable source (e.g., cholecystitis, cholangitis, and diverticulitis).

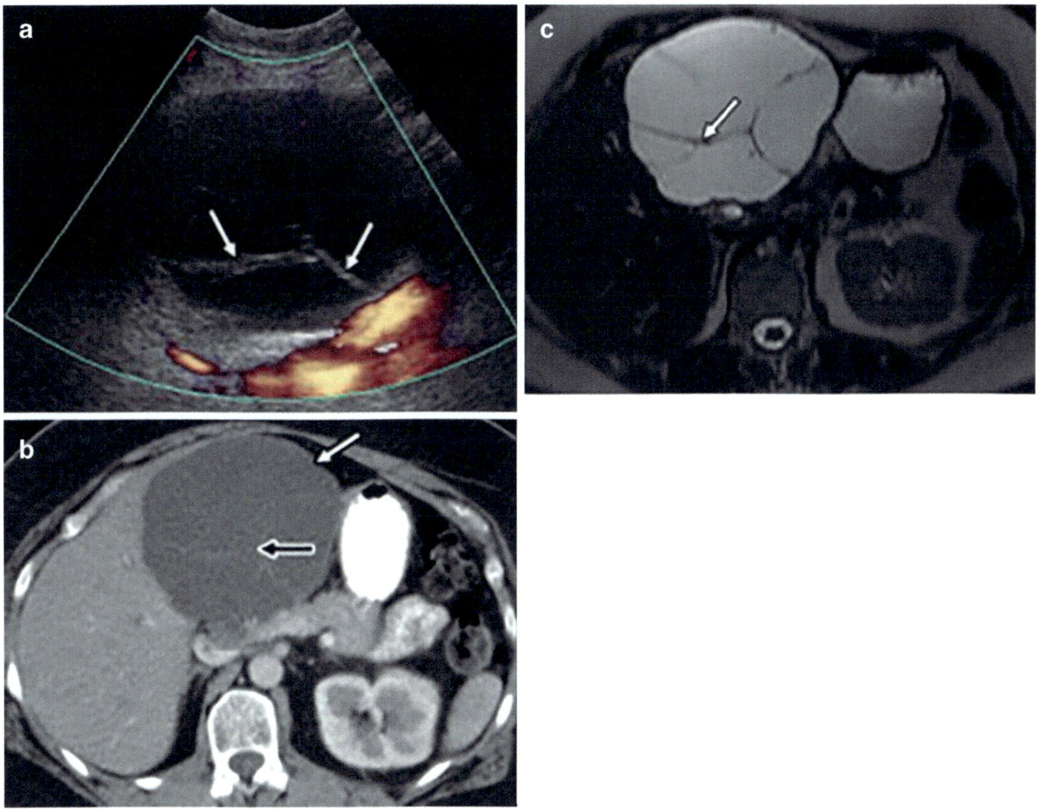

Fig. 5.1 US, CT, and MRI features of mucinous cystic neoplasm (MCN) of the liver. (**a**) Doppler US image of the liver shows a large multiloculate cystic mass with echogenic septa (arrows). The septa are of varying thickness and are centrally located and arise from the cyst wall without external indentation or macrolobulation. (**b**) Axial contrast-enhanced CT image shows a solitary cystic mass (white arrow) with thin central internal septa (black arrow) in hepatic segment IV. (**c**) Axial T2-weighted image shows a circumscribed fluid-hyperintense mass with hypointense internal septa (arrow). The septa are centrally located and arise from the cyst wall without associated external indentation or macrolobulation. (Used with permission) [6]

Magnetic resonance imaging (MRI) is another important tool to characterize different cystic lesions of the liver. On MRI, cyst fluid will have different signal intensities depending on the protein content, which can be useful when trying to differentiate MCNs from hemorrhagic cysts. On MRI, classic MCNs will have a homogeneous low-intensity T1 signal and a high-intensity T2 signal (Figs. 5.1c and 5.2). In contrast, due to clot formation within the cyst, hemorrhagic cysts will have a high-intensity T1 signal and a low-intensity T2 signal [1]. Magnetic resonance cholangiopancreatography (MRCP) can further delineate whether a cyst communicates with the biliary tree and demonstrate internal septations not seen on CT scan. MRCP also allows imaging of the biliary tree proximal to an obstruction that may be difficult to evaluate with an ERCP. ERCP is useful for obtaining tissue sample and relieving extrahepatic biliary obstruction due to a cyst [1].

5.4.2 MCN Versus IPMN-BD

When discerning the differential diagnosis, it can be difficult to separate MCNs from IPMN-BD. Both are rare tumors that produce mucin and have a similar appearance on imaging yet are distinct entities (Table 5.2). Of note, MCNs are classified as liver tumors, and IPMN-BD are classified as biliary duct tumors [6]. IPMN-BD occur equally in men and women and, on average, present at an older age than patients with MCN [2]. IPMN-BD also tend to have a higher incidence of malignant potential (40–80%) [6]. Differentiating IPMN-BD subtypes prior to treatment can be important as these lesions have different growth patterns. For example, IPMN-BD will spread superficially along the bile ducts, which may be important to consider relative to the margin status during the resection [19]. Given the rarity of both of these tumors,

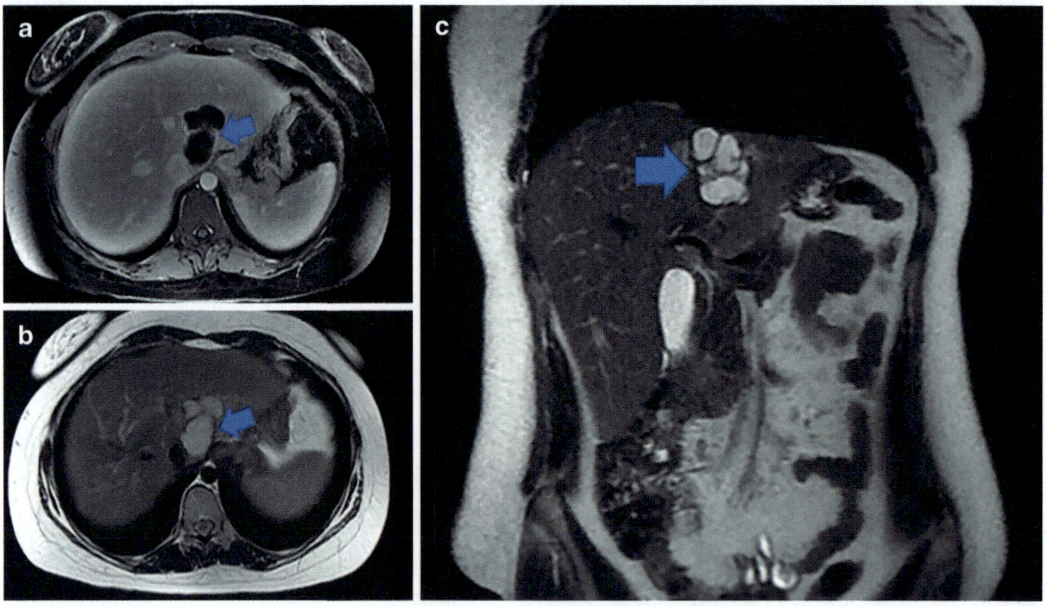

Fig. 5.2 Mucinous cystic neoplasm (MCN) of the liver findings on magnetic resonance imaging showing a septate and multilobulated lesion on T1-weighted imaging (**a**) and hyperintense signaling on T2-weighted imaging (**b**, **c**). (Used with permission) [5]

Table 5.2 Comparison of mucinous cystic neoplasm (MCN) of the liver and intraductal papillary neoplasm of the biliary duct (IPMN-BD)

Features	MCN	IPMN-B
Distinguishing features	Subepithelial OLS, required for diagnosis	Bile duct communication, bile duct mass or masses, upstream and downstream ductal dilatation, absent OLS
Prior nomenclature	Biliary cystadenoma (benign), biliary cystadenocarcinoma (malignant), biliary cystic neoplasm	Biliary papilloma, biliary papillomatosis, mucin-hypersecreting bile duct tumor, mucin-producing cholangiocarcinoma, intraductal papillary mucinous neoplasm of the bile duct (IPMN-B), biliary tract IPMN, IPMN of the biliary tract, IPMN-B or IPMN-BD-M for IPMN-BD with mucin secretion, IPMN-BD-NM for IPMN-BD without mucin secretion
Demographics	Patients almost exclusively female, middle-aged or older, typically younger than for IPMN-BD	Patients slightly more often male than female, middle-aged or older, typically older than for MCN
Pancreatic counterpart	MCN-P; MCN has less malignant potential than MCN-P	IPMN; IPMN-BD has more malignant potential and less mucin hypersecretion than IPMN
Geographic differences	More common in Western countries than in East Asia	More common in East Asia than in Western countries East Asia: IHD more often than EHD Western countries: EHD more often than IHD
Common imaging findings	Large, often solitary, multiloculate cystic mass Commonly occurs in the left hepatic lobe Septa arising from a cyst wall without external indentation or macrolobulation Septa and mural calcification on CT, septal enhancement on MRI No bile duct communication	Mass within disproportionately dilated bile ducts, upstream and downstream ductal dilatation, bile duct communication Complex cystic mass with or without solid enhancing masses, bile duct dilatation Ductal dilatation without mass, parenchymal atrophy Thread sign on the MRCP
Malignant potential	Majority benign, 6% with invasive carcinoma (typically older patients)	Higher than in MCN, 40%–80% with invasive carcinoma at presentation
Treatment	Enucleation, hepatic resection	Surgical resection with tumor-free margins

Used with permission [6]
OLS ovarian-like stroma, *MRCP* magnetic resonance cholangiopancreatography, *MCN-P* mucinous cystic neoplasm of the pancreas, *IHD* intrahepatic duct, *EHD* extrahepatic duct

there are only small case series comparing the two clinical entities. On imaging, one of the best ways to differentiate an MCN from an IPMN-BD is that the latter lesion has communication with the bile duct [3]. MCNs are also more likely to have smooth walls with septa, whereas IPMN-BD will have papillary projections [19]. On pathology, the presence of ovarian-type stroma will confirm the diagnosis of MCN since this is not present in IPMN-BD.

5.4.3 Diagnosing BCA Versus BCAC

Imaging can differentiate MCNs from other cystic liver lesions, but distinguishing benign (BCA) from invasive (BCAC) disease can be more challenging. Both lesions often appear as solitary, multiloculate cystic lesions. The presence of mural nodules (especially those greater than 1 cm) and irregular cyst walls is more likely to suggest malignancy [2, 6]. Often, the final diagnosis is made only on pathological examination following surgical resection.

Wang et al. proposed a scoring system to distinguish between BCA and BCAC in the preoperative setting. The authors performed a retrospective review of 20 patients with BCA and 10 patients with BCAC who underwent resection. Based on the analysis, a scoring system using age, gender, duration of symptoms, and lesion location to diagnose BCA versus BCAC was proposed. Patients who were older and male and had symptoms for less than 4 months, with a hypervascular lesion in the left lobe of the liver, were at the highest risk of BCAC. The score was validated with a patient cohort from another hospital and demonstrated 100% sensitivity and 87.5% specificity [20]. While it is difficult to interpret data from such a small case series, these findings have generally been consistent with other small case series in the literature regarding the risk factors for malignancy. Of note, patients without ovarian-type stroma (older patients and men) tend to have a worse prognosis.

5.4.4 Role of Biopsy in Diagnosing MCN

In some instances, aspiration of MCNs can provide additional insights regarding the diagnosis and will demonstrate bile-tinged mucin. Although rare, cytology can sometimes identify malignant cells to suggest BCAC. Several studies have evaluated the role of testing cyst fluid for cancer antigen (CA) 19-9 and carcinoembryonic antigen (CEA). Unfortunately, these studies have demonstrated conflicting results and provide little diagnostic insight into the role of tumor markers in MCNs [21–23]. Given that it is rare to identify BCA versus BCAC on a fine-needle aspiration and biopsies have been associated with pleural and peritoneal dissemination, the biopsy of MCNs is generally not recommended [12, 21, 24, 25]. Avoidance of biopsy is particularly true since the treatment for BCA and BCAC is the same regardless of the diagnosis.

5.4.5 Pathological Diagnosis

On pathology, the cyst wall of MCNs is composed of a single layer of cuboidal-to-columnar, mucin-producing epithelium with some dense fibrosis and calcifications (Fig. 5.3). The defining characteristic of MCNs is the ovarian-type stroma characterized by estrogen and progesterone receptors (Figs. 5.3c and 5.4a) [2, 14]. MCNs do not always have ovarian-type stroma, but when present, it will be seen as a mesenchymal stroma layer between the epithelial, mucin-producing layer and the outer connective tissue [5]. Ovarian-type stroma is characterized using immunohistochemical staining for progesterone and estrogen receptors. This finding was initially documented by Wheeler and Edmondson in the 1980s [2]. MCNs also stain for α-inhibin [6]. The presence of ovarian-type stroma may explain why MCNs are commonly seen in women and may increase in size during pregnancy or with estrogen-based contraception [2].

When ovarian-type stroma is absent, a hyaline (pale, glassy, and acellular) stroma layer is present in place of the mesenchymal stroma layer. The absence of ovarian-like stroma (OLS) is associated with a worse prognosis and a higher rate of recurrence [5]. In a large series of patients with MCN, individuals with BCAC and no ovarian-type stroma had a median survival of 3 years, whereas patients with BCAC and ovarian-type stroma were still alive at the time of follow-up between 4 and 8 years [11]. Some authors have also suggested that ovarian-type stroma may regress during malignant transformation [26].

MCNs are classified as low-, intermediate-, or high-grade dysplasia, carcinoma in situ, or invasive carcinoma (commonly referred to as BCAC) [3]. While difficult to distinguish from BCAs, BCACs are defined by the presence of malignant characteristics. These features include the presence of cellular pleomorphism, frequent mitotic figures, loss of polarity/tissue disorganization, and/or infiltration of the underlying fibrous stroma (Fig. 5.4b) [1, 5]. On immunohistochem-

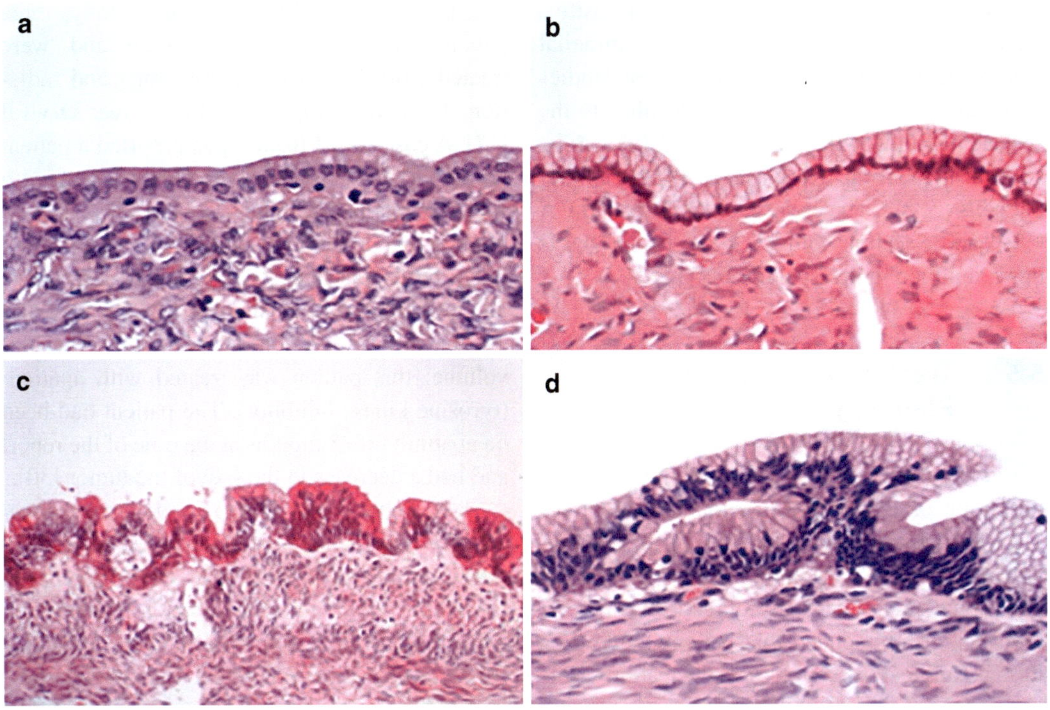

Fig. 5.3 Histopathology of hepatic mucinous cystic neoplasms. Benign mucinous cystadenomas show a single-layered biliary-type epithelium (**a**) with occasional foci of mucin-containing cells (**b**). Borderline tumors exhibit cellular atypia such as nuclear enlargement and stratification (**c**, **d**). Original magnification: **a**, **b**, **d**, ×400; **c**, ×200. (Used with permission) [14]

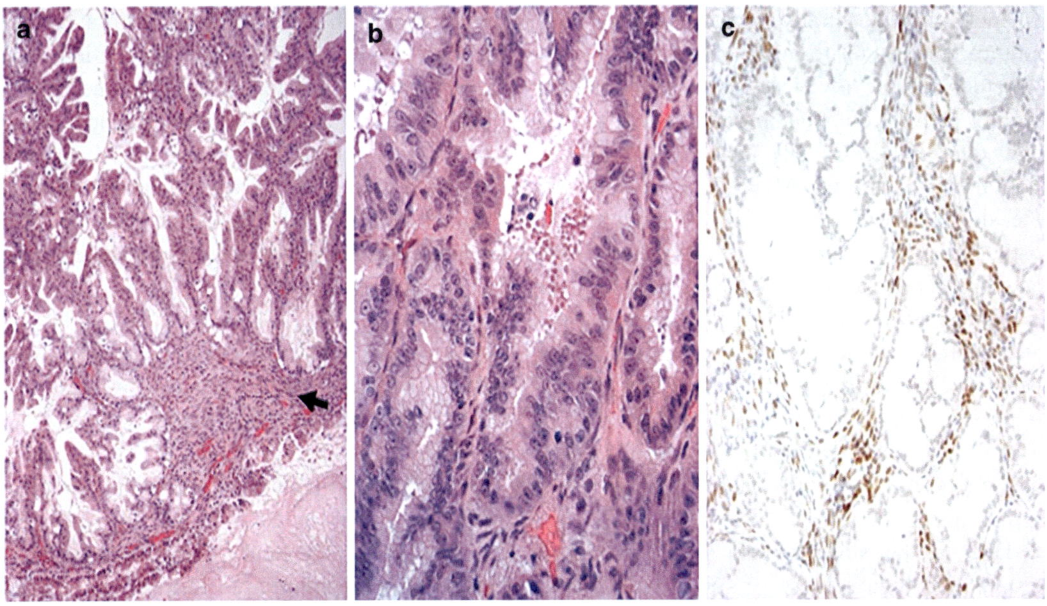

Fig. 5.4 A carcinoma in situ case of hepatic mucinous cystic neoplasm. (**a**) There is papillary proliferation of atypical epithelium with fibrovascular cores. Ovarian-like stroma (OLS) is noted (arrow). (**b**) Nuclear enlargement with occasional foci of loss of polarity is seen. (**c**) Immunostaining for the progesterone receptor reveals a stroma positive for progesterone receptor in the fibrovascular cores of the papillary lesion. Original magnification: **a**, ×100; **b**, **c**, ×400. (Used with permission) [14]

istry (IHC), both BCA and BCAC stain positive for cytokeratins CAM5.2, AE1, AE3, epithelial membrane antigen, and CEA. Small case studies have demonstrated that CEA will localize to the surface of BCA epithelial cells, but CEA can be seen throughout the cytoplasm of BCAC epithelial cells [5, 27]. The expression of CEA and CA 19-9 can be seen in both BCA and BCAC but is more common in invasive MCN [1].

5.5 Treatment and Surgical Planning

Given that there is a 20% risk of malignant transformation of BCAs, the first-line treatment for MCNs is complete resection [2]. With fenestration, aspiration, marsupialization, or partial resection, there is a high risk of recurrence; therefore, it is recommended that patients undergo a formal surgical resection or enucleation. It is important not to rupture the cyst during resection and that a rim of normal liver tissue is taken as a margin to ensure complete resection. The decision to resect versus enucleate is often based on the anatomic location of the MCN. Peripheral lesions can undergo a nonanatomic resection, whereas more centrally located lesions may require enucleation to avoid vascular or biliary structures. If the MCN is extrahepatic, it may require a liver resection in combination with a bile duct resection and hepaticojejunostomy. Depending on the underlying liver disease and the size of the resection that is required, the patient may need to undergo volumetric liver assessment prior to an operation. Laparoscopic or open surgery can be performed. When appropriate, laparoscopic surgery often carries with it the benefit of shorter hospital length of stay (LOS), improved pain control, and quicker recovery [2]. There are a few case reports in which patients have required a liver transplant for unresectable, symptomatic MCNs [12, 28].

Due to the slow-growing nature of these lesions and high success of surgical treatment, there is very little information regarding the role of chemotherapy or radiation therapy for invasive MCN. Lauffer et al. performed a meta-analysis of 112 patients with BCAC. In this study, three patients had unresectable disease and were treated with definitive chemotherapy and radiation. The authors reported a 33% 2-year survival [12]. A case report from Japan reported a patient with metastatic BCAC who was treated with 5-fluorouracil (5FU) and cisplatin. The authors noted a reduction in the patient's CEA level and tumor burden/ascites [29]. One report described a patient with recurrent invasive MCN who could not undergo a resection due to insufficient liver volume; this patient was treated with apatinib (tyrosine kinase inhibitor). The patient had been on apatinib for 48 months at the time of the report and had a decrease in the size of the tumor [30].

A few groups have also tried local/regional therapy with hepatic artery infusion pump and interventional radiology. One case report discussed the use of a hepatic artery infusion pump with cisplatin in a woman with an unresectable BCAC. The authors reported a dramatic decrease in the size of the lesion (from 12 cm to 2 cm) after 8 months [31]. A recent case report described a 75-year-old woman with unresectable BCAC who underwent cryoablation and microwave ablation, in combination with sclerotherapy. At 6 months, there was no enhancement of most of the lesions on the arterial phase, with a volume reduction ratio of 70%, and the patient had improvement in her abdominal pain and distention [32]. To date, data on chemotherapy, radiation, or regional treatments are based on case reports. In turn, patients with metastatic disease or unresectable disease should be presented at a multidisciplinary tumor board since there are no clear guidelines.

5.6 Follow-Up/Recommendations

The incidence of recurrence following complete surgical excision of BCA is low (5–10%) [2]. BCAs have an excellent prognosis, which has been confirmed in multiple case series. Patients rarely had a recurrence after resection or enucleation, and survival was near 100% on long-term follow-up [33–36]. In contrast, because BCAC is a malignant process, this type of cystic liver lesion has a higher risk of recurrence and metastatic spread, whether locally in the liver or in more rare circumstances at extrahepatic sites. While there are no set guidelines for surveillance, imaging once a year, with plans to lengthen the interval between scans after a few years, is generally recommended. Overall survival and recurrence rates are difficult to predict, given the rarity of BCA/BCAC. In a series of seven patients with BCAC, the 1-, 3-, and 5-year disease-free survival rates after resection were 100%, 85.7%, and 57.1%, respectively [36]. Another case series with 12 BCAC patients reported 5- and 10-year survival after surgical resection of 72.9% and 60.9%, respectively [37].

5.7 Conclusion

MCNs are rare hepatic lesions that account for less than 5% of liver cysts. Often found incidentally, MCNs are usually benign, slow-growing lesions with a low potential for malignant transformation. A subset of patients will, however, harbor cystic tumors with malignant potential, such as BCAC. In turn, surgical resection is the recommended treatment option for most patients with MCNs.

References

1. Soni S, Pareek P, Narayan S, Varshney V. Mucinous cystic neoplasm of the liver (MCN-L): a rare presentation and review of the literature. Med Pharm Rep. 2021;94(3):366–71.
2. Soares KC, Arnaoutakis DJ, Kamel I, Anders R, Adams RB, Bauer TW, et al. Cystic neoplasms of the liver: biliary cystadenoma and cystadenocarcinoma. J Am Coll Surg. 2014;218(1):119–28.
3. Kunovsky L, Kala Z, Svaton R, Moravcik P, Mazanec J, Husty J, et al. Mucinous cystic neoplasm of the liver or intraductal papillary mucinous neoplasm of the bile duct? A case report and a review of literature. Ann Hepatol. 2018;17(3):519–24.
4. Dhali A, Ray S, Dhali GK, Khamrui S, Ghosh R. Extrahepatic mucinous biliary cystadenoma: a rare cause of gastric outlet obstruction. Clin Case Rep. 2022;10(3):e05531.
5. Averbukh LD, Wu DC, Cho WC, Wu GY. Biliary mucinous cystadenoma: a review of the literature. J Clin Transl Hepatol. 2019;7(2):149–53.
6. Lee MH, Katabathina VS, Lubner MG, Shah HU, Prasad SR, Matkowskyj KA, et al. Mucin-producing cystic hepatobiliary neoplasms: updated nomenclature and clinical, pathologic, and imaging features. Radiographics. 2021;41(6):1592–610.
7. Erdogan D, Kloek J, Lamers WH, Offerhaus GJA, Busch ORC, Gouma DJ, et al. Mucinous cystadenomas in liver: management and origin. Dig Surg. 2010;27(1):19–23.
8. Van Treeck BJ, Lotfalla M, Czeczok TW, Mounajjed T, Moreira RK, Allende DS, et al. Molecular and immunohistochemical analysis of mucinous cystic neoplasm of the liver. Am J Clin Pathol. 2020;154(6):837–47.
9. Suyama Y, Horie Y, Suou T, Hirayama C, Ishiguro M, Nishimura O, et al. Oral contraceptives and intrahepatic biliary cystadenoma having an increased level of estrogen receptor. Hepato-Gastroenterology. 1988;35(4):171–4.
10. Akwari OE, Tucker A, Seigler HF, Itani KM. Hepatobiliary cystadenoma with mesenchymal stroma. Ann Surg. 1990;211(1):18–27.
11. Devaney K, Goodman ZD, Ishak KG. Hepatobiliary cystadenoma and cystadenocarcinoma. A light microscopic and immunohistochemical study of 70 patients. Am J Surg Pathol. 1994;18(11):1078–91.
12. Läuffer JM, Baer HU, Maurer CA, Stoupis C, Zimmerman A, Büchler MW. Biliary cystadenocarcinoma of the liver: the need for complete resection. Eur J Cancer. 1998;34(12):1845–51.
13. Kubota K, Nakanuma Y, Kondo F, Hachiya H, Miyazaki M, Nagino M, et al. Clinicopathological features and prognosis of mucin-producing bile duct tumor and mucinous cystic tumor of the liver: a multi-institutional study by the Japan Biliary Association. J Hepatobiliary Pancreat Sci. 2014;21(3):176–85.
14. Zen Y, Pedica F, Patcha VR, Capelli P, Zamboni G, Casaril A, et al. Mucinous cystic neoplasms of the liver: a clinicopathological study and comparison with intraductal papillary neoplasms of the bile duct. Mod Pathol. 2011;24(8):1079–89.
15. Xu X, Peng C, Tong R, Dong M, Deng J. An extremely rare phenomenon of mucinous cystic neoplasm of the liver: spontaneous rupture. Hepatobiliary Surg Nutr. 2021;10(3):424–7.
16. Xu HX. Contrast-enhanced ultrasound in the biliary system: potential uses and indications. World J Radiol. 2009;1(1):37–44.
17. Yu FC, Chen JH, Yang KC, Wu CC, Chou YY. Hepatobiliary cystadenoma: a report of two cases. J Gastrointestin Liver Dis. 2008;17(2):203–6.
18. Xu MY, Shi XJ, Wan T, Liang YR, Wang HG, Zhang WZ, et al. Clinicopathological characteristics and prognostic factors of intrahepatic biliary cystadenocarcinoma. Chin Med J. 2015;128(9):1177–83.

19. Lim JH, Jang KT, Rhim H, Kim YS, Lee KT, Choi SH. Biliary cystic intraductal papillary mucinous tumor and cystadenoma/cystadenocarcinoma: differentiation by CT. Abdom Imaging. 2007;32(5):644–51.
20. Wang C, Miao R, Liu H, Du X, Liu L, Lu X, et al. Intrahepatic biliary cystadenoma and cystadenocarcinoma: an experience of 30 case. Dig Liver Dis. 2012;44(5):426–31.
21. Hai S, Hirohashi K, Uenishi T, Yamamoto T, Shuto T, Tanaka H, et al. Surgical management of cystic hepatic neoplasms. J Gastroenterol. 2003;38(8):759–64.
22. Choi HK, Lee JK, Lee KH, Lee KT, Rhee JC, Kim KH, et al. Differential diagnosis for intrahepatic biliary cystadenoma and hepatic simple cyst: significance of cystic fluid analysis and radiologic findings. J Clin Gastroenterol. 2010;44(4):289–93.
23. Seo JK, Kim SH, Lee SH, Park JK, Woo SM, Jeong JB, et al. Appropriate diagnosis of biliary cystic tumors: comparison with atypical hepatic simple cysts. Eur J Gastroenterol Hepatol. 2010;22(8):989–96.
24. Ahanatha Pillai S, Velayutham V, Perumal S, Ulagendra Perumal S, Lakshmanan A, Ramaswami S, et al. Biliary cystadenomas: a case for complete resection. HPB Surg. 2012;2012:501705.
25. Teoh AY, Ng SS, Lee KF, Lai PB. Biliary cystadenoma and other complicated cystic lesions of the liver: diagnostic and therapeutic challenges. World J Surg. 2006;30(8):1560–6.
26. Ishibashi Y, Ojima H, Hiraoka N, Sano T, Kosuge T, Kanai Y. Invasive biliary cystic tumor without ovarian-like stroma. Pathol Int. 2007;57(12):794–8.
27. Tomioka T, Tsuchiya R, Harada N, Tsunoda T, Matsuo T. Cystadenoma and cystadenocarcinoma of the liver: localization of carcinoembryonic antigen. Jpn J Surg. 1986;16(1):62–7.
28. Romagnoli R, Patrono D, Paraluppi G, David E, Tandoi F, Strignano P, et al. Liver transplantation for symptomatic centrohepatic biliary cystadenoma. Clin Res Hepatol Gastroenterol. 2011;35(5):408–13.
29. Iyama S, Takahashi Y, Shintani N, Fujikawa K, Ohkubo S, Sato Y, et al. A case of recurrent biliary cystadenocarcinoma successfully treated with 5FU/CDDP systemic chemotherapy. Nihon Shokakibyo Gakkai Zasshi. 2006;103(10):1163–8.
30. Yang Y, Mai W, Chen W, Yang C, Li M, Liu L. Case report: low-dose apatinib in the treatment of intrahepatic biliary cystadenoma with recurrence and malignant transformation. Front Oncol. 2021;11:676092.
31. Hanazaki K, Yoshizawa K, Mori H. Hepatic arterial infusion chemotherapy of cisplatin for biliary cystadenocarcinoma. Hepatogastroenterology. 1999;46(25):462–4.
32. Zhu JE, Li JX, Zhang HL, Li XL, Sun LP, Yu SY, et al. Sequential thermal ablation in combination with sclerotherapy using lauromacrogol as a successful translative therapy for an unresectable huge biliary cystadenocarcinoma: the first experience assisted by contrast-enhanced ultrasound. Clin Hemorheol Microcirc. 2022;82(1):95–105.
33. Wheeler DA, Edmondson HA. Cystadenoma with mesenchymal stroma (CMS) in the liver and bile ducts. A clinicopathologic study of 17 cases, 4 with malignant change. Cancer. 1985;56(6):1434–45.
34. Strasberg SM, Chapman WC. Enucleation of biliary cystadenomas: a review. J Gastrointest Surg. 2021;25(10):2700–6.
35. Treska V, Ferda J, Daum O, Liska V, Skalicky T, Bruha J. Intrahepatic biliary cystadenoma-diagnosis and treatment options. Turk J Gastroenterol. 2016;27(3):252–6.
36. Jwa EK, Hwang S. Clinicopathological features and post-resection outcomes of biliary cystadenoma and cystadenocarcinoma of the liver. Ann Hepatobiliary Pancreat Surg. 2017;21(3):107–13.
37. Song Y, Kang MJ, Jang JY, Lee KU, Suh KS, Kim SW. Clinical outcome and long term results after surgical treatment of biliary cystadenoma and cystadenocarcinoma. Korean J Hepatobiliary Pancreat Surg. 2012;16(1):24–8.

Embryological Rare Liver Tumors

6

Pin-Jung Chen and Ju Dong Yang

6.1 Lipoma

6.1.1 Incidence

Lipomas are focal areas of mature fat cells surrounded by a thin fibrous capsule. They can occur anywhere throughout the body, most frequently in the subcutaneous tissues. Lipomas of the liver are very uncommon, with only a small number of cases reported. The first description was an incidental finding on an autopsy study in 1970 [1, 2].

6.1.2 Clinical Presentation

Patients are typically asymptomatic at presentation [3–5]. Rarely, vague abdominal pain has been reported, which is likely secondary to mass effect and stretching of the hepatic capsule [6].

P.-J. Chen
Samuel Oschin Comprehensive Cancer Institute, Cedars-Sinai Medical Center, Los Angeles, CA, USA
e-mail: pin-jung.chen@cshs.org

J. D. Yang (✉)
Samuel Oschin Comprehensive Cancer Institute, Cedars-Sinai Medical Center, Los Angeles, CA, USA

Karsh Division of Gastroenterology and Hepatology, Cedars-Sinai Medical Center, Los Angeles, CA, USA

Comprehensive Transplant Center, Cedars-Sinai Medical Center, Los Angeles, CA, USA
e-mail: judong.yang@cshs.org

6.1.3 Workup Investigation

Ultrasound demonstrates a homogeneous, hyperechoic mass. It is typically solitary with a well-demarcated border and posterior acoustic enhancement. A phenomenon of apparent discontinuity of the diaphragm, secondary to refractive effects at the interface between the lipoma and normal hepatic tissue, has been described [6]. Hepatic lipomas on CT are well-demarcated, homogeneous, hypoattenuating masses, with attenuation values less than −20 Hounsfield units (HU). The lesions do not enhance. If enhancement is present, it indicates the presence of an adenomatous or angiomatous component [3, 7, 8]. MRI demonstrates a hyperintense mass on T1-weighted sequences, with signal reduction on out-of-phase imaging [3]. Lipomas have the same signal intensity as retroperitoneal or subcutaneous fat on all sequences [9].

Histologically, lipomas are composed of mature adipose tissue. The adipocytes are uniform in size and without nuclear atypia. Rarely, they can be admixed with other benign soft tissue elements, such as fibrous tissue in fibrolipomas. Lipomas are S100-positive and are negative for murine double minute 2 (MDM2) amplification (MDM2 amplification is found in many well-differentiated liposarcomas).

The ultrasound, CT, and MRI findings are characteristic. More aggressive diagnostic procedures are not necessary.

T. Hackert, A. Gulla (eds.), *Rare Liver and Biliary Tract Diseases*,
https://doi.org/10.1007/978-3-032-15076-9_6

6.1.4 Differential Diagnosis

Before a diagnosis of lipoma is made, other liver tumors should also be excluded. In case of a solitary tumor containing fat in the liver, the most common diagnoses are hepatocellular carcinoma (HCC) and hepatocellular adenoma. In case of multiple lesions containing fat, the most common diagnoses are fatty adenomatosis and multifocal nodular steatosis [9].

6.1.5 Treatment, Follow-Up, and Recommendations

Malignant degeneration of lipoma to liposarcoma is exceedingly rare in lesions found elsewhere in the body and is never described in hepatic lipomas [10]. Imaging appearances should allow a diagnosis, with no biopsy or surgery typically warranted [7].

6.2 Mesenchymal Hamartoma

6.2.1 Incidence

Mesenchymal hamartoma is an uncommon benign tumor of the liver, with a reported incidence of 0.7 per million population per year [11]. It is the second most common benign liver tumor in children, after hemangioma [12, 13]. It is composed of loosely organized mesenchymal tissue, bile ducts, and hepatic parenchyma. Unencapsulated fluid accumulates, giving the characteristic cystic appearance. The lesion is most commonly seen in patients less than 2 years old, with a male preponderance [14].

6.2.2 Clinical Presentation

Patients commonly present with an asymptomatic enlarging mass. Other symptoms such as vomiting, fever, diarrhea, respiratory distress, and weight loss are less common [14]. The prognosis is generally good, with rare fatal complications reported secondary to fetal hydrops, respiratory distress, compression of vital vessels, and congestive cardiac failure secondary to arteriovenous shunting within the mass. Laboratory tests may demonstrate an elevated serum alpha (α)-fetoprotein (AFP); however, liver function tests are usually normal.

6.2.3 Workup Investigation

The diagnosis requires a high index of suspicion on clinical and radiological bases, but histopathology is the gold standard for definitive diagnosis.

Imaging typically demonstrates a cystic lesion in the right liver, with both solid and solid/cystic lesions rarely identified [15]. Sonography demonstrates a cystic mass with thick septations [16]. Rarely, a solid mass has been described [17]. The mass is well-defined and heterogeneous on noncontrast CT, with heterogeneous enhancement of the solid components post administration of iodinated contrast [16–18]. MRI demonstrates a multiloculate cystic mass, with internal low signal on T1-weighted sequences and high signal on T2-weighted sequences. The signal may vary depending on the protein content of the fluid [7, 19].

Histologically, mesenchymal hamartomas are composed of loose, edematous mesenchymal tissue, often with cystic degeneration. The mesenchymal tissue contains cytologically bland spindled cells as well as occasional clusters of benign hepatocytes. Hyalinized portal tract–like areas can also be found, more commonly at the periphery of the tumor. In some cases, the bile ducts in the portal tract–like areas can show a ductal plate malformation pattern. Rarely, the bile ducts in these portal tract–like areas become dilated, forming a small biliary cyst.

6.2.4 Differential Diagnosis

Patients can present with varied clinical, imaging, and histological findings. Thus, mesenchymal hamartomas can mimic various benign and malignant neoplasms of the liver. It is important to recognize this rare entity to avoid unnecessary overmanagement. Common differential diagnoses include mixed epithelial–mesenchymal hepatoblastoma, infantile hemangioendothelioma, and embryonal sarcoma.

Mixed epithelial–mesenchymal hepatoblastoma is the most similar to mesenchymal hamartoma. On histology, the distinguishing features are the presence of fetal/embryonal patterns, high cellularity, and cartilaginous and osteoid-type mesenchymal elements, which are absent in mesenchymal hamartoma.

6.2.5 Treatment, Follow-Up, and Recommendations

Surgical resection is the predominant mode of therapy, with excellent survival in those in whom surgical resection is possible [15]. Marsupialization or even aspiration has been reported in unresectable cases [20]. After complete surgical resection, the prognosis is good; however, incomplete excision may be associated with malignant transformation to undifferentiated embryonal sarcoma. Spontaneous regression has also been reported [12, 21].

6.3 Hepatic Lymphangioma

6.3.1 Incidence

Hepatic lymphangioma is a rare tumor characterized by cystic dilatation of lymphatic vessels in the hepatic parenchyma [22]. The mass is believed to develop secondary to congenital obstruction of the lymphatic system with resultant dilatation [22]. Intra-abdominal lesions account for only 5% of all lymphangiomas [23]. Solitary hepatic lymphangiomas are rare, with lesions usually occurring with other masses in multiple organs, and occur predominantly in children or adolescents [24–26].

6.3.2 Clinical Presentation

Patients are typically asymptomatic, with symptoms, when present, usually nonspecific, such as abdominal pain, fever, nausea, and vomiting [27–29]. Laboratory tests such as liver function tests and tumor markers are typically negative [29–31].

6.3.3 Workup Investigation

On ultrasound, the masses are multiloculate cystic masses with echogenic debris. On CT or MRI, hepatic lymphangioma may appear as a cystic or multicystic mass with internal septations. Hyperechoic lesions have also been described [32]. MRI demonstrates a heterogeneous mass, low signal intensity on T1-weighted images, and high signal on T2-weighted images. Septal enhancement can occur and may mimic a solid lesion in the microcystic variant [31, 33].

Microscopically, hepatic lymphangiomas consist of variably sized cyst-like spaces lined by benign endothelial cells. The cyst-like spaces often contain a thin proteinaceous fluid. In most cases, lymphangiomas are not isolated to the liver, and there is systemic involvement, with similar lesions in the spleen, skeleton, and other organs.

6.3.4 Differential Diagnosis

Laboratory and imaging results have been of limited use for the preoperative diagnosis of lymphangioma. On imaging, it is difficult to differentiate it from other cystic diseases such as bile duct cyst, biliary cystadenoma and cystadenocarcinoma, or hepatic hydatidosis, while MRI is very helpful in differentiating lymphangioma from a true solid tumor [32, 33]. The lack of specificity of these preoperative investigations and the rarity of hepatic lymphangioma have made it very challenging to give an accurate preoperative diagnosis. The correct diagnosis often remains elusive until tissue is obtained.

6.3.5 Treatment, Follow-Up, and Recommendations

Surgical resection is the treatment of choice, with a complete cure possible [27]. Recurrence has been described post resection of lymphangiomas elsewhere at a rate of 0–27% for complete resection and 10–100% for incomplete resection [34]. When complete resection is not possible, percutaneous ablation using alcohol and OK-432 has been described in lesions outside of the liver [35–37].

6.4 Hepatic Angiomyolipoma

6.4.1 Incidence

Angiomyolipomas (AMLs) are rare mesenchymal tumors characterized by the presence of variable mixtures of adipose tissue, smooth muscle cells, and thick-walled blood vessels. AMLs belong to a group of perivascular epithelioid cell (PEC) tumors known as "PEComa." This entity is defined by the World Health Organization as a "mesenchymal tumor composed of histologically and immunohistochemically distinctive perivascular epithelioid cells" [38], including tumors such as pulmonary lymphangioleiomyomatosis, clear-cell "sugar" tumor (CCST), clear-cell myomelanocytic tumor of the falciform ligament, and AMLs [39].

Hepatic angiomyolipoma (HAML) is a very rare mesenchymal liver tumor, assumed to be predominantly benign. These tumors were first described in 1976 [40]. Only approximately 600 cases were reported up until 2016 [41–43]. The incidence of HAML is higher in females, with a large age range from 8 to 86 years [44–56]. There are limited data to suggest any viral or genetic association; however, AMLs have been associated with certain genetic variants of tuberous sclerosis [52, 57]. HAMLs are only seen in 6% of patients with tuberous sclerosis, whereas renal AMLs are more commonly present in 20% of tuberous sclerosis patients [58].

6.4.2 Clinical Presentation

The clinical presentation is predominantly of an asymptomatic hepatic lesion found incidentally on imaging. When symptoms arise, they are generally secondary to mass effect and take the form of abdominal discomfort and fullness [44, 49]. Liver tests, viral serology, and tumor markers are generally normal [48, 49]. It usually follows a benign clinical course, while some patients have visited hospitals with nonspecific symptoms [59].

However, malignant behaviors, which occur mostly in epithelioid-type HAML [60, 61], have been described in approximately 4% of patients [43, 59], including growth in size, recurrence after surgical resection, metastasis, and invasive growth pattern into the parenchyma and along the vessels [46, 47, 54, 62–64]. In general, a favorable prognosis can be expected for HAMLs since the majority of the tumors are benign. Human melanoma black-45 (HMB-45) staining, Ki-67, and p53 reactivity following fine-needle biopsy (FNB) might be useful to establish the diagnosis of the tumor and assess its malignant potential.

6.4.3 Workup Investigation

HAML may easily be misdiagnosed as a malignancy [65]. When an HAML diagnosis is considered on cross-sectional imaging, biopsy is indicated and may provide valuable additional information, especially when surgical resection imposes a risk of complications.

The appearance of HAMLs on imaging is inconsistent, given the variation in the proportions of tumor components [66]. Intralesional fat is seen in only 50% of HAMLs in comparison to renal AMLs, where it is more commonly seen [44]. The sonographic appearance is generally of a solitary, echogenic lesion, ranging from 5 to 6 cm in size [52, 67]. Unless features such as speed propagation artifact and refraction artifact are present, HAMLs are virtually identical to hemangiomas [50, 68]. On CT, the lesions demonstrate varying amounts of intralesional fat from obvious fat attenuation to a more heterogeneous mixed attenuation appearance. When fat is present, the lesion can be described as two specific components: a peripheral angiomyomatous component and a central fatty component with a CT number less than −20 HU [69]. On MRI, HAMLs demonstrate high signal on T1- and T2-weighted images, with signal decrease on opposed-phase imaging when fat is present.

In histological and cytological examinations, HAMLs are composed of neoplastic cells that show a mixture of steatosis, smooth muscle (myoid) differentiation, and large, thick-walled vessels. The myoid cells can be either spindled or epithelioid. The proportion of each component varies considerably between tumors, leading to difficulties in diagnosis [44, 70]. A small number of HAMLs can have marked lymphoplasmacyte-rich inflammation, mimicking inflammatory pseudotumors [44]. Other rare histological findings include striking peliotic changes, hemorrhage, and necrosis. Incidentally, HAMLs can be clinically aggressive. Findings that raise concern for a more malignant phenotype include vascular invasion [71], coagulative necrosis [72], and marked cytological atypia associated with increased mitotic activity [73]. Because of the diagnostic challenges in recognizing HAMLs on H&E, in most cases, the diagnosis is confirmed by immunohistochemistry. AMLs are negative for both cytokeratins and markers of hepatic differentiation but are positive for HMB-45, Melan A, and smooth muscle actin, with the strongest staining in the myoid components [49, 74, 75].

6.4.4 Differential Diagnosis

The differential diagnoses include HCC, focal nodular hyperplasia (FNH), hepatic adenoma, leiomyoma, hepatoblastoma, and metastases of gastrointestinal stromal tumor, colon carcinoma, and melanoma.

Although imaging is an essential component of the diagnostic evaluation, a definitive conclusion is only achieved in approximately 5% of cases, with the lesions often misdiagnosed as HCC or FNH [66]. Features such as intense arterial enhancement later than that of HCC, a peripheral rim of contrast washout on equilibrium and delayed phases, and the presence of an early draining vein on CT or MRI are more specific to HAML [66]. The fatty areas are also generally hypervascular in HAMLs and relatively hypovascular in HCCs [76]. HAML occurring in a patient with chronic liver disease might have easily been misdiagnosed and treated as HCC in the past, as biopsy confirmation is often not required for making the diagnosis of HCC. With an increase in the number of case reports showing detailed imaging studies and immunohistochemical staining of the tumor with HMB-45 [39], the diagnostic accuracy is also increasing [59].

6.4.5 Treatment, Follow-Up, and Recommendations

When cross-sectional imaging shows a lesion with intralesional fat and washout in a non-cirrhotic liver, a diagnostic biopsy should be performed to avoid missing HAML. Conservative management with regular imaging follow-up is justified when biopsy confirms (classic type) HAML, given the rarity of malignant behavior. Surgical resection with long-term follow-up is warranted if there is diagnostic uncertainty, if the lesion is symptomatic, or if the size is greater than 5 cm or enlarging over a short period of observation [43, 46, 61, 62, 65].

6.5 Hepatic Epithelioid Hemangioendothelioma

6.5.1 Incidence

Hepatic epithelioid hemangioendothelioma (HEHE) is a rare, malignant vascular endothelial cell tumor in the liver with unknown etiology. The term epithelioid hemangioendothelioma (EHE) was first defined as a distinct entity in 1982 as a soft tissue vascular tumor of endothelial origin, with a clinical course between benign hemangioma and angiosarcoma [77, 78]. HEHE was first reported in 1984 by Ishak et al. in a series of 32 patients [79, 80]. The incidence is about 1 per one million people [80–82]. HEHE most commonly occurs between the ages of 30 and 50 years, with a male-to-female incidence ratio of 2:3 [27, 80, 81]. The etiological factors remain unclear.

6.5.2 Clinical Presentation

The clinical presentation of HEHE varies from asymptomatic patients to patients with portal hypertension or hepatic failure. The most common clinical manifestations are right upper quadrant pain, hepatomegaly, and weight loss [80]. Extrahepatic involvement at the time of diagnosis is observed in about one-third of the cases, with the lungs, peritoneum, lymph nodes, and bones being the most common sites of extrahepatic involvement. Liver function tests can be normal or elevated, but tumor markers (e.g., α-fetoprotein, carcinoembryonic antigen (CEA), and carcinoantigen (CA) 19-9) are usually normal. Hence, the value of tumor markers is only to rule out other primary or metastatic liver tumors. Patients are commonly initially misdiagnosed due to nonspecific presentations [77, 83]. The clinical course and prognosis of HEHE are variable and unpredictable.

6.5.3 Workup Investigation

HEHE can be classified into three types: solitary, multifocal, and diffuse. Most patients present with multifocal tumors that involve both lobes of the liver. On ultrasound, lesions typically appear as hypoechoic. Contrast-enhanced ultrasound (CEUS) can provide enhanced detection ability for multifocal HEHE, which shows hyperenhancement in the arterial phase and hypoenhancement in the portal venous and late phases [84]. The CT findings include low-density or heterogeneous-signal-intensity lesions on non-contrast scans, centripetal enhancement in the arterial phase, and homogeneous enhancement in the portal venous and delay phases [85]. On MRI, T1-weighted images show a low signal at the tumor, and T2-weighted images show a high signal. Characteristic imaging features include capsular retraction, the white target sign (a centrally enhancing core surrounded by a low-signal-intensity halo) and black target sign (peripheral ring-like enhancement with central low signal intensity) on contrast-enhanced imaging, and the lollipop sign, in which an enhancing tumor is associated with truncation or encasement of a hepatic or portal venous branch extending to the edge of the lesion [85–88].

Imaging studies can lead to a strong suspicion regarding the presence of HEHE and its pattern. However, definitive diagnosis still requires a histopathological analysis. Histologically, the tumors are composed of nests and cords of dendritic and epithelioid cells that often contain vacuoles representing intracellular lumina [89, 90]. The stroma is fibrous, with myxohyaline areas. Immunohistochemically, the detection of endothelial markers, including CD34, CD31, CD10, and factor VIII–related antigen (FVIII-Rag), is the basis of diagnosis [90, 91]. A t(1;3) (p36.3;q25) translocation resulting in the WWTR1–CAMTA1 fusion gene is reported in about 90% of cases. Nuclear CAMTA1 expression can be identified in the majority of HEHE tumors and is specific to HEHE [92–94].

6.5.4 Differential Diagnosis

Due to the rarity of the disease, pathologists' awareness is essential. The most common misdiagnoses are angiosarcoma, intrahepatic cholangiocarcinoma, HCC, metastatic carcinoma, and sclerosing adenocarcinoma or hemangioma. The major difference between HEHE and angiosarcoma is the greater tendency of the angiosarcoma to have a destructive growth pattern. HEHE preserves the portal tracts more than angiosarcoma and sclerosing adenocarcinoma [80]. HEHE can also be confused with mixed hamartoma, spindle-cell neoplasm, inflammatory pseudotumors, bile duct adenoma, FNH, carcinoma with chondromyxoid change, veno-occlusive disease, fibrolamellar carcinoma, and postnecrotic fibrosis [77, 79, 81]. Immunohistochemical staining and nuclear staining of CAMTA1 are helpful for the differentiation of HEHE from mimics [92].

6.5.5 Treatment, Follow-Up, and Recommendations

Surgical intervention, including liver transplantation (LT) and resection, is the first choice for treatment. Since the tumor is often multifocal and widespread within the parenchyma, complete resection may not be possible. LT is by far the most common treatment modality. The survival after successful liver resection or LT is good compared with other malignant tumors [80, 82, 95]. Macrovascular invasion, pre-LT waiting time of 120 days or less, and hilar lymph node invasion but not pre-LT extrahepatic disease [96] are significant risk factors for recurrence [97].

For patients who are not fit for surgical treatment, radiation; ablation therapy; vascular endothelial growth factor (VEGF) inhibitors, such as sorafenib [98, 99], pazopanib [100], and bevacizumab; and chemotherapeutic drugs, such as thalidomide, pegylated liposomal doxorubicin, and metronomic cyclophosphamide, are reportedly effective [81].

6.6 Primary Hepatic Lymphoma

6.6.1 Incidence

Primary hepatic lymphoma (PHL) is a rare entity, first described in 1965 [101]. It is defined as a lymphoproliferative disorder confined to the liver, without disease involvement elsewhere [102–104]. Typically, distal disease should not be present for approximately 6 months after the onset of hepatic lesions [105]. Lymphomas that originate from any site in the body can eventually spread to the liver, and most lymphomas involving the liver are not primary to the liver [106]. The distinction between primary and secondary hepatic lymphoma is important, as the treatment and prognosis vary considerably [106, 107]. PHL corresponds to about 0.02% of non-Hodgkin's lymphomas and 0.4% of extranodal lymphomas [108]. The median age is 61.7 years, with a male-to-female ratio of around 1.6:1.0 [109]. PHL is rare, but the incidence has been steadily increasing over the past four decades [110].

The factors leading to PHL are not completely understood. Various etiological factors such as chronic hepatitis, cirrhosis, treatment with immunosuppressive therapy, systemic lupus erythematosus, continuous post-transplant B-cell proliferation, and acquired immune deficiency syndrome have been implicated [111–126]. However, most associations are based on case reports, and no unifying etiological factors have been identified.

The most common primary lymphomas of the liver are diffuse large B-cell lymphoma, which comprises approximately 59.8% of cases, and marginal zone lymphoma [110, 116, 127]. The major known risk factors for diffuse large B-cell lymphoma of the liver are immunosuppression and chronic hepatitis C [128]. The major known risk factors for primary marginal zone lymphomas of the liver are primary biliary cirrhosis, autoimmune hepatitis, and chronic hepatitis B and C [116].

6.6.2 Clinical Presentation

Patients typically present with abdominal pain, jaundice, and other nonspecific symptoms, such as fever, weight loss, night sweats, nausea, and vomiting [103, 109, 129]. On clinical examination, hepatomegaly is the most common finding, seen in approximately 50% [103, 109, 130, 131]. Liver tests are inconsistently elevated, predominantly alkaline phosphatase and lactate dehydrogenase (LDH) [110, 132]. The level of LDH, as a prognostic marker, increases in 30–80% of all cases [103]. Serum calcium and tumor markers such as alpha-fetoprotein (AFP) and carcinoembryonic antigen may also be raised [132–135].

6.6.3 Workup Investigation

On imaging, PHL can present with a solitary mass, multiple lesions, or diffuse infiltration [136–138]. A single solitary mass is reported to be the most common, occurring in 55–60% of presentations [103]. The mass may grow into the hepatic veins, inferior vena cava, and the right atrium, mimicking an HCC. Approximately 35–40% of patients have multiple lesions [139]. Diffuse infiltration is rare [140]. On ultrasound, lesions are typically solid and hypoechoic or anechoic, often resembling cysts [105, 140]. A target lesion has also been described [102]. In the infiltrating form of the disease, the only imaging feature is often hepatomegaly [141]. Focal hepatic lymphoma lesions are hypoattenuating on non-contrast CT, with rim enhancement often seen with contrast administration. A target-type lesion can also occur on CT, with lesions consisting of central necrosis, rim enhancement, and a peripheral ill-defined hypoattenuating area [102].

On MRI, focal lesions are hypointense on T1-weighted images and hyperintense on T2-weighted images. Increased signal on diffusion-weighted imaging (DWI) and decreased signal on apparent diffusion coefficient (ADC) would indicate decreased diffusion of water or "restricted diffusion" within that volume of tissue. Primary hepatic lymphoma (PHL) typically demonstrates marked diffusion restriction, with signal on ADC mapping typically lower than most other benign and malignant hepatic lesions. In the arterial and portal venous phases, the lesions typically demonstrate heterogeneous but predominantly decreased enhancement compared to the surrounding hepatic parenchyma. In the hepatobiliary phase, however, hepatic lymphoma is markedly and homogeneously hypointense [142].

Positron emission tomography (PET) with fluorine-18-fluoro-2-deoxyglucose is often used to assess distant disease. Increased disease activity often correlates with increased radiotracer uptake [143]. PET/CT is an excellent modality for the diagnosis, staging, and follow-up of tumors.

Because PHL is often misdiagnosed as many other liver diseases, the diagnosis should be established by pathological analysis. Liver tissue can be obtained by fine-needle biopsy (FNB), image-guided percutaneous biopsy, laparoscopic biopsy, or open biopsy [144–146].

Microscopically, diffuse large B-cell lymphomas are composed of sheets of atypical B cells that are more than twice the size of normal lymphocytes, with prominent nucleoli and increased or atypical mitotic figures [104, 147]. Most diffuse large B-cell lymphomas are mass-forming lesions associated with destruction of the normal liver architecture. In primary hepatic mucosa-associated lymphoid tissue (MALT) lymphoma, the atypical lymphoid cells are small in size, with mildly irregular nucleoli, dense chromatin, and scant cytoplasm, without germinal center differentiation [104, 148]. Lymphoepithelial lesions involving the bile ducts are common but are neither sensitive nor specific for the diagnosis of lymphoma. PHLs are always diagnosed and further subtyped using immunostains and fluorescence in situ hybridization (FISH) [138].

6.6.4 Differential Diagnosis

The main differential diagnoses considered are HCC, inflammatory hepatocellular adenoma, hypervascular metastasis (renal cell carcinoma, thyroid carcinoma, neuroendocrine, sarcomas, melanoma), and infection. The imaging features of more common hepatic diseases may overlap with those of hepatic lymphoma. Combining the imaging features with clinical manifestations and laboratory findings can facilitate a correct diagnosis. A definite diagnosis can only be made after pathological analysis.

6.6.5 Treatment, Follow-Up, and Recommendations

Treatment modalities include chemotherapy, radiation therapy, and, perhaps, surgery. Surgical resection may be attempted if the disease is localized or for debulking prior to chemotherapy [125, 131, 149–151]. Chemotherapy or chemotherapy with radiotherapy is often utilized, with varying degrees of success [103, 131, 152, 153]. Most of the patients received CHOP-like (cyclophosphamide, doxorubicin, vincristine, and prednisone) regimens. The overall prognosis is poor, with reported 1-, 5-, and 10-year overall survival (OS) rates of 50.85%, 39.6%, and 30.4%, respectively [110, 131]. Age, sex, race, marital status, histological subtype, stage, surgery, and chemotherapy are independent prognostic factors for survival.

6.7 Primary Hepatic Neuroendocrine Neoplasm

6.7.1 Incidence

Neuroendocrine neoplasms (NENs) are primary malignant tumors that arise from neuroendocrine cells, which grow throughout the body. The most common primary organ for these tumors is the gastrointestinal tract, followed by the bronchopulmonary system and the thymus [154]. Primary hepatic neuroendocrine neoplasms (PHNENs) are rare, with about 150 cases reported in the English literature up until 2012; however, the incidence is increasing [155–159]. There is no documented relationship to underlying liver disease [160].

6.7.2 Clinical Presentation

More than 10% of cases are asymptomatic. Presenting symptoms include right upper quadrant pain, fatigue, and weight loss. Carcinoid syndrome can occur but is rare [156]. Laboratory tests demonstrate high 24-h urine 5-hydroxyindoleacetic acid [161] and elevated serum chromogranin A. An elevated chromogranin A level has a good sensitivity and specificity in diagnosing NENs [162]. Tumor markers such as carcinoembryonic antigen, CA19-9, and AFP may also be elevated; however, their specificity is poor.

6.7.3 Workup Investigation

NENs arise from neuroendocrine cells in the endocrine tissues, which demonstrate various characteristics depending on the hormonal profile of the cell [163–166]. The classification is based on tumor grade using a system developed by the World Health Organization, which was most recently updated in 2019. The system differentiates gastroenteropancreatic NENs into well-differentiated neuroendocrine tumors (NETs), consisting of low (G1)-, intermediate (G2)-, and high (G3)-grade neoplasms, and poorly differentiated neuroendocrine carcinomas (NECs), consisting of high-grade carcinomas that resemble small cell carcinoma or large cell NEC of the lung. Grading is based on mitotic count and Ki-67 index [167, 168].

Imaging demonstrates a focal mass or masses typically in the right liver, which vary in appearance depending on histological grade [160]. Lesions on ultrasound can be variable, ranging from solid hypoechoic masses to heterogeneous or hyperechoic masses [160].

Low-grade PHNENs typically demonstrate a single mass on CT and MRI. On CT, the lesions are homogeneously hypoattenuating, with enhancement in the arterial phase post administration of contrast. Necrosis, hemorrhage, or calcification is infrequently present [160, 169]. Low-grade PHNENs on MRI demonstrate a low signal intensity on T1-weighted sequences and high signal intensity on T2-weighted sequences, with homogeneous arterial phase hyperenhancement on postcontrast images. On delayed postcontrast sequences, an enhancing capsule is commonly seen [169].

Intermediate-grade PHNENs on CT are more heterogeneous, with necrotic change and peripheral nodular enhancement on postcontrast images. MRI also demonstrates heterogeneity on T1- and T2-weighted sequences, with peripheral nodular enhancement.

High-grade PHNEN lesions demonstrate further progression in heterogeneity on CT and MRI, with peripheral nodular enhancement [160, 169]. MRI demonstrates increased necrosis and hemorrhagic change, with progressive restricted diffusion and decreasing mean ADC values [169].

Multiple radiopharmaceuticals have been employed in the detection of neuroendocrine neoplasms. Scintigraphy using 111In-pentetreotide or octreotide scanning has demonstrated a sensitivity of 90% and specificity of 83% [170, 171]. PET/CT with gallium-68-

labeled somatostatin analogs has improved diagnostic performance, with 68 Ga-DOTATATE and 68Ga-DOTATOC demonstrating sensitivities of 96% and 93%, respectively, and specificities of 100% and 85%, respectively [172]. PET/CT is now the preferred functional imaging study for neuroendocrine neoplasms.

6.7.4 Differential Diagnosis

Differential diagnoses include hepatic adenoma, HCC, cholangiocarcinoma, congenital liver hemangioma, focal nodular hyperplasia, primary hepatic angiosarcoma, secondary hepatic neuroendocrine carcinoma, and hepatic metastases from any other primary cancer site.

Diagnoses of PHNENs are dependent on pathological examination. However, it is very difficult to use pathological techniques to prove that a neuroendocrine tumor is primary to the liver, as there are no morphological, immunostain, or molecular findings that indicate that a neuroendocrine tumor is likely to be primary to the liver. Thus, the final diagnosis requires (1) establishing that the tumor in the liver is a neuroendocrine tumor through morphology and immunostain findings and (2) ruling out another primary site through imaging findings.

6.7.5 Treatment, Follow-Up, and Recommendations

Treatment depends on presentation. The role of chemotherapy is limited [158]. Radical resection of the tumor remains the most effective treatment of choice. Liver transplantation is also possible for liver-confined disease [158, 173, 174]. Transcatheter arterial embolization can provide excellent outcomes for unresectable tumors, given the sensitivity of neuroendocrine neoplasms to an alteration in blood flow [175]. Percutaneous ablation and somatostatin analogs may also be utilized [176–178]. The therapeutic application of lutetium-177 has been employed with promising results in advanced disease [179–181]. R0 resection and a G1/G2 histological classification are favorable prognostic factors for this disease [182].

6.8 Desmoplastic Small Round Cell Tumor

6.8.1 Incidence

Desmoplastic small round cell tumors (DSRCTs) are rare tumors of young adults first described in 1989 [183]. They belong to a family of small round blue cell tumors with other malignancies such as non-Hodgkin's lymphoma, rhabdomyosarcoma, Ewing sarcoma, Wilms tumor, poorly differentiated synovial cell sarcoma, small cell osteosarcoma, and neuroectodermal tumor. They are most commonly present in males, with a ratio to females of approximately 5:1. The mean age at presentation is 22 years, with a mean survival time of less than 3 years [184–187]. Because of limited published data, the incidence of DSRCT is inadequately understood.

6.8.2 Clinical Presentation

DSRCT most commonly originates in the mesothelium of the abdomen, involving the omentum and peritoneum. Organ involvement, including the liver and lungs, is infrequent and likely represents metastatic disease. In the majority of cases, patients remain asymptomatic for extended periods of time, and the diagnosis is made when the tumor burden is significant [188]. Patients present with abdominal mass, abdominal pain, weight loss, ascites, jaundice, diaphoresis, back pain, and lethargy [187]. About one-half of the patients will present extraperitoneal metastasis at the time of diagnosis [189–191]. The liver and lungs are the two most common sites for distant metastasis [188, 190, 192, 193].

6.8.3 Workup Investigation

Imaging commonly demonstrates a large intra-abdominal mass involving the peritoneum, with multifocal peritoneal masses. Hepatic involvement is often associated with a retrovesical or rectouterine space mass in approximately 85% of patients [194]. Hepatic masses are heterogeneously hypoattenuating on contrast-enhanced CT [187, 195]. MRI can be helpful in delineating the extent of the disease if surgical resection is considered [195]. MRI demonstrates lesions of high signal intensity on T2-weighted sequences and low signal intensity on T1-weighted images. Heterogeneous enhancement is seen post administration of gadolinium. Areas of internal hemorrhage or necrosis may be present [187, 196].

Histologically, DSRCTs are primitive tumors composed of small round blue cells that elicit a desmoplastic response. The tumor cells are uniform in appearance and grow in cords and nests surrounded by fibrotic stroma. Other cytological changes can include spindled areas, signet ring-like cells, pseudorosette formation, and cystic degeneration [197]. The tumors are positive for keratin, a marker of epithelial differentiation, and desmin, a marker of rhabdoid differentiation [184]. A molecular hallmark of DSRCT is a reciprocal translocation (t(11;22) (p13;q12)) resulting in an EWS–WT1 gene fusion [198]. It is the driver of tumorigenesis of DSRCT, and it acts by upregulating the expression of several genes [199].

6.8.4 Differential Diagnosis

The differential diagnosis of DSRCTs can be made with a spectrum of other round cell neoplasms, which include Ewing sarcoma, rhabdomyosarcoma, small cell carcinoma, and mesothelioma [200]. The diagnosis of DSRCT is made by a combination of the histological appearance and immunohistochemical staining results. DSRCT is distinguished from the other neoplasms by the presence of EWS–WT1 translocation, ideally performed by PCR or FISH or by immunohistochemistry staining if the former are not available.

6.8.5 Treatment, Follow-Up, and Recommendations

Treatment involves debulking surgery, hyperthermic intraperitoneal chemotherapy (HIPEC), combination cytotoxic chemotherapy, and radiation therapy in varying proportions [201]. Improved survival is demonstrated with radiotherapy and surgical resection for localized disease [194, 202]. DSRCT remains a challenging disease and needs prospective clinical trials, although this is a challenge in such a rare tumor type.

6.9 Hepatic Angiosarcoma

6.9.1 Incidence

Hepatic angiosarcoma is a high-grade, malignant neoplasm of endothelial cells of the blood or lymphatic vessels. The incidence is about 200 cases diagnosed per year worldwide [203] and 0.5–2.5 cases every 10,000,000 persons [204, 205]. The most important etiological factors are exposure to vinyl chloride monomer [206, 207] or other chemical carcinogens, e.g., iatrogenic exposure to colloidal thorium dioxide (Thorotrast) [208, 209], androgenic steroid use, and chronic arsenic ingestion [210], but around 75% of tumors have no known etiology [206, 211]. Hepatic angiosarcoma due to environmental exposure has a prolonged latency period of 10–40 years. It usually occurs in older men, with a peak incidence in the sixth or seventh decade of life. Males are more frequently affected than females, with a ratio of 3–4:1 [203].

6.9.2 Clinical Presentation

Patients present with vague symptoms like abdominal pain, weight loss, distension, or fatigue or are asymptomatic [205]. The physical examination commonly reveals jaundice, ascites, and hepatomegaly [212]. Laboratory studies show elevated alanine transaminase and aspartate transaminase, as well as thrombocytopenia and anemia. Tumor markers like AFP, CEA, CA19-9, and CA125 are in the normal range or only slightly elevated. They can also present with symptoms of hemoperitoneum due to tumor rupture or develop features of acute liver failure or disseminated intravascular coagulation [213]. Tumor rupture with hemoperitoneum is a sudden, severe complication and is reported to be seen in 17–27% of patients [205, 214]. Such a presentation is associated with high morbidity and mortality.

6.9.3 Workup Investigation

Ultrasonography shows multiple nodules or a solitary mass with varying echogenicity due to necrosis and hemorrhage. Contrast-enhanced CT is the best reference technique for diagnosis [203, 215]. Hepatic angiosarcoma is usually multicentric and involves both lobes; the entire liver may also be involved. Lesions appear to be hypodense, with variable patterns of enhancement on contrast, and become partly or completely isodense in comparison with the hepatic tissue postcontrast [216]. MRI shows dominant masses with heterogeneous intensity, including heterogeneous hypointense T1-weighted imaging and homogeneous or heterogeneous hyperintense T2-weighted imaging. Hemorrhage shows higher hyperintensity, with spot or patchy signals [217, 218]. However, hepatic angiosarcoma lacks specific features on imaging, so pathological diagnosis is still necessary.

Histologically, the malignancy is composed of spindle or pleomorphic cells with hyperchromatic nuclei that infiltrate various patterns of vascular channels. Solid areas that resemble fibrosarcoma, central necrosis, and smaller satellite lesions may also be seen. Parenchymal loss causes scarring, and occlusion of preexisting vessels can result in fibrosis, areas of infarction, and atrophy. CD31, CD34, *Ulex europaeus* agglutinin I, FVIII-Rag, and ETS-related gene (ERG) are immunohistochemical markers that can be used to aid diagnosis [219]. Due to the highly vascular nature of the tumor, liver biopsy has a high risk of morbidity and mortality. Open biopsy is currently recommended by most of the studies [203, 220].

6.9.4 Differential Diagnosis

Differential diagnoses include inflammatory or benign vascular diseases of the liver, Kaposi sarcoma, liver metastases from a primary tumor of other origin, epithelioid hemangioendothelioma, hepatocellular carcinoma, and fibrosarcoma. It is difficult to differentiate hepatic angiosarcoma from other hepatic tumors radiologically, and it is not uncommon to diagnose hepatic angiosarcoma on autopsy [203].

6.9.5 Treatment, Follow-Up, and Recommendations

Hepatic angiosarcoma is a rapidly fatal tumor. Complete hepatic resection or radical resection of the tumor is the most effective treatment for a single lesion; however, it is not always feasible in multifocal masses or metastatic disease [213, 221, 222]. Liver transplantation is not recommended due to the high rate of recurrence and the rapid progression of the disease. No effective chemotherapy or radiotherapy has been established. Transcatheter arterial chemoembolization (TACE) can also be used with palliative intention or to control bleeding [213]. Unfortunately, there are no established guidelines on optimal treatment modalities regarding surgery, chemotherapy, and radiation because of the low incidence and aggressive nature of the disease. The majority of patients die within 6 months from liver failure or hemorrhage, and even after surgical resection, most die within a year [203, 217].

6.10 Hepatoblastoma

6.10.1 Incidence

Hepatoblastoma is the most common primary hepatic malignancy in children. The overall age-adjusted incidence was 0.19 patients per 100,000 children, with a statistically significant increase per year [223]. The increasing rate in the United States was 4%, reported between 1992 and 2004 [224]. There is a slight male preponderance, and hepatoblastoma is associated with a number of genetic syndromes, such as familial adenomatous polyposis, Beckwith–Wiedemann syndrome, isolated hemihyperplasia, and trisomy 18 [225–229]. The prognosis is generally poor compared to other pediatric cancers, with an overall survival at 1, 3, and 5 years for all patients in the United States of 89.3%, 84.6%, and 81.9%, respectively [223].

6.10.2 Clinical Presentation

Patients generally present with an enlarging abdominal mass, with weight loss and decreased appetite. Rarely, excess β-human chorionic gonadotropin may lead to precocious puberty [230]. Serum AFP is generally elevated and is an important clinical marker. Hepatoblastoma without a raised AFP carries a worse prognosis and is often associated with small cell undifferentiated morphology [231].

6.10.3 Workup Investigation

Imaging typically demonstrates a large, well-defined, mass most commonly in the right lobe of the liver [232]. Ultrasound demonstrates an echogenic mass, which increases in heterogeneity as the tumor size increases. Increased vascularity may be appreciated on color Doppler imaging [233, 234]. On contrast-enhanced CT, the mass is heterogeneous and largely hypoattenuating, with areas of necrosis. Calcifications are visualized in up to 50% [232, 235]. Hepatoblastomas are predominantly of low signal on T1-weighted images and high signal on T2-weighted sequences, with heterogeneity depending on the extent of hemorrhage and necrosis. Heterogeneous enhancement post administration of gadolinium is also commonly seen, and a variable degree of washout may be seen in the delayed phases. MRI may also allow for a better appreciation of hepatic segmental involvement, leading to improved staging [232]. A large heterogeneous liver mass, with heterogeneous enhancement occurring in a child, along with an elevated serum AFP, is characteristic of hepatoblastoma.

Histologically, hepatoblastomas are epithelial malignancies. An epithelial component is required, but the tumors can be composed entirely of epithelial cells or can have both epithelial and mesenchymal components. Hepatoblastomas are further classified into eight histological subtypes based on the extent of hepatic differentiation and, for cases with fetal growth patterns, the amount of cytological atypia and mitotic count: well-differentiated fetal (pure fetal) with minimal mitotic activity, crowded or mitotically active fetal, pleomorphic fetal, anaplastic fetal, embryonal, macrotrabecular, small cell undifferentiated, and cholangioblastic [236]. Currently, the most clinically important patterns are the small cell undifferentiated pattern because it requires more aggressive chemotherapy and the well-differentiated fetal pattern with minimal mitotic activity because it is cured with complete excision and does not require chemotherapy.

Staging by imaging is based on the pretreatment extent of disease (PRETEXT) system. The PRETEXT group (I, II, III, and IV) describes the parenchymal tumor involvement of hepatic segments before any therapy and has a close correlation with the prognosis [237]. PRETEXT annotation factors include metastatic disease, macrovascular involvement of all hepatic veins or portal bifurcation, contiguous extrahepatic tumor, multifocality, and spontaneous rupture and have evolved over time. In the past decades, increasing amounts of prognostic data of this rare cancer have emerged [238–241]. Four major cooperative trial groups—International Childhood Liver Tumours Strategy Group (SIOPEL), Children's Oncology Group (COG), German Society for Paediatric Oncology and Haematology (GPOH), and Japanese Study Group for Pediatric Liver Tumors (JPLT)—have combined the data of published clinical trials. The Children's Hepatic tumors International Collaboration (CHIC) was formed in hopes of developing a more cooperative global approach to the staging and risk stratification of hepatoblastoma. The most prognostic factors are PRETEXT staging and annotation factors, age, and the AFP level. Metastatic disease, higher age (>8 years), and low AFP (<100 ng/ml) at diagnosis are associated with the worst outcome [242, 243].

6.10.4 Differential Diagnosis

There can be diagnostic challenges at both ends of the tumor differentiation spectrum. Small cell undifferentiated hepatoblastoma can mimic other small round blue cell tumors on small biopsies, and additional stains are usually needed to confirm the diagnosis and exclude other entities in the differential. On the other hand, tumors with a pure fetal growth pattern can closely resemble conventional HCC. There are no molecular or immunostain findings that have high diagnostic value in distinguishing these two possibilities, so the diagnosis is made based on morphological and clinical findings. Underlying liver disease and/or advanced fibrosis strongly favor conventional HCC. Embryonal or mesenchymal components strongly favor hepatoblastoma. Mesenchymal components are found in up to 40% of cases. The mesenchymal component usually consists of nondescript spindled cells, but osteoid material, skeletal muscle, or cartilage can also be found.

6.10.5 Treatment, Follow-Up, and Recommendations

Surgical resection is the cornerstone of treatment. Approximately 30% of tumors are resectable on presentation, which increases significantly with neoadjuvant chemotherapy [244, 245]. Orthotopic liver transplantation (OLT) is the only curative treatment option for unresectable hepatoblastoma. OLT can be considered the primary surgery when there is at least a partial response to neoadjuvant chemotherapy and no evidence of metastatic or extrahepatic disease. Patients who have had intrahepatic relapse after a previous partial hepatectomy with no metastatic or extrahepatic disease and patients who have had an incomplete resection (rescue OLT) are also eligible for transplantation [82, 246]. The prognosis of the resection group is similar to that of the transplant group [223, 247, 248].

Few conventional chemotherapy agents have demonstrated activity in progressive or relapsed hepatoblastoma [249]. Doxorubicin, carboplatin, etoposide, irinotecan, and ifosfamide have been incorporated in upfront therapy for high-risk patients or used as part of rescue strategies [250–252]. High-dose chemotherapy with stem cell transplantation is used in the setting of progressive or relapsed hepatoblastoma [253]. Hepatic intra-arterial chemoembolization can also be efficacious in shrinking tumors and allowing complete surgical resection after initial systemic chemotherapy [254, 255].

6.11 Undifferentiated Embryonal Sarcoma of the Liver

6.11.1 Incidence

Undifferentiated embryonal sarcoma of the liver, first described in 1978, is an extremely rare, highly malignant, undifferentiated mesenchymal neoplasm, with peak incidence between 6 and 10 years of age [256]. It was ranked the third common primary liver malignancy after hepatoblastoma and HCC in children [257]. The tumor is rare in adults, with a female preponderance [258, 259]. The incidence is unclear because there are no reports on large patient series.

6.11.2 Clinical Presentation

Patients present with an enlarging abdominal mass. Abdominal pain may or may not be present. Features such as fever, decreased appetite, weight loss, vomiting, and diarrhea are less frequent [256, 260, 261]. Laboratory tests are not useful with liver function tests, tumor markers, and inflammatory markers typically within normal ranges. Cases have been reported of elevated aminotransferases, leukocytosis, increased erythrocyte sedimentation rate, and increased AFP or CA-125 [256, 262, 263].

6.11.3 Workup Investigation

Imaging typically presents a large, well-circumscribed mass in the liver. The sonographic appearance is variable. A complex cystic mass with multiple septations and mural nodularity is most commonly described, with a solid echogenic lesion also possible [264]. CT and MRI demonstrate a well-defined mass with necrotic and hemorrhagic change to varying degrees. The lesion is hypoattenuating on non-contrast CT, with MRI demonstrating low signal on T1-weighted sequences and high signal on T2-weighted sequences. At times, the mass may resemble a cystic lesion due to the high water content of the myxoid stroma [264, 265]. Minimal enhancement is noted on early postcontrast phase imaging, with subtle enhancement in delayed phases [266].

Histologically, embryonal sarcomas are high-grade sarcomas with high cellularity and numerous anaplastic cells, frequently with giant cell transformation. Tumor cells often contain cytoplasmic hyaline globules, but this finding is neither highly sensitive nor specific. The stroma can vary from loose and myxoid to dense and collagenized. Embryonal sarcomas can arise from mesenchymal hamartomas, so some cases will have residual mesenchymal hamartomas at their edges.

6.11.4 Differential Diagnosis

Diagnosis of undifferentiated embryonal sarcoma of the liver is made by a constellation of demographic information; clinical history; a panel of undifferentiated pathological markers, including vimentin, desmin, CD68, α1 antitrypsin, and CD10; and ruling out of other pathologies [267]. The main differential diagnoses in the pediatric population are mesenchymal hamartoma, hepatoblastoma, and embryonal rhabdomyosarcoma of the biliary tree. HCC, gastrointestinal stromal tumor, angiolipoma, leiomyosarcoma, liposarcoma, angiosarcoma, epithelioid hemangioendothelioma, and malignant melanoma are more commonly seen in adults [268].

The diagnosis of mesenchymal hamartoma and embryonal sarcoma of the liver is often mistaken, leading to inadequate management [269]. If feasible, complete surgical resection of solid–cystic liver masses in the pediatric age group must be aimed for to get a definitive, final diagnosis, followed by an adequate treatment strategy.

6.11.5 Treatment, Follow-Up, and Recommendations

Surgical resection is the treatment of choice in undifferentiated embryonal sarcoma. Survival is poor, with a reported 37% 3-year survival in 1990 [270]. With improved multimodal treatment in the form of neoadjuvant chemotherapy and radiation therapy, more recently, survival rates have improved to 70–100% over a follow-up period of 21–68 months [260, 271–273].

References

1. Newman KD. Malignant liver tumors of children. Semin Pediatr Surg. 1992;1(2):145–51.
2. Ramchand S, Ahmed Y, Baskerville L. Lipoma of the liver. Arch Pathol. 1970;90(4):331–3.
3. Martí-Bonmatí L, Menor F, Vizcaino I, Vilar J. Lipoma of the liver: US, CT, and MRI appearance. Gastrointest Radiol. 1989;14(2):155–7. https://doi.org/10.1007/bf01889182.
4. Roberts JL, Fishman EK, Hartman DS, Sanders R, Goodman Z, Siegelman SS. Lipomatous tumors of the liver: evaluation with CT and US. Radiology. 1986;158(3):613–7. https://doi.org/10.1148/radiology.158.3.3511497.
5. Reading CC, Charboneau JW. Case of the day. Ultrasound hepatic lipoma. Radiographics. 1990;10(3):511–2. https://doi.org/10.1148/radiographics.10.3.2188310.
6. Puljiz Z, Petričević M, Bratanić A, Barišić I, Puljiz M, Karin Z. An unusually large liver lipoma. Med Glas (Zenica). 2012;9(2):411–4.

7. Horton KM, Bluemke DA, Hruban RH, Soyer P, Fishman EK. CT and MR imaging of benign hepatic and biliary tumors. Radiographics. 1999;19(2):431–51. https://doi.org/10.1148/radiographics.19.2.g99mr04431.
8. Bruneton JN, Kerboul P, Drouillard J, Menu Y, Normand F, Santini N. Hepatic lipomas: ultrasound and computed tomographic findings. Gastrointest Radiol. 1987;12(4):299–303. https://doi.org/10.1007/bf01885166.
9. Valls C, Iannacconne R, Alba E, Murakami T, Hori M, Passariello R, et al. Fat in the liver: diagnosis and characterization. Eur Radiol. 2006;16(10):2292–308. https://doi.org/10.1007/s00330-006-0146-0.
10. Dalal KM, Antonescu CR, Singer S. Diagnosis and management of lipomatous tumors. J Surg Oncol. 2008;97(4):298–313. https://doi.org/10.1002/jso.20975.
11. Rosado E, Cabral P, Campo M, Tavares A. Mesenchymal hamartoma of the liver-a case report and literature review. J Radiol Case Rep. 2013;7(5):35–43.
12. Apellaniz-Ruiz M, Segni M, Kettwig M, Glüer S, Pelletier D, Nguyen V-H, et al. Mesenchymal hamartoma of the liver and DICER1 syndrome. N Engl J Med. 2019;380(19):1834–42. https://doi.org/10.1056/NEJMoa1812169.
13. Goodman Z, Terracciano LM. Tumours and tumour-like lesions of the liver. In: MacSween's pathology of the liver. Edinburgh: Churchill Livingstone/Elsevier; 2006.
14. Stocker JT, Ishak KG. Mesenchymal hamartoma of the liver: report of 30 cases and review of the literature. Pediatr Pathol. 1983;1(3):245–67. https://doi.org/10.3109/15513818309040663.
15. Isaacs H Jr. Fetal and neonatal hepatic tumors. J Pediatr Surg. 2007;42(11):1797–803. https://doi.org/10.1016/j.jpedsurg.2007.07.047.
16. Stanley P, Hall TR, Woolley MM, Diament MJ, Gilsanz V, Miller JH. Mesenchymal hamartomas of the liver in childhood: sonographic and CT findings. AJR Am J Roentgenol. 1986;147(5):1035–9. https://doi.org/10.2214/ajr.147.5.1035.
17. Kim SH, Kim WS, Cheon JE, Yoon HK, Kang GH, Kim IO, et al. Radiological spectrum of hepatic mesenchymal hamartoma in children. Korean J Radiol. 2007;8(6):498–505. https://doi.org/10.3348/kjr.2007.8.6.498.
18. Thampy R, Elsayes KM, Menias CO, Pickhardt PJ, Kang HC, Deshmukh SP, et al. Imaging features of rare mesenychmal liver tumours: beyond haemangiomas. Br J Radiol. 2017;90(1079):20170373. https://doi.org/10.1259/bjr.20170373.
19. Roberts EA, Liu P, Stringer D, Superina RA, Mancer K. Mesenchymal hamartoma in a 10-month-old infant: appearance by magnetic resonance imaging. Can Assoc Radiol J. 1989;40(4):219–21.
20. Ito H, Kishikawa T, Toda T, Arai M, Muro H. Hepatic mensenchymal hamartoma of an infant. J Pediatr Surg. 1984;19(3):315–7. https://doi.org/10.1016/s0022-3468(84)80197-9.
21. Stringer MD, Alizai NK. Mesenchymal hamartoma of the liver: a systematic review. J Pediatr Surg. 2005;40(11):1681–90. https://doi.org/10.1016/j.jpedsurg.2005.07.052.
22. Asch MJ, Cohen AH, Moore TC. Hepatic and splenic lymphangiomatosis with skeletal involvement: report of a case and review of the literature. Surgery. 1974;76(2):334–9.
23. Losanoff JE, Richman BW, El-Sherif A, Rider KD, Jones JW. Mesenteric cystic lymphangioma. J Am Coll Surg. 2003;196(4):598–603. https://doi.org/10.1016/s1072-7515(02)01755-6.
24. Stavropoulos M, Vagianos C, Scopa CD, Dragotis C, Androulakis J. Solitary hepatic lymphangioma. A rare benign tumour: a case report. HPB Surg. 1994;8(1):33–6. https://doi.org/10.1155/1994/63638.
25. Koh CC, Sheu JC. Hepatic lymphangioma—a case report. Pediatr Surg Int. 2000;16(7):515–6. https://doi.org/10.1007/s003839900327.
26. O'Sullivan DA, Torres VE, de Groen PC, Batts KP, King BF, Vockley J. Hepatic lymphangiomatosis mimicking polycystic liver disease. Mayo Clin Proc. 1998;73(12):1188–92. https://doi.org/10.4065/73.12.1188.
27. Allen JG, Riall TS, Cameron JL, Askin FB, Hruban RH, Campbell KA. Abdominal lymphangiomas in adults. J Gastrointest Surg. 2006;10(5):746–51. https://doi.org/10.1016/j.gassur.2005.10.015.
28. Matsumoto T, Ojima H, Akishima-Fukasawa Y, Hiraoka N, Onaya H, Shimada K, et al. Solitary hepatic lymphangioma: report of a case. Surg Today. 2010;40(9):883–9. https://doi.org/10.1007/s00595-010-4255-7.
29. Liu Q, Sui CJ, Li BS, Gao A, Lu JY, Yang JM. Solitary hepatic lymphangioma: a one-case report. Springerplus. 2014;3:314. https://doi.org/10.1186/2193-1801-3-314.
30. Biondi A, Malaguarnera G, Vacante M, Berretta M, D'Agata V, Malaguarnera M, et al. Elevated serum levels of Chromogranin A in hepatocellular carcinoma. BMC Surg. 2012;12 Suppl 1(Suppl 1):S7. https://doi.org/10.1186/1471-2482-12-s1-s7.
31. Choi WJ, Jeong WK, Kim Y, Kim J, Pyo JY, Oh YH. MR imaging of hepatic lymphangioma. Korean J Hepatol. 2012;18(1):101–4. https://doi.org/10.3350/kjhep.2012.18.1.101.
32. Levy AD, Cantisani V, Miettinen M. Abdominal lymphangiomas: imaging features with pathologic correlation. AJR Am J Roentgenol. 2004;182(6):1485–91. https://doi.org/10.2214/ajr.182.6.1821485.
33. Siegel MJ, Glazer HS, St Amour TE, Rosenthal DD. Lymphangiomas in children: MR imaging. Radiology. 1989;170(2):467–70. https://doi.org/10.1148/radiology.170.2.2911671.
34. Roisman I, Manny J, Fields S, Shiloni E. Intra-abdominal lymphangioma. Br J Surg.

1989;76(5):485–9. https://doi.org/10.1002/bjs.1800760519.
35. Stein M, Hsu RK, Schneider PD, Ruebner BH, Mina Y. Alcohol ablation of a mesenteric lymphangioma. J Vasc Interv Radiol. 2000;11(2 Pt 1):247–50. https://doi.org/10.1016/s1051-0443(07)61473-0.
36. De Santis M, Calò GF, Trombini P, Romagnoli R. Percutaneous sclerosing treatment with ethanol of a large cystic lymphangioma of the neck in an adult. Radiol Med. 2003;105(1–2):127–30.
37. Banieghbal B, Davies MR. Guidelines for the successful treatment of lymphangioma with OK-432. Eur J Pediatr Surg. 2003;13(2):103–7. https://doi.org/10.1055/s-2003-39581.
38. Fletcher CD, Unni K, Mertens F. World Health Organization classification of tumours. Pathology and genetics of tumours of soft tissue and bone. Lyon: IARC Press; 2002.
39. Petrolla AA, Xin W. Hepatic angiomyolipoma. Arch Pathol Lab Med. 2008;132(10):1679–82. https://doi.org/10.5858/2008-132-1679-ha.
40. Ishak KG. Mesenchymal tumors of the liver. Hepatocellular carcinoma. New York: John Wiley & Sons; 1976. p. 247–307.
41. Jiang TA, Zhao QY, Chen MY, Wang LJ, Ao JY. Diagnostic analysis of hepatic angiomyolipoma. Hepatobiliary Pancreat Dis Int. 2005;4(1):152–5.
42. Talati H, Radhi J, Popovich S, Marcaccio M. Hepatic epithelioid angiomyolipoma: case series. Gastroenterology Res. 2010;3(6):293–5. https://doi.org/10.4021/gr273w.
43. Klompenhouwer AJ, Verver D, Janki S, Bramer WM, Doukas M, Dwarkasing RS, et al. Management of hepatic angiomyolipoma: a systematic review. Liver Int. 2017;37(9):1272–80. https://doi.org/10.1111/liv.13381.
44. Tsui WM, Colombari R, Portmann BC, Bonetti F, Thung SN, Ferrell LD, et al. Hepatic angiomyolipoma: a clinicopathologic study of 30 cases and delineation of unusual morphologic variants. Am J Surg Pathol. 1999;23(1):34–48. https://doi.org/10.1097/00000478-199901000-00004.
45. Terris B, Fléjou JF, Picot R, Belghiti J, Hénin D. Hepatic angiomyolipoma. A report of four cases with immunohistochemical and DNA-flow cytometric studies. Arch Pathol Lab Med. 1996;120(1):68–72.
46. Ren N, Qin LX, Tang ZY, Wu ZQ, Fan J. Diagnosis and treatment of hepatic angiomyolipoma in 26 cases. World J Gastroenterol. 2003;9(8):1856–8. https://doi.org/10.3748/wjg.v9.i8.1856.
47. Nonomura A, Enomoto Y, Takeda M, Tamura T, Kasai T, Yosikawa T, et al. Invasive growth of hepatic angiomyolipoma; a hitherto unreported ominous histological feature. Histopathology. 2006;48(7):831–5. https://doi.org/10.1111/j.1365-2559.2006.02427.x.
48. Wang SN, Tsai KB, Lee KT. Hepatic angiomyolipoma with trace amounts of fat: a case report and literature review. J Clin Pathol. 2006;59(11):1196–9. https://doi.org/10.1136/jcp.2005.027227.
49. Xu AM, Zhang SH, Zheng JM, Zheng WQ, Wu MC. Pathological and molecular analysis of sporadic hepatic angiomyolipoma. Hum Pathol. 2006;37(6):735–41. https://doi.org/10.1016/j.humpath.2006.01.028.
50. Prasad SR, Wang H, Rosas H, Menias CO, Narra VR, Middleton WD, et al. Fat-containing lesions of the liver: radiologic-pathologic correlation. Radiographics. 2005;25(2):321–31. https://doi.org/10.1148/rg.252045083.
51. Agaimy A, Vassos N, Croner RS, Strobel D, Lell M. Hepatic angiomyolipoma: a series of six cases with emphasis on pathological-radiological correlations and unusual variants diagnosed by core needle biopsy. Int J Clin Exp Pathol. 2012;5(6):512–21.
52. Black ME, Hedgire SS, Camposano S, Paul E, Harisinghani M, Thiele EA. Hepatic manifestations of tuberous sclerosis complex: a genotypic and phenotypic analysis. Clin Genet. 2012;82(6):552–7. https://doi.org/10.1111/j.1399-0004.2012.01845.x.
53. Butte JM, Do RK, Shia J, Gönen M, D'Angelica MI, Getrajdman GI, et al. Liver angiomyolipomas: a clinical, radiologic, and pathologic analysis of 22 patients from a single center. Surgery. 2011;150(3):557–67. https://doi.org/10.1016/j.surg.2011.03.006.
54. Ding G-H, Liu Y, Wu M-C, Yang G-S, Yang J-M, Cong W-M. Diagnosis and treatment of hepatic angiomyolipoma. J Surg Oncol. 2011;103(8):807–12. https://doi.org/10.1002/jso.21814.
55. Du S, Li Y, Mao Y, Sang X, Lu X, Wang W, et al. Diagnosis and treatment of hepatic angiomyolipoma. Hepatobiliary Surg Nutr. 2012;1(1):19–24.
56. Flemming P, Lehmann U, Becker T, Klempnauer J, Kreipe H. Common and epithelioid variants of hepatic angiomyolipoma exhibit clonal growth and share a distinctive immunophenotype. Hepatology. 2000;32(2):213–7. https://doi.org/10.1053/jhep.2000.9142.
57. Dabora SL, Jozwiak S, Franz DN, Roberts PS, Nieto A, Chung J, et al. Mutational analysis in a cohort of 224 tuberous sclerosis patients indicates increased severity of TSC2, compared with TSC1, disease in multiple organs. Am J Hum Genet. 2001;68(1):64–80. https://doi.org/10.1086/316951.
58. Cha I, Cartwright D, Guis M, Miller TR, Ferrell LD. Angiomyolipoma of the liver in fine-needle aspiration biopsies: its distinction from hepatocellular carcinoma. Cancer. 1999;87(1):25–30.
59. Kamimura K, Nomoto M, Aoyagi Y. Hepatic angiomyolipoma: diagnostic findings and management. Int J Hepatol. 2012;2012:410781. https://doi.org/10.1155/2012/410781.
60. Garoufalia Z, Machairas N, Kostakis ID, Liakea A, Tsaparas P, Liapis G. Malignant potential of epithelioid angiomyolipomas of the liver: a case report and comprehensive review of the literature. Mol Clin Oncol. 2018;9(2):226–30.
61. Zhu J, Wang G, Sun G, Xie B, Xiao W, Li Y. Primary hepatic epithelioid angiomyolipoma: a small case

series. ANZ J Surg. 2022;92(7–8):1803–8. https://doi.org/10.1111/ans.17777.

62. Yang C-Y, Ho M-C, Jeng Y-M, Hu R-H, Wu Y-M, Lee P-H. Management of hepatic angiomyolipoma. J Gastrointest Surg. 2007;11(4):452–7. https://doi.org/10.1007/s11605-006-0037-3.
63. Zhi-Gang C, Jin-Ming Z, Jiao-Qian Y, Yu-Ping G. Characteristics and treatment strategy of hepatic angiomyolipoma: a series of 94 patients collected from four institutions. J Gastrointest Liver Dis. 2011;20(1):65–9.
64. Kamimura K, Oosaki A, Sugahara S, Mori S, Moroda T, Satoh O, et al. Malignant potential of hepatic angiomyolipoma: case report and literature review. Clin J Gastroenterol. 2010;3(2):104–10. https://doi.org/10.1007/s12328-010-0136-2.
65. Klompenhouwer AJ, Dwarkasing RS, Doukas M, Pellegrino S, Vilgrain V, Paradis V, et al. Hepatic angiomyolipoma: an international multicenter analysis on diagnosis, management and outcome. HPB. 2020;22(4):622–9. https://doi.org/10.1016/j.hpb.2019.09.004.
66. Cai PQ, Wu YP, Xie CM, Zhang WD, Han R, Wu PH. Hepatic angiomyolipoma: CT and MR imaging findings with clinical-pathologic comparison. Abdom Imaging. 2013;38(3):482–9. https://doi.org/10.1007/s00261-012-9932-0.
67. Wang Z, Xu HX, Xie XY, Xie XH, Kuang M, Xu ZF, et al. Imaging features of hepatic angiomyolipomas on real-time contrast-enhanced ultrasound. Br J Radiol. 2010;83(989):411–8. https://doi.org/10.1259/bjr/81174247.
68. Musante F, Derchi LE, Zappasodi F, Bazzocchi M, Riviezzo GC, Banderali A, et al. Myelolipoma of the adrenal gland: sonographic and CT features. AJR Am J Roentgenol. 1988;151(5):961–4. https://doi.org/10.2214/ajr.151.5.961.
69. Ahmadi T, Itai Y, Takahashi M, Onaya H, Kobayashi T, Tanaka YO, et al. Angiomyolipoma of the liver: significance of CT and MR dynamic study. Abdom Imaging. 1998;23(5):520–6. https://doi.org/10.1007/s002619900391.
70. Nonomura A, Minato H, Kurumaya H. Angiomyolipoma predominantly composed of smooth muscle cells: problems in histological diagnosis. Histopathology. 1998;33(1):20–7. https://doi.org/10.1046/j.1365-2559.1998.00426.x.
71. Dalle I, Sciot R, de Vos R, Aerts R, van Damme B, Desmet V, et al. Malignant angiomyolipoma of the liver: a hitherto unreported variant. Histopathology. 2000;36(5):443–50. https://doi.org/10.1046/j.1365-2559.2000.00891.x.
72. Nguyen TT, Gorman B, Shields D, Goodman Z. Malignant hepatic angiomyolipoma: report of a case and review of literature. Am J Surg Pathol. 2008;32(5):793–8. https://doi.org/10.1097/PAS.0b013e3181607349.
73. Deng YF, Lin Q, Zhang SH, Ling YM, He JK, Chen XF. Malignant angiomyolipoma in the liver: a case report with pathological and molecular analysis. Pathol Res Pract. 2008;204(12):911–8. https://doi.org/10.1016/j.prp.2008.06.007.
74. Makhlouf HR, Remotti HE, Ishak KG. Expression of KIT (CD117) in angiomyolipoma. Am J Surg Pathol. 2002;26(4):493–7. https://doi.org/10.1097/00000478-200204000-00012.
75. Xie L, Jessurun J, Manivel JC, Pambuccian SE. Hepatic epithelioid angiomyolipoma with trabecular growth pattern: a mimic of hepatocellular carcinoma on fine needle aspiration cytology. Diagn Cytopathol. 2012;40(7):639–50. https://doi.org/10.1002/dc.21703.
76. Yan F, Zeng M, Zhou K, Shi W, Zheng W, Da R, et al. Hepatic angiomyolipoma: various appearances on two-phase contrast scanning of spiral CT. Eur J Radiol. 2002;41(1):12–8. https://doi.org/10.1016/s0720-048x(01)00392-8.
77. Makhlouf HR, Ishak KG, Goodman ZD. Epithelioid hemangioendothelioma of the liver. Cancer. 1999;85(3):562–82. https://doi.org/10.1002/(SICI)1097-0142(19990201)85:3<562::AID-CNCR7>3.0.CO;2-T.
78. Weiss SW, Enzinger FM. Epithelioid hemangioendothelioma a vascular tumor often mistaken for a carcinoma. Cancer. 1982;50(5):970–81. https://doi.org/10.1002/1097-0142(19820901)50:5<970::AID-CNCR2820500527>3.0.CO;2-Z.
79. Ishak KG, Sesterhenn IA, Goodman MZD, Rabin L, Stromeyer FW. Epithelioid hemangioendothelioma of the liver: a clinicopathologic and follow-up study of 32 cases. Hum Pathol. 1984;15(9):839–52. https://doi.org/10.1016/S0046-8177(84)80145-8.
80. Mehrabi A, Kashfi A, Fonouni H, Schemmer P, Schmied BM, Hallscheidt P, et al. Primary malignant hepatic epithelioid hemangioendothelioma. Cancer. 2006;107(9):2108–21. https://doi.org/10.1002/cncr.22225.
81. Kou K, Chen YG, Zhou JP, Sun XD, Sun DW, Li SX, et al. Hepatic epithelioid hemangioendothelioma: update on diagnosis and therapy. World J Clin Cases. 2020;8(18):3978–87. https://doi.org/10.12998/wjcc.v8.i18.3978.
82. Hertl M, Cosimi AB. Liver transplantation for malignancy. Oncologist. 2005;10(4):269–81. https://doi.org/10.1634/theoncologist.10-4-269.
83. Neofytou K, Chrysochos A, Charalambous N, Dietis M, Petridis C, Andreou C, et al. Hepatic epithelioid hemangioendothelioma and the danger of misdiagnosis: report of a case. Case Rep Oncol Med. 2013;2013:243939. https://doi.org/10.1155/2013/243939.
84. Dong Y, Wang WP, Cantisani V, D'Onofrio M, Ignee A, Mulazzani L, et al. Contrast-enhanced ultrasound of histologically proven hepatic epithelioid hemangioendothelioma. World J Gastroenterol. 2016;22(19):4741–9. https://doi.org/10.3748/wjg.v22.i19.4741.
85. Luo L, Cai Z, Zeng S, Wang L, Kang Z, Yang N, et al. CT and MRI features of hepatic epitheli-

oid haemangioendothelioma: a multi-institutional retrospective analysis of 15 cases and a literature review. Insights Imaging. 2023;14(1):2. https://doi.org/10.1186/s13244-022-01344-y.
86. Paolantonio P, Laghi A, Vanzulli A, Grazioli L, Morana G, Ragozzino A, et al. MRI of hepatic epithelioid hemangioendothelioma (HEH). J Magn Reson Imaging. 2014;40(3):552–8. https://doi.org/10.1002/jmri.24391.
87. Zhou L, Cui M-Y, Xiong J, Dong Z, Luo Y, Xiao H, et al. Spectrum of appearances on CT and MRI of hepatic epithelioid hemangioendothelioma. BMC Gastroenterol. 2015;15(1):69. https://doi.org/10.1186/s12876-015-0299-x.
88. Gan L, Chang R, Jin H, Yang L. Typical CT and MRI signs of hepatic epithelioid hemangioendothelioma. Oncol Lett. 2016;11(3):1699–706. https://doi.org/10.3892/ol.2016.4149.
89. Choi KH, Moon WS. Epithelioid hemangioendothelioma of the liver. Clin Mol Hepatol. 2013;19(3):315–9. https://doi.org/10.3350/cmh.2013.19.3.315.
90. Deyrup AT, Tighiouart M, Montag AG, Weiss SW. Epithelioid hemangioendothelioma of soft tissue: a proposal for risk stratification based on 49 cases. Am J Surg Pathol. 2008;32(6):924–7. https://doi.org/10.1097/PAS.0b013e31815bf8e6.
91. Fujii T, Zen Y, Sato Y, Sasaki M, Enomae M, Minato H, et al. Podoplanin is a useful diagnostic marker for epithelioid hemangioendothelioma of the liver. Mod Pathol. 2008;21(2):125–30. https://doi.org/10.1038/modpathol.3800986.
92. Doyle LA, Fletcher CDM, Hornick JL. Nuclear expression of CAMTA1 distinguishes epithelioid hemangioendothelioma from histologic mimics. Am J Surg Pathol. 2016;40(1):94–102. https://doi.org/10.1097/pas.0000000000000511.
93. Errani C, Zhang L, Sung YS, Hajdu M, Singer S, Maki RG, et al. A novel WWTR1-CAMTA1 gene fusion is a consistent abnormality in epithelioid hemangioendothelioma of different anatomic sites. Genes Chromosom Cancer. 2011;50(8):644–53. https://doi.org/10.1002/gcc.20886.
94. Mendlick MR, Nelson M, Pickering D, Johansson SL, Seemayer TA, Neff JR, et al. Translocation t(1;3)(p36.3;q25) is a nonrandom aberration in epithelioid hemangioendothelioma. Am J Surg Pathol. 2001;25(5):684–7.
95. Remiszewski P, Szczerba E, Kalinowski P, Gierej B, Dudek K, Grodzicki M, et al. Epithelioid hemangioendothelioma of the liver as a rare indication for liver transplantation. World J Gastroenterol. 2014;20(32):11333–9. https://doi.org/10.3748/wjg.v20.i32.11333.
96. Madariaga JR, Marino IR, Karavias DD, Nalesnik MA, Doyle HR, Iwatsuki S, et al. Long-term results after liver transplantation for primary hepatic epithelioid hemangioendothelioma. Ann Surg Oncol. 1995;2(6):483–7. https://doi.org/10.1007/BF02307080.
97. Lai Q, Feys E, Karam V, Adam R, Klempnauer J, Oliverius M, et al. Hepatic epithelioid hemangioendothelioma and adult liver transplantation: proposal for a prognostic score based on the analysis of the ELTR-ELITA Registry. Transplantation. 2017;101(3):555–64. https://doi.org/10.1097/tp.0000000000001603.
98. Sangro B, Iñarrairaegui M, Fernández-Ros N. Malignant epithelioid hemangioendothelioma of the liver successfully treated with Sorafenib. Rare Tumors. 2012;4(2):106–9.
99. Chevreau C, Le Cesne A, Ray-Coquard I, Italiano A, Cioffi A, Isambert N, et al. Sorafenib in patients with progressive epithelioid hemangioendothelioma: a phase 2 study by the French Sarcoma Group (GSF/GETO). Cancer. 2013;119(14):2639–44.
100. Bally O, Tassy L, Richioud B, Decouvelaere A-V, Blay J-Y, Derbel O. Eight years tumor control with pazopanib for a metastatic resistant epithelioid hemangioendothelioma. Clin Sarcoma Res. 2015;5(1):12. https://doi.org/10.1186/s13569-014-0018-3.
101. Ata AA, Kamel IA. Primary reticulum cell sarcoma of the liver. A case report. J Egypt Med Assoc. 1965;48(7):514–21.
102. Elsayes KM, Menias CO, Willatt JM, Pandya A, Wiggins M, Platt J. Primary hepatic lymphoma: imaging findings. J Med Imaging Radiat Oncol. 2009;53(4):373–9. https://doi.org/10.1111/j.1754-9485.2009.02081.x.
103. Noronha V, Shafi NQ, Obando JA, Kummar S. Primary non-Hodgkin's lymphoma of the liver. Crit Rev Oncol Hematol. 2005;53(3):199–207. https://doi.org/10.1016/j.critrevonc.2004.10.010.
104. Choi WT, Gill RM. Hepatic lymphoma diagnosis. Surg Pathol Clin. 2018;11(2):389–402. https://doi.org/10.1016/j.path.2018.02.003.
105. Tomasian A, Sandrasegaran K, Elsayes KM, Shanbhogue A, Shaaban A, Menias CO. Hematologic malignancies of the liver: spectrum of disease. Radiographics. 2015;35(1):71–86. https://doi.org/10.1148/rg.351130008.
106. Peng Y, Qing AC, Cai J, Yue C, French SW, Qing X. Lymphoma of the liver: clinicopathological features of 19 patients. Exp Mol Pathol. 2016;100(2):276–80. https://doi.org/10.1016/j.yexmp.2016.02.001.
107. Chiang I, Wang RC, Lai YC, Chang CC, Chen CH, Hsu CY, et al. Clinicopathologic features of lymphoproliferative neoplasms involving the liver. Medicina (Kaunas). 2022;58(1). https://doi.org/10.3390/medicina58010072.
108. Loddenkemper C, Longerich T. Lymphoma of the liver. In: Cavalli F, Stein H, Zucca E, editors. Extranodal lymphomas, pathology and management. Abingdon: CRC Press; 2008. p. 277–88.
109. Ugurluer G, Miller RC, Li Y, Thariat J, Ghadjar P, Schick U, et al. Primary Hepatic lymphoma: a retrospective, multicenter rare cancer network study. Rare

Tumors. 2016;8(3):6502. https://doi.org/10.4081/rt.2016.6502.
110. Zhang SL, Chen C, Rao QW, Guo Z, Wang X, Wang ZM, et al. Incidence, prognostic factors and survival outcome in patients with primary hepatic lymphoma. Front Oncol. 2020;10:750. https://doi.org/10.3389/fonc.2020.00750.
111. Lisker-Melman M, Pittaluga S, Pluda JM, Kleiner DE, Thompson P, Martin P, et al. Primary lymphoma of the liver in a patient with acquired immune deficiency syndrome and chronic hepatitis B. Am J Gastroenterol. 1989;84(11):1445–8.
112. Mohan C, Alurkar SS, Sharma OP, Advani SH. Primary liver lymphoma: a diagnostic dilemma. AJR Am J Roentgenol. 1991;157(2):413. https://doi.org/10.2214/ajr.157.2.1853833.
113. Mohamed M, Fernando R. Diagnostic and therapeutic quandaries in a patient with primary hepatic lymphoma and concurrent hepatitis C infection. Indian J Hematol Blood Transfus. 2014;30(Suppl 1):394–7. https://doi.org/10.1007/s12288-014-0431-z.
114. Sekiguchi Y, Yoshikawa H, Shimada A, Imai H, Wakabayashi M, Sugimoto K, et al. Primary hepatic circumscribed Burkitt's lymphoma that developed after acute hepatitis B: report of a case with a review of the literature. J Clin Exp Hematop. 2013;53(2):167–73. https://doi.org/10.3960/jslrt.53.167.
115. Somaglino C, Pramaggiore P, Polastri R. Primary hepatic lymphoma in a patient with chronic hepatitis B and C infection: diagnostic pitfalls and therapeutic challenge. Updat Surg. 2014;66(1):89–90. https://doi.org/10.1007/s13304-013-0208-1.
116. Kikuma K, Watanabe J, Oshiro Y, Shimogama T, Honda Y, Okamura S, et al. Etiological factors in primary hepatic B-cell lymphoma. Virchows Arch. 2012;460(4):379–87. https://doi.org/10.1007/s00428-012-1199-x.
117. Nagata S, Harimoto N, Kajiyama K. Primary hepatic mucosa-associated lymphoid tissue lymphoma: a case report and literature review. Surg Case Rep. 2015;1:87. https://doi.org/10.1186/s40792-015-0091-8.
118. Sato S, Masuda T, Oikawa H, Satoh T, Suzuki Y, Takikawa Y, et al. Primary hepatic lymphoma associated with primary biliary cirrhosis. Am J Gastroenterol. 1999;94(6):1669–73. https://doi.org/10.1111/j.1572-0241.1999.01160.x.
119. Chowdhary VR, Crowson CS, Poterucha JJ, Moder KG. Liver involvement in systemic lupus erythematosus: case review of 40 patients. J Rheumatol. 2008;35(11):2159–64. https://doi.org/10.3899/jrheum.080336.
120. Sutton E, Malatjalian D, Hayne OA, Hanly JG. Liver lymphoma in systemic lupus erythematosus. J Rheumatol. 1989;16(12):1584–8.
121. Honda H, Franken EA Jr, Barloon TJ, Smith JL. Hepatic lymphoma in cyclosporine-treated transplant recipients: sonographic and CT findings. AJR Am J Roentgenol. 1989;152(3):501–3. https://doi.org/10.2214/ajr.152.3.501.
122. Palazzo JP, Lundquist K, Mitchell D, Mittal KR, Hann HW, Munoz S, et al. Rapid development of lymphoma following liver transplantation in a recipient with hepatitis B and primary hemochromatosis. Am J Gastroenterol. 1993;88(1):102–4.
123. Rostaing L, Suc B, Fourtanier G, Baron E, Lloveras JJ, Durand D. Liver B cell lymphoma after liver transplantation. Transplant Proc. 1995;27(2):1781–2.
124. Caccamo D, Pervez NK, Marchevsky A. Primary lymphoma of the liver in the acquired immunodeficiency syndrome. Arch Pathol Lab Med. 1986;110(6):553–5.
125. Yang XW, Tan WF, Yu WL, Shi S, Wang Y, Zhang YL, et al. Diagnosis and surgical treatment of primary hepatic lymphoma. World J Gastroenterol. 2010;16(47):6016–9. https://doi.org/10.3748/wjg.v16.i47.6016.
126. Zhao Q, Liu HP, Gu YJ, Cong WM. Clinicopathological and survival features of primary hepatic lymphoma: an analysis of 35 cases. Zhonghua Zhong Liu Za Zhi. 2013;35(9):689–92.
127. Swadley MJ, Deliu M, Mosunjac MB, Gunthel CJ, Nguyen ML, Hanley KZ. Primary and secondary hepatic lymphomas diagnosed by image-guided fine-needle aspiration: a retrospective study of clinical and cytomorphologic findings. Am J Clin Pathol. 2014;141(1):119–27. https://doi.org/10.1309/ajcpe58escqdzfkx.
128. Bronowicki JP, Bineau C, Feugier P, Hermine O, Brousse N, Oberti F, et al. Primary lymphoma of the liver: clinical-pathological features and relationship with HCV infection in French patients. Hepatology. 2003;37(4):781–7. https://doi.org/10.1053/jhep.2003.50121.
129. Farag F, Morcus R, Ramachandran P, Pasrija UR, Wang JC. Fever of unknown origin due to primary hepatic diffuse large B-cell lymphoma: a case report. Cureus. 2019;11(3):e4220. https://doi.org/10.7759/cureus.4220.
130. Lei KI. Primary non-Hodgkin's lymphoma of the liver. Leuk Lymphoma. 1998;29(3–4):293–9. https://doi.org/10.3109/10428199809068566.
131. Avlonitis VS, Linos D. Primary hepatic lymphoma: a review. Eur J Surg. 1999;165(8):725–9. https://doi.org/10.1080/11024159950189474.
132. Page RD, Romaguera JE, Osborne B, Medeiros LJ, Rodriguez J, North L, et al. Primary hepatic lymphoma: favorable outcome after combination chemotherapy. Cancer. 2001;92(8):2023–9. https://doi.org/10.1002/1097-0142(20011015)92:8<2023::aid-cncr1540>3.0.co;2-b.
133. Seymour JF, Gagel RF, Hagemeister FB, Dimopoulos MA, Cabanillas F. Calcitriol production in hypercalcemic and normocalcemic patients with non-Hodgkin lymphoma. Ann Intern Med. 1994;121(9):633–40. https://doi.org/10.7326/0003-4819-121-9-199411010-00001.

134. Ali AM, Omore I, Riaz MF, Paliou M, Simon K. Primary hepatic lymphoma masquerading as symptomatic hypercalcemia. Cureus. 2020;12(9):e10633. https://doi.org/10.7759/cureus.10633.
135. Hsu A, Gagnier M, Ryer E, Salhab M, Rosmarin AG. Hypercalcemia due to primary hepatic lymphoma. Case Rep Hematol. 2016;2016:1876901. https://doi.org/10.1155/2016/1876901.
136. Maher MM, McDermott SR, Fenlon HM, Conroy D, O'Keane JC, Carney DN, et al. Imaging of primary non-Hodgkin's lymphoma of the liver. Clin Radiol. 2001;56(4):295–301. https://doi.org/10.1053/crad.2000.0649.
137. Kelekis NL, Semelka RC, Siegelman ES, Ascher SM, Outwater EK, Woosley JT, et al. Focal hepatic lymphoma: magnetic resonance demonstration using current techniques including gadolinium enhancement. Magn Reson Imaging. 1997;15(6):625–36. https://doi.org/10.1016/s0730-725x(97)00111-2.
138. Wang Q, Wu K, Zhang X, Liu Y, Sun Z, Wei S, et al. Primary hepatopancreatobiliary lymphoma: pathogenesis, diagnosis, and management. Front Oncol. 2022;12:951062. https://doi.org/10.3389/fonc.2022.951062.
139. Emile JF, Azoulay D, Gornet JM, Lopes G, Delvart V, Samuel D, et al. Primary non-Hodgkin's lymphomas of the liver with nodular and diffuse infiltration patterns have different prognoses. Ann Oncol. 2001;12(7):1005–10. https://doi.org/10.1023/a:1011131930409.
140. Gazelle GS, Lee MJ, Hahn PF, Goldberg MA, Rafaat N, Mueller PR. US, CT, and MRI of primary and secondary liver lymphoma. J Comput Assist Tomogr. 1994;18(3):412–5. https://doi.org/10.1097/00004728-199405000-00013.
141. Rajesh S, Bansal K, Sureka B, Patidar Y, Bihari C, Arora A. The imaging conundrum of hepatic lymphoma revisited. Insights Imaging. 2015;6(6):679–92. https://doi.org/10.1007/s13244-015-0437-6.
142. Colagrande S, Calistri L, Grazzini G, Nardi C, Busoni S, Morana G, et al. MRI features of primary hepatic lymphoma. Abdom Radiol (NY). 2018;43(9):2277–87. https://doi.org/10.1007/s00261-018-1476-5.
143. Goldberg MA, Lee MJ, Fischman AJ, Mueller PR, Alpert NM, Thrall JH. Fluorodeoxyglucose PET of abdominal and pelvic neoplasms: potential role in oncologic imaging. Radiographics. 1993;13(5):1047–62. https://doi.org/10.1148/radiographics.13.5.8210589.
144. Ippolito D, Porta M, Maino C, Pecorelli A, Ragusi M, Giandola T, et al. Diagnostic approach in hepatic lymphoma: radiological imaging findings and literature review. J Cancer Res Clin Oncol. 2020;146(6):1545–58. https://doi.org/10.1007/s00432-020-03205-x.
145. Nishikawa K, Katsuta K, Tanaka S, Fujibe K, Hattori A, Shiono Y, et al. Primary hepatic lymphoma diagnosed using endoscopic ultrasound-guided liver biopsy: a case report. J Med Case Rep. 2021;15(1):199. https://doi.org/10.1186/s13256-021-02791-9.
146. Loddenkemper C, Longerich T, Hummel M, Ernestus K, Anagnostopoulos I, Dienes HP, et al. Frequency and diagnostic patterns of lymphomas in liver biopsies with respect to the WHO classification. Virchows Arch. 2007;450(5):493–502. https://doi.org/10.1007/s00428-007-0384-9.
147. Xing AY, Dong XZ, Zhu LQ, Liu L, Sun D, Guo S. Clinicopathological characteristics and molecular phenotypes of primary hepatic lymphoma. Front Oncol. 2022;12:906245. https://doi.org/10.3389/fonc.2022.906245.
148. Grewe S, Shahid M, Zhang L, Jiang K. Clinically unsuspected primary hepatic mucosa-associated lymphoid tissue lymphoma collision with an intrahepatic cholangiocarcinoma: a case report and literature review. SAGE Open Med Case Rep. 2021;9:2050313x211041838. https://doi.org/10.1177/2050313x211041838.
149. Scoazec JY, Degott C, Brousse N, Barge J, Molas G, Potet F, et al. Non-Hodgkin's lymphoma presenting as a primary tumor of the liver: presentation, diagnosis and outcome in eight patients. Hepatology. 1991;13(5):870–5.
150. Bouliaris K, Christodoulidis G, Koukoulis G, Mamaloudis I, Ioannou M, Bouronikou E, et al. A primary hepatic lymphoma treated with liver resection and chemotherapy. Case Rep Surg. 2014;2014:749509. https://doi.org/10.1155/2014/749509.
151. Cesaretti M, Loustau M, Robba C, Senescende L, Zarzavadjian Le Bian A. Reappraisal of primary hepatic lymphoma: is surgical resection underestimated? Crit Rev Oncol Hematol. 2018;123:1–6. https://doi.org/10.1016/j.critrevonc.2018.01.004.
152. Chowla A, Malhi-Chowla N, Chidambaram A, Surick B. Primary hepatic lymphoma in hepatitis C: case report and review of the literature. Am Surg. 1999;65(9):881–3.
153. Coiffier B, Lepage E, Briere J, Herbrecht R, Tilly H, Bouabdallah R, et al. CHOP chemotherapy plus rituximab compared with CHOP alone in elderly patients with diffuse large-B-cell lymphoma. N Engl J Med. 2002;346(4):235–42. https://doi.org/10.1056/NEJMoa011795.
154. Bosman FT, Carneiro F, Hruban RH, Theise ND. WHO classification of tumours of the digestive system, vol. 3. 4th ed. Lyon: World Health Organization; 2010.
155. Iwao M, Nakamuta M, Enjoji M, Kubo H, Fukutomi T, Tanabe Y, et al. Primary hepatic carcinoid tumor: case report and review of 53 cases. Med Sci Monit. 2001;7(4):746–50.
156. Donadon M, Torzilli G, Palmisano A, Del Fabbro D, Panizzo V, Maggioni M, et al. Liver resection for primary hepatic neuroendocrine tumours: report of three cases and review of the literature. Eur J Surg

Oncol. 2006;32(3):325–8. https://doi.org/10.1016/j.ejso.2005.11.017.
157. Huang YQ, Xu F, Yang JM, Huang B. Primary hepatic neuroendocrine carcinoma: clinical analysis of 11 cases. Hepatobiliary Pancreat Dis Int. 2010;9(1):44–8.
158. Park CH, Chung JW, Jang SJ, Chung MJ, Bang S, Park SW, et al. Clinical features and outcomes of primary hepatic neuroendocrine carcinomas. J Gastroenterol Hepatol. 2012;27(8):1306–11. https://doi.org/10.1111/j.1440-1746.2012.07117.x.
159. Yao JC, Hassan M, Phan A, Dagohoy C, Leary C, Mares JE, et al. One hundred years after "carcinoid": epidemiology of and prognostic factors for neuroendocrine tumors in 35,825 cases in the United States. J Clin Oncol. 2008;26(18):3063–72. https://doi.org/10.1200/jco.2007.15.4377.
160. Yang K, Cheng YS, Yang JJ, Jiang X, Guo JX. Primary hepatic neuroendocrine tumors: multimodal imaging features with pathological correlations. Cancer Imaging. 2017;17(1):20. https://doi.org/10.1186/s40644-017-0120-x.
161. Sippel RS, Chen H. Carcinoid tumors. Surg Oncol Clin N Am. 2006;15(3):463–78. https://doi.org/10.1016/j.soc.2006.05.002.
162. Campana D, Nori F, Piscitelli L, Morselli-Labate AM, Pezzilli R, Corinaldesi R, et al. Chromogranin A: is it a useful marker of neuroendocrine tumors? J Clin Oncol. 2007;25(15):1967–73. https://doi.org/10.1200/jco.2006.10.1535.
163. Cho MY, Kim JM, Sohn JH, Kim MJ, Kim KM, Kim WH, et al. Current trends of the incidence and pathological diagnosis of gastroenteropancreatic neuroendocrine tumors (GEP-NETs) in Korea 2000–2009: multicenter study. Cancer Res Treat. 2012;44(3):157–65. https://doi.org/10.4143/crt.2012.44.3.157.
164. Klimstra DS, Modlin IR, Coppola D, Lloyd RV, Suster S. The pathologic classification of neuroendocrine tumors: a review of nomenclature, grading, and staging systems. Pancreas. 2010;39(6):707–12. https://doi.org/10.1097/MPA.0b013e3181ec124e.
165. Klöppel G, Perren A, Heitz PU. The gastroenteropancreatic neuroendocrine cell system and its tumors: the WHO classification. Ann N Y Acad Sci. 2004;1014:13–27. https://doi.org/10.1196/annals.1294.002.
166. Klöppel G, Couvelard A, Perren A, Komminoth P, McNicol AM, Nilsson O, et al. ENETS Consensus Guidelines for the Standards of Care in Neuroendocrine Tumors: towards a standardized approach to the diagnosis of gastroenteropancreatic neuroendocrine tumors and their prognostic stratification. Neuroendocrinology. 2009;90(2):162–6. https://doi.org/10.1159/000182196.
167. Yang Z. Pathology, classification, and grading of neuroendocrine neoplasms arising in the digestive system. In: Goldberg RM, editor. UpToDate. Waltham: UpToDate; 2022.
168. Nagtegaal ID, Odze RD, Klimstra D, Paradis V, Rugge M, Schirmacher P, et al. The 2019 WHO classification of tumours of the digestive system. Histopathology. 2020;76(2):182–8. https://doi.org/10.1111/his.13975.
169. Wang L-X, Liu K, Lin G-W, Jiang T. Primary hepatic neuroendocrine tumors: comparing CT and MRI features with pathology. Cancer Imaging. 2015;15(1):13. https://doi.org/10.1186/s40644-015-0046-0.
170. Critchley M. Octreotide scanning for carcinoid tumours. Postgrad Med J. 1997;73(861):399–402. https://doi.org/10.1136/pgmj.73.861.399.
171. Knox CD, Anderson CD, Lamps LW, Adkins RB, Pinson CW. Long-term survival after resection for primary hepatic carcinoid tumor. Ann Surg Oncol. 2003;10(10):1171–5. https://doi.org/10.1245/aso.2003.04.533.
172. Yang J, Kan Y, Ge BH, Yuan L, Li C, Zhao W. Diagnostic role of Gallium-68 DOTATOC and Gallium-68 DOTATATE PET in patients with neuroendocrine tumors: a meta-analysis. Acta Radiol. 2014;55(4):389–98. https://doi.org/10.1177/0284185113496679.
173. Fenwick SW, Wyatt JI, Toogood GJ, Lodge JP. Hepatic resection and transplantation for primary carcinoid tumors of the liver. Ann Surg. 2004;239(2):210–9. https://doi.org/10.1097/01.sla.0000109155.89514.42.
174. de Liguori Carino N, Manzia TM, Tariciotti L, Berlanda M, Orlando G, Tisone G. Liver transplantation in primary hepatic carcinoid tumor: case report and literature review. Transplant Proc. 2009;41(4):1386–9. https://doi.org/10.1016/j.transproceed.2009.03.011.
175. Kress O, Wagner HJ, Wied M, Klose KJ, Arnold R, Alfke H. Transarterial chemoembolization of advanced liver metastases of neuroendocrine tumors—a retrospective single-center analysis. Digestion. 2003;68(2–3):94–101. https://doi.org/10.1159/000074522.
176. Yao KA, Talamonti MS, Nemcek A, Angelos P, Chrisman H, Skarda J, et al. Indications and results of liver resection and hepatic chemoembolization for metastatic gastrointestinal neuroendocrine tumors. Surgery. 2001;130(4):677–82; discussion 82–5. https://doi.org/10.1067/msy.2001.117377.
177. Gamblin TC, Christians K, Pappas SG. Radiofrequency ablation of neuroendocrine hepatic metastasis. Surg Oncol Clin N Am. 2011;20(2):273–9, vii–viii. https://doi.org/10.1016/j.soc.2010.11.002.
178. Kvols LK, Moertel CG, O'Connell MJ, Schutt AJ, Rubin J, Hahn RG. Treatment of the malignant carcinoid syndrome. Evaluation of a long-acting somatostatin analogue. N Engl J Med. 1986;315(11):663–6. https://doi.org/10.1056/nejm198609113151102.

179. Das T, Banerjee S. Theranostic applications of lutetium-177 in radionuclide therapy. Curr Radiopharm. 2016;9(1):94–101. https://doi.org/10.2174/1874471008666150313114644.
180. Kam BL, Teunissen JJ, Krenning EP, de Herder WW, Khan S, van Vliet EI, et al. Lutetium-labelled peptides for therapy of neuroendocrine tumours. Eur J Nucl Med Mol Imaging. 2012;39 Suppl 1(Suppl 1):S103–12. https://doi.org/10.1007/s00259-011-2039-y.
181. Claringbold PG, Turner JH. NeuroEndocrine tumor therapy with lutetium-177-octreotate and everolimus (NETTLE): a phase I study. Cancer Biother Radiopharm. 2015;30(6):261–9. https://doi.org/10.1089/cbr.2015.1876.
182. Shi C, Zhao Q, Dai B, Xie F, Yang J. Primary hepatic neuroendocrine neoplasm: long-time surgical outcome and prognosis. Medicine (Baltimore). 2018;97(31):e11764. https://doi.org/10.1097/md.0000000000011764.
183. Gerald WL, Rosai J. Case 2. Desmoplastic small cell tumor with divergent differentiation. Pediatr Pathol. 1989;9(2):177–83. https://doi.org/10.3109/15513818909022347.
184. Gerald WL, Ladanyi M, Alava ED, Cuatrecasas M, Kushner BH, LaQuaglia MP, et al. Clinical, pathologic, and molecular spectrum of tumors associated with t(11;22)(p13;q12): desmoplastic small round-cell tumor and its variants. J Clin Oncol. 1998;16(9):3028–36. https://doi.org/10.1200/jco.1998.16.9.3028.
185. Kushner BH, LaQuaglia MP, Wollner N, Meyers PA, Lindsley KL, Ghavimi F, et al. Desmoplastic small round-cell tumor: prolonged progression-free survival with aggressive multimodality therapy. J Clin Oncol. 1996;14(5):1526–31. https://doi.org/10.1200/jco.1996.14.5.1526.
186. Quaglia MP, Brennan MF. The clinical approach to desmoplastic small round cell tumor. Surg Oncol. 2000;9(2):77–81. https://doi.org/10.1016/s0960-7404(00)00024-4.
187. Thomas R, Rajeswaran G, Thway K, Benson C, Shahabuddin K, Moskovic E. Desmoplastic small round cell tumour: the radiological, pathological and clinical features. Insights Imaging. 2013;4(1):111–8. https://doi.org/10.1007/s13244-012-0212-x.
188. Dufresne A, Cassier P, Couraud L, Marec-Bérard P, Meeus P, Alberti L, et al. Desmoplastic small round cell tumor: current management and recent findings. Sarcoma. 2012;2012:714986. https://doi.org/10.1155/2012/714986.
189. Lettieri CK, Garcia-Filion P, Hingorani P. Incidence and outcomes of desmoplastic small round cell tumor: results from the surveillance, epidemiology, and end results database. J Cancer Epidemiol. 2014;2014:680126. https://doi.org/10.1155/2014/680126.
190. Honoré C, Amroun K, Vilcot L, Mir O, Domont J, Terrier P, et al. Abdominal desmoplastic small round cell tumor: multimodal treatment combining chemotherapy, surgery, and radiotherapy is the best option. Ann Surg Oncol. 2015;22(4):1073–9. https://doi.org/10.1245/s10434-014-4123-6.
191. Gani F, Goel U, Canner JK, Meyer CF, Johnston FM. A national analysis of patterns of care and outcomes for adults diagnosed with desmoplastic small round cell tumors in the United States. J Surg Oncol. 2019;119(7):880–6. https://doi.org/10.1002/jso.25426.
192. Bulbul A, Fahy BN, Xiu J, Rashad S, Mustafa A, Husain H, et al. Desmoplastic small round blue cell tumor: a review of treatment and potential therapeutic genomic alterations. Sarcoma. 2017;2017:1278268. https://doi.org/10.1155/2017/1278268.
193. Stiles ZE, Dickson PV, Glazer ES, Murphy AJ, Davidoff AM, Behrman SW, et al. Desmoplastic small round cell tumor: a nationwide study of a rare sarcoma. J Surg Oncol. 2018;117(8):1759–67. https://doi.org/10.1002/jso.25071.
194. Bellah R, Suzuki-Bordalo L, Brecher E, Ginsberg JP, Maris J, Pawel BR. Desmoplastic small round cell tumor in the abdomen and pelvis: report of CT findings in 11 affected children and young adults. AJR Am J Roentgenol. 2005;184(6):1910–4. https://doi.org/10.2214/ajr.184.6.01841910.
195. Kis B, O'Regan KN, Agoston A, Javery O, Jagannathan J, Ramaiya NH. Imaging of desmoplastic small round cell tumour in adults. Br J Radiol. 2012;85(1010):187–92. https://doi.org/10.1259/bjr/57186741.
196. Pickhardt PJ, Fisher AJ, Balfe DM, Dehner LP, Huettner PC. Desmoplastic small round cell tumor of the abdomen: radiologic-histopathologic correlation. Radiology. 1999;210(3):633–8. https://doi.org/10.1148/radiology.210.3.r99mr42633.
197. Ordóñez NG. Desmoplastic small round cell tumor: I: a histopathologic study of 39 cases with emphasis on unusual histological patterns. Am J Surg Pathol. 1998;22(11):1303–13. https://doi.org/10.1097/00000478-199811000-00001.
198. Gerald WL, Rosai J, Ladanyi M. Characterization of the genomic breakpoint and chimeric transcripts in the EWS-WT1 gene fusion of desmoplastic small round cell tumor. Proc Natl Acad Sci USA. 1995;92(4):1028–32. https://doi.org/10.1073/pnas.92.4.1028.
199. Gedminas JM, Chasse MH, McBrairty M, Beddows I, Kitchen-Goosen SM, Grohar PJ. Desmoplastic small round cell tumor is dependent on the EWS-WT1 transcription factor. Oncogene. 2020;9(4):41. https://doi.org/10.1038/s41389-020-0224-1.
200. Machado I, Navarro L, Pellin A, Navarro S, Agaimy A, Tardío JC, et al. Defining Ewing and Ewing-like small round cell tumors (SRCT): the need for molecular techniques in their categorization and differential diagnosis. A study of 200 cases. Ann Diagn Pathol. 2016;22:25–32. https://doi.org/10.1016/j.anndiagpath.2016.03.002.

201. Mello CA, Campos FAB, Santos TG, Silva MLG, Torrezan GT, Costa FDA, et al. Desmoplastic small round cell tumor: a review of main molecular abnormalities and emerging therapy. Cancer. 2021;13(3):498.
202. Wong HH, Hatcher HM, Benson C, Al-Muderis O, Horan G, Fisher C, et al. Desmoplastic small round cell tumour: characteristics and prognostic factors of 41 patients and review of the literature. Clin Sarcoma Res. 2013;3(1):14. https://doi.org/10.1186/2045-3329-3-14.
203. Chaudhary P, Bhadana U, Singh RAK, Ahuja A. Primary hepatic angiosarcoma. Eur J Surg Oncol. 2015;41(9):1137–43. https://doi.org/10.1016/j.ejso.2015.04.022.
204. Zocchetti C. Liver angiosarcoma in humans: epidemiologic considerations. Med Lav. 2001;92(1):39–53.
205. Molina E, Hernandez A. Clinical manifestations of primary hepatic angiosarcoma. Dig Dis Sci. 2003;48(4):677–82. https://doi.org/10.1023/A:1022868221670.
206. Mark L, Delmore F, Creech J Jr, Ogden L II, Fadell EH, Songster CL, Clanton J, Johnson MN, Christopherson WM. Clinical and morphologic features of hepatic angiosarcoma in vinyl chloride workers. Cancer. 1976;37(1):149–63.
207. Elliott P, Kleinschmidt I. Angiosarcoma of the liver in Great Britain in proximity to vinyl chloride sites. Occup Environ Med. 1997;54(1):14–8.
208. Ito Y, Kojiro M, Nakashima T, Mori T. Pathomorphologic characteristics of 102 cases of thorotrast-related hepatocellular carcinoma, cholangiocarcinoma, and hepatic angiosarcoma. Cancer. 1988;62(6):1153–62.
209. Kojiro M, Nakashima T, Ito Y, Ikezaki H, Mori T, Kido C. Thorium dioxide-related angiosarcoma of the liver. Pathomorphologic study of 29 autopsy cases. Arch Pathol Lab Med. 1985;109(9):853–7.
210. Salgado M, Sans M, Forns X, Bruguera M, Castells A, Navasa M, et al. Hepatic angiosarcoma: a report of a case associated with treatment with arsenic salts and a review of the literature. Gastroenterol Hepatol. 1995;18(3):132–5.
211. Falk H, Popper H, Thomas L, Ishak K. Hepatic angiosarcoma associated with androgenic-anabolic steroids. Lancet. 1979;314(8152):1120–3. https://doi.org/10.1016/S0140-6736(79)92515-7.
212. Forbes A, Portmann B, Johnson P, Williams R. Hepatic sarcomas in adults: a review of 25 cases. Gut. 1987;28(6):668–74. https://doi.org/10.1136/gut.28.6.668.
213. Zheng Y-w, Zhang X-w, Zhang J-l, Hui Z-z, Du W-j, Li R-m, et al. Primary hepatic angiosarcoma and potential treatment options. J Gastroenterol Hepatol. 2014;29(5):906–11. https://doi.org/10.1111/jgh.12506.
214. Leowardi C, Hormann Y, Hinz U, Wente MN, Hallscheidt P, Flechtenmacher C, et al. Ruptured angiosarcoma of the liver treated by emergency catheter-directed embolization. World J Gastroenterol. 2006;12(5):804–8. https://doi.org/10.3748/wjg.v12.i5.804.
215. Park Y, Kim J, Kim K, Lee I, Yoon H-K, Ko G-Y, et al. Primary hepatic angiosarcoma: imaging findings and palliative treatment with transcatheter arterial chemoembolization or embolization. Clin Radiol. 2009;64(8):779–85.
216. Koyama T, Fletcher JG, Johnson CD, Kuo MS, Notohara K, Burgart LJ. Primary hepatic angiosarcoma: findings at CT and MR imaging. Radiology. 2002;222(3):667–73.
217. Yi LL, Zhang JX, Zhou SG, Wang J, Huang YQ, Li J, et al. CT and MRI studies of hepatic angiosarcoma. Clin Radiol. 2019;74(5):406.e1–8. https://doi.org/10.1016/j.crad.2018.12.013.
218. Bruegel M, Muenzel D, Waldt S, Specht K, Rummeny EJ. Hepatic angiosarcoma: cross-sectional imaging findings in seven patients with emphasis on dynamic contrast-enhanced and diffusion-weighted MRI. Abdom Imaging. 2013;38:745–54.
219. Wang Z-B, Yuan J, Chen W, Wei L-X. Transcription factor ERG is a specific and sensitive diagnostic marker for hepatic angiosarcoma. World J Gastroenterol: WJG. 2014;20(13):3672.
220. Locker GY, Doroshow JH, Zwelling LA, Chabner BA. The clinical features of hepatic angiosarcoma: a report of four cases and a review of the English literature. Medicine (Baltimore). 1979;58(1):48–64.
221. Chi T, Yang Z, Xue H, Lü K, Feng R, Xu H, et al. Diagnosis and treatment of primary hepatic angiosarcoma: a report of 7 cases with a literature review. Zhonghua Yi Xue Za Zhi. 2011;91(24):1694–7.
222. Timaran CH, Grandas OH, Bell JL. Hepatic angiosarcoma: long-term survival after complete surgical removal. Am Surg. 2000;66(12):1153–7.
223. Feng TC, Zai HY, Jiang W, Zhu Q, Jiang B, Yao L, et al. Survival and analysis of prognostic factors for hepatoblastoma: based on SEER database. Ann Transl Med. 2019;7(20):555. https://doi.org/10.21037/atm.2019.09.76.
224. Linabery AM, Ross JA. Trends in childhood cancer incidence in the U.S. (1992–2004). Cancer. 2008;112(2):416–32. https://doi.org/10.1002/cncr.23169.
225. Ries LAG, Smith MA, Gurney JG, Linet M, Tamra T, Young JL, Bunin GR, editors. Cancer incidence and survival among children and adolescents: United States SEER Program 1975–1995. Bethesda: National Cancer Institute, SEER Program. NIH Pub No 99-4649; 1999.
226. Giardiello FM, Offerhaus GJ, Krush AJ, Booker SV, Tersmette AC, Mulder JW, et al. Risk of hepatoblastoma in familial adenomatous polyposis. J Pediatr. 1991;119(5):766–8. https://doi.org/10.1016/s0022-3476(05)80297-5.
227. DeBaun MR, Tucker MA. Risk of cancer during the first four years of life in children from The Beckwith-Wiedemann Syndrome Registry. J Pediatr.

1998;132(3 Pt 1):398–400. https://doi.org/10.1016/s0022-3476(98)70008-3.
228. Kitanovski L, Ovcak Z, Jazbec J. Multifocal hepatoblastoma in a 6-month-old girl with trisomy 18: a case report. J Med Case Rep. 2009;3(1):8319. https://doi.org/10.4076/1752-1947-3-8319.
229. Hoyme HE, Seaver LH, Jones KL, Procopio F, Crooks W, Feingold M. Isolated hemihyperplasia (hemihypertrophy): report of a prospective multicenter study of the incidence of neoplasia and review. Am J Med Genet. 1998;79(4):274–8. https://doi.org/10.1002/(SICI)1096-8628(19981002)79:4<274::AID-AJMG8>3.0.CO;2-M.
230. Hiyama E. Pediatric hepatoblastoma: diagnosis and treatment. Transl Pediatr. 2014;3(4):293–9. https://doi.org/10.3978/j.issn.2224-4336.2014.09.01.
231. De Ioris M, Brugieres L, Zimmermann A, Keeling J, Brock P, Maibach R, et al. Hepatoblastoma with a low serum alpha-fetoprotein level at diagnosis: the SIOPEL group experience. Eur J Cancer. 2008;44(4):545–50. https://doi.org/10.1016/j.ejca.2007.11.022.
232. Adeyiga AO, Lee EY, Eisenberg RL. Focal hepatic masses in pediatric patients. AJR Am J Roentgenol. 2012;199(4):W422–40. https://doi.org/10.2214/ajr.11.7581.
233. Dachman AH, Pakter RL, Ros PR, Fishman EK, Goodman ZD, Lichtenstein JE. Hepatoblastoma: radiologic-pathologic correlation in 50 cases. Radiology. 1987;164(1):15–9. https://doi.org/10.1148/radiology.164.1.3035605.
234. Gubernick JA, Rosenberg HK, Ilaslan H, Kessler A. US approach to jaundice in infants and children. Radiographics. 2000;20(1):173–95. https://doi.org/10.1148/radiographics.20.1.g00ja25173.
235. King SJ, Babyn PS, Greenberg ML, Phillips MJ, Filler RM. Value of CT in determining the resectability of hepatoblastoma before and after chemotherapy. AJR Am J Roentgenol. 1993;160(4):793–8. https://doi.org/10.2214/ajr.160.4.8384403.
236. López-Terrada D, Alaggio R, de Dávila MT, Czauderna P, Hiyama E, Katzenstein H, et al. Towards an international pediatric liver tumor consensus classification: proceedings of the Los Angeles COG liver tumors symposium. Mod Pathol. 2014;27(3):472–91. https://doi.org/10.1038/modpathol.2013.80.
237. Roebuck DJ, Aronson D, Clapuyt P, Czauderna P, de Ville de Goyet J, Gauthier F, et al. 2005 PRETEXT: a revised staging system for primary malignant liver tumours of childhood developed by the SIOPEL group. Pediatr Radiol. 2007;37(2):123–32; quiz 249–50. https://doi.org/10.1007/s00247-006-0361-5.
238. Fuchs J, Rydzynski J, Von Schweinitz D, Bode U, Hecker H, Weinel P, et al. Pretreatment prognostic factors and treatment results in children with hepatoblastoma: a report from the German Cooperative Pediatric Liver Tumor Study HB 94. Cancer. 2002;95(1):172–82. https://doi.org/10.1002/cncr.10632.
239. Aronson DC, Schnater JM, Staalman CR, Weverling GJ, Plaschkes J, Perilongo G, et al. Predictive value of the pretreatment extent of disease system in hepatoblastoma: results from the International Society of Pediatric Oncology Liver Tumor Study Group SIOPEL-1 study. J Clin Oncol. 2005;23(6):1245–52. https://doi.org/10.1200/jco.2005.07.145.
240. Meyers RL, Rowland JR, Krailo M, Chen Z, Katzenstein HM, Malogolowkin MH. Predictive power of pretreatment prognostic factors in children with hepatoblastoma: a report from the Children's Oncology Group. Pediatr Blood Cancer. 2009;53(6):1016–22. https://doi.org/10.1002/pbc.22088.
241. Maibach R, Roebuck D, Brugieres L, Capra M, Brock P, Dall'Igna P, et al. Prognostic stratification for children with hepatoblastoma: the SIOPEL experience. Eur J Cancer. 2012;48(10):1543–9. https://doi.org/10.1016/j.ejca.2011.12.011.
242. Czauderna P, Haeberle B, Hiyama E, Rangaswami A, Krailo M, Maibach R, et al. The Children's Hepatic tumors International Collaboration (CHIC): novel global rare tumor database yields new prognostic factors in hepatoblastoma and becomes a research model. Eur J Cancer. 2016;52:92–101. https://doi.org/10.1016/j.ejca.2015.09.023.
243. Meyers RL, Maibach R, Hiyama E, Häberle B, Krailo M, Rangaswami A, et al. Risk-stratified staging in paediatric hepatoblastoma: a unified analysis from the Children's Hepatic tumors International Collaboration. Lancet Oncol. 2017;18(1):122–31. https://doi.org/10.1016/s1470-2045(16)30598-8.
244. Venkatramani R, Stein JE, Sapra A, Genyk Y, Jhaveri V, Malogolowkin M, et al. Effect of neoadjuvant chemotherapy on resectability of stage III and IV hepatoblastoma. Br J Surg. 2015;102(1):108–13. https://doi.org/10.1002/bjs.9681.
245. Ortega JA, Douglass EC, Feusner JH, Reynolds M, Quinn JJ, Finegold MJ, et al. Randomized comparison of cisplatin/vincristine/fluorouracil and cisplatin/continuous infusion doxorubicin for treatment of pediatric hepatoblastoma: a report from the Children's Cancer Group and the Pediatric Oncology Group. J Clin Oncol. 2000;18(14):2665–75. https://doi.org/10.1200/jco.2000.18.14.2665.
246. Otte JB, Pritchard J, Aronson DC, Brown J, Czauderna P, Maibach R, et al. Liver transplantation for hepatoblastoma: results from the International Society of Pediatric Oncology (SIOP) study SIOPEL-1 and review of the world experience. Pediatr Blood Cancer. 2004;42(1):74–83. https://doi.org/10.1002/pbc.10376.
247. McAteer JP, Goldin AB, Healey PJ, Gow KW. Surgical treatment of primary liver tumors in children: outcomes analysis of resection and transplantation in the SEER database. Pediatr Transplant.

2013;17(8):744–50. https://doi.org/10.1111/petr.12144.
248. Czauderna P, Lopez-Terrada D, Hiyama E, Häberle B, Malogolowkin MH, Meyers RL. Hepatoblastoma state of the art: pathology, genetics, risk stratification, and chemotherapy. Curr Opin Pediatr. 2014;26(1):19–28. https://doi.org/10.1097/mop.0000000000000046.
249. Semeraro M, Branchereau S, Maibach R, Zsiros J, Casanova M, Brock P, et al. Relapses in hepatoblastoma patients: clinical characteristics and outcome—experience of the International Childhood Liver Tumour Strategy Group (SIOPEL). Eur J Cancer. 2013;49(4):915–22. https://doi.org/10.1016/j.ejca.2012.10.003.
250. Malogolowkin MH, Katzenstein HM, Krailo M, Chen Z, Quinn JJ, Reynolds M, et al. Redefining the role of doxorubicin for the treatment of children with hepatoblastoma. J Clin Oncol. 2008;26(14):2379–83. https://doi.org/10.1200/jco.2006.09.7204.
251. Katzenstein HM, London WB, Douglass EC, Reynolds M, Plaschkes J, Finegold MJ, et al. Treatment of unresectable and metastatic hepatoblastoma: a pediatric oncology group phase II study. J Clin Oncol. 2002;20(16):3438–44. https://doi.org/10.1200/jco.2002.07.400.
252. Qayed M, Powell C, Morgan ER, Haugen M, Katzenstein HM. Irinotecan as maintenance therapy in high-risk hepatoblastoma. Pediatr Blood Cancer. 2010;54(5):761–3. https://doi.org/10.1002/pbc.22408.
253. Niwa A, Umeda K, Awaya T, Yui Y, Matsubara H, Hiramatsu H, et al. Successful autologous peripheral blood stem cell transplantation with a double-conditioning regimen for recurrent hepatoblastoma after liver transplantation. Pediatr Transplant. 2009;13(2):259–62. https://doi.org/10.1111/j.1399-3046.2008.00948.x.
254. Malogolowkin MH, Stanley P, Steele DA, Ortega JA. Feasibility and toxicity of chemoembolization for children with liver tumors. J Clin Oncol. 2000;18(6):1279–84. https://doi.org/10.1200/jco.2000.18.6.1279.
255. Czauderna P, Zbrzezniak G, Narozanski W, Korzon M, Wyszomirska M, Stoba C. Preliminary experience with arterial chemoembolization for hepatoblastoma and hepatocellular carcinoma in children. Pediatr Blood Cancer. 2006;46(7):825–8. https://doi.org/10.1002/pbc.20422.
256. Stocker JT, Ishak KG. Undifferentiated (embryonal) sarcoma of the liver: report of 31 cases. Cancer. 1978;42(1):336–48. https://doi.org/10.1002/1097-0142(197807)42:1<336::aid-cncr2820420151>3.0.co;2-v.
257. Weinberg AG, Finegold MJ. Primary hepatic tumors of childhood. Hum Pathol. 1983;14(6):512–37. https://doi.org/10.1016/s0046-8177(83)80005-7.
258. Lenze F, Birkfellner T, Lenz P, Hussein K, Länger F, Kreipe H, et al. Undifferentiated embryonal sarcoma of the liver in adults. Cancer. 2008;112(10):2274–82. https://doi.org/10.1002/cncr.23431.
259. Nishio J, Iwasaki H, Sakashita N, Haraoka S, Isayama T, Naito M, et al. Undifferentiated (embryonal) sarcoma of the liver in middle-aged adults: smooth muscle differentiation determined by immunohistochemistry and electron microscopy. Hum Pathol. 2003;34(3):246–52. https://doi.org/10.1053/hupa.2003.44.
260. Bisogno G, Pilz T, Perilongo G, Ferrari A, Harms D, Ninfo V, et al. Undifferentiated sarcoma of the liver in childhood: a curable disease. Cancer. 2002;94(1):252–7. https://doi.org/10.1002/cncr.10191.
261. Pachera S, Nishio H, Takahashi Y, Yokoyama Y, Oda K, Ebata T, et al. Undifferentiated embryonal sarcoma of the liver: case report and literature survey. J Hepato-Biliary-Pancreat Surg. 2008;15(5):536–44. https://doi.org/10.1007/s00534-007-1265-y.
262. Wei ZG, Tang LF, Chen ZM, Tang HF, Li MJ. Childhood undifferentiated embryonal liver sarcoma: clinical features and immunohistochemistry analysis. J Pediatr Surg. 2008;43(10):1912–9. https://doi.org/10.1016/j.jpedsurg.2008.06.016.
263. Almogy G, Lieberman S, Gips M, Pappo O, Edden Y, Jurim O, et al. Clinical outcomes of surgical resections for primary liver sarcoma in adults: results from a single centre. Eur J Surg Oncol. 2004;30(4):421–7. https://doi.org/10.1016/j.ejso.2004.01.004.
264. Ros PR, Olmsted WW, Dachman AH, Goodman ZD, Ishak KG, Hartman DS. Undifferentiated (embryonal) sarcoma of the liver: radiologic-pathologic correlation. Radiology. 1986;161(1):141–5. https://doi.org/10.1148/radiology.161.1.3532179.
265. Buetow PC, Buck JL, Pantongrag-Brown L, Marshall WH, Ros PR, Levine MS, et al. Undifferentiated (embryonal) sarcoma of the liver: pathologic basis of imaging findings in 28 cases. Radiology. 1997;203(3):779–83. https://doi.org/10.1148/radiology.203.3.9169704.
266. Psatha EA, Semelka RC, Fordham L, Firat Z, Woosley JT. Undifferentiated (embryonal) sarcoma of the liver (USL): MRI findings including dynamic gadolinium enhancement. Magn Reson Imaging. 2004;22(6):897–900. https://doi.org/10.1016/j.mri.2004.02.003.
267. Kiani B, Ferrell LD, Qualman S, Frankel WL. Immunohistochemical analysis of embryonal sarcoma of the liver. Appl Immunohistochem Mol Morphol. 2006;14(2):193–7. https://doi.org/10.1097/01.pai.0000173052.37673.95.
268. Putra J, Ornvold K. Undifferentiated embryonal sarcoma of the liver: a concise review. Arch Pathol Lab Med. 2015;139(2):269–73. https://doi.org/10.5858/arpa.2013-0463-RS.

269. Wildhaber BE, Montaruli E, Guérin F, Branchereau S, Martelli H, Gauthier F. Mesenchymal hamartoma or embryonal sarcoma of the liver in childhood: a difficult diagnosis before complete surgical excision. J Pediatr Surg. 2014;49(9):1372–7. https://doi.org/10.1016/j.jpedsurg.2014.04.005.
270. Leuschner I, Schmidt D, Harms D. Undifferentiated sarcoma of the liver in childhood: morphology, flow cytometry, and literature review. Hum Pathol. 1990;21(1):68–76. https://doi.org/10.1016/0046-8177(90)90077-i.
271. May LT, Wang M, Albano E, Garrington T, Dishop M, Macy ME. Undifferentiated sarcoma of the liver: a single institution experience using a uniform treatment approach. J Pediatr Hematol Oncol. 2012;34(3):e114–6. https://doi.org/10.1097/MPH.0b013e3182331fbe.
272. Plant AS, Busuttil RW, Rana A, Nelson SD, Auerbach M, Federman NC. A single-institution retrospective cases series of childhood undifferentiated embryonal liver sarcoma (UELS): success of combined therapy and the use of orthotopic liver transplant. J Pediatr Hematol Oncol. 2013;35(6):451–5. https://doi.org/10.1097/MPH.0b013e318271c948.
273. Weitz J, Klimstra DS, Cymes K, Jarnagin WR, D'Angelica M, La Quaglia MP, et al. Management of primary liver sarcomas. Cancer. 2007;109(7):1391–6. https://doi.org/10.1002/cncr.22530.

7 Hepatobiliary Sarcoma

Jan Lerut, Jean de Ville de Goyet, and Quirino Lai

Abbreviations

BERMS	Biliary embryonal rhabdomyosarcoma
CCC	Cholangiocellular cancer
DFS	Disease-free survival
ELTR-ELITA	European Liver Transplant Registry-European Liver Intestine Transplant Association
H&E	Haematoxylin and eosine
HCC	Hepatocellular cancer
(H)EHE	(Hepatic) epithelioid haemangioendothelioma
HHS	Hepatic haemangiosarcoma
HIHE	Hepatic infantile haemangioendothelioma
HPC	Haemangiopericytoma
HSVN	Hepatic small vessel neoplasm
IHC	Immunohistochemistry
(LD)LT	(Living-donor) liver transplantation
LMS	Leiomyosarcoma
LPS	Liposarcoma
MMT	Malignant mesenchymal tumour
OS	Overal survival
PS	Patient survival
RMS	Rhabdomyosarcoma
SaHCC	Sarcomatous HCC
UELS	Undifferentiated embryonal liver sarcoma
UNOS	United network organ sharing

J. Lerut (✉)
Institute for Experimental and Clinical Research (IREC), Université catholique de Louvain – UCL, Brussels, Belgium
e-mail: jan.lerut@saintluc.uclouvain.be

J. d. V. de Goyet
Department of Paediatrics, IRCCS-ISMETT (Institute for Scientific-Based Care and Research-Mediterranean Institute for Transplantation and Advanced Specialized Therapies), Palermo, Italy
e-mail: jdeville@ismett.edu

Q. Lai
General Surgery and Organ Transplantation Unit, Sapienza University of Rome, AOU Policlinico Umberto I, Rome, Italy
e-mail: quirino.lai@uniroma1.it

7.1 Introduction

In contrast to hepatocellular cancers (HCCs) and cholangiocellular cancers (CCCs), the diagnostic and therapeutic algorithms of hepatobiliary sarcomas are not yet standardized due to the variability of clinical, morphological, and histopathological presentations and also due to the limited awareness of the medical community about these 'orphan' diseases (defined as a disease occurring in less than 6/pmp) [1–9]. This chapter gives an up-to-date 'view' of these tumours based on a recent literature review and

T. Hackert, A. Gulla (eds.), *Rare Liver and Biliary Tract Diseases*,
https://doi.org/10.1007/978-3-032-15076-9_7

data collected by the European Liver Transplant Registry (ELTR) [10–13]. Special attention is given to the role of liver transplantation (LT) in treating hepatobiliary sarcomas.

Vascular tumours were seen for a long time as a continuum ranging from the most benign lesion—the hepatic haemangioma (HA)—to the less aggressive hepatic epithelioid haemangioendothelioma (HEHE) and the most aggressive tumour, the hepatic haemangiosarcoma (HHS). Molecular biology recently showed that these different tumours are associated with different genetic mutations and do not form a continuum [14–16].

7.2 Vascular Sarcomas

7.2.1 Hepatic Epithelioid Haemangioendothelioma (HEHE)

Epithelioid haemangioendothelioma (EHE) is a rare (<1/pmp), low-grade malignancy with an epithelioid and histiocytoid appearance, originating from vascular endothelial or pre-endothelial cells [3, 16, 17].

Dail and Liebow first recognized this as a lung tumour; later, EHE was found in the soft tissues, head and neck region, pleura, bones, and many other organs. The first liver series was reported in 1984 by Makhlouf [17, 18]. The Haemangioendothelioma, Epithelioid haemangioendothelioma And Related vascular Disorders (HEARD) support group showed that EHE is most commonly located in the liver (alone in 21% and combined with lung lesions in 18% of the cases), followed by the primary site in the bone (14%) or lungs (12%) [19]. Pulmonary and hepatic lesions behave similarly [17]. HEHE is more frequent in middle-aged women (female/male ratio: 4/1) and is rare in children [20]. Although a relationship between chronic *Bartonella* infection and HEHE has been *suggested* through the induction of vaso-proliferation, no definitive aetiological factor has been identified so far [21].

The clinical manifestation is highly variable and non-specific, ranging from an asymptomatic status (25% of patients) to (infrequent) hepatic failure. Upper abdominal discomfort or pain (60%), weight loss (20%), poor general condition (weakness and fatigue) (20%), and dyspnoea (5%) are the dominating symptoms. Hepatosplenomegaly (30%) is frequent; jaundice, portal hypertension, and Budd–Chiari syndrome due to tumour compression or venous infiltration are rare (5%). One-third of the patients present with cholestasis and cytolysis. Kasabach–Merritt syndrome (with severe thrombocytopenia) is exceptional. Serum tumour markers are almost never increased.

Imaging is initially characterized by peripheral, nodular, usually bi-lobar, and subcapsular lesions ('peripheral pattern'), which progressively become confluent ('diffuse pattern') (Fig. 7.1a, b). Macrovascular invasion, remodelling of the non-tumoural parenchyma (due to the vascular restructuring, the liver may even have a 'cirrhotic outlook'), capsular retraction, and focal calcifications (due to central tumour necrosis) may all develop with time. Several lesions present with the halo and lollipop signs. Larger HEHE lesions may present on contrast MRI a dealyed, peripheral, arterial, rim, with progressive enhancement towards the centre (targetoid appearance) [22, 23].

Angiography (if done) reveals moderate vascularization only, with a displacement of the intrahepatic vascular trees by the tumour masses. Therefore, liver biopsy is not, per se, contraindicated—and it is a requisite for the definitive diagnosis of HEHE and for excluding angiosarcoma. Thoracic CT scan, scintigraphy, and Fluorodeoxyglucose (FDG) PET scan are indispensable for staging [24]. Chest lesions can be pulmonary, pleural, and mediastinal. Three major different thoracic patterns exist. The most frequent (60%) are bilateral multiple or solitary pulmonary nodules (measuring up to 5 cm in 10–20% of cases) or multiple pulmonary reticulonodular opacities; the (less favourable) pleural invasion presents as a diffuse infiltrative thickening (Fig. 7.2). Bone metastases appear as osteolytic lesions [25, 26].

HEHE diagnosis is based on a *high index of suspicion*, integrating clinical manifestation and imaging: (a) the presence of numerous intrahe-

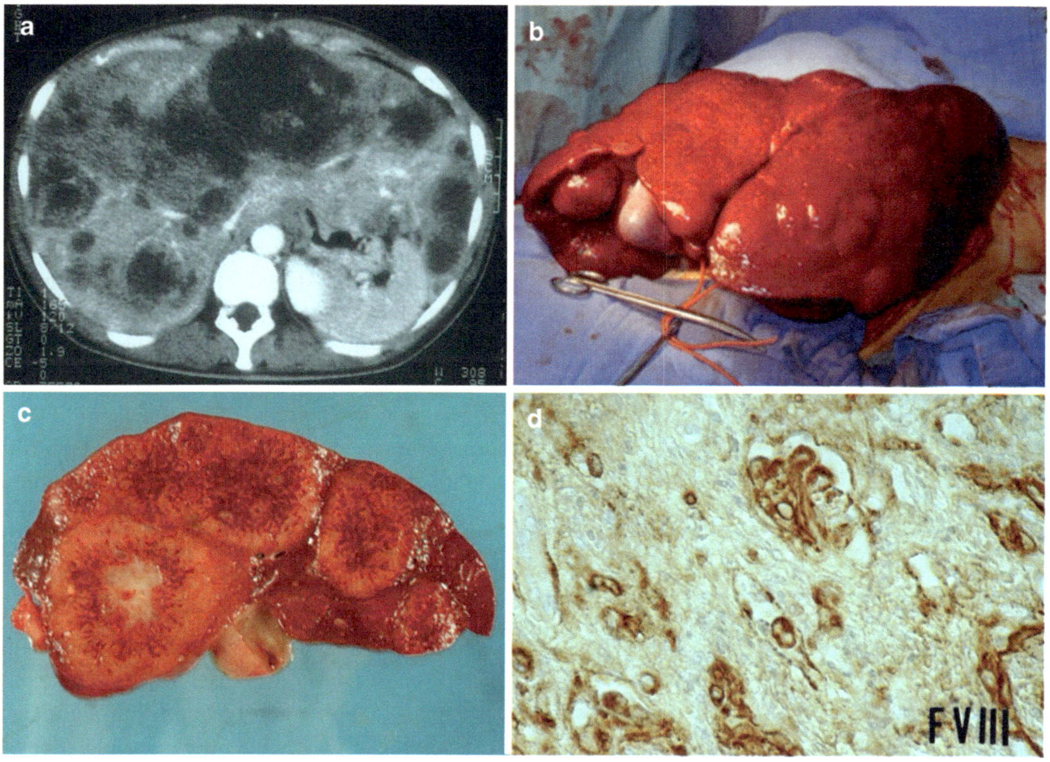

Fig. 7.1 Symptomatic hepatic epithelioid haemangioendothelioma (HEHE). (**a**) Typical CT scan findings of multiple confluent, peripheral bi-lobar lesions. (**b**) Macroscopic appearance: the massive tumour occupying the whole abdominal cavity was responsible for an inferior vena cava compression syndrome. (**c**) Fibrous mass formation due to the sarcoma-type tumour growth with central necrosis. (**d**) FVIII antigen staining confirming the vascular nature of the tumour. This patient is alive and immunosuppression-free 26 years post-LT, without any evidence of disease recurrence

patic tumours, (b) in a young, merely female adult presenting a good condition, (c) despite (a usually) long-lasting clinical history points to the direction of the diagnosis [9, 10, 12]. Histopathology, including Haematoxylin & Eosin (H&E) and immunohistochemical (IHC) staining, and molecular biology are required to confirm the diagnosis. Cytology may contribute to the diagnosis, but histology on larger (laparoscopically procured) samples is usually needed to differentiate HEHE from HHS, secondary malignancies, and other rare tumours [9, 27, 28]. Sometimes even large biopsies have been shown unable to make the correct diagnosis. Gross examination reveals several fibrous masses with characteristic, necrosis-related, central zoning; microscopy shows pleomorphic, medium-sized, and large-sized epithelioid cells spreading within sinusoids and small veins but, importantly, preserved portal tract landmarks (Fig. 7.1c). Lymph nodes can be negative for metastases on H&E staining but positive on IHC. Cellular atypia, nuclear fission, presence of spindle cells, necrotic tumour changes, and Ki-67 index >10–15% indicate a more aggressive tumour [17, 27, 29–31]. IHC of the vascular endothelial markers, factor VIII (FVIII)-related antigen, Fli-1 (a protein expressed by the endothelium), CD31, CD34, and an erythroblast transformation specific–related gene (ERG), expressed on endothelial cells, will further confirm the diagnosis (Fig. 7.1d) [14, 32]. Concordant clinical presentation, radiology, histopathology, cytology, IHC, and molecular biology will definitively confirm the diagnosis. Despite all progress in imaging and histopathology, it can still be challenging to differentiate HEHE from HHS [11, 13, 27, 33].

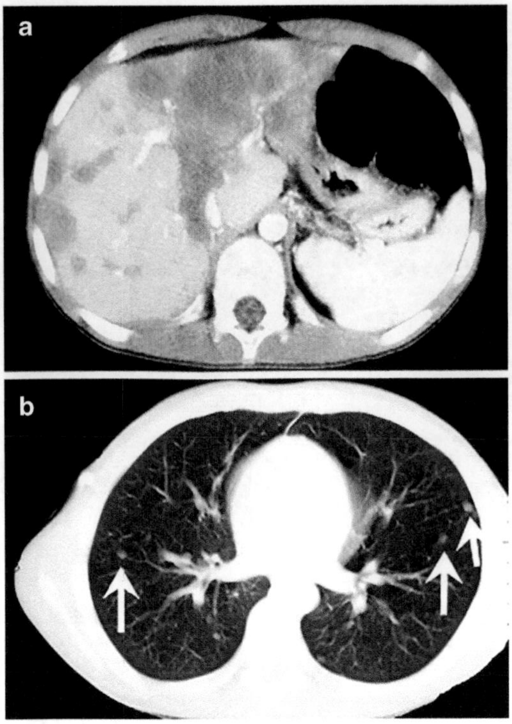

Fig. 7.2 Incidental hepatic epithelioid haemangioendothelioma. (**a**) The CT scan shows the typical findings of multiple confluent, peripheral bi-lobar liver lesions. (**b**) Multiple synchronous, bilateral, small pulmonary metastases. As he was asymptomatic and had no hepatic dysfunction nor portal hypertension, chemotherapy was proposed

The treatment algorithm of HEHE is complicated because of its rarity and unpredictable behaviour. The well-documented 'spontaneous long-term' (up to 28 years) survivals, the frequent absence of symptoms (25%), the synchronous presence of extrahepatic lesions (45%), the lack of prognostic clinical or histological criteria, the high recurrence rate after surgery (33%), and the lack of detailed long-term outcomes troubled the attitude of the medical community towards the role of surgery [10, 12, 16, 18, 31, 34]. Several smaller experiences and the 2006 review by Mehrabi et al. (including 286 patients) favoured partial and total liver resection as the treatment of choice [16, 35–37]. Unfortunately, partial resection is only possible in less than 10% of patients harbouring single or a few (≤4) lesions. A Mayo experience based on 11 patients reported a 62% five-year patient survival (PS) after partial resection [37]. The 2007 and 2017 'ELTR-ELITA HEHE reports', including 149 HEHE patients with a long-term follow-up, changed the 'medical awareness' towards these patients, as shown by the steep rise in patients reported to the registry and the high number of (personal) online consults since then [10, 12, 13]. The place of LT became validated, based on the 5- and 10-year post-transplant PS rates of 81 and 77% and, most importantly, disease-free survival (DFS) rates of 79 and 73%. Pre-LT treatment (28%), lymph node invasion (27%), and limited extrahepatic disease (26.8%) did not significantly influence the outcome, whereas micro- and macrovascular invasion (13 and 48%) did. Presence of multiple osseous metastases is also a poor prognostic factor (personal communication J. Heimbach). The Leuven group even reported successful sequential (lung after liver) or simultaneous liver–lung transplantation in four cases of multifocal chest and liver disease. In the two cases of the sequential approach, 8 and 10 years of post-transplant survival were reached despite the evidence of pleural and diaphragmatic invasion at transplantation. In the two cases of simultaneous approach, 1 and 7 years of post-transplant survival were observed without signs of disease progression despite bone metastases at the time of transplantation [38]. Recurrent disease, observed in and outside the graft in 25% of liver recipients, remains of concern. Aggressive treatment is suggested in case of recurrence due to the possibility of reaching prolonged and tumour-free survivals. The value of re-LT remains to be determined [27].

Prognostic scores and efficacious neo-adjuvant and adjuvant oncologic therapies are still missing. Lau et al. identified the presence of pulmonary lesions, multi-organ involvement, disease progression, ascites, age ≥55 years, and male gender as poor prognostic factors [19]. The ELTR-ELITA HEHE study proposed a therapeutic algorithm based on a tentative prognostic score, including macrovascular and hilar lymph node invasion and waiting time. Low (0–2), intermediate [3–5], and high [6–10] scores resulted in 5-year DFS rates of 94%, 77%, and 38.5%, respectively [13] (Fig. 7.3). An observation (on the LT list) is a useful 'help', besides different

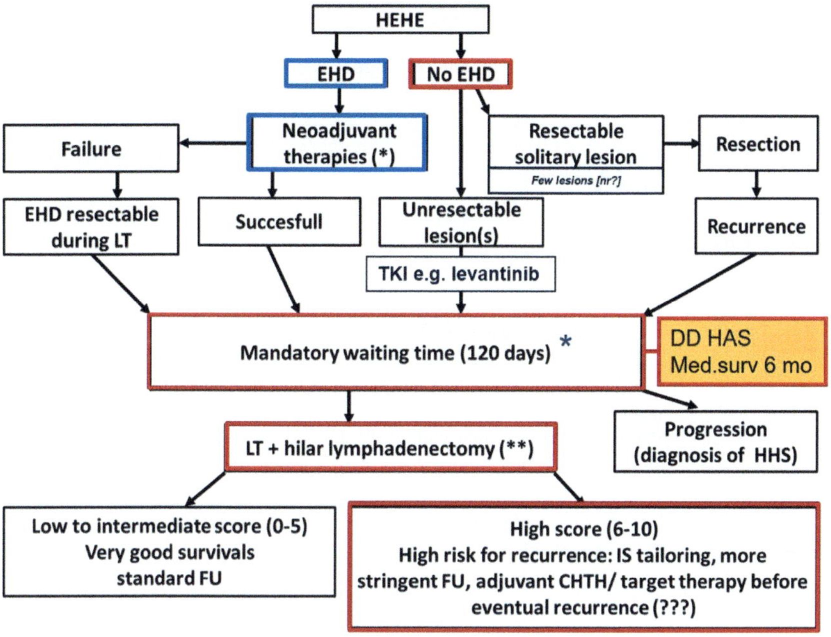

Fig. 7.3 Therapeutic algorithm for hepatic epithelioid haemangioendothelioma. In case of unresectable and/or extrahepatic disease localization, neo-adjuvant therapy may be warranted. The proposed waiting time is an additional tool to differentiate unclear lesions from angiosarcoma. *: non-standardized neo-adjuvant approach, **: histological examination combining IHC and H&E staining. Abbreviations: CHTH: chemotherapy, EHD: extrahepatic disease, FU: follow-up, IS: immunosuppression, HHS: hepatic haemangiosarcoma, LT: liver transplantation

clinical, biochemical, and imaging characteristics, to differentiate HEHE from HHS, as the latter invariably progresses within some months of diagnosis (Table 7.1).

The value of the various non-surgical treatments, radiotherapy, tumour ablation, trans-arterial (chemo-) embolization (TA(C)E), hormone treatment, systemic or locoregional radio-chemotherapy, and anti-angiogenic or anti-tumour pharmacotherapy is difficult to judge because of small, heterogeneous patient cohorts and a lack of uniformity and long-term follow-up. Radiotherapy is helpful for local pain control. Besides drugs aiming at counteracting angiogenic pathways [bevacizumab and oral tyrosine kinase inhibitors (sorafenib, lenvatinib, sunitinib, pazopanib, and paclitaxel)] or non-vascular endothelial growth factor (non-VEGF) angiogenic pathways (angiopoietin peptibody, platelet derived growth factor receptor (PDGFR), and endoglin inhibitors), several other vascular target agents (thalidomide, lenalidomide, interferon, and beta-blockers) and chemotherapies (cyclophosphamide, doxorubicin, and carboplatin-etoposide) have all been tried. As these vascular tumours contain VEGF receptors, treatments based on anti-VEGF antibodies seem logical. Higher contents of VEGF and beta-adrenergic receptors might improve outcomes [39–46]. The phase II trials of the French sarcoma group (sorafenib) and the Eastern Cooperative Oncology Group (bevacizumab), including advanced, non-resectable, metastatic diseases in 15 and seven HEHE patients, is, however, somewhat disappointing as a temporary stabilizing effect and a 6-month partial response were obtained in 20–40% and 10% of patients only [47, 48].

A better understanding of the biochemical, histological (mitotic index and pleomorphism), and molecular behaviour is thus required to develop more effective neo-adjuvant and adju-

Table 7.1 Clues to differential diagnosis between hepatic epithelioid haemangioendothelioma and hepatic haemangiosarcoma

Variables	Epithelioid haemangioendothelioma	Haemangiosarcoma
Sex	Female (3/4)	Male (2/3)
Mean age	40	60
Risk factors	Aspecific	Exposure to carcinogens (25%)
Clinical presentation	Aspecific	Aspecific More aggressive: sicker
Biochemical presentation	Aspecific	More anaemia and thrombocytopenia
Liver function	Aspecific	More compromised (International normalized ratio (INR) and albumin)
Radiological presentation	Rarely unique lesion (<10%) Multinodular (>15 lesions) Confluent lesions Heterogeneous lesions Persistent enhancement without filling; halo and lollipop sign	Unique Multinodular Diffuse infiltrating Heterogeneous lesions Persistent and complete filling in the portal venous phase
Pathology	Preserved architecture Calcification and fibrosis	Destruction of lobular/acinar architecture
Immunohistochemistry staining	FVIII Ag–positive	FVIII Ag-positive ERG-positive
Gold therapy	Surgery Partial liver resection (rarely possible) Liver transplantation	Symptomatic Partial liver resection (rarely possible)
Medical therapy	Some results	No clear evidence
Outcome natural evolution	Very variable	Poor: very aggressive tumour
Outcome post-transplantation	Good (70–80% survival)	Poor (0% survival at 2 years)

vant treatments and identify the aggressive tumour subtypes [16, 35, 49, 50]. The confirmation of the monoclonal nature of all the different lesions of a multifocal HEHE in the same patient is also crucial because it points to the fact that multifocality and extrahepatic spread are metastatic implants of the same neoplastic clone rather than (as thought for a long time) the synchronous occurrence of multiple different clones. If confirmed, (neo-)adjuvant medical treatment will be equally effective for both hepatic and extrahepatic lesions [51].

7.2.2 Hepatic Infantile Haemangioendothelioma (HIHE)

HIHE, the most common hepatic tumour in the infant age group, is usually diagnosed during the first 6 months of life (Fig. 7.4). HIHE is more frequent in females and presents with (a)symptomatic hepatosplenomegaly, failure to thrive, intra-tumour arteriovenous shunting (with possible secondary congestive cardiac failure in 15% of cases), and associated cutaneous haemangiomas (20–40%) (Fig. 7.5a–d). Though the natural history of HIHE is benign in most cases that remain asymptomatic, there is a broad spectrum of clinical presentation, and the prognosis may be severe in those who are symptomatic early after birth. Up to two-thirds of severely symptomatic infants die of complications such as heart failure [19, 35]. Histopathology identifies two HIHE types: the 'benign' type I and the more pleomorphic type II. Type II HIHE is nowadays considered a pre-malignant lesion evolving to HHS in childhood, and pre-emptive resection has been proposed for that reason. On immunohistochemistry (IHC) staining, this tumour is GLUT1-negative [52]. Pathology of several cases in the ELTR-ELITA study revealed HHS foci in a 'supposed HEHE' (Fig. 7.6). These children all died due to early tumour recurrence. Treatment

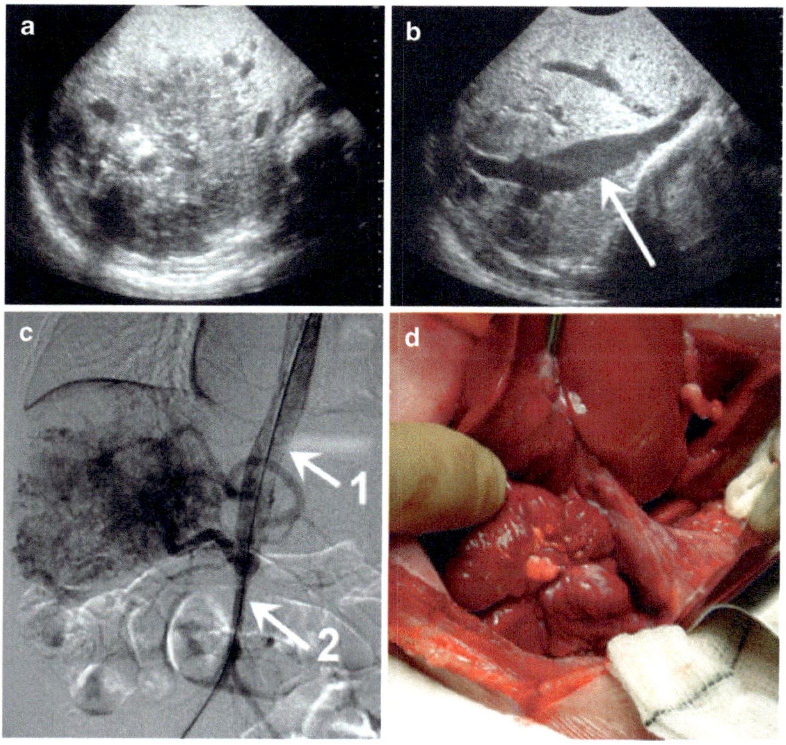

Fig. 7.4 Hepatic infantile haemangioma. (**a**, **b**) Doppler ultrasound identified a large unifocal lesion with multiple vascular signals and enlarged hepatic veins. (**c**) Angiography confirmed the typical presence of arteriovenous fistulae and enlarged hepatic arteries. Of note, the major discrepancy between the diameters of the supra- and infracoeliac aorta (arrows 1 and 2, respectively). (**d**) The intraoperative view shows a huge tumour occupying the whole right liver. This patient was cured by RO hepatectomy

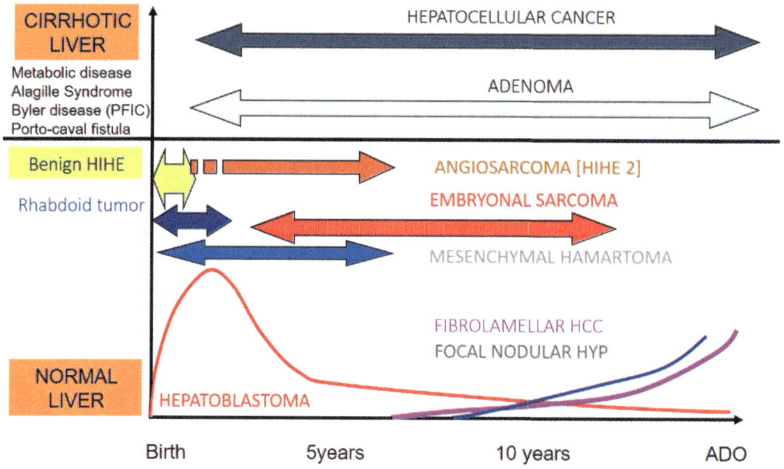

Fig. 7.5 Timeline of hepatobiliary tumours in childhood

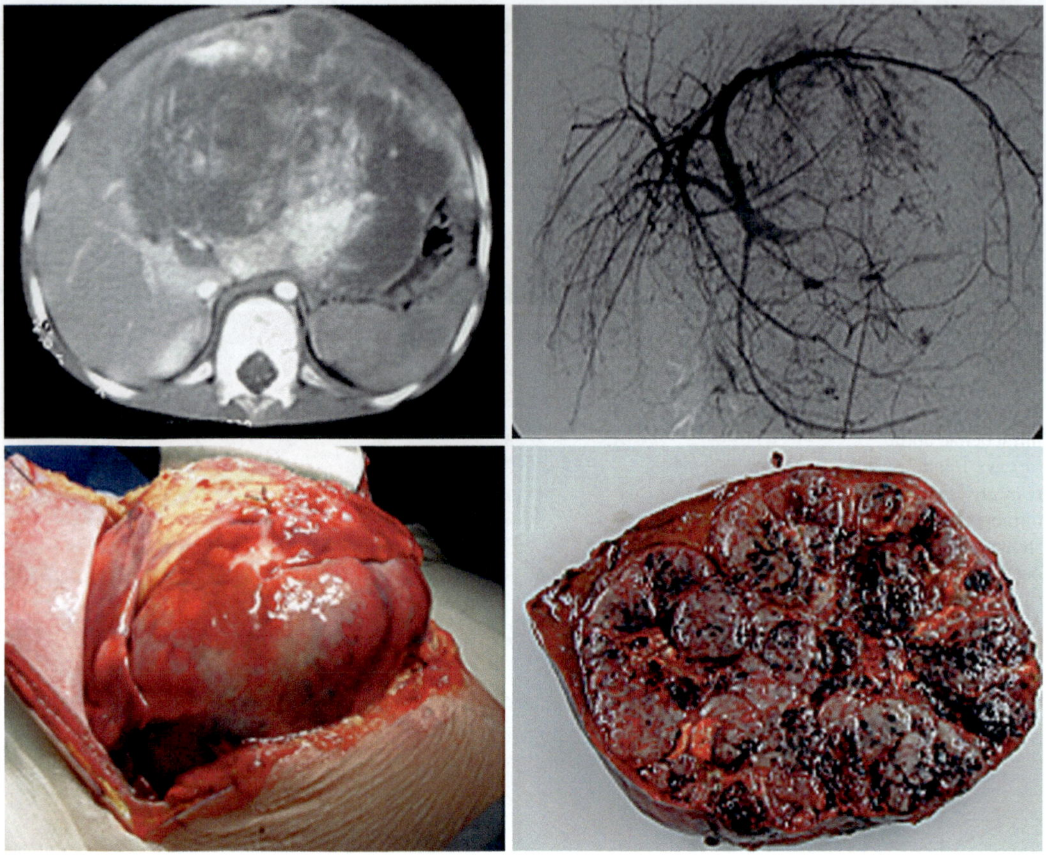

Fig. 7.6 Six-year-old young girl diagnosed with hepatic epithelioid haemangioendothelioma and finding of haemangiosarcoma features on final histology. An RO ex situ resection, followed by an autotransplantation of the right posterior sector, was performed. This extended liver resection was done ex situ after the instauration of a temporary internal bypass, portocaval shunt, and replacement of the inferior vena cava using a GORE-TEX graft. At 48 months post-surgery, she was disease-free and well

modalities include anti-angiogenic therapies (using or combining high-dose steroids, interferon, and chemo- or radiotherapy), interventional radiology, and surgery [19, 53, 54]. The Boston group developed an algorithm for treating HIHE children [19]. Partial hepatectomy is indicated in the case of solitary lesions or lesions confined to one liver lobe; LT is required in diffuse lesions and non-response to steroid therapy. In rapid tumour growth, HHS should be excluded to avoid a futile LT [55].

7.2.3 Hepatic Haemangiosarcoma (HHS)

HHS is the most common primary liver sarcoma, accounting for up to 2% of all primary liver tumours. It occurs mainly during the sixth and seventh decades of life and is more frequent in males (M/F ratio: 3/1). It is exceptional in children [35, 56–58]. Most HHSs are sporadic. Many environmental carcinogens (thorium dioxide, vinyl chloride monomer, radium, pesticides, external radiation, cyclophosphamide, arsenical compounds, the use of androgenic/anabolic steroids, and iron) lead to the development of HHS [9, 16, 17, 59, 60].

The delay between toxic exposure and tumour development may be extremely long (up to 65 years!) [59, 60]. The diagnosis can be challenging despite modern imaging and pathology [6, 33, 61–64]. Macroscopically, HHS presents as ill-defined spongy haemorrhagic nodule(s) involving the whole liver as multiple nodules, a sizeable dominant mass, and, more rarely, diffuse infiltrating macro-nodular tumours [3, 16]. At diagnosis, 40% of patients already present extrahepatic lesions, mainly in the lungs, spleen, bones, and adrenal glands. The 'ELTR HHS study' based on 20 LT recipients identified several differences among HEHE and HHS patients (Table 7.1). HHS patients are sicker than HEHE patients. Weakness and fatigue (75%), upper abdominal pain and discomfort due to hepatosplenomegaly (60%), anorexia and nausea (50%), and weight loss (60%) are dominating symptoms. Signs and symptoms of portal hypertension [thrombocytopenia, jaundice, ascites (45%), and peripheral oedema (25%)], liver failure (10%), and acute abdominal pain due to tumour rupture are frequent [11, 56]. MRI imaging commonly shows progressive, heterogeneous nodular enhancement towards the centre and haemorrhage [7]. Pathology reveals diffuse bi-lobar involvement in most cases. Despite surgical resection being able to somewhat prolong survival, the outcome after partial or total hepatectomy (LT) is highly disappointing [16]. After LT, all recipients present an early lethal recurrence [11]. HHS, therefore, represents an absolute contraindication to LT [11, 56, 57, 65–90] (Table 7.2). Controversy persists about the possible role and success of LT for children with HHS [79, 83, 88, 91–93].

Combining efficient primary adjuvant chemotherapy and secondary surgery is likely necessary to improve outcomes [94, 95]. Though HHS has been refractory to many chemotherapy regimens in the past, encouraging chemotherapy results have been reported in some cases of multinodular, metastasized HHS [96]. Radiotherapy is not helpful due to the radio-resistant character of the tumour [97]. TAE is an excellent symptomatic treatment in the case of bleeding due to tumour rupture [98]. Similar to HEHE, adequate medical therapies, mainly based on the expression of

Table 7.2 Literature review of LT for hepatic haemangiosarcoma

Author	Year	Ref.	Country	Article type	Age	Nr	Donor type	Death	Post-LT FU mo	Recurrence
Ringe	1989	[65]	Germany	Case series	Adult	1	DDLT	Yes	5	Yes
Penn	1991	[66]	Penn ITTS, USA	Registry	–	14	DDLT	$n = 14$ (100%)	<27.5	9/14 (64.3%)
Von Schönfeld	1992	[67]	Germany	Case report	65	1	DDLT	Yes	***14***	***No***
Moreno-González	1993	[68]	Spain	Case series	–	1	DDLT	Yes	5	Yes
Rojter	1995	[69]	USA	Case series	59	1	DDLT	Yes	6	Yes
Awan	1996	[70]	UK	Case series	Paediatric	1	DDLT	Yes	***4***	***No***
Vennarecci	1997	[71]	UK	Case series	–	2	DDLT	$n = 2$	3 and 5	Yes
Pichlmayr	1997	[72]	Germany	Case series	Adult	1	DDLT	Yes	***0***	***No***
Pimentel Cauduro	2002	[73]	USA	Case report	70	1	DDLT	Yes	***0.5***	***No***
Dimashkieh	2004	[74]	USA	Case report	5	1	LT	No	14	Yes
Walsh	2004	[75]	USA	Case report	3 months	1	Split	No	***17***	***No***
Maluf	2005	[57]	USA	Case report	61	1	DDLT	No	12	Yes
			UNOS, USA	Registry	–	7	LT	–	8.7 (mean)	–
Husted	2006	[76]	Penn ITTS, USA	Registry	53.3 (med) (35–66.8)	6	DDLT	$n = 6$	5.7 (med) 2.6–15.4	Yes (6)
Bismuth	2009	[77]	France	Case report	44	1	DDLT	Yes	30	Yes
Matthaei	2009	[78]	Germany	Case series	19	2	DDLT	Yes	73	Yes
					51		DDLT	No	141	Yes
Geramizadeh	2011	[79]	Iran	Case report	Paediatric	7	LDLT	Yes	***3***	***No***
Orlando	2013	[11]	ELTR Europe	Registry	$n = 6 < 15$ year 35.3 ± 22.6 year (med: 41) (range: 1–65)	22	DDLT	$n = 22$	7.2 (med)	$n = 17$ (77.3%)

Terzi	2014	[80]	Turkey	Case series	–	2	LT	$n = 1$ yes $n = 1$ lost FU	18 -	Yes (1) Lost FU (1)
Xue	2014	[81]	USA	Case report	5	1		No	***27***	***No***
Huerta-Orozco	2015	[82]	Mexico	Case report	41	1	LDLT	Yes	6	Yes
Pilbeam	2018	[83]	USA	Case report	2	1	DDLT	No	***24***	***No***
Konstantinidis	2018	[84]	National Cancer Database, USA	Registry	–	24	LT	–	6 (med)	–
Mont'Alverne Pierre	2019	[85]	Brazil	Case series	69	1	DDLT	Yes	10	Yes
Zeng	2020	[86]	China	Systematic review	≤60 = 11 >60 = 2	13	LT	–	5.8 (med)	–
Dhaliwal	2021	[87]	USA	Case report	61	1	DDLT	No	***16***	***No***
Pire	2021	[88]	Belgium	Case series	4	1	DDLT	No	***126***	***No***
Aldén	2021	[89]	Sweden	Case series	4 and 4	2	DDLT	Yes (1)	16 and 6	Yes (1)
Kim	2021	[90]	Korea	Case series	2 and 60	2	LDLT	Yes	31 and 13	Yes (2)

Abbreviations: *Ref.* reference, *Nr* number, *FU* follow-up, *DD/LDLT* deceased-donor/living-donor liver transplantation angiogenic growth factor receptors and vascular-targeted agents, are needed to improve the outcome. Some drug combinations and immunotherapy (anti-PD1), occasionally combined with standard chemotherapy, have been reported to generate a sporadic, partial response [56, 99, 100].

7.3 Haemangiopericytoma (HPC)

HPC, an uncommon vascular tumour comprising less than 2% of soft tissue sarcomas, arises from Zimmermann's pericytes, the small oval cells surrounding the capillaries. This tumour is rare and is usually seen in adults of both genders as a painless mass. The upper and lower limbs, abdomen, retroperitoneal space, skull, head, neck, and central nervous system are most commonly affected, while primary liver involvement is rare. HPC can present as solitary and multiple lesions. Imaging features are not distinctive; contrast imaging shows heterogeneous and persistent enhancement without filling, as is often the case in malignant sarcomatous lesions. The diagnosis can only be confirmed with a biopsy and IHC staining. Pathology shows hyper-vascular, well-circumscribed lesion(s) containing spindle-shaped cells; half of them are malignant. Large tumour size (> 20 cm), more than four mitoses per ten high-power fields, pleomorphic cells with a chromatin pattern, and central necrosis or intra-tumour haemorrhage indicate malignant transformation. Histology, molecular biology, and IHC allow its differentiation from other sarcomas [101–103].

The clinical presentation is again very variable, ranging from the absence of symptoms to paraneoplastic syndromes at diagnosis or at the time of development of metastases. Hypoglycaemia, secondary to the release of insulin-like growth factors, appears in the later stage of the disease. Although aggressive surgery is the treatment of choice for both primary and metastatic lesions, two-thirds of patients recur even after R0 resection. The role of chemo- and radiotherapy is still open. Detection of recurrence is difficult because of the diversity of the tumour size and the lack of specific markers. A PET scan is helpful for diagnosis and follow-up if the initial tumour had tracer uptake. After R0 resection, the 5-year DFS reaches 50%. Long-term follow-up is necessary as 10% of tumours recur *after* 5 years. Repetitive surgery may be helpful in the case of paraneoplastic syndromes, in particular when invalidating hypoglycaemia is present [103]. Four patients were identified in the ELTR vascular tumour study, two each with primary or metastatic HPC. One (metastatic) patient had a DFS of 12 years after LT and multiple abdominal, thoracic, and orthopaedic re-interventions [104]. Radio- and chemotherapy are unsuccessful. Some partial responses have been obtained using combination therapies such as temozolomide and bevacizumab. Again, the search for specific molecular tumour markers will be needed to improve the outlook [105].

7.4 Hepatic Small Vessel Neoplasm (HSVN)

HSVN has recently been described as an infiltrative hepatic neoplasm. Despite its infiltrative nature (mimicking HHS) and its share of GNAQ and GNA14 mutations (which are also seen in some types of HHS and Kaposiform HE), HSVN is considered a benign or low-grade tumour because it lacks cellular atypia and increased proliferation [106, 107]. Diagnosis again needs detailed histological and molecular biology examinations. Resection is the proposed treatment. Given its rarity, infiltrative nature, and insufficient long-term follow-up, the nature of this tumour is questioned (benign vs. low-grade malignant) [108]. Recently, a patient has been transplanted because of a low-grade HSVN in the presence of stable osseous metastases; 2.5 years post-LT, she was alive and in good condition. She underwent three vertebroplasties for spine metastases following a treatment with tyrosine kinase inhibitor [109]. As for all vascular tumours, efficacious medical (neo-)adjuvant treatment targeting the 'diseased' vessels is needed to improve outcomes [110].

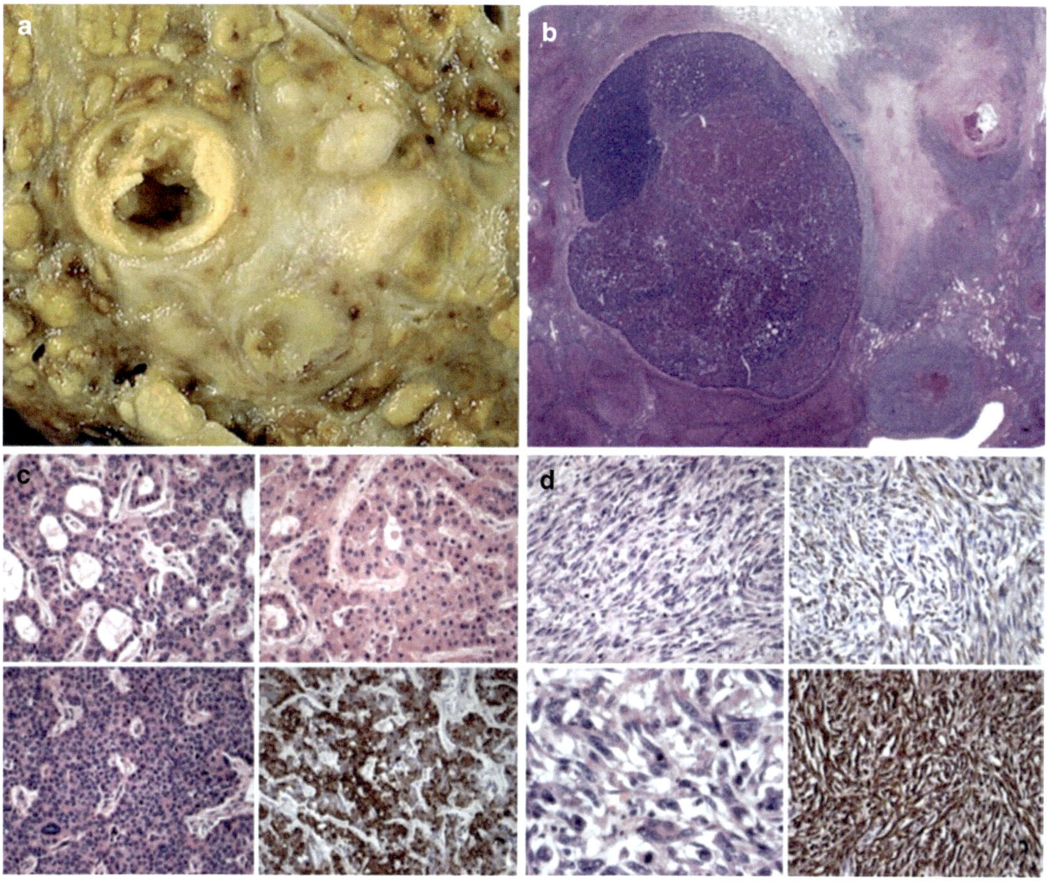

Fig. 7.7 Combined sarcomatous hepatocellular cancer (SaHCC) developed in an hepatitis C virus (HCV)-infected cirrhotic liver. (**a**) Macroscopy of a 4-cm tumour reveals two distinct zones corresponding to an HCC, with bud formation, surrounded by a sarcomatous lesion. (**b**) Microscopy shows the different glandular and spindle cell types corresponding to the two different tumour components. (**c**) IHC staining of the HCC part was positive for alfo-foetoprotein (AFP) antigen. (**d**) Immunohistochemistry of the sarcomatous part of the tumour was negative for other different stains. (From Refs. [115, 120], with permission)

7.5 Sarcomatous Hepatocellular Cancer (SaHCC)

SaHCC, a rare variant of HCC, combines HCC and spindle-cell components [111] (Fig. 7.7a–d). SaHCC is also known as spindle-cell carcinoma, sarcomatoid carcinoma, pseudo-sarcoma, and carcinosarcoma [112]. This tumour represents a mosaic of components with distinct histogenesis and carcinogenic pathways. The behaviour and natural history of SaHCC are still poorly understood. In recent years, SaHCC has been more frequently diagnosed due to the rising incidence of LT for HCC and the more detailed examination of total hepatectomy specimens, including extensive IHC and molecular biology. Pre-LT locoregional therapies, such as chemo-embolization, nowadays applied in around 80% of potential HCC transplant recipients, seem to play an important role in the development of these combined tumours. The diagnosis remains challenging as serological tumour markers are not increased, and typical imaging findings are missing. The sarcomatous component of HCC likely derives from de-differentiated anaplastic cells. Intra- and extrahepatic metastases are frequent. The prognosis is poor due to aggressive tumour biology. Response to locoregional treatment such

Table 7.3 Literature review of LT for sarcomatous hepatocellular cancer (SaHCC)

Author	Year	Ref.	Country	Article type	Age	DD/LDLT	Nr	Death	FU mo	Recurrence
Garcez-Silva	2006	[120]	Brazil	Case report	40	DDLT	1	Yes	5	Yes
Hwang	2008	[115]	S. Korea	Case series	54	LDLT	4	Yes	3	Yes
					59	LDLT		No	***58***	***No***
					46	LDLT		Yes	27	Yes
					56	DDLT		No	22	Yes
Kaneko	2010	[112]	Japan	Case report	53	LDLT	1	Yes	12	Yes
Orlando	2020	[113]	Belgium	Case report	65	DDLT	1	Yes	7	Yes

Abbreviations: *Ref.* reference, *DD/LDLT* deceased-donor/living-donor liver transplantation, *Nr* number, *FU* follow-up

as TACE is poor, and early (metastatic) recurrence is the rule after both partial resection and LT [113, 114].

Similar to combined HCC–CCC tumours, the prognosis is steered by the most aggressive (thus sarcomatous) tumour component [72, 113–117]. In order to avoid futile LT, percutaneous biopsy should, despite its poor sensitivity, be more deliberately used in case of unspecific, 'targetoid', liver tumour findings, as it is the only method to differentiate SaHCC from HCC [113, 118]. Only seven (six in Eastern countries) LT cases have been reported [113, 115, 119, 120] (Table 7.3). All recipients were adults. As all but one recurred early, LT should be omitted.

7.6 Undifferentiated Embryonal Liver Sarcoma (UELS)

UELS is a rare tumour accounting for 9–15% of paediatric liver malignancies [121]. UELS represents children's third most common malignant liver tumour, following hepatoblastoma and HCC [122]. The peak incidence of UELS is between 6 and 10 years of age ('not yet teenagers'), but this tumour has also been reported in predominantly female young adults [123, 124]. UELS arises more commonly in the right liver lobe and presents as a large (10–30 cm) mass [125]. This either cystic or solid mass formation explains the clinical presentation with non-specific symptoms of abdominal pain, (high) fever (due to tumour necrosis), weight loss, nausea, and anorexia [121, 123, 125]. Occasionally, post-traumatic abdominal pain may lead to an erroneous diagnosis of haematoma. MRI imaging typically shows cystic and solid components [126, 127] (Fig. 7.8). The combination of cystic lesions and high fever (due to tumour necrosis) may lead to the erroneous diagnosis of liver abscess. As tumour markers are usually not increased, a liver biopsy is indicated to confirm the diagnosis. UELS is a mesenchymal tumour with sarcomatous features. Histologically, the tumour cells appear variable with spindle-, oval-, and stellate-shaped cells in a myxoid background; mitotic indices are usually high, and anisonucleosis with hyperchromasia is often marked [125]. Chromosomal aberrations, such as the breakpoint at t19q13.4 that is sometimes present, suggest that UESL may result from a malignant transformation of a benign mesenchymal hamartoma (precursor lesion) [128, 129].

Today, the standard of care for UELS consists of aggressive adjuvant therapies (malignant mesenchymal tumour chemotherapy, radiotherapy, and R0 resection allow not only for prolonged survival but also for curing adult patients) [121, 130–132]. Partial resection is the gold standard, but when the tumour remains unresectable despite aggressive chemotherapy, LT can be of value [124, 133–147] (Fig. 7.9a–h). The UELS-LT literature comprises 19 recipients described in case reports/case series; three US registry series composed of 12, 10, and 17 patients [142, 143, 145]; and two systematic reviews based on 14 and 28 patients [146, 147] (Table 7.4). Most patients were paediatric, with only four patients aged over 20 years. Results of the most extensive United Network for Organ

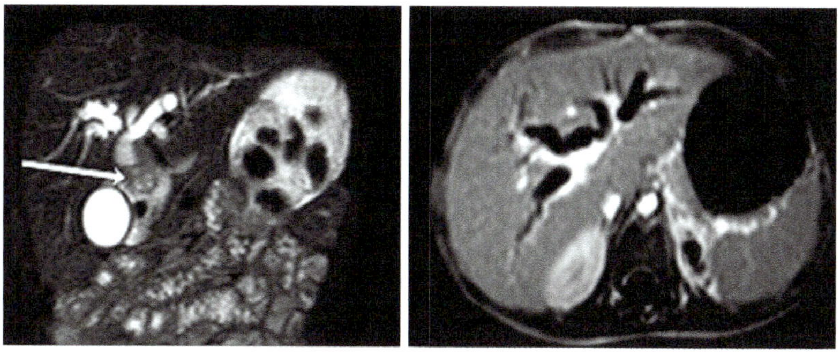

Fig. 7.8 Undifferentiated embryonal liver sarcoma (UELS). Typical CT scan showing the combined presence of solid and cystic areas. This tumour was amenable to radical liver resection after very successful neo-adjuvant chemotherapy

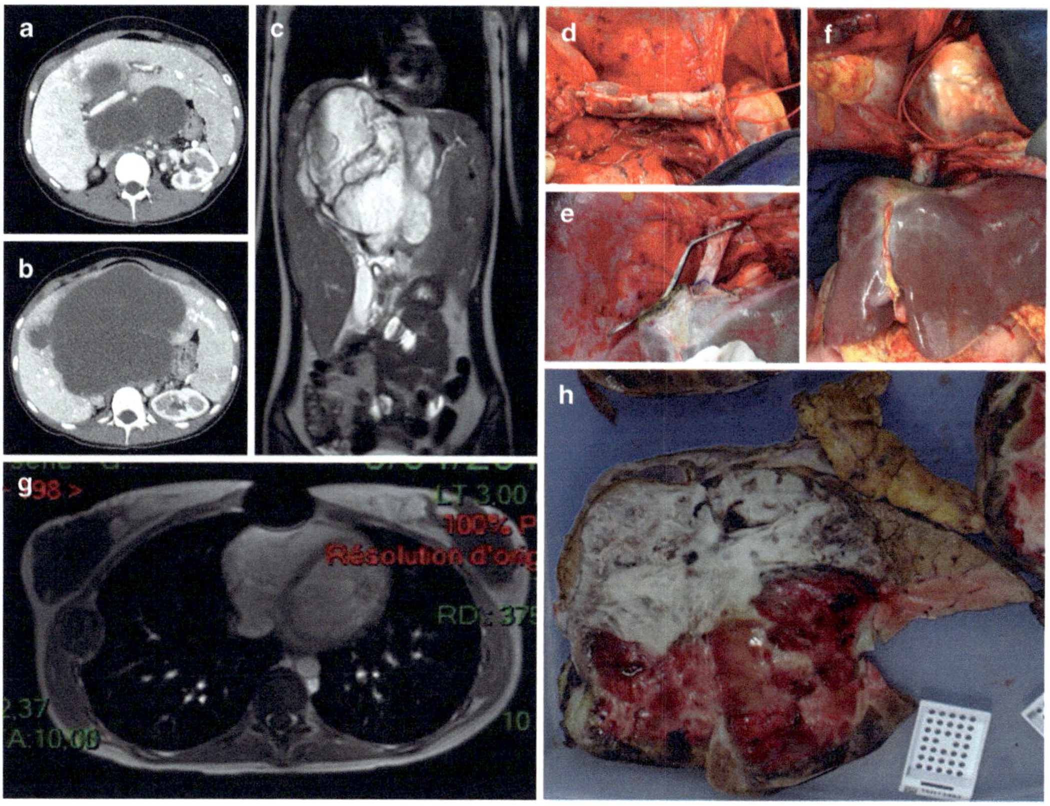

Fig. 7.9 Undifferentiated embryonal sarcoma (UELS) in an adolescent. (**a–c**) CT scan shows a huge central hepatic tumour englobing the hilar structures and the inferior vena cava. This female young adult presented with high-grade fever until the day of LT, explained by an extended tumour necrosis. (**d–f**) Left-liver living-donor LT with the replacement of the inferior vena cava using a free iliac vessel graft from a post-mortem donor. (**g**) Thirty months post-LT, an extensive thoracic wall reconstruction was done because of the development of a large rib metastasis. She died of a recurrent tumour 39 months post-LT. (**h**) Macroscopy of the 3.5-kg-weighing hepatectomy specimen shows a 16 × 13.5 × 13-cm-large myxoid mass with a large central necrosis and pseudocyst formations and invasion of the gall bladder. IHC staining was positive for CD34 and glypican-3. All lymph nodes were tumour-free

Table 7.4 Literature review of LT for undifferentiated embryonal liver sarcoma (UELS)

Author	Year	Ref.	Country	Article type	Adult/paediatric	DD/LDLT	Nr	Death	FU mo	Recurrence
Otte	1996	[133]	Belgium	Case series	Paediatric	DDLT	2	Yes	<6	Yes
						LDLT		Yes	***<6***	***No***
Chen	2006	[134]	USA	Case series	6 year	DDLT	2	No	***45***	***No***
					7 year	DDLT		No	***29***	***No***
Okajima	2009	[135]	Japan	Case series	15 year	LDLT	1	No	***18***	***No***
Kelly	2009	[136]	USA	Case report	9 year	DDLT	1	No	***60***	***No***
Dhanasekaran	2012	[137]	USA	Case report	54 year	DDLT	1	No	***123***	***No***
Plant	2013	[138]	USA	Case series	<19 year	DDLT	1	No	61	Yes
Ismail	2013	[139]	Poland	Case series	4 year	DDLT	1	Yes	***4***	***No***
Walther	2014	[140]	USA	Case series	13 year	DDLT	3	No	***24***	***No***
					11 year	DDLT		No	***24***	***No***
					7 year	DDLT		No	***84***	***No***
Schluckebier	2016	[141]	Switzerland	Case report	10 year	DDLT	1	No	***36***	***No***
Techavichit	2016	[142]	USA	Case series	22 year	DDLT	1	No	***28***	***No***
			UNOS, USA	Registry	Paediatric	DDLT	12	*n* = 1 (8.3%)	–	–
Shi	2017	[143]	USA	Registry	Paediatric	LT	10	No	>60	–
Khan	2017	[124]	Pakistan	Case report	21 year	LT	1	No	***18***	***No***
Vinayak	2017	[145]	UNOS, USA	Registry	Paediatric	LT	17	5-year: 67%	–	2/17
			USA	Case series	3.6 (1–7) year	3 DDLT	3	No	***>60***	***No***
Lerut	2019	[144]	Belgium	Case	21 year	LDLT and IVC replacement	1	Yes	39	Yes
Wu	2020	[146]	China	Systematic review	Paediatric = 10 Adult = 4	LT	14	*n* = 3	5-year OS: 78.9%	–
Babu	2021	[147]	Canada	Systematic review	Paediatric = 8 year (med) Adult = 27 year (med)	LT	28	*n* = 1	28.5 (8–123)	*n* = 2

Two children reported to the ELTR died at 5 and 12 months due to tumour recurrence and post-operative complications; one 24-year-old adult is alive and disease-free at 12 years (personal communication)

Abbreviations: *Ref.* reference, *DD/LDLT* deceased-donor/living-donor liver transplantation, *Nr* number, *FU* follow-up

Sharing (UNOS) series ($n = 17$) are encouraging, with a 5-year patient survival rate of 67.2% and a DFS of 88.0% [145].

7.7 Rhabdomyosarcoma (RMS)

Rhabdomyosarcoma (RMS) is the most common, ubiquitous, soft tissue sarcoma in childhood, accounting for 5% of childhood malignancies. Five subgroups of RMS have been reported: embryonal, alveolar, pleomorphic, epithelioid, and botryoid. Embryonal RMS is the most frequent type of RMS in young children, alveolar RMS is the most frequent type in patients older than 10 years, and pleomorphic and epithelioid RMS are the most frequent types in advanced-aged adults [148, 149].

7.7.1 Biliary Embryonal Rhabdomyosarcoma (BERMS)

BERMS is very rare but represents the most common biliary tumour in children. It usually presents with obstructive jaundice and cholangitis. The diagnosis remains difficult; when suspected on biliary imaging based on bile duct dilatation, malformation, and suspicious intraluminal material/tissue, a biopsy with biliary drainage (percutaneous or endoscopic) should be performed to allow the prompt start of neo-adjuvant chemotherapy (Fig. 7.9).

7.7.2 Hepatic Rhabdomyosarcoma

Hepatic RMS is rare in adults [148]. Typical imaging and symptoms are missing. This tumour also presents as a large heterogeneous mass containing cystic and solid components (Fig. 7.10). Histopathology again needs a large IHC staining panel, looking into these tumours specifically for the mutation or loss of NF-1 [150]. Therapeutic modalities have been well-studied by the European, German, and Italian soft tissue sarcoma consortia [151–153]. The rarity of the disease has not yet allowed putting forward clear guidelines. However, the results have already been markedly improved by combining neo-adjuvant chemotherapy and RO surgery. The chemotherapy regimen is adapted to the risk identification specified by the Intergroup Rhabdomyosarcoma Study Group. Age over 10 years, botryoid histology, large tumour (>5 cm), lymph node involvement, and primary and R1 surgery are all unfavourable prognostic factors [152, 153]. Depending on the obtained result, the patient is oriented towards a surgical resection. RO resectability should be assessed preoperatively and guided by an intraoperative frozen section. Delayed surgery allowed a significantly higher incidence of RO resection (12/16 patients) than primary surgery (1/8 patients). The role of adjuvant external beam radiotherapy could not be fully proven. Five-year PS and DFS can nowadays reach 85% and 76%, respectively [151]. The prognosis is dependent on the response to chemotherapy and the quality of the hepatobiliary resection, sometimes needing even a combined or sequential liver–pancreas resection. Age is also a critical prognostic factor. The outcome in adults is poor; most

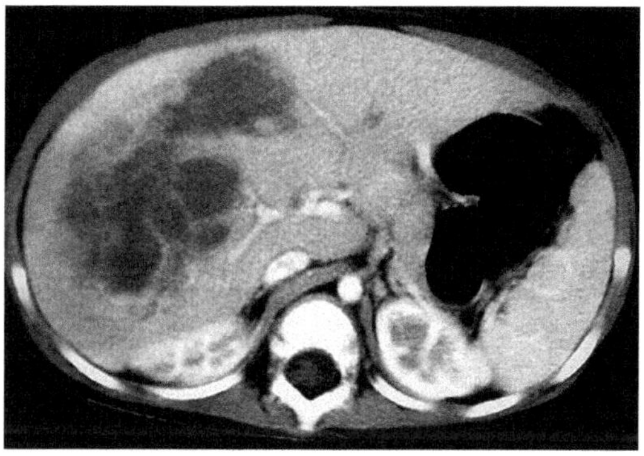

Fig. 7.10 Biliary rhabdomyosarcoma (BERMS) in a young child. The lesion of the biliary bifurcation mimicked a choledochal cyst. The arrow shows the following: (**a**) a dilated bile duct with the typical botryoides aspect of the tumour, and (**b**) the intrahepatic bile ducts are markedly dilated due to the obstruction of the biliary bifurcation. Conventional neo-adjuvant chemotherapy resulted in a shrinkage of the tumour to a very tiny mass; afterwards, an en bloc mesohepatectomy with resection of the bile duct bifurcation and the extrahepatic bile duct was successfully performed

Table 7.5 Literature review of LT for biliary embryonal rhabdomyosarcoma (BERMS)

Author	Year	Ref.	51.91 pt	Article type	Age	Nr	DD/LDLT	Death	Post-LT FU mo	Recurrence
Lerut	2011	[157]	Belgium	Case report	18	1	LDLT	Yes (suicide) No recurrence	60	No
Paganelli	2014	[155]	Canada	Case report	2	1	DDLT	No	48	No
Shen	2017	[156]	China	Case report	8	1	DDLT	No	6	No
Perruccio	2017	[152]	Italy	Case series	Paediatric	2	LT	$n = 2$	2 and 9	Yes: 1 pat
Vinayak	2017	[145]	USA	Case series	Paediatric	1	LT	No	60	No
Guerin	2019	[151]	Europe	Registry	Paediatric	1	LT	Yes	Early death	No
Namgoong	2022	[158]	Korea	Case report	6	1	LDLT	No	26	No

Two more adults were reported to the ELTR; one is alive and disease-free at 2 years; the other died at 1 month due to post-operative complications (personal communication)

Abbreviations: *Ref.* reference, *Nr* number, *FU* follow-up, *DD/LDLT* deceased-donor/living-donor liver transplantation patients die within 1 year from the onset of initial symptoms [148]. In case of complete remission after chemotherapy, surgery should be advocated to mitigate a high recurrence rate with a poor outcome [154]. The role of LT is restricted to unresectable BERMS or patients presenting with local relapse. The BERS-LT literature identified eight cases [145, 151, 152, 155–158]. The obtained results are encouraging (Table 7.5). Four children were transplanted because of RMS. Three died at 9, 13, and 36 months due to tumour recurrence, and one died at day 7 because of graft failure (personal communication).

7.8 Leiomyosarcoma

LMS is a malignant mesenchymal neoplasm deriving from smooth muscle cells. LMS is the second most frequent malignant soft tissue tumour in adults after liposarcoma. LMS can derive directly from the liver, the round ligament, and the intrahepatic vessels. These tumours have a poor prognosis due to their high aggressivity, leading to a high incidence of recurrence.

7.8.1 Vascular Leiomyosarcoma

Vascular LMS represents 2% of all LMSs. Only a few hundred cases have been reported. They occur only in the inferior vena cava (50%), the hepatic veins, and rarely (only five cases reported) in the portal vein [159–161]. Radical RO resection is the most important prognostic factor allowing us to obtain a 30–60% 5-year survival. (Neo-)adjuvant therapies are recommended. There is no consensus yet on the value of chemotherapy [159]. Of note is the fact that the two resected portal vein LMSs presented a recurrence in the liver only, thereby questioning the possible role of (a rescue) LT [160].

Although frequently linked to extensive liver surgery, including caval replacement using prosthetic, allo-, or autologous vascular or peritoneal grafts, the vena cava LMS should, per se, not be considered a hepatic sarcoma [161, 162].

7.8.2 Hepatic Leiomyosarcoma

Hepatic LMS tumour is also extremely rare; till 2020, only 76 cases were reported [163, 164]. Diagnostic workup, including FDG-PET, needs to exclude an extrahepatic source of the lesion, as well as extrahepatic metastases. These are most frequently located in the lungs. The patients commonly present with large (often >10 cm), (often right) liver masses, which explain the symptoms of abdominal pain and distention, weight loss, appetite loss, and weakness; fever, back pain, and jaundice are less common symptoms. Small tumours may be asymptomatic. No aetiological factor has been identified, but hepatic LMS has been reported in several immunosuppressed (organ transplant recipients) and immunodeficient patients. The diagnosis is challenging due to the non-specific presentation and absence of tumour markers. IHC staining for the smooth muscle markers actin, desmin, and vimentin and smooth muscle antibodies is essential for diagnosis. Imaging is non-specific. CT scan reveals a hypodense, well-defined, and heterogeneous mass, eventually presenting with internal and peripheral enhancement. Cystic variants may have an enhancing thick wall and, therefore, may lead to the erroneous diagnosis of liver abscess. MRI reveals homo- or heterogeneously hypointense lesions on T1 weighting, which are hyperintense on T2 scans. The rarity of the disease goes along with the absence of clear therapeutic guidelines. Unfortunately, many published cases lack long-term follow-up. The therapy includes resection, chemotherapy, chemo-embolization, and radiotherapy. As for every type of sarcoma, radical R0 resection offers the best long-term survival. The five-year survival rate reaches 40%. The place of LT is controversial due to the high recurrence rate and the low long-term survival rate. LT has only been anecdotally reported for these uncommon sarcomas: one for Kupffer cell sarcoma [165] and 12 for LMS [78, 145, 166–169] (Table 7.6). Seven LMS patients were children; the ages of the five adults ranged from 19 to 68 years. Three adults presented with a lethal LMS recurrence several years after LT. The UNOS data reported only

Table 7.6 Literature review of LT for leiomyosarcoma (LMS)

Author	Year	Ref.	Country	Article type	Age	Nr	DD/LDLT	Death	Post-LT FU mo	Recurrence
Saint-Paul	1993	[166]	France	Case report	68	1	DDLT	Yes	***0.5***	***No***
Matthaei	2009	[78]	Germany	Case series	19	1	DDLT	Yes	73	Yes
					51	1	DDLT	Yes	141 disease-free	Partial resection of chest wall
Liang	2010	[167]	China	Case report	44	1	DDLT	Yes	34	Yes
Vinayak	2017	[145]	UNOS, USA	Registry	Paediatric	6	LT	5-year: 62.5%	NA	Yes: 1 pat
Xie	2017	[168]	China	Case report	10	1	LT	NA	NA	Na
Gunasekaran	2018	[169]	India	Case report	39	1	LDLT	No	24	No

Abbreviations: *Ref.* reference, *Nr* number, *FU* follow-up, *DD/LDLT* deceased-donor/living-donor liver transplantation, *NA* non-available one recurrence out of six children. LT guaranteed satisfactory results, with a 5-year patient survival rate of 62.5% [145]. The role of neoadjuvant and adjuvant chemo(-radio)therapy should be further elucidated, although this is difficult, given the rarity of transplantable patients. It is likely that the wider application of living-donor liver transplantation (LDLT) will increase the number of patients transplanted for these sarcomas [144, 157, 158, 168].

7.9 Hepatic Liposarcoma (LPS)

Hepatic liposarcoma is exceedingly rare; only 12 cases were reported till 2018 [170, 171]. Histologically, there are four subtypes of LPS: well-differentiated, de-differentiated, myxoid-round cell, and pleomorphic LPS. Hepatic myxoid LPS accounts for half of liver LPSs. Symptoms include abdominal pain, nausea, vomiting, jaundice, weight loss, and eventual symptoms due to the compression of neighbouring organs. Tumour markers are normal. Diagnostic workup includes comprehensive imaging, including CT, MRI, and PET-CT scan, and molecular biology. CT shows a well-defined hypo-attenuating mass with cystic degeneration, occasional bleeding, and margin enhancement; MRI reveals T1 and T2 weigthed (T1WI and T2WI) hyperintensity of the fat-containing components. Contrast MRI of hepatic myxoid LPS containing myxoid components and nonfat, non-myxoid components shows heterogeneous enhancement. PET-CT scan is of help to further confirm the diagnosis and exclude the frequently present extrahepatic lesions. Fine-needle aspiration biopsy has been shown to not be of great diagnostic help. Molecular biology reveals, in the case of myxoid LPS, a reciprocal chromosomal translocation of t(12;16)(q13;p11), and the affected genes include DNA damage inducible transcript (DDIT3) [cyclophosphamide, doxorubicin hydrochloride, vincristine and prednisone (CHOP)] (CHOP) and fused in sarcoma (FUS) [tumor lysis syndrome (TLS)]. Radical surgical resection, and even re-resection in case of localized recurrence, is the treatment of choice [171]. LT is contraindicated due to the very high recurrence rates after R0 resection. Radiotherapy is only moderately effective. The 5-year survival rate of hepatic LPS after surgery or radiotherapy is around 50%. Older age (>45 years), necrosis, and high grading are all associated with a poorer prognosis in myxoid liposarcoma patients [170].

7.10 Conclusion

Hepatobiliary sarcomas represent a rare entity. Due to their low incidence, protean clinical presentation, heterogeneous imaging characteristics, and insufficient clinical awareness, unequivocal diagnostic and therapeutic algorithms are still lacking. Multimodal therapies, combining neoadjuvant and adjuvant chemo-radiotherapy and liver resection, including liver transplantation (because the best R0 resection therapy), have already allowed us to make significant advances in the care of these merely, young patients. More progress is needed to identify more reliable prognostic parameters and efficacious anti-tumour drugs. The hepatologic, paediatric, oncologic, and liver 'resection and transplantation' surgical communities should focus on developing this underrated part of hepatobiliary and transplant oncology. By enlarging the different sarcoma cohorts through international collaboration of expert hepatobiliary and sarcoma centres, more knowledge can be gathered, thereby allowing us to discuss fundamental issues in treating these different hepatobiliary 'orphan diseases'. Long-term follow-up, missing in the great majority of reports, is another essential item in order to obtain insights into the real value of the different medical and surgical therapies applied to these rare hepatobiliary lesions.

References

1. Bridgewater J, Galle PR, Khan SA, et al. Guidelines for the diagnosis and management of intrahepatic cholangiocarcinoma. J Hepatol. 2014;60:1268–89.
2. European Association for the Study of the Liver. EASL clinical practice guidelines: manage-

ment of hepatocellular carcinoma. J Hepatol. 2018;69:182–236.
3. Ishak K, Goodman Z, Stocker J. Tumours of the liver and intrahepatic bile ducts. In: Atlas of tumour pathology. Third series, fascicle 31. Washington: Armed Forces Institute of Pathology; 1999.
4. Sempoux C, Balabaud C, Paradis V, et al. Hepatocellular nodules in vascular liver diseases. Virchows Arch. 2018;473:33–44.
5. Valla DC, Cazals-Hatem D. Vascular liver diseases on the clinical side: definitions and diagnosis, new concepts. Virchows Arch. 2018;473:3–13.
6. Thampy R, Elsayes KM, Menias CO, et al. Imaging features of rare mesenychmal liver tumours: beyond haemangiomas. Br J Radiol. 2017;90:20170373.
7. Semelka RC, Nimojan N, Chandana S, et al. MRI features of primary rare malignancies of the liver: a report from four university centres. Eur Radiol. 2018;28:1529–39.
8. Ehman EC, Torbenson MS, Wells ML, et al. Hepatic tumours of vascular origin: imaging appearances. Abdom Radiol (NY). 2018;43:1978–90.
9. Studer LL, Selby DM. Hepatic epithelioid haemangioendothelioma. Arch Pathol Lab Med. 2018;142:263–7.
10. Lerut JP, Orlando G, Adam R, et al. The place of liver transplantation in the treatment of hepatic epithelioid haemangioendothelioma: report of the European Liver Transplant Registry. Ann Surg. 2007;246:949–57.
11. Orlando G, Adam R, Mirza D, et al. Hepatic haemangiosarcoma: an absolute contraindication to liver transplantation—the European Liver Transplant Registry experience. Transplantation. 2013;95:872–7.
12. Lerut JP, Weber M, Orlando G, et al. Vascular and rare liver tumours: a good indication for liver transplantation? J Hepatol. 2007;47:466–75.
13. Lai Q, Feys E, Karam V, et al. Hepatic epithelioid haemangioendothelioma and adult liver transplantation: proposal for a prognostic score based on the analysis of the ELTR-ELITA Registry. Transplantation. 2017;101:555–64.
14. Flucke U, Vogels RJ, de Saint Aubain Somerhausen N, et al. Epithelioid haemangioendothelioma: clinicopathologic, immunhistochemical, and molecular genetic analysis of 39 cases. Diagn Pathol. 2014;9:131.
15. Antonescu CR, Le Loarer F, Mosquera JM, et al. Novel YAP1-TFE3 fusion defines a distinct subset of epithelioid haemangioendothelioma. Genes Chromosomes Cancer. 2013;52:775–84.
16. Martínez C, Lai JK, Ramai D, et al. Cancer registry study of malignant hepatic vascular tumours: hepatic angiosarcomas and hepatic epithelioid haemangioendotheliomas. Cancer Med. 2021;10:8883–90.
17. Ishak KG, Sesterhenn IA, Goodman ZD, et al. Epithelioid haemangioendothelioma of the liver: a clinicopathologic and follow-up study of 32 cases. Hum Pathol. 1984;15:839–52.
18. Makhlouf HR, Ishak KG, Goodman ZD. Epithelioid haemangioendothelioma of the liver: a clinicopathologic study of 137 cases. Cancer. 1999;85:562–82.
19. Lau K, Massad M, Pollak C, et al. Clinical patterns and outcome in epithelioid haemangioendothelioma with or without pulmonary involvement: insights from an internet registry in the study of a rare cancer. Chest. 2011;140:1312–8.
20. Sharif K, English M, Ramani P, et al. Management of hepatic epithelioid haemangio-endothelioma in children: what option? Br J Cancer. 2004;90:1498–501.
21. Mascarelli PE, Iredell JR, Maggi RG, et al. Bartonella species bacteremia in two patients with epithelioid haemangioendothelioma. J Clin Microbiol. 2011;49:4006–12.
22. Lee JH, Jeong WK. Magnetic resonance findings of hepatic epithelioid haemangioendothelioma: emphasis on hepatobiliary phase using Gd-EOB-DTPA. Abdom Radiol (NY). 2017;42:2261–71.
23. Zhou Y, Hou P, Wang F, et al. Primary hepatic malignant vascular tumours: a follow-up study of imaging characteristics and clinicopathological features. Cancer Imaging. 2020;20:59.
24. Nguyen BD. Epithelioid haemangioendothelioma of the liver with F-18 FDG PET imaging. Clin Nucl Med. 2004;29:828–30.
25. Bagan P, Hassan M, Le Pimpec Barthes F, et al. Prognostic factors and surgical indications of pulmonary epithelioid haemangioendothelioma: a review of the literature. Ann Thorac Surg. 2006;82:2010–3.
26. Duarte Mesquita R, Sousa M, Trinidad C, et al. New insights about pulmonary epithelioid haemangioendothelioma: review of the literature and two case reports. Case Rep Radiol. 2017;2017:5972940.
27. Demetris AJ, Minervini M, Raikow RB, et al. Hepatic epithelioid haemangioendothelioma: biological questions based on pattern of recurrence in an allograft and tumour immunophenotype. Am J Surg Pathol. 1997;21:263–70.
28. Campione S, Cozzolino I, Mainenti P, et al. Hepatic epithelioid haemangioendothelioma: pitfalls in the diagnosis on fine needle cytology and "small biopsy" and review of the literature. Pathol Res Pract. 2015;211:702–5.
29. Dong K, Wang XX, Feng JL, et al. Pathological characteristics of liver biopsies in eight patients with hepatic epithelioid haemangioendothelioma. Int J Clin Exp Pathol. 2015;8:11015–23.
30. Kitaichi M, Nagai S, Nishimura K, et al. Pulmonary epithelioid haemangioendothelioma in 21 patients, including three with partial spontaneous regression. Eur Respir J. 1998;12:89–96.
31. Rodriguez JA, Becker NS, O'Mahony CA, et al. Long-term outcomes following liver transplantation for hepatic haemangioendothelioma: the UNOS experience from 1987 to 2005. J Gastrointest Surg. 2008;12:110–6.
32. Miettinen M, Wang ZF, Paetau A, et al. ERG transcription factor as an immunohistochemical marker

for vascular endothelial tumours and prostatic carcinoma. Am J Surg Pathol. 2011;35:432–41.
33. Madariaga JR, Marino IR, Karavias DD, et al. Long-term results after liver transplantation for primary hepatic epithelioid haemangioendothelioma. Ann Surg Oncol. 1995;2:483–7.
34. Nudo CG, Yoshida EM, Bain VG, et al. Liver transplantation for hepatic epithelioid haemangioendothelioma: the Canadian multicentre experience. Can J Gastroenterol. 2008;22:821–4.
35. Mehrabi A, Kashfi A, Fonouni H, et al. Primary malignant hepatic epithelioid haemangioendothelioma: a comprehensive review of the literature with emphasis on the surgical therapy. Cancer. 2006;107:2108–21.
36. Jung DH, Hwang S, Hong SM, et al. Clinicopathological features and prognosis of hepatic epithelioid haemangioendothelioma after liver resection and transplantation. Ann Transplant. 2016;21:784–90.
37. Grotz TE, Nagorney D, Donohue J, et al. Hepatic epithelioid haemangioendothelioma: is transplantation the only treatment option? HPB (Oxford). 2010;12:546–53.
38. Desie N, Van Raemdonck DE, Ceulemans LJ, et al. Combined or serial liver and lung transplantation for epithelioid haemangioendothelioma: a case series. Am J Transplant. 2015;15:3247–54.
39. Pallotti MC, Nannini M, Agostinelli C, et al. Long-term durable response to lenalidomide in a patient with hepatic epithelioid haemangioendothelioma. World J Gastroenterol. 2014;20:7049–54.
40. Mascarenhas RC, Sanghvi AN, Friedlander L, et al. Thalidomide inhibits the growth and progression of hepatic epithelioid haemangioendothelioma. Oncology. 2004;67:471–5.
41. Soape MP, Verma R, Payne JD, et al. Treatment of hepatic epithelioid haemangioendothelioma: finding uses for thalidomide in a new era of medicine. Case Rep Gastroenterol Med. 2015;2015:326795.
42. Semenisty V, Naroditsky I, Keidar Z, et al. Pazopanib for metastatic pulmonary epithelioid haemangioendothelioma-a suitable treatment option: case report and review of anti-angiogenic treatment options. BMC Cancer. 2015;15:402.
43. Kelly H, O'Neil BH. Response of epithelioid haemangioendothelioma to liposomal doxorubicin. Lancet Oncol. 2005;6:813–5.
44. Lakkis Z, Kim S, Delabrousse E, et al. Metronomic cyclophosphamide: an alternative treatment for hepatic epithelioid haemangioendothelioma. J Hepatol. 2013;58:1254–7.
45. Kayler LK, Merion RM, Arenas JD, et al. Epithelioid haemangioendothelioma of the liver disseminated to the peritoneum treated with liver transplantation and interferon alpha-2B. Transplantation. 2002;74:128–30.
46. Stiles JM, Amaya C, Rains S, et al. Targeting of beta adrenergic receptors results in therapeutic efficacy against models of haemangioendothelioma and angiosarcoma. PLoS One. 2013;8:e60021.
47. Chevreau C, Le Cesne A, Ray-Coquard I, et al. Sorafenib in patients with progressive epithelioid haemangioendothelioma: a phase 2 study by the French Sarcoma Group (GSF/GETO). Cancer. 2013;119:2639–44.
48. Agulnik M, Yarber JL, Okuno SH, et al. An open-label, multicenter, phase II study of bevacizumab for the treatment of angiosarcoma and epithelioid haemangioendotheliomas. Ann Oncol. 2013;24:257–63.
49. Theurillat JP, Vavricka SR, Went P, et al. Morphologic changes and altered gene expression in an epithelioid haemangioendothelioma during a ten-year course of disease. Pathol Res Pract. 2003;199:165–70.
50. Miller MA, Sandler AD. Elevated plasma vascular endothelial growth factor levels in 2 patients with haemangioendothelioma. J Pediatr Surg. 2005;40:e17–9.
51. Errani C, Sung YS, Zhang L, et al. Monoclonality of multifocal epithelioid haemangioendothelioma of the liver by analysis of WWTR1-CAMTA1 breakpoints. Cancer Genet. 2012;205:12–7.
52. Calder CJ, Raafat F, Buckels JAC, et al. Orthotopic liver transplantation for type 2 hepatic infantile haemangioendothelioma. Histopathology. 1996;28:271–3.
53. Daller JA, Bueno J, Gutierrez J, et al. Hepatic haemangioendothelioma: clinical experience and management strategy. J Pediatr Surg. 1999;34:98–105; discussion 105–6.
54. Selby DM, Stocker JT, Waclawiw MA, et al. Infantile haemangioendothelioma of the liver. Hepatology. 1994;20:39–45.
55. Zhang Z, Chen HJ, Yang WJ, et al. Infantile hepatic haemangioendothelioma: a clinicopathologic study in a Chinese population. World J Gastroenterol. 2010;16:4549–57.
56. Li DB, Si XY, Wan T, et al. A pooled analysis of treatment and prognosis of hepatic angiosarcoma in adults. Hepatobiliary Pancreat Dis Int. 2018;17:198–203.
57. Maluf D, Cotterell A, Clark B, et al. Hepatic angiosarcoma and liver transplantation: case report and literature review. Transplant Proc. 2005;37:2195–9.
58. Grassia KL, Peterman CM. Clinical case series of paediatric hepatic angiosarcoma. Pediatr Blood Cancer. 2017;64:11.
59. Coulier B, Pierard F, Gielen I, et al. Hepatic angiosarcoma occurring 65 years after thorium dioxide (Thorotrast) exposure: imaging, surgical and histopathologic findings of a historical case. JBR-BTR. 2014;97:254–8.
60. Collins JJ, Jammer B, Sladeczek FM, et al. Surveillance for angiosarcoma of the liver among vinyl chloride workers. J Occup Environ Med. 2014;56:1207–9.
61. Saleh HA, Tao LC. Hepatic angiosarcoma: aspiration biopsy cytology and immunocytochemical contribution. Diagn Cytopathol. 1998;18:208–11.

62. Kim B, Byun JH, Lee JH, et al. Imaging findings of primary hepatic angiosarcoma on gadoxetate disodium-enhanced liver MRI: comparison with hepatic haemangiomas of similar size. Clin Radiol. 2018;73:244–53.
63. Pickhardt PJ, Kitchin D, Lubner MG, et al. Primary hepatic angiosarcoma: multi-institutional comprehensive cancer centre review of multiphasic CT and MR imaging in 35 patients. Eur Radiol. 2015;25:315–22.
64. Groeschl RT, Miura JT, Oshima K, et al. Does histology predict outcome for malignant vascular tumours of the liver? J Surg Oncol. 2014;109:483–6.
65. Ringe B, Wittekind C, Bechstein WO, et al. The role of liver transplantation in hepatobiliary malignancy. A retrospective analysis of 95 patients with particular regard to tumour stage and recurrence. Ann Surg. 1989;209:88–98.
66. Penn I. Hepatic transplantation for primary and metastatic cancers of the liver. Surgery. 1991;110:726–34.
67. von Schönfeld J, Erhard J, Donhuijsen K, Breuer N. Haemangiosarcoma of the liver. The diagnostic difficulties and therapeutic possibilities. Dtsch Med Wochenschr. 1992;117:211–5.
68. Moreno-González E, Loinaz C, Gómez R, et al. Orthotopic liver transplantation in primary liver tumours. J Surg Oncol Suppl. 1993;3:74–7.
69. Rojter S, Villamil FG, Petrovic LM, et al. Malignant vascular tumours of the liver presenting as liver failure and portal hypertension. Liver Transpl Surg. 1995;1:156–61.
70. Awan S, Davenport M, Portmann B, Howard ER. Angiosarcoma of the liver in children. J Pediatr Surg. 1996;31:1729–32.
71. Vennarecci G, Ismail T, Gunson B, McMaster P. Primary angiosarcoma of the liver. Minerva Chir. 1997;52:1141–6.
72. Pichlmayr R, Weimann A, Tusch G, Schlitt HJ. Indications and role of liver transplantation for malignant tumours. Oncologist. 1997;2:164–70.
73. Pimentel Cauduro SK, Petrovic LM, Sodeman TC, et al. Unsuspected primary hepatic angiosarcoma associated with portal vein thrombosis complicating cirrhosis. Liver Transpl. 2002;8:1080–1.
74. Dimashkieh HH, Mo JQ, Wyatt-Ashmead J, Collins MH. Paediatric hepatic angiosarcoma: case report and review of the literature. Pediatr Dev Pathol. 2004;7:527–32.
75. Walsh R, Harrington J, Beneck D, Ozkaynak MF. Congenital infantile hepatic haemangioendothelioma type II treated with orthotopic liver transplantation. J Pediatr Hematol Oncol. 2004;26:121–3.
76. Husted TL, Neff G, Thomas MJ, et al. Liver transplantation for primary or metastatic sarcoma to the liver. Am J Transplant. 2006;6:392–7.
77. Bismuth B, Castel H, Boleslawski E, et al. Primary sarcoma of the liver and transplantation: a case study and literature review. Rare Tumors. 2009;1:e31.
78. Matthaei H, Krieg A, Schmelzle M, et al. Long-term survival after surgery for primary hepatic sarcoma in adults. Arch Surg. 2009;144:339–44.
79. Geramizadeh B, Safari A, Bahador A, et al. Hepatic angiosarcoma of childhood: a case report and review of literature. J Pediatr Surg. 2011;46:e9–11.
80. Terzi A, Deniz EE, Haberal N, et al. Hepatic angiosarcoma and liver transplant: a report of 2 cases with diagnostic difficulties. Exp Clin Transplant. 2014;12:126–8.
81. Xue M, Masand P, Thompson P, et al. Angiosarcoma successfuly treated with liver transplantation and sirolimus. Pediatr Transplant. 2014;18:E114–9.
82. Huerta-Orozco LD, Leonher-Ruezga KL, Ramírez-González LR, et al. Hepatic angiosarcoma and liver transplantation: case report and literature review. Cir Cir. 2015;83:510–5.
83. Pilbeam K, Eidenschink B, Sulciner M, et al. Success of chemotherapy and a liver transplant in a paediatric patient with hepatic angiosarcoma: a case report. Pediatr Transplant. 2019;23:e13410.
84. Konstantinidis IT, Nota C, Jutric Z, et al. Primary liver sarcomas in the modern era: resection or transplantation? J Surg Oncol. 2018;117:886–91.
85. Mont Alverne Pierre AM, Veras CM, Esmeraldo TM, et al. Liver transplantation for non-hepatocellular carcinoma malignancy: a single-center experience. Transplant Proc. 2019;51:3355–9.
86. Zeng D, Cheng J, Gong Z, et al. A pooled analysis of primary hepatic angiosarcoma. Jpn J Clin Oncol. 2020;50:556–67.
87. Dhaliwal A, Braseth A, Dhindsa BS, Ramai D, Rochling FA. Liver transplantation in a patient with hepatic angiosarcoma. Cureus. 2021;13:e12609.
88. Pire A, Tambucci R, De Magnée C, et al. Living donor liver transplantation for hepatic malignancies in children. Pediatr Transplant. 2021;25:e14047.
89. Aldén J, Baecklund F, Psaros Einberg A, et al. Is primary hepatic angiosarcoma in children an indication for liver transplantation?-A single-centre experience and review of the literature. Pediatr Transplant. 2021;25:e14095.
90. Kim SJ, Rhu J, Kim JM, Choi GS, Joh JW. Surgical treatment outcomes of primary hepatic sarcomas: a single-center experience. World J Hepatol. 2021;13:584–94.
91. Potanos KM, Hodgkinson N, Fullington NM, et al. Long term survival in paediatric hepatic angiosarcoma (PHAS): a case report and review of the literature. J Pediatr Surg Case Rep. 2015;3:410–3.
92. Alden J, Baecklund F, Einberg AP, et al. Is primary hepatic angiosarcoma in children an indication for liver transplantation?-A single-centre experience and review of the literature. Pediatr Transplant. 2021;25:e14095.
93. Grimaldi C, de Ville de Goyet J, Bici K, Cianci MC, Callea F, Morabito A. The role of liver transplantation in the care of primary hepatic vascular tumours in children. Front Oncol. 2022;12:1026232.

94. Tripke V, Heinrich S, Huber T, et al. Surgical therapy of primary hepatic angiosarcoma. BMC Surg. 2019;19:5.
95. Katou S, Di Pietro Martinelli C, Silveira C, et al. Liver resection for primary hepatic angiosarcoma: bicentric analysis of a challenging entity. J Clin Med. 2022;11:2990.
96. Huang NC, Kuo YC, Chiang JC, et al. Hepatic angiosarcoma may have fair survival nowadays. Medicine (Baltimore). 2015;94:e816.
97. Zhu YP, Chen YM, Matro E, et al. Primary hepatic angiosarcoma: a report of two cases and literature review. World J Gastroenterol. 2015;21:6088–96.
98. Pierce DB, Johnson GE, Monroe E, et al. Safety and efficacy outcomes of embolization in hepatic sarcomas. AJR Am J Roentgenol. 2018;210:175–82.
99. Young RJ, Woll PJ. Anti-angiogenic therapies for the treatment of angiosarcoma: a clinical update. Memo. 2017;10:190–3.
100. Sindhu S, Gimber LH, Cranmer L, et al. Angiosarcoma treated successfuly with anti-PD-1 therapy – a case report. J Immunother Cancer. 2017;5:58.
101. McMaster MJ, Soule EH, Ivins JC. Hemangiopericytoma. A clinicopathologic study and long-term follow-up of 60 patients. Cancer. 1975;36:2232–44.
102. Enzinger FM, Smith BH. Hemangiopericytoma. An analysis of 106 cases. Hum Pathol. 1976;7:61–82.
103. Flores-Stadler EM, Chou P, Walterhouse D, et al. Hemangiopericytoma of the liver: immunohistochemical observations, expression of angiogenic factors, and review of the literature. J Pediatr Hematol Oncol. 1997;19:449–54.
104. Adams J, Lodge JP, Parker D. Liver transplantation for metastatic hemangiopericytoma associated with hypoglycemia. Transplantation. 1999;67:488–9.
105. Park MS, Patel SR, Ludwig JA, et al. Activity of temozolomide and bevacizumab in the treatment of locally advanced, recurrent, and metastatic hemangiopericytoma and malignant solitary fibrous tumour. Cancer. 2011;117:4939–47.
106. Gill RM, Buelow B, Mather C, et al. Hepatic small vessel neoplasm, a rare infiltrative vascular neoplasm of uncertain malignant potential. Hum Pathol. 2016;54:143–51.
107. Joseph NM, Brunt EM, Marginean C, et al. Frequent GNAQ and GNA14 mutations in hepatic small vessel neoplasm. Am J Surg Pathol. 2018;42:1201–7.
108. Walcott-Sapp S, Tang E, Kakar S, et al. Resection of the largest reported hepatic small vessel neoplasm. Hum Pathol. 2018;78:159–62.
109. Di Renzo C, D'Amico F, Finotti M, et al. A novel entity among vascular liver tumours: the first reported liver transplantation. Is it feasible? Transplant Proc. 2021;53:1690–3.
110. Lazăr DC, Avram MF, Romoşan I, et al. Malignant hepatic vascular tumours in adults: characteristics, diagnostic difficulties and current management. World J Clin Oncol. 2019;10:110–35.
111. Ishak KG. Mesenchymal tumour of the liver. In: Okuda K, RLP, editors. Hepatocellular carcinoma. New York: John Wiley & Sons; 1976. p. 247–308.
112. Li DB, Si XY, Wan T, Zhou YM. A pooled analysis of treatment and prognosis of hepatic angiosarcoma in adults. Hepatobiliary Pancreat Dis Int. 2018;17:198–2036.
113. Hwang S, Lee SG, Lee YJ, et al. Prognostic impact of sarcomatous change of hepatocellular carcinoma in patients undergoing liver resection and liver transplantation. J Gastrointest Surg. 2008;12:718–24.
114. Nishi H, Taguchi K, Asayama Y, et al. Sarcomatous hepatocellular carcinoma: a special reference to ordinary hepatocellular carcinoma. J Gastroenterol Hepatol. 2003;18:415–23.
115. Kaneko J, Sugawara Y, Togashi J, et al. Sarcomatous change of hepatocellular carcinoma in a patient undergoing living donor liver transplantation. Biosci Trends. 2010;4:279–82.
116. Sapisochin G, Fidelman N, Roberts JP, Yao FY. Mixed hepatocellular cholangiocarcinoma and intrahepatic cholangiocarcinoma in patients undergoing transplantation for hepatocellular carcinoma. Liver Transpl. 2011;17:934–42.
117. Park SE, Lee SH, Yang JD, et al. Clinicopathological characteristics and prognostic factors in combined hepatocellular carcinoma and cholangiocarcinoma. Korean J Hepatobiliary Pancreat Surg. 2013;17:152–6.
118. Bruix J, Sherman M. Management of hepatocellular carcinoma: an update. Hepatology. 2011;53:1020–2.
119. Garcez-Silva MH, Gonzalez AM, Moura RA, Linhares MM, Lanzoni VP, Trivino T. Carcinosarcoma of the liver: a case report. Transplant Proc. 2006;38:1918–9.
120. Orlando G, Lai Q, Lerut J. Composite hepatocellular and haemangiosarcomatous tumour: the prognosis is determined by the sarcomatous component. Hepatobiliary Pancreat Dis Int. 2019. pii: S1499-3872(19)30253-X.
121. Stocker JT, Ishak KG. Undifferentiated (embryonal) sarcoma of the liver: report of 31 cases. Cancer. 1978;42:336–48.
122. Weinberg AG, Finegold MJ. Primary hepatic tumours of childhood. Hum Pathol. 1983;14:512–37.
123. Webber EM, Morrison KB, Pritchard SL, Sorensen PH. Undifferentiated embryonal sarcoma of the liver: results of clinical management in one center. J Pediatr Surg. 1999;34:1641–4.
124. Khan ZH, Ilyas K, Khan HH, et al. Unresectable undifferentiated embryonal sarcoma of the liver in an adult male treated with chemotherapy and orthotopic liver transplantation. Cureus. 2017;9:e1759.
125. Wei ZG, Tang LF, Chen ZM, Tang HF, Li MJ. Childhood undifferentiated embryonal liver sarcoma: clinical features and immunohistochemistry analysis. J Pediatr Surg. 2008;43:1912–9.
126. Joshi SW, Merchant NH, Jambhekar NA. Primary multilocular cystic undifferentiated (embryonal) sar-

coma of the liver in childhood resembling hydatid cyst of the liver. Br J Radiol. 1997;70:314–6.
127. Buetow PC, Buck JL, Pantongrag-Brown L, et al. Undifferentiated (embryonal) sarcoma of the liver: pathologic basis of imaging findings in 28 cases. Radiology. 1997;203:779–83.
128. Shehata BM, Gupta NA, Katzenstein HM, et al. Undifferentiated embryonal sarcoma of the liver is associated with mesenchymal hamartoma and multiple chromosomal abnormalities: a review of eleven cases. Pediatr Dev Pathol. 2011;14:111–6.
129. Mathews J, Duncavage EJ, Pfeifer JD. Characterization of translocations in mesenchymal hamartoma and undifferentiated embryonal sarcoma of the liver. Exp Mol Pathol. 2013;95:319–24.
130. Weitz J, Klimstra DS, Cymes K, et al. Management of primary liver sarcomas. Cancer. 2007;109:1391–6.
131. Kim D-Y, Kim K-H, Jung S-E, Lee S-C, Park K-W, Kim W-K. Undifferentiated (embryonal) sarcoma of the liver: combination treatment by surgery and chemotherapy. J Pediatr Surg. 2002;37:1419–23.
132. Lenze F, Birkfellner T, Lenz P, et al. Undifferentiated embryonal sarcoma of the liver in adults. Cancer. 2008;112:2274–82.
133. Otte JB, Aronson D, Vraux H, et al. Preoperative chemotherapy, major liver resection, and transplantation for primary malignancies in children. Transplant Proc. 1996;28:2393–4.
134. Chen LE, Shepherd RW, Nadler ML, Chapman WC, Kotru A, Lowell JA. Liver transplantation and chemotherapy in children with unresectable primary hepatic malignancies: development of a management algorithm. J Pediatr Gastroenterol Nutr. 2006;43:487–93.
135. Okajima H, Ohya Y, Lee KJ, et al. Management of undifferentiated sarcoma of the liver including living donor liver transplantation as a backup procedure. J Pediatr Surg. 2009;44:e33–8.
136. Kelly MJ, Martin L, Alonso M, Altura RA. Liver transplant for relapsed undifferentiated embryonal sarcoma in a young child. J Pediatr Surg. 2009;44:e1–3.
137. Dhanasekaran R, Hemming A, Salazar E, Cabrera R. Rare case of adult undifferentiated (embryonal) sarcoma of the liver treated with liver transplantation: excellent long-term survival. Case Rep Hepatol. 2012;2012:519741.
138. Plant AS, Busuttil RW, Rana A, Nelson SD, Auerbach M, Federman NC. A single-institution retrospective cases series of childhood undifferentiated embryonal liver sarcoma (UELS): success of combined therapy and the use of orthotopic liver transplant. J Pediatr Hematol Oncol. 2013;35:451–5.
139. Ismail H, Dembowska-Bagińska B, Broniszczak D, et al. Treatment of undifferentiated embryonal sarcoma of the liver in children—single center experience. J Pediatr Surg. 2013;48:2202–6.
140. Walther A, Geller J, Coots A, et al. Multimodal therapy including liver transplantation for hepatic undifferentiated embryonal sarcoma. Liver Transpl. 2014;20:191–9.
141. Schluckebier D, McLin VA, Kanavaki I, Ansari M, Wildhaber BE. The role of liver transplantation in undifferentiated embryonal sarcoma of the liver in children. J Pediatr Hematol Oncol. 2016;38:495–6.
142. Techavichit P, Masand PM, Himes RW, et al. Undifferentiated embryonal sarcoma of the liver: a single-center experience and review of the literature. J Pediatr Hematol Oncol. 2016;38:261–8.
143. Shi Y, Rojas Y, Zhang W, et al. Characteristics and outcomes in children with undifferentiated embryonal sarcoma of the liver: a report from the National Cancer Database. Pediatr Blood Cancer. 2017;64:e26272.
144. Lerut J, Iesari S, Inostroza Núñez ME, et al. Adult-to-adult living-donor liver transplantation: the experience of the Université catholique de Louvain. Hepatobiliary Pancreat Dis Int. 2019;18:132–42.
145. Vinayak R, Cruz RJ Jr, Ranganathan S, et al. Paediatric liver transplantation for hepatocellular cancer and rare liver malignancies: US multicenter and single-center experience (1981–2015). Liver Transpl. 2017;23:1577–88.
146. Wu Z, Wei Y, Cai Z, Zhou Y. Long-term survival outcomes of undifferentiated embryonal sarcoma of the liver: a pooled analysis of 308 patients. ANZ J Surg. 2020;90:1615–20.
147. Babu BI, Bigam DL, Gilmour SM, et al. Liver transplantation in locally unresectable, undifferentiated embryonal cell sarcoma. Transplant Direct. 2021;7:e654.
148. Okazaki M, Tajima H, Ohbatake Y, et al. Pleomorphic rhabdomyosarcoma of the liver in an adult: a rare case report. BMC Surg. 2020;20:81.
149. Nakamura H, Koyanagi Y, Kitamura M, et al. Primary epithelioid rhabdomyosarcoma of the liver: case report of an unusual histological variant. Int J Surg Pathol. 2022;30:331–4.
150. Alhashem F, Yilmaz E, Ozdemir MA, et al. Biliary rhabdomyosarcoma in an infant male with neurofibromatosis type 1. J Pediatr Hematol Oncol. 2019;41:e24–6.
151. Guérin F, Minard-Colin TRV, Gaze MN, et al. Outcome of localized liver-bile duct rhabdomyosarcoma according to local therapy: a report from the European Paediatric Soft-Tissue Sarcoma Study Group (EpSSG)-RMS 2005 study. Pediatr Blood Cancer. 2019;66:e27725.
152. Perruccio K, Cecinati V, Scagnellato A, et al. Biliary tract rhabdomyosarcoma: a report from the Soft Tissue Sarcoma Committee of the Associazione Italiana Ematologia Oncologia Paediatrica. Tumori J. 2018;104:232–7.
153. Urla C, Warmann SW, Sparber-Sauer M, et al. Treatment and outcome of the patients with rhabdomyosarcoma of the biliary tree: experience of

the Cooperative Weichteilsarkom Studiengruppe (CWS). BMC Cancer. 2019;19:945.
154. Vaarwerk B, van der Lee JH, Breunis WB, et al. Prognostic relevance of early radiologic response to induction chemotherapy in paediatric rhabdomyosarcoma: a report from the International Society of Paediatric Oncology Malignant Mesenchymal Tumour 95 Study. Cancer. 2018;124:1016–24.
155. Paganelli M, Beaunoyer M, Samson Y, et al. A child with unresectable biliary rhabdomyosarcoma: 48-month disease-free survival after liver transplantation. Pediatr Transplant. 2014;18:E146–51.
156. Shen CH, Dong KR, Tao YF, et al. Liver transplantation for biliary rhabdomyosarcoma with liver metastasis: report of one case. Transplant Proc. 2017;49:185–7.
157. Apestegui CA, Julliard O, Ciccarelli O, et al. Energy drinks: another red flag for the liver allograft. Liver Transpl. 2011;17:1117–8.
158. Namgoong JM, Hwang S, Park GC, et al. Paediatric living donor liver transplantation for biliary embryonal rhabdomyosarcoma: a case report of a case showing disease-free survival over 2 years. Korean J Transplant. 2022;36:148–53.
159. Schettini AV, Coubeau L, Mazzeo F, Lerut J. Leiomyosarcoma of the inferior vena cava level II including both renal veins: surgical approach. Acta Chir Belg. 2015;115:96–8164.
160. Gaignard E, Bergeat D, Stock N, et al. Portal vein leiomyosarcoma: a rare case of hepatic hilar tumour with review of the literature. Indian J Cancer. 2019;56:83–5.
161. Tzedakis S, Heithem Jeddou H, Triki H, et al. Right hepatectomy with vascular and biliary reconstruction for a portal vein leiomyosarcoma. Ann Surg Oncol. 2021;28:1699.
162. Coubeau L, Rico Juri JM, Ciccarelli O, et al. The use of autologous peritoneum for complete caval replacement following resection of major intra-abdominal malignancies. World J Surg. 2017;41:1005–11.
163. Feretis T, Kostakis ID, Damaskos C, et al. Primary hepatic leiomyosarcoma: a case report and review of the literature. Acta Med (Hradec Kralove). 2018;61:153–7.
164. Vella S, Cortis K, Pisani D, et al. Case of primary hepatic leiomyosarcoma successfuly treated with laparoscopic right hepatectomy. BMJ Case Rep. 2020;13:e233567.
165. Calne RY, Williams R. Orthotopic liver transplantation: the first 60 patients. Br Med J. 1977;1:471–6.
166. Saint-Paul MC, Gugenheim J, Hofman P, et al. Leiomyosarcoma of the liver: a case treated by transplantation. Gastroenterol Clin Biol. 1993;17:218–22. French.
167. Liang X, Xiao-Min S, Jiang-Ping X, et al. Liver transplantation for primary hepatic leiomyosarcoma: a case report and review of the literatures. Med Oncol. 2010;27:1269–72.
168. Xie P, Zhuang H. FDG PET/CT findings of primary hepatic leiomyosarcoma in an immunocompetent pediatric patient. Clin Nucl Med. 2017;42:323–4.
169. Gunasekaran V, Rammohan A, Reddy SM, Rela M. Liver transplantation for inferior vena cava leiomyosarcoma: from a Maslow's hammer to the Occam's razor. BMJ Case Rep. 2018;2018:bcr2018225827.
170. Nelson V, Fernandes NF, Wool GM, et al. Primary liposarcoma of the liver a case report and review of the literature. Arch Pathol Lab Med. 2001;125:410–2.
171. Liu W, Liang W, Peng Z, et al. Positron emission tomography/computed tomography manifestations of primary hepatic myxoid liposarcoma. A case report. Medicine. 2018;97(39):e12307.

8 Caroli's Disease

Kevin Ka-Wan Chu and Jin He

8.1 Introduction

Caroli's disease is a rare congenital hepatobiliary disease, characterized by macroscopic, multifocal, saccular, or segmental dilatation of intrahepatic bile ducts. It was named after a French physician, Jacques Caroli, in 1958 [1]. Two varieties were described: a pure form (Caroli's disease) characterized by ectasias of the intrahepatic bile ducts without further histological abnormalities and a combined form (Caroli's syndrome) in which Caroli's disease is associated with peripor-

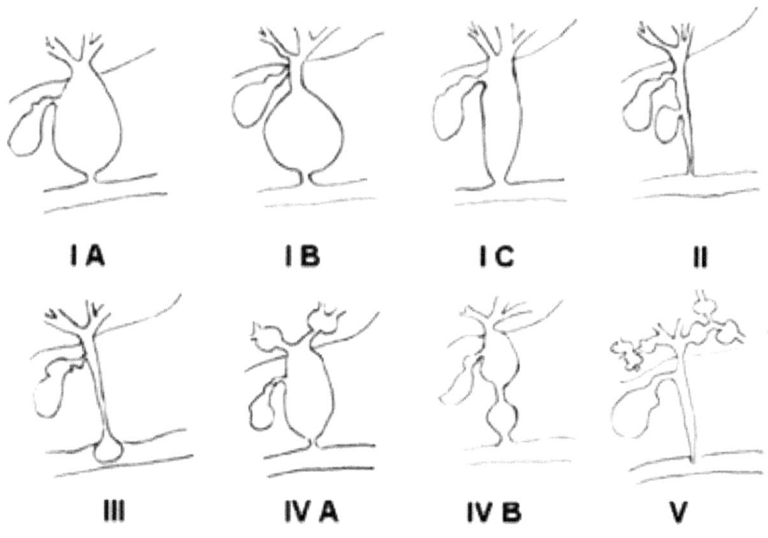

Fig. 8.1 Todani classification of choledochal cysts: types I–IV and type V. Caroli's disease featured with saccular dilatation of intrahepatic bile ducts

K. K.-W. Chu
Department of Surgery, Queen Mary Hospital, The University of Hong Kong, Hong Kong, China

J. He (✉)
Department of Surgery, Johns Hopkins University School of Medicine, Baltimore, MD, USA
e-mail: jhe11@jhmi.edu

T. Hackert, A. Gulla (eds.), *Rare Liver and Biliary Tract Diseases*,
https://doi.org/10.1007/978-3-032-15076-9_8

tal fibrosis corresponding to congenital hepatic fibrosis [2]. Both of them were described as distinct entities in 1964 [3]. They also correspond to the type V choledochal cyst, as classified by Todani [4] (Fig. 8.1).

8.2 Embryology of Intrahepatic Bile Duct Disease

Caroli's disease was believed to involve a total or partial arrest of the remodeling of the ductal plate of the larger intrahepatic bile ducts, which was a form of ductal plate malformation [5]. During the fourth week of human gestation, the liver arises as a bud of cells (hepatic diverticulum) from the ventral wall of the most cephalad portion of the foregut [5]. Bile duct formation in the developing liver begins around the eighth gestational week. The intrahepatic biliary system is believed to derive from hepatocyte precursor cells, which transform into ductules and ducts to join the extrahepatic biliary bud at the hilum [6]. In the simple variety (Caroli's disease), the abnormality consists of moniliform or saccular dilatation of the larger intrahepatic ducts, with predominant involvement of segmental ducts [3]. The dilated parts are in continuity with the rest of the biliary system and contain bile. The dilatations of the ducts are a predisposing factor in the stagnation of bile and, in this way, are the root of biliary sludge formation and intraductal lithiasis, which are often complicated by superimposed infection. In the combined form of Caroli's syndrome, the abnormalities of the larger ducts are associated with lesions of congenital hepatic fibrosis. These two varieties may occur in the same family, and both are inherited in an autosomal recessive manner and associated with kidney abnormalities corresponding to autosomal recessive polycystic kidney disease [3]. However, the exact cause of Caroli's disease remains unknown. Most authors believe the two variants are one disease with different stages and associated with the autosomal recessive polycystic kidney disease [7].

8.3 Incidence

Most early literature only contained case reports. Systematic reviews, including up to more than 500 patients, have been published recently [8]. However, the true incidence of Caroli's disease remains unknown. Due to its rarity, it is estimated to have a prevalence of one in 1,000,000 [9]. Males and females are equally affected, and more than 80% of patients present before 30 years of age [10].

8.4 Clinical Presentation

Bile ductal plate malformation starts in the intrauterine period, and the biliary tract is continuously destroyed over decades [5, 11]. Patients with Caroli's disease can be asymptomatic for the first 5–20 years, or symptoms can occur infrequently throughout their life [12]. It was reported that 14% of patients could be diagnosed during a routine health examination. On the other hand, patients could develop symptoms of Charcot's triad (cholangitis), including upper abdominal discomfort, jaundice, and fever. Other manifestations can include weight loss, anorexia, nausea, vomiting, pancreatitis, and biliary colic.

As intrahepatic ductal dilatation predisposes to the stagnation of bile flow and stone formation, cholangitis is the main mode of presentation, reported in 64% of patients [13]. In Caroli's syndrome, cystic biliary disease coexists with congenital or primary hepatic fibrosis. Clinical presentations of hepatic insufficiency and portal hypertension can develop, including splenomegaly, ascites, peripheral edema, coagulopathy, and esophageal varices [14, 15].

With recurrent episodes of cholangitis and the development of biliary stones, malignant transformation could happen. The risk of developing intrahepatic cholangiocarcinoma in Caroli's disease or Caroli's syndrome increased 100-fold compared with healthy individuals [16]. Although the mechanism of carcinogenesis is unknown, postulated theories include the carcinogenic component of bile during prolonged biliary stasis, permanent stone irritation and formation of carcinogens [17], and cellular predisposition for the neoplastic change of congenital cystic formation of the biliary tract [16].

Despite the known carcinogenic tendency of Caroli's disease, preoperative diagnosis of malignant transformation is difficult; the diagnosis is typically made during pathological examination of the surgical specimen and, less commonly, in preoperative liver biopsy. An overall incidence of 6.6% of malignant transformation for Caroli's disease or Caroli's syndrome, more likely in older patients, was reported [8].

8.5 Clinical Investigations

Caroli's disease or Caroli's syndrome has no pathognomic clinical symptoms or signs [18]. The cardinal step to achieve a diagnosis is a cholangiogram of typical appearance, showing multifocal segmental dilatation. A cholangiogram can be obtained with different techniques, namely, endoscopic retrograde cholangiopancreatography (ERCP), magnetic resonance cholangiopancreatography (MRCP), or percutaneous transhepatic cholangiography (PTC). Most patients can have the diagnosis established by combining ultrasonography, computed tomography (CT) studies, and cholangiogram. CT scan shows central dot signs in Caroli's disease patients. The fibrovascular bundles containing portal vein pedicles and the hepatic artery bridging the saccule appear as central dots or linear streaks. The central dot sign described on CT could also be demonstrated on ultrasonography (Fig. 8.2). ERCP or PTC are considered to be a direct cholangiography but with potential serious complications, such as sepsis, bile leakage, pancreatitis, bleeding, and death. These complications were reported with an overall incidence of approximately 3%, while the noninvasive alternative would be MRCP [19].

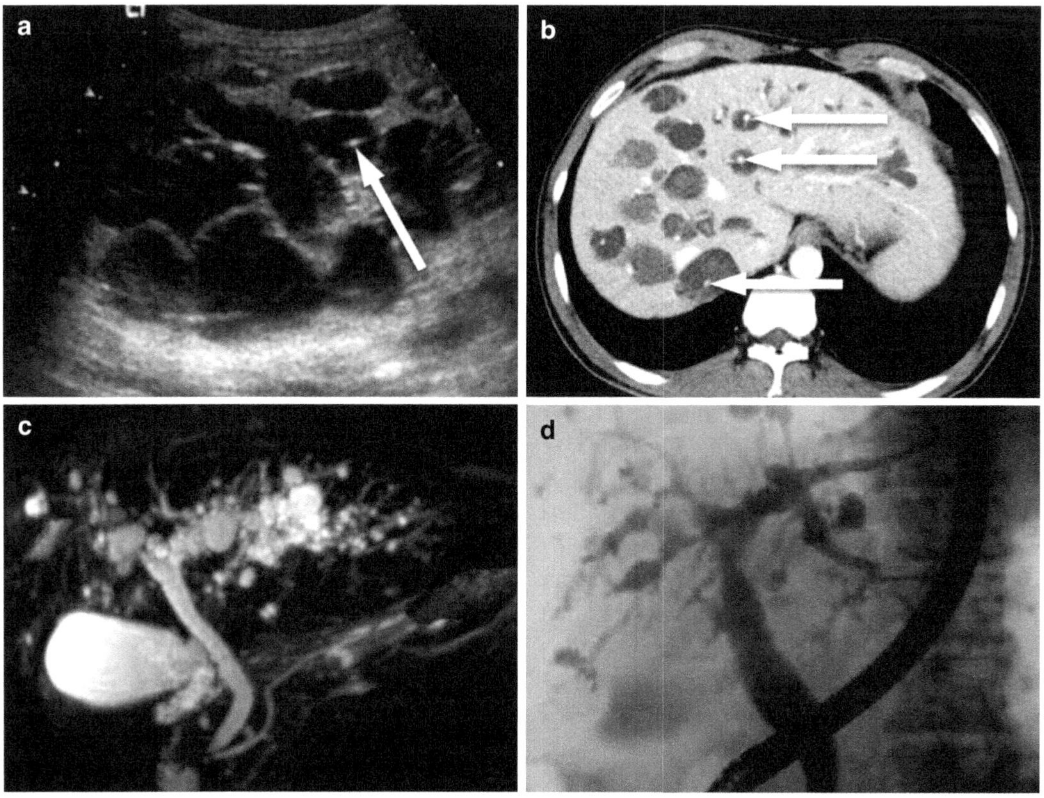

Fig. 8.2 Typical imaging findings of Caroli's disease. (**a**) Ultrasonography with central dot sign. (**b**) Central dot sign in computed tomography. (**c**) Magnetic resonance cholangiopancreatography (MRCP). (**d**) Endoscopic retrograde cholangiopancreatography (ERCP)

As liver resection and liver transplantation are the potential surgical treatment options for Caroli's disease [19], treatment-specific workup may be relevant. For liver resection, indocyanine green retention test [20] and liver volumetry for future liver remnant [21] should be included as pre-resection workup to reduce post-hepatectomy liver failure, while cardiac workup and malignancy screening may be relevant for liver transplantation.

Prenatal diagnosis of Caroli's disease was reported, though uncommon [22–24]. A detailed investigation should be prompted because of cystic liver masses detected by routine prenatal ultrasound at the second or third trimester. Mutation screening was reported in one of the studies for the family and was concluded to be consistent with a recessive pattern of inheritance [23]. However, investigation at the genetic level is still in the stage of academic interest.

8.6 Differential Diagnosis

Caroli's disease could sometimes be confused with other diseases that demonstrate abnormal liver function and imaging findings of cystic lesions in the liver. The differential diagnosis for patients exhibiting the symptoms of Caroli's disease is broad and includes but is not limited to primary sclerosing cholangitis, recurrent pyogenic cholangitis, polycystic liver disease, choledochal cysts, biliary papillomatosis, and, occasionally, obstructive biliary dilatation, biliary hamartomas, etc.

Primary sclerosing cholangitis (PSC) is a chronic disease characterized by inflammation and scarring of bile ducts. Seventy percent of individuals with PSC also have inflammatory bowel disease, most often ulcerative colitis [25]. Historically, a cholangiogram would be obtained via ERCP, which typically reveals "beading" (alternating strictures and dilatation) of intra- or extrahepatic bile ducts. Currently, the preferred option for diagnostic cholangiography is MRCP because of its strength of high spatial resolution. Caroli's disease can be distinguished from PSC through imaging findings (CT, MRCP, or cholangiography) because of the difference in ductal dilatation. PSC is isolated and fusiform, while Caroli's disease is saccular and segmental. Most patients with PSC have evidence of autoantibodies and abnormal immunoglobulin levels, including antineutrophil cytoplasmic antibodies (ANCAs), antinuclear antibodies (ANAs), and anti-smooth muscle antibodies (ASMAs) [26].

Polycystic liver disease is commonly seen in association with autosomal dominant polycystic kidney disease, with a prevalence of 1 in 400–1000, and accounts for 8–10% of all cases of end-stage renal disease [27]. The cysts rarely communicate with bile ducts and typically appear as multiple homogeneous and hypodense lesions with a regular outline on CT and without wall or content enhancement on contrast-enhanced image. At the same time, Caroli's disease is related to autosomal recessive polycystic kidney disease.

Recurrent pyogenic cholangitis (RPC), also known as Hong Kong disease, Oriental cholangitis, and Oriental infestational cholangitis, is a chronic infection characterized by recurrent bouts of bacterial cholangitis, with primary hepatolithiasis [28]. Cholangiography could be diagnostic with a typical arrow sign [29]. Other key cholangiographic features of recurrent pyogenic cholangitis include dilated common bile duct and hepatic ducts, intrahepatic biliary calculi, and preferential involvement of the left lateral section [30].

Choledochal cysts are congenital conditions involving cystic dilatation of the bile duct. They are uncommon in Western countries but not as rare in East Asian nations [31]. Choledochal cyst is frequently associated (64%) with the anomalous union of pancreaticobiliary duct (AUPBD), and AUPBD has been regarded to be the etiological factor for choledochal cysts. AUPBD was found only in types I and IV, according to Todani's classification of choledochal cysts [32]. Although Todani included Caroli's disease in the classification, they are often regarded as two diagnostic identities [33].

In any case of diagnostic difficulty, histopathologic examination of the liver tissue would be the gold standard. Features of Caroli disease include intensive portal fibrosis, numerous ductal plate remnants, hyperplastic and dilated bile ducts and cholestasis, and foci of microabscesses [34]. The pathological finding of congenital hepatic fibrosis and proliferative dilated bile ducts suggested the diagnosis of Caroli's syndrome [35].

8.7 Treatment

No guidelines exist for Caroli's disease, and given the scarcity of case reports, there are no randomized trials on different treatment modalities. The treatment of Caroli's disease depends on the clinical features and the location of the biliary abnormalities (Fig. 8.3). The proposed therapy should be tailored to individual patients and be contingent on clinical presentation, the site of lesions, and the extent of biliary abnormality. The major aim of medical therapy for Caroli's disease is to reduce and treat the severity of recurrent cholangitis, hepatic abscess, and biliary obstruction. Episodes of cholangitis require treatment with antibiotics and relief of biliary obstruction. Ursodeoxycholic acid is a useful treatment for hepatolithiasis [36]. Endoscopic treatment with sphincterotomy, extraction of intrahepatic and common bile duct calculi, and stent insertion into the affected ducts helps in the resolution of the bile duct condition [37]. Therapeutic interventional radiologists can help in bile drainage and hepatolithiasis removal [19]. Liver resection could be contemplated if patients present with a relatively spared part of healthy liver. For example, if the main disease is localized in the right lobe and the remnant left lobe is sizable, right hepatectomy, with or without hepaticojejunostomy, could be contemplated. Orthotopic liver transplantation should be considered in patients with a diffuse form of the disease, causing frequent cholangitis or secondary biliary cirrhosis [38].

8.8 Surgical Planning and Management

Different forms of hepatectomy were reported for localized Caroli's disease [19]. A high-quality cholangiogram is critical for planning any surgical treatment. ERCP and MRCP are useful to demonstrate the communication between the saccular ectasia and the normal biliary tract. Liver resection follows the basic principle of surgery. The patients have to be fully assessed for performance status and anesthesiology fitness. Assessment of the size and function of the future liver remnant is critical. Caroli's syndrome patients may have different degrees of liver fibrosis and cirrhosis. It is important that patients with poor liver function reserve should not receive excessive removal of the liver parenchyma in order to avoid postoperative liver failure [39]. Indocyanine green retention rate at 15 min is recommended for a safe major and minor hepatectomy at 14% and 22%, respectively. Liver volumetry is most commonly estimated with 3D

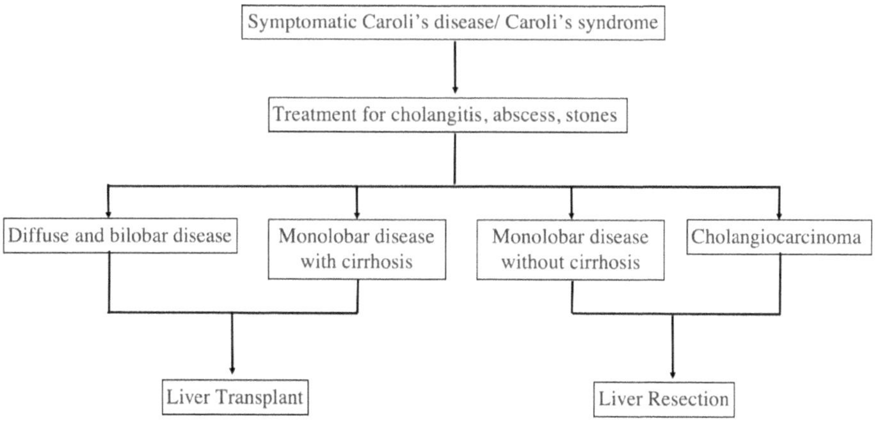

Fig. 8.3 Treatment algorithm for Caroli's disease or syndrome

volume CT calculation. The critical residual liver volume for patients with a normal liver has been reported to be 20–30%, according to different studies [40–43].

For patients with multilobar disease, together with hepatic cirrhosis, liver transplantation should be considered. And for patients with autosomal recessive polycystic kidney disease with indication, combined liver–kidney transplantation may be the option [44]. Careful malignancy screening is also essential, as Caroli's disease could be associated with cholangiocarcinoma. Despite most cholangiocarcinomas associated with Caroli disease being diagnosed in the early stage, the 3-year survival is only 30% [45]. Better results could be achieved with a more stringent protocol, and the 5-year survival rate could reach 73% if only tumors smaller than 2 cm are included [46].

The long-term outcome of the diffuse form of Caroli disease is poor, even after major hepatectomy. The lack of therapeutic means to prevent a recurrence of cholangitis is considered to be the main reason [47]. Due to the rarity of the disease, large series and outcome reporting of Caroli disease are scarce. One study that included 155 patients was the largest cohort for surgical outcomes. They reported no postoperative mortality after liver resection, 15.3% with grade 3 or higher postoperative morbidity, and 88.5% 5-year overall survival [48]. However, for patients with coexistent cholangiocarcinoma, the outcome was dismal, with only 33.3% 1-year survival being reported.

Contrary to liver resection, liver transplantation is a curative therapy for Caroli disease with a slightly higher reported morbidity (39% major complications) [48]. Patient series with combined liver and kidney transplants have also been reported [11]. At the same time, the American United Network for Organ Sharing/Organ Procurement and Transplantation Network and the European Liver Transplant Registry provided data for surgical outcomes after liver transplant. Excellent results with 80.9% 5-year patient survival and 70.6% 5-year graft survival could be achieved [49, 50]. Due to their low priority on the waiting list for liver transplant, patients might benefit from living-donor liver transplantation, with shorter waiting times and fewer cumulative episodes of septic complications [44].

8.9 Follow-Up

Purposeful follow-up and surveillance of patients with Caroli's disease after surgery is important. For patients who have undergone resection, recurrent biliary sepsis, development of cholangiocarcinoma in the remnant liver, and progression of liver cirrhosis are the key events to be picked up. Among these adverse events, recurrence of cholangitis is common and often hard to control without therapeutic means to prevent it from happening [19]. While tumor markers such as Cancer Antigen 19-9 (CA19-9) can be used to detect cancer, false elevation of CA19–9 can be caused by local cholestasis with hyperbilirubinemia [51].

References

1. Caroli J, Soupault R, Kossakowski J, Plocker L, Paradowska. Congenital polycystic dilation of the intrahepatic bile ducts; attempt at classification. La semaine des hopitaux: organe fonde par l'Association d'enseignement medical des hopitaux de Paris. 1958;34(8/2):488–95/SP.
2. Mall JC, Ghahremani GG, Boyer JL. Caroli's disease associated with congenital hepatic fibrosis and renal tubular ectasia. A case report. Gastroenterology. 1974;66(5):1029–35.
3. Caroli J, Corcos V. Congenital dilatation of the intrahepatic bile ducts. Rev Med Chir Mal Foie. 1964;39:1–70.
4. Todani T, Watanabe Y, Narusue M, Tabuchi K, Okajima K. Congenital bile duct cysts: classification, operative procedures, and review of thirty-seven cases including cancer arising from choledochal cyst. Am J Surg. 1977;134(2):263–9. https://doi.org/10.1016/0002-9610(77)90359-2.
5. Desmet VJ. Congenital diseases of intrahepatic bile ducts: variations on the theme "ductal plate malformation". Hepatology. 1992;16(4):1069–83. https://doi.org/10.1002/hep.1840160434.
6. Blankenberg TA, Lund JK, Ruebner BH. Normal and abnormal development of human intrahepatic bile ducts. An immunohistochemical perspective. Perspect Pediatr Pathol. 1991;14:143–67.
7. Taylor AC, Palmer KR. Caroli's disease. Eur J Gastroenterol Hepatol. 1998;10(2):105–8. https://doi.org/10.1097/00042737-199802000-00001.

8. Fahrner R, Dennler SG, Inderbitzin D. Risk of malignancy in Caroli disease and syndrome: a systematic review. World J Gastroenterol. 2020;26(31):4718–28. https://doi.org/10.3748/wjg.v26.i31.4718.
9. Acevedo E, Lainez SS, Caceres Cano PA, Vivar D. Caroli's syndrome: an early presentation. Cureus. 2020;12(10):e11029. https://doi.org/10.7759/cureus.11029.
10. Habib S, Shakil O, Couto OF, Demetris AJ, Fung JJ, Marcos A, et al. Caroli's disease and orthotopic liver transplantation. Liver Transpl. 2006;12(3):416–21. https://doi.org/10.1002/lt.20719.
11. Millwala F, Segev DL, Thuluvath PJ. Caroli's disease and outcomes after liver transplantation. Liver Transpl. 2008;14(1):11–7. https://doi.org/10.1002/lt.21366.
12. Wu KL, Changchien CS, Kuo CM, Chuah SK, Chiu YC, Kuo CH. Caroli's disease - a report of two siblings. Eur J Gastroenterol Hepatol. 2002;14(12):1397–9. https://doi.org/10.1097/00042737-200212000-00019.
13. Giovanardi RO. Monolobar Caroli's disease in an adult. Case report. Hepatogastroenterology. 2003;50(54):2185–7.
14. Ananthakrishnan AN, Saeian K. Caroli's disease: identification and treatment strategy. Curr Gastroenterol Rep. 2007;9(2):151–5. https://doi.org/10.1007/s11894-007-0010-7.
15. Yonem O, Bayraktar Y. Clinical characteristics of Caroli's syndrome. World J Gastroenterol. 2007;13(13):1934–7. https://doi.org/10.3748/wjg.v13.i13.1934.
16. Dayton MT, Longmire WP Jr, Tompkins RK. Caroli's disease: a premalignant condition? Am J Surg. 1983;145(1):41–8. https://doi.org/10.1016/0002-9610(83)90164-2.
17. Flanigan DP. Biliary carcinoma associated with biliary cysts. Cancer. 1977;40(2):880–3. https://doi.org/10.1002/1097-0142(197708)40:2<880::aid-cncr2820400242>3.0.co;2-x.
18. Wang ZX, Li YG, Wang RL, Li YW, Li ZY, Wang LF, et al. Clinical classification of Caroli's disease: an analysis of 30 patients. HPB (Oxford). 2015;17(3):278–83. https://doi.org/10.1111/hpb.12330.
19. Kassahun WT, Kahn T, Wittekind C, Mossner J, Caca K, Hauss J, et al. Caroli's disease: liver resection and liver transplantation. Experience in 33 patients. Surgery. 2005;138(5):888–98. https://doi.org/10.1016/j.surg.2005.05.002.
20. Cheung TT, Chan SC, Chok KS, Chan AC, Yu WC, Poon RT, et al. Rapid measurement of indocyanine green retention by pulse spectrophotometry: a validation study in 70 patients with Child-Pugh A cirrhosis before hepatectomy for hepatocellular carcinoma. Hepatobiliary Pancreat Dis Int. 2012;11(3):267–71. https://doi.org/10.1016/s1499-3872(12)60159-3.
21. Shirabe K, Shimada M, Gion T, Hasegawa H, Takenaka K, Utsunomiya T, et al. Postoperative liver failure after major hepatic resection for hepatocellular carcinoma in the modern era with special reference to remnant liver volume. J Am Coll Surg. 1999;188(3):304–9. https://doi.org/10.1016/s1072-7515(98)00301-9.
22. Stringer MD, Dhawan A, Davenport M, Mieli-Vergani G, Mowat AP, Howard ER. Choledochal cysts: lessons from a 20 year experience. Arch Dis Child. 1995;73(6):528–31. https://doi.org/10.1136/adc.73.6.528.
23. Sgro M, Rossetti S, Barozzino T, Toi A, Langer J, Harris PC, et al. Caroli's disease: prenatal diagnosis, postnatal outcome and genetic analysis. Ultrasound Obstet Gynecol. 2004;23(1):73–6. https://doi.org/10.1002/uog.943.
24. Bratu I, Laberge JM, Khalife S, Sinsky A. Regression of antenatally diagnosed localized Caroli's disease. J Pediatr Surg. 2000;35(9):1390–3. https://doi.org/10.1053/jpsu.2000.9349.
25. Mertz A, Nguyen NA, Katsanos KH, Kwok RM. Primary sclerosing cholangitis and inflammatory bowel disease comorbidity: an update of the evidence. Ann Gastroenterol. 2019;32(2):124–33. https://doi.org/10.20524/aog.2019.0344.
26. Tabibian JH, Enders F, Imam MH, Kolar G, Lindor KD, Talwalkar JA. Association between serum IgE level and adverse clinical endpoints in primary sclerosing cholangitis. Ann Hepatol. 2014;13(3):384–9.
27. Zhang ZY, Wang ZM, Huang Y. Polycystic liver disease: classification, diagnosis, treatment process, and clinical management. World J Hepatol. 2020;12(3):72–83. https://doi.org/10.4254/wjh.v12.i3.72.
28. Tsui WM, Chan YK, Wong CT, Lo YF, Yeung YW, Lee YW. Hepatolithiasis and the syndrome of recurrent pyogenic cholangitis: clinical, radiologic, and pathologic features. Semin Liver Dis. 2011;31(1):33–48. https://doi.org/10.1055/s-0031-1272833.
29. Co M, Pang SY, Wong KY, Ip WK, Yuen WK. Surgical management of recurrent pyogenic cholangitis: 10 years of experience in a tertiary referral centre in Hong Kong. HPB (Oxford). 2014;16(8):776–80. https://doi.org/10.1111/hpb.12185.
30. Lee KH, Ho YC. The arrowhead appearance of bile ducts in recurrent pyogenic cholangitis. Abdom Radiol. 2017;42(12):2964–5. https://doi.org/10.1007/s00261-017-1234-0.
31. Liu YB, Wang JW, Devkota KR, Ji ZL, Li JT, Wang XA, et al. Congenital choledochal cysts in adults: twenty-five-year experience. Chin Med J. 2007;120(16):1404–7.
32. Song HK, Kim MH, Myung SJ, Lee SK, Kim HJ, Yoo KS, et al. Choledochal cyst associated the with anomalous union of pancreaticobiliary duct (AUPBD) has a more grave clinical course than choledochal cyst alone. Korean J Intern Med. 1999;14(2):1–8. https://doi.org/10.3904/kjim.1999.14.2.1.
33. Visser BC, Suh I, Way LW, Kang SM. Congenital choledochal cysts in adults. Arch Surg. 2004;139(8):855–60. discussion 60–2. https://doi.org/10.1001/archsurg.139.8.855.

34. Mavlikeev M, Titova A, Saitburkhanova R, Abyzova M, Sayfutdinov I, Gizzatullina N, et al. Caroli syndrome: a clinical case with detailed histopathological analysis. Clin J Gastroenterol. 2019;12(2):106–11. https://doi.org/10.1007/s12328-018-0917-6.
35. Nakanuma Y, Terada T, Ohta G, Kurachi M, Matsubara F. Caroli's disease in congenital hepatic fibrosis and infantile polycystic disease. Liver. 1982;2(4):346–54. https://doi.org/10.1111/j.1600-0676.1982.tb00833.x.
36. Ros E, Navarro S, Bru C, Gilabert R, Bianchi L, Bruguera M. Ursodeoxycholic acid treatment of primary hepatolithiasis in Caroli's syndrome. Lancet. 1993;342(8868):404–6. https://doi.org/10.1016/0140-6736(93)92817-d.
37. Ciambotti GF, Ravi J, Abrol RP, Arya V. Right-sided monolobar Caroli's disease with intrahepatic stones: nonsurgical management with ERCP. Gastrointest Endosc. 1994;40(6):761–4.
38. Schiano TD, Fiel MI, Miller CM, Bodenheimer HC Jr, Min AD. Adult presentation of Caroli's syndrome treated with orthotopic liver transplantation. Am J Gastroenterol. 1997;92(10):1938–40.
39. Fan ST. Liver functional reserve estimation: state of the art and relevance for local treatments: the eastern perspective. J Hepatobiliary Pancreat Sci. 2010;17(4):380–4. https://doi.org/10.1007/s00534-009-0229-9.
40. Abdalla EK, Adam R, Bilchik AJ, Jaeck D, Vauthey JN, Mahvi D. Improving resectability of hepatic colorectal metastases: expert consensus statement. Ann Surg Oncol. 2006;13(10):1271–80. https://doi.org/10.1245/s10434-006-9045-5.
41. Abdalla EK, Barnett CC, Doherty D, Curley SA, Vauthey JN. Extended hepatectomy in patients with hepatobiliary malignancies with and without preoperative portal vein embolization. Arch Surg. 2002;137(6):675–80; discussion 80–1. https://doi.org/10.1001/archsurg.137.6.675.
42. Shoup M, Gonen M, D'Angelica M, Jarnagin WR, DeMatteo RP, Schwartz LH, et al. Volumetric analysis predicts hepatic dysfunction in patients undergoing major liver resection. J Gastrointest Surg. 2003;7(3):325–30. https://doi.org/10.1016/s1091-255x(02)00370-0.
43. Vauthey JN, Chaoui A, Do KA, Bilimoria MM, Fenstermacher MJ, Charnsangavej C, et al. Standardized measurement of the future liver remnant prior to extended liver resection: methodology and clinical associations. Surgery. 2000;127(5):512–9. https://doi.org/10.1067/msy.2000.105294.
44. Lai Q, Lerut J. Proposal for an algorithm for liver transplantation in Caroli's disease and syndrome: putting an uncommon effort into a common task. Clin Transpl. 2016;30(1):3–9. https://doi.org/10.1111/ctr.12640.
45. Casavilla FA, Marsh JW, Iwatsuki S, Todo S, Lee RG, Madariaga JR, et al. Hepatic resection and transplantation for peripheral cholangiocarcinoma. J Am Coll Surg. 1997;185(5):429–36. https://doi.org/10.1016/s1072-7515(97)00088-4.
46. Sapisochin G, Rodriguez de Lope C, Gastaca M, Ortiz de Urbina J, Suarez MA, Santoyo J, et al. "Very early" intrahepatic cholangiocarcinoma in cirrhotic patients: should liver transplantation be reconsidered in these patients? Am J Transplant. 2014;14(3):660–7. https://doi.org/10.1111/ajt.12591.
47. Landen S, Bardaxoglou E, Maddern GJ, Delugeau V, Gosselin M, Launois B. Caroli's disease: a surgical dilemma. Acta Chir Belg. 1993;93(5):224–6.
48. Mabrut JY, Kianmanesh R, Nuzzo G, Castaing D, Boudjema K, Letoublon C, et al. Surgical management of congenital intrahepatic bile duct dilatation, Caroli's disease and syndrome: long-term results of the French Association of Surgery Multicenter Study. Ann Surg. 2013;258(5):713–21; discussion 21. https://doi.org/10.1097/SLA.0000000000000269.
49. Harring TR, Nguyen NT, Liu H, Goss JA, O'Mahony CA. Caroli disease patients have excellent survival after liver transplant. J Surg Res. 2012;177(2):365–72. https://doi.org/10.1016/j.jss.2012.04.022.
50. De Kerckhove L, De Meyer M, Verbaandert C, Mourad M, Sokal E, Goffette P, et al. The place of liver transplantation in Caroli's disease and syndrome. Transpl Int. 2006;19(5):381–8. https://doi.org/10.1111/j.1432-2277.2006.00292.x.
51. Mery CM, Duarte-Rojo A, Paz-Pineda F, Gomez E, Robles-Diaz G. Does cholestasis change the clinical usefulness of CA 19-9 in pacreatobiliary cancer? Rev Investig Clin. 2001;53(6):511–7.

Cryptogenic Cirrhosis

9

Grey Leonard and Perry Shen

9.1 Key Points

- Cryptogenic cirrhosis (CC) is a diagnosis of exclusion.
- The incidence of CC is decreasing over time as alternative diagnoses increase (metabolic-associated steatotic liver disease (MASLD) and autoimmune hepatitis (AIH)).
- Management begins with a thorough diagnostic investigation.
- Treatments and outcomes for CC are broadly similar to other causes of cirrhosis (Table 9.1).

Table 9.1 Possible alternative diagnoses to cryptogenic cirrhosis [1–5]

Metabolic	Nonalcoholic fatty liver disease (NAFLD) Nonalcoholic steatohepatitis (NASH)
Autoimmune	Autoimmune hepatitis (AIH) Primary sclerosing cholangitis (PSC)
Infectious	Hepatitis viruses
Exposure	Alcohol
Rare	Celiac disease Wilson disease Hemochromatosis Alpha-1-antitrypsin deficiency Systemic lupus erythematosus

9.2 Definition

Cryptogenic means "of obscure or unknown origin," and generally, cryptogenic cirrhosis (CC) is described as a diagnosis of exclusion in a patient with cirrhosis. Cirrhosis is a diffuse process characterized by progressive fibrosis and structurally abnormal nodules in the liver [1, 2]. Adding to the confusion, CC has carried several different names, including "nonspecific," "indeterminate," "bland," and "cirrhosis of uncertain cause" [3]. As such, this entity is somewhat dependent upon the extent and sophistication of diagnostic inquiry, including histopathologic examination, antibody testing, viral panels, and exhaustive personal history of alcohol intake, among others. This is complicated further by several studies finding alternative diagnoses using such methods for previously labeled CC cases [2, 3, 6–8]. While the unknown causes of cirrhosis dwindle, the predominant definition remains unchanged, making true CC more distinct from other conditions [9].

9.3 Epidemiology

CC likely represents between 5% and 10% of cirrhosis cases [10] and approximately 4% of liver transplant listings [4]. For a perspective on the evolution of this entity, CC represented 50% of all cirrhosis cases prior to 1965 [2]. In a study by Thuluvath et al. [9], outcomes after liver

G. Leonard
Fort Sanders Regional, Knoxville, TN, USA

P. Shen (✉)
Department of General Surgery, Surgical Oncology Division, Medical Center Boulevard, Winston-Salem, NC, USA
e-mail: Perry.Shen@advocatehealth.org

T. Hackert, A. Gulla (eds.), *Rare Liver and Biliary Tract Diseases*,
https://doi.org/10.1007/978-3-032-15076-9_9

transplant were compared between CC and nonalcoholic steatohepatitis (NASH) cirrhosis. During the study period between 2002 and 2016, the incidence of CC decreased from 8% of listings to 4%, while the NASH listing increased from 1% to 16%. It must be recognized that the incidence of diagnosis of exclusion is contingent upon the frequency of excluded diagnoses. It is likely that the rate of CC will decrease in the future with better diagnostic techniques. For this, some knowledge of alternative causes is necessary.

9.4 Diagnosis of Exclusion

The bulk of the understanding of CC comes from understanding what it is *not*. Seeking an answer to this question, Ayata et al. [11] examined 27 explanted livers between 1983 and 1999 from patients with a diagnosis of CC after transplantation and found that in 85% of this population, a more definite diagnosis was possible. The most common alternative diagnoses included NASH (33%), autoimmune hepatitis AIH (22%), and alcohol abuse (15%). The authors noted that prior to their analysis, 5% of their transplants were of presumed CC, but after analysis, only 0.7% remained truly cryptogenic. More recently, Heringlake et al. [8] examined 126 patients with a diagnosis of CC and reanalyzed each with new clinical, laboratory, and histological data. After discovery of other definitive diagnoses, only 42, exactly one-third, of patients remained cryptogenic. Alternative diagnoses included seronegative autoimmune hepatitis (33%), NASH (17%), and exogenous liver damage (15%). Furthermore, this process was aided without the convenience of an explanted liver to examine. The importance of accurate diagnosis was highlighted in the study by the benefit sustained in the autoimmune group to immunosuppressive therapy, whereas the CC group did not respond. In addition to NASH, AIH, hepatitis viruses, and alcohol, rarer alternatives include celiac disease, Wilson disease, hemochromatosis, alpha-1-antitrypsin disorder, and systemic lupus erythematosus [3]. While these rarer diagnoses must be ruled out, it is important to distinguish CC from NASH cirrhosis, an entity that is quickly rising in proportion.

9.5 Alternatives

Metabolic-associated steatotic liver disease (MASLD) is a subset of nonalcoholic fatty liver disease (NAFLD). NAFLD encompasses nonalcoholic fatty liver (NAFL) and NASH. Metabolic-associated steatotic liver disease (MASLD) is characterized by the presence of steatosis, whereas NASH includes steatosis, in addition to inflammation [12, 13]. NASH categorization has seen the development of several scoring systems to enhance diagnostic accuracy [14, 15]. The disease is typically characterized by >5% of hepatocytes with steatosis, lobular and portal inflammation, cellular ballooning, and various degrees of fibrosis [16]. During the evolution of this disease process, similarities in NASH, both in patient population characteristics and outcomes, have been noted [5, 17].

Caldwell et al. [18], in 1999, examined 70 consecutive patients diagnosed with CC and reevaluated them for alcoholic intake, hepatitis virus exposure, and risk factors for NASH. They compared the CC group with other causes of cirrhosis, including NASH, Hepatitis C virus (HCV), and primary biliary cirrhosis (PBC). They found that CC patients tended to be older and female, with a high propensity for type 2 diabetes mellitus (DM) and/or obesity (73%). This proportion was similar to the NASH group (70%) but different from the HCV (28%) and PBC (33%) cohorts. While rates of metabolic risk factors were similar in the CC and NASH groups, the CC patients were about a decade older (63 vs. 49 years) than the NASH group. This important detail suggests that CC may be a form of late-stage NASH. This is plausible, given the known loss of steatosis and other distinctive histological features occurring within the natural history of NASH [19].

Poonawala et al. [20], in 2000, published a case control study of 65 patients with CC and a Child–Pugh score of at least 7, who were listed for transplant. CC was defined as cirrhosis with "undetermined etiology." They compared this cohort in a 1:2 ratio with other patients from the transplant list, who were age- and gender-matched controls. Consistent with other studies, the authors removed 16 CC patients, who, under further review, were found to have an alternative diagnosis. They found higher rates of obesity (55% vs. 24%), type 2 DM (47% vs. 22%), and obesity with concurrent DM (23% vs. 5%). Notably, this study's explicit design was to exclude NASH patients in comparison to CC in order to demonstrate CC's distinctiveness from age- and sex-matched patients with liver disease marked by more well-defined clinical characteristics, such as HCV and primary biliary cirrhosis (PBC). The recurring theme of metabolic disease in CC was again demonstrated.

In 2008, Tellez-Avila et al. [21] designed another study to characterize CC compared with other cirrhotic liver diseases, this time in a group of 134 Mexican Mestizo patients. Similar to the prior studies, they found higher rates of metabolic syndrome, obesity, and diabetes in the CC cohort, compared to HCV, alcoholic, and autoimmune liver diseases. This study was retrospective, only had histopathologic data on 43% of their CC patients, and did not include patients with a diagnosis of NASH for comparison. This study provided more evidence that CC is associated with metabolic disturbances, similar to NASH.

Building upon the idea of a spectrum, including NAFLD, NASH, and CC, Younossi et al. [22] examined 247 patients with cirrhosis and compared NASH (103) with CC (144). Histopathologic data were available, and patients were considered to have CC if no other clear diagnosis was identified and they had less than 5% hepatic steatosis. This study found similar metabolic characteristics between the two groups, including BMI (34.8 vs. 33.6) and type 2 diabetes (72.2% vs. 64.1%). Additionally, the age of the two groups was similar between NASH and CC (56 vs. 54 years). The authors included time to liver-related event data (decompensation, liver transplantation, achieving a model for end-stage liver disease (MELD) score of greater than or equal to 15, and death) and found CC to have an increased hazard of these events (HR 1.76, CI 1.02–3.06; $p = 0.043$). Median event time was not reached. They found the hazard ratio to remain significant when the model included age, sex, BMI, and type 2 DM but not when the MELD score was used. This may be interpreted as the entity of CC being associated with increased hazard but not being independent from the MELD score. This is reasonable, given that MELD is a common scoring system of liver disease. This study provided more evidence that NASH and CC are similar in terms of risk factors but that CC may either be a more severe disease in itself or the more hazardous end stage on the spectrum of NAFLD.

To compare CC to other liver diseases requiring transplantation, Thuluvath et al. [4] in 2018 analyzed the United Network for Organ Sharing (UNOS) database. In this subset of patients, they found that NASH patients tended to be more commonly obese (65% vs. 33%) and diabetic (53% vs. 29%) than the CC group. A logistic regression model built upon this database found that the strongest predictors of NASH were type 2 DM, obesity, female gender, and white race. There was also a higher proportion of patients with NASH who later developed hepatocellular carcinoma (HCC), regardless of obesity or diabetes diagnosis. In matched analysis, the authors demonstrated distinctiveness between NASH and CC while taking obesity and type 2 DM into account. They concluded that NASH and CC should be seen as separate entities rather than as two parts of the same spectrum. The disparities between CC and NASH in this study may be attributable to the severity of liver disease inherent to those listed for transplantation. While NAFLD and NASH mortality increases exponentially with the stage of fibrosis [23], only a small proportion of patients become cirrhotic and are listed for transplant [24]. It may be that the metabolic differences between CC and NASH only exist in the most severe cases.

Further complicating this distinction is the realization that pathological features defining NAFLD and NASH fade away with time and disease progression [19]. Along the lines of the spectrum hypothesis, CC may represent a form of "burned-out" NASH. Using another transplant database, Ong et al. [17] assessed the incidence of NAFLD in post-transplant patients with a pre-transplant diagnosis of CC. Among the 25 patients for whom post-transplant pathological specimen review was available, 25.4% had NAFLD, and 15.7% had NASH. The factors associated with post-transplant NAFLD were pre- and post-transplant type 2 DM and elevated fasting triglycerides. It was noted that those patients who did not have NAFLD posttransplant showed a decrease in BMI compared with pre-transplant levels, hypothetically decreasing the risk of NAFLD development. These data give credence to the spectrum hypothesis such that the causal process in these presumed CC patients with post-transplant NAFLD also existed prior to transplantation.

While associations or at least an overlap between CC and the spectrum of NAFLD likely exists, autoimmune hepatitis is another entity that may share a proportion with CC. As mentioned above, Heringlake et al. did an extensive reevaluation of CC patients, and only a third maintained their prior diagnosis, while another third was designated as seronegative AIH. Masior et al. [25], in 2009, examined long-term outcomes for liver transplantation for CC at a single center in Warsaw, Poland. Using a comprehensive review, 55 patients transplanted between 1994 and 2013 were determined to have CC, and the authors took great pains to exclude NASH. Consistent with this, patients had a lower BMI (23.7) and lower rates of DM (23.6%) than were typically seen in NASH. Similar to Ayata et al. [11], the authors submitted the explanted livers for pathological review. Of the explanted livers, 43.1% could not provide an alternative diagnosis to CC. Of the diseased livers, 31.4% were deemed to be so from immunologic causes. While NASH and CC likely have an overlap, it is plausible that the remaining non-NASH instances of CC may actually be a form of autoimmune hepatitis.

9.6 Outcomes

Analysis of outcomes in CC must be seen in the light of this condition's diagnostic uncertainty, overlapping alternatives, and evolution as a distinct entity. For example, outcomes in CC today, with more rigorous exclusion processes, may be (and often are) different from outcomes where true CC was mixed with NASH, AIH, and others.

Ratziu et al. [26] retrospectively compared the survival rate and incidence of HCC among 37 patients with CC, 27 of them designated as overweight (CC-O) and ten as lean (CC-L), with 391 age-matched patients with HCV cirrhosis. Consistent with other studies, CC was diagnosed later in life than HCV patients. Most of the differences in outcomes were observed between the CC-O group and the HCV group, including 30-month survival and median survival (6.3 vs. 28 months). CC-0 patients were also more likely to be obese and diabetic. There were no observed survival differences between the CC-L and HCV groups. This was an older study, published in 2002. The distinction between NASH cirrhosis and CC was not made; rather, there was a tacit understanding that CC-O at least contained a substantial portion of actual NASH patients. As such, it is difficult to elicit conclusions about the natural history of true CC from this study.

The transplant experience for CC has evolved with time as well. Charlton et al. [27] compared the results from 560 liver transplantation cases between 1985 and 1994. Thirty-nine (6.9%) of these met the authors' criteria for CC. Notably excluded from pathology review were indicators of NASH, such as steatosis. The 1- and 5-year actuarial survival rates between CC and the rest of the cohort were 72% and 58% vs. 89% and 80%, these differences being statistically significant. This is in contrast with a study by Thuluvath, Hanish, and Savva [9] who reported transplant outcomes in 2018. In their study, there was similar graft and patient survival among patients diagnosed with CC, NASH, alcoholic cirrhosis, and AIH. Additionally, the patient characteristics between the CC and NASH group were different, including BMI (29 vs. 32) and type 2 DM (25% vs. 45%), indicating that there was a more accurate differentiation between the two entities. While the outcomes were the same, the authors indicated that the compared diseases were distinct and that their patients with CC had a truly cryptogenic etiology.

Development of HCC is a known potential sequela of cirrhosis. Gianni et al. [28] compared 45 consecutive patients with CC, diagnosed with HCC, to 426 HCV patients between 1992 and 2006. They found similar rates of Child–Pugh A patients. However, they also found that HCC in the CC cohort was greater in size, more advanced, and less likely to receive curative treatment than those with HCV. This is likely an effect of less rigorous screening and surveillance in the CC group. HCC was less likely to be discovered during surveillance in CC vs. HCC (29% vs. 64%, $p = 0.001$). It is unlikely that the increased severity of HCC was due to a greater carcinogenic cause among the cryptogenic patients.

9.7 Treatment

Due to the nature of cryptogenic cirrhosis as a diagnosis of exclusion, there exists no specific treatment for this condition. Most beneficial for these patients would be an exhaustive search for alternative diagnoses that may have specific treatments (AIH, HCV, NASH, etc.). Otherwise, treatment for CC includes standard cirrhosis protocols, such as managing complications, avoiding alcohol, optimizing nutrition, and, eventually, liver transplantation for the most severe cases.

9.8 Conclusion

Cryptogenic cirrhosis is a diagnosis of exclusion that is decreasing in incidence as diagnostic techniques increase in sophistication and alternative diagnoses such as NASH and AIH become better understood. It is likely that many patients with NASH have been given a diagnosis of CC due to absent histopathologic features after disease progression. It is also likely that a considerable portion of CC is truly some form of AIH. While a causative and explainable mechanistic process that leads to cirrhosis of the liver, heretofore known as CC, remains elusive, modern technology has greatly narrowed and refined this category. Until this entity is either elucidated or ceases to exist, clinicians should not fear the shadow of cryptogenic cirrhosis, as treatments and prognosis continue to improve, along with those of other cirrhotic liver diseases.

References

1. Anthony PP, Ishak KG, Nayak NC, Poulsen HE, Scheuer PJ, Sobin LH. The morphology of cirrhosis. Recommendations on definition, nomenclature, and classification by a working group sponsored by the World Health Organization. J Clin Pathol. 1978;31(5):395–414. https://doi.org/10.1136/jcp.31.5.395.
2. Desai HG. Cryptogenic cirrhosis: a vanishing entity. J Assoc Physicians India. 2009;57(751–4):759.
3. Caldwell S. Cryptogenic cirrhosis: what are we missing? Curr Gastroenterol Rep. 2010;12(1):40–8. https://doi.org/10.1007/s11894-009-0082-7.
4. Thuluvath PJ, Kantsevoy S, Thuluvath AJ, Savva Y. Is cryptogenic cirrhosis different from NASH cirrhosis? J Hepatol. 2018;68(3):519–25. https://doi.org/10.1016/j.jhep.2017.11.018.
5. Caldwell SH, Crespo DM. The spectrum expanded: cryptogenic cirrhosis and the natural history of non-alcoholic fatty liver disease. J Hepatol. 2004;40(4):578–84. https://doi.org/10.1016/j.jhep.2004.02.013.
6. Kaymakoglu S, Cakaloglu Y, Demir K, et al. Is severe cryptogenic chronic hepatitis similar to autoimmune hepatitis? J Hepatol. 1998;28(1):78–83. https://doi.org/10.1016/s0168-8278(98)80205-5.
7. Tardu A, Karagul S, Yagci MA, et al. Histopathological examination of explanted liver after transplantation in patients with cryptogenic cirrhosis. Transplant Proc. 2015;47(5):1450–2. https://doi.org/10.1016/j.transproceed.2015.04.020.
8. Heringlake S, Schütte A, Flemming P, Schmiegel W, Manns MP, Tillmann HL. Presumed cryptogenic liver disease in Germany: high prevalence of autoantibody-negative autoimmune hepatitis, low prevalence of NASH, no evidence for occult viral etiology. Z Gastroenterol. 2009;47(5):417–23. https://doi.org/10.1055/s-0028-1109146.
9. Thuluvath PJ, Hanish S, Savva Y. Liver transplantation in cryptogenic cirrhosis: outcome comparisons between NASH, alcoholic, and AIH cirrhosis. Transplantation. 2018;102(4):656–63. https://doi.org/10.1097/tp.0000000000002030.
10. Nalbantoglu I, Jain D. Cryptogenic cirrhosis: old and new perspectives in the era of molecular and genomic medicine. Semin Diagn Pathol. 2019;36(6):389–94. https://doi.org/10.1053/j.semdp.2019.07.003.

11. Ayata G, Gordon FD, Lewis WD, et al. Cryptogenic cirrhosis: clinicopathologic findings at and after liver transplantation. Hum Pathol. 2002;33(11):1098–104. https://doi.org/10.1053/hupa.2002.129419.
12. Ludwig J, Viggiano TR, McGill DB, Oh BJ. Nonalcoholic steatohepatitis: Mayo Clinic experiences with a hitherto unnamed disease. Mayo Clin Proc. 1980;55(7):434–8.
13. Sheth SG, Gordon FD, Chopra S. Nonalcoholic steatohepatitis. Ann Intern Med. 1997;126(2):137–45. https://doi.org/10.7326/0003-4819-126-2-199701150-00008.
14. Brunt EM, Janney CG, Di Bisceglie AM, Neuschwander-Tetri BA, Bacon BR. Nonalcoholic steatohepatitis: a proposal for grading and staging the histological lesions. Am J Gastroenterol. 1999;94(9):2467–74. https://doi.org/10.1111/j.1572-0241.1999.01377.x.
15. Kleiner DE, Brunt EM, Van Natta M, et al. Design and validation of a histological scoring system for nonalcoholic fatty liver disease. Hepatology. 2005;41(6):1313–21. https://doi.org/10.1002/hep.20701.
16. Takahashi Y, Dungubat E, Kusano H, Fukusato T. Artificial intelligence and deep learning: new tools for histopathological diagnosis of nonalcoholic fatty liver disease/nonalcoholic steatohepatitis. Comput Struct Biotechnol J. 2023;21:2495–501. https://doi.org/10.1016/j.csbj.2023.03.048.
17. Ong J, Younossi ZM, Reddy V, et al. Cryptogenic cirrhosis and posttransplantation nonalcoholic fatty liver disease. Liver Transpl. 2001;7(9):797–801. https://doi.org/10.1053/jlts.2001.24644.
18. Caldwell SH, Oelsner DH, Iezzoni JC, Hespenheide EE, Battle EH, Driscoll CJ. Cryptogenic cirrhosis: clinical characterization and risk factors for underlying disease. Hepatology. 1999;29(3):664–9. https://doi.org/10.1002/hep.510290347.
19. Powell EE, Cooksley WG, Hanson R, Searle J, Halliday JW, Powell LW. The natural history of nonalcoholic steatohepatitis: a follow-up study of forty-two patients for up to 21 years. Hepatology. 1990;11(1):74–80. https://doi.org/10.1002/hep.1840110114.
20. Poonawala A, Nair SP, Thuluvath PJ. Prevalence of obesity and diabetes in patients with cryptogenic cirrhosis: a case-control study. Hepatology. 2000;32(4 Pt 1):689–92. https://doi.org/10.1053/jhep.2000.17894.
21. Tellez-Avila FI, Sanchez-Avila F, García-Saenz-de-Sicilia M, et al. Prevalence of metabolic syndrome, obesity and diabetes type 2 in cryptogenic cirrhosis. World J Gastroenterol. 2008;14(30):4771–5. https://doi.org/10.3748/wjg.14.4771.
22. Younossi Z, Stepanova M, Sanyal AJ, et al. The conundrum of cryptogenic cirrhosis: adverse outcomes without treatment options. J Hepatol. 2018;69(6):1365–70. https://doi.org/10.1016/j.jhep.2018.08.013.
23. Dulai PS, Singh S, Patel J, et al. Increased risk of mortality by fibrosis stage in nonalcoholic fatty liver disease: systematic review and meta-analysis. Hepatology. 2017;65(5):1557–65. https://doi.org/10.1002/hep.29085.
24. Younossi ZM, Stepanova M, Rafiq N, et al. Pathologic criteria for nonalcoholic steatohepatitis: interprotocol agreement and ability to predict liver-related mortality. Hepatology. 2011;53(6):1874–82. https://doi.org/10.1002/hep.24268.
25. Masior Ł, Grąt M, Krasnodębski M, Patkowski W, Krawczyk M. Liver transplantation in patients with cryptogenic cirrhosis provides excellent long-term outcome. Ann Transplant. 2016;21:160–6. https://doi.org/10.12659/aot.894686.
26. Ratziu V, Bonyhay L, Di Martino V, et al. Survival, liver failure, and hepatocellular carcinoma in obesity-related cryptogenic cirrhosis. Hepatology. 2002;35(6):1485–93. https://doi.org/10.1053/jhep.2002.33324.
27. Charlton MR, Kondo M, Roberts SK, Steers JL, Krom RA, Wiesner RH. Liver transplantation for cryptogenic cirrhosis. Liver Transpl Surg. 1997;3(4):359–64. https://doi.org/10.1002/lt.500030402.
28. Giannini EG, Marabotto E, Savarino V, et al. Hepatocellular carcinoma in patients with cryptogenic cirrhosis. Clin Gastroenterol Hepatol. 2009;7(5):580–5. https://doi.org/10.1016/j.cgh.2009.01.001.

10 Wilson Disease and Hemochromatosis

Uta Merle

10.1 Wilson Disease

10.1.1 Introduction

Wilson disease (WD) is a rare autosomal-recessively inherited copper overload disorder, with a prevalence of ~1:30,000. The manifestation of this disease is typically between the ages of 5 and 35 but can be also at younger and older ages. The disease is characterized by hepatic and/or neuropsychiatric symptoms, and clinical presentation can vary widely. The key features of Wilson disease are liver disease (ranging from asymptomatic elevation of aminotransferase levels to cirrhosis), neuropsychiatric disturbances, and Kayser–Fleischer rings in the Descemet membrane of the cornea. Without treatment, Wilson disease is assumed to be progressive and fatal. Therefore, knowledge of the symptoms, diagnostic criteria, and treatment options is important.

10.1.2 Etiology and Pathogenesis

Approximately 50% of dietary copper (~0.8–2 mg/d) is absorbed in the upper small intestine. After uptake by hepatocytes, biliary excretion is the main pathway for the elimination of excess copper. In Wilson disease, the export of copper into bile is impaired. Impaired copper excretion leads to pathological copper accumulation, primarily within the liver and subsequently in the brain (particularly in the basal ganglia) and other tissues (e.g., kidneys and cornea). Wilson disease is caused by mutations of the Wilson disease gene ATP7B, which codes for a copper-transporting, transmembrane P-type ATPase, primarily expressed in the liver [1, 2]. To date, about 750 polymorphisms of the ATP7B gene have been described, with several of them of unknown clinical significance [3]. Most Wilson disease patients are compound heterozygotes, possessing alleles with different mutations in both parental genes. In general, the mutation variability has no relevant impact on the phenotypic expression in individual Wilson disease patients [4].

U. Merle (✉)
University Hospital Heidelberg, Department of Gastroenterology, Hepatology and Infectious Diseases, Heidelberg, Germany
e-mail: uta.merle@med.uni-heidelberg.de

T. Hackert, A. Gulla (eds.), *Rare Liver and Biliary Tract Diseases*,
https://doi.org/10.1007/978-3-032-15076-9_10

Impaired ATP7B function leads to reduced biliary copper excretion and, in addition, a disturbed incorporation of copper into apoceruloplasmin. Failure to incorporate copper during holo-ceruloplasmin biosynthesis results in the secretion of an apoprotein that is devoid of enzymatic activity and is rapidly degraded. The resulting low serum ceruloplasmin level is a diagnostic hallmark of Wilson disease. Because ceruloplasmin accounts for binding most of the serum copper, total serum copper is typically reduced in Wilson disease.

10.1.3 Clinical Presentation

Although the biochemical copper metabolism defect is already present at birth, the manifestation of Wilson disease typically occurs between 5 and 35 years of age. Of note, Wilson disease is increasingly diagnosed in children who are less than 5 years old. Clinical findings may be nonspecific in children who are less than 2 years old [5, 6]. In addition to younger presentation, first manifestations at older ages than typically assumed are also possible. Although the majority of patients manifest disease-related symptoms until the age of 35, the evaluation for Wilson disease should also be carried out in older individuals [7].

Table 10.1 Clinical symptoms in Wilson disease patients

Manifestation	Clinical symptom
Hepatic	Asymptomatic hepatomegaly
	Isolated splenomegaly
	Acute hepatitis of variable severity
	Chronic hepatitis
	Hepatic steatosis
	Liver cirrhosis, compensated or decompensated
	Acute-on-chronic liver failure
	Acute liver failure, typically with Coombs-negative hemolysis, high bilirubin level, and high bilirubin: alkaline phosphatase (ALP) level
Neurological	Dysarthria
	Movement disorders (tremors and involuntary movements)
	Akinetic-rigid syndrome similar to Parkinson's disease
	Gait abnormality, ataxia
	Dystonia
	Chorea, athetosis
	Drooling, oropharyngeal dystonia, transfer dysphagia
	Dysautonomia
	Seizures
	Sleep disorder, insomnia
Psychiatric	Depression
	Bipolar spectrum disorder
	Neurotic behaviors
	Personality and behavioral changes
	Psychosis
	Subtle cognitive dysfunction
Eye	Kayser–Fleischer rings, sunflower cataract

10.1.4 Hepatic Presentation

Most pediatric patients with Wilson disease present with hepatic disease, whereas adults present with hepatic disease with or without a concurrent neuropsychiatric disease. Hepatic symptoms in Wilson disease patients can be highly variable. Therefore, Wilson disease is often misdiagnosed, and the average time from symptom onset to diagnostic treatment is long, about 12 months [8].

Clinical presentations include clinically asymptomatic states with only biochemical abnormalities, chronic hepatitis, steatosis, splenomegaly, hepatomegaly, and compensated or decompensated liver cirrhosis (Table 10.1) [9, 10]. The features of hepatitis can be similar to other causes of hepatitis, such as chronic viral hepatitis, chronic autoimmune hepatitis, chronic steatohepatitis, or drug-related hepatitis. Transient episodes of hemolysis presenting as intermittent jaundice can occur in some patients.

10.1.5 Acute Liver Failure

Acute hepatic failure as the first disease manifestation occurs in about 5% of patients. In these patients, liver fibrosis or cirrhosis is usually already present, although acute hepatic failure in these patients typically occurs as the first manifestation of the disease. The diagnosis of Wilson disease presenting as acute hepatic failure can be challenging. Wilson disease should be suspected in every patient presenting with acute liver failure with jaundice and only a slight elevation of the activity of transaminases. Despite massive hepatic necrosis, which is responsible for the deleterious clinical course, especially in the presence of hepatic encephalopathy, serum aminotransferases are usually less than ten times normal and, thus, much lower than the values commonly seen in acute severe hepatitis of other etiologies. Further characteristic features are low hemoglobin concentrations resulting from Coombs-negative hemolytic anemia (due to the massive release of copper from dying hepatocytes), hyperbilirubinemia, low alkaline phosphatase, and highly elevated urinary copper concentrations. Renal insufficiency due to copper-associated tubular injury is frequently present but is, in general, reversible. Prognosis of acute liver failure due to Wilson disease is usually poor, and the need for transplantation can be predicted with the Revised Wilson Disease Prognostic Index in children and adults [11, 12].

10.1.6 Neuropsychiatric Presentation

Neurological symptoms usually develop later than hepatic symptoms, most often in the twenties (Table 10.1). The initial symptoms may be very subtle, such as behavioral changes, deterioration in school performance, and speech and writing problems with micrography. Other common findings are tremors, lack of motor coordination, drooling, dysarthria, dystonia, and spasticity.

Psychiatric abnormalities in Wilson disease patients are more common than generally acknowledged. Approximately 50%–70% of patients have psychiatric symptoms at the beginning or at the later stages of their illness, with or without hepatic or neurological findings [13, 14]. These psychiatric symptoms include depression, bipolar disorder, neurotic behaviors, personality changes, anxiety, labile mood, and even frank psychosis (Table 10.1). Many of the individuals with neuropsychiatric symptoms may have concomitant but frequently asymptomatic liver disease.

Kayser–Fleischer rings represent the corneal deposition of copper within the Descemet's membrane and have a golden-brown appearance. They are present in nearly all patients with neurological symptoms but only in about 50% of Wilson disease patients with liver disease. In addition, in the early stages of the disease and in asymptomatic siblings, they are commonly absent.

10.1.7 Other Manifestations

In addition to the common hepatic and neuropsychiatric presentations, symptoms may arise as a result of the dysfunction of any organ in which excess copper is deposited. Clinical manifestations may include abnormalities of the kidney (aminoaciduria and nephrolithiasis), the endocrine system (hypoparathyroidism, infertility, secondary amenorrhea, and repeated miscarriages), the heart (cardiac arrhythmias and cardiomyopathy), and the skeleton (premature osteoporosis and arthritis) (Table 10.1).

10.1.8 Liver Malignancies in Wilson Disease

Based on the data from a retrospective multicenter cohort study, the rate of hepatobiliary malignancies in Wilson disease is commonly assumed to be very low, even in cirrhotic patients [15]. In this retrospective analysis of 1186 patients, 14 developed hepatobiliary malignancies (eight hepatocellular carcinomas (HCCs) and six intrahepatic cholangiocellular carcinomas (ICCs)). The prevalence of hepatobiliary malignancies in the cohort was 1.2%, and the incidence was 0.28 per 1000 person-years. Similar results were obtained from a Dutch retrospective cohort study in 130 patients with WD, who were followed during a median follow-up of 15 years (range of 0.1–51.2) [16]. Although data do not support regular HCC surveillance in patients with WD [16], the risk of carcinogenesis is increased in these patients. HCC occurrence has been reported both in cirrhotic [17, 18] and

Table 10.2 Biochemical tests for the diagnosis of Wilson disease

Test	Typical finding	False "negative"	False "positive"
Serum ceruloplasmin	Decreased by 50% of the lower normal value	Inflammation, Measurement by immunological assay, Pregnancy, contraceptive/ estrogen therapy	Malabsorption, Protein-losing nephropathy, aceruloplasminemia, Heterozygous carriers, Acquired copper deficiency
24-h urinary copper	>1.6 μmol/24 h	Incorrect/incomplete collection, kidney failure	Hepatocellular necrosis, cholestasis, sample contamination, heterozygous carriers
Serum "free" copper	>1.6 μmol/L >10.2 μg/dl	Normal if ceruloplasmin overestimated by an immunological assay	
To date, not in clinical routine: relative exchangeable copper (REC)	>18.5%	Not reported	Not reported
Hepatic copper content	>250 μg/g dry weight	Sampling error, especially in patients with active liver disease and in patients with regenerative nodules	Cholestatic syndromes
Kayser–Fleischer rings	Present in examination by slit lamp	Absent in up to 50% of Wilson disease patients with hepatic presentation, absent in most asymptomatic siblings	Chronic cholestatic disorders like primary biliary cholestasis

Adapted to EASL Wilson disease guideline [9]

non-cirrhotic WD patients [19]. As a result of the occurrence of not only HCC but also ICC, histological analysis through surgical resection or biopsy should be mandatory when a suspicious liver lesion is detected.

10.1.9 Diagnostic Findings

Diagnosis is usually established on the basis of clinical findings and laboratory abnormalities. Diagnosis is straightforward if two or more of the following symptoms are present: Kayser–Fleischer rings, typical neurological symptoms, low serum ceruloplasmin levels (<20 mg/dL), and increased hepatic copper content (>250 μg/g dry weight). In patients presenting with liver disease, diagnostic markers are in ~20% in the normal range and, therefore, misleading. To establish the diagnosis in most patients, a combination of various parameters is necessary, as not a single test is per se specific (Table 10.2). A diagnostic score based on several available tests was proposed by the Working Party at the 8th International Meeting on Wilson disease, Leipzig, 2001—commonly named the "Leipzig score" (Table 10.3) [20]. This score provides a good diagnostic accuracy and was also reevaluated for children with liver disease [21].

10.1.10 Kayser–Fleischer Rings

Kayser–Fleischer rings are found in most neurological Wilson disease patients and in ~50% of hepatic patients [8, 22]. Slit lamp examination is necessary to confirm the presence or absence of Kayser–Fleischer rings, although, sometimes, Kayser–Fleischer rings can be visible to the naked eye. They are not pathognomonic for Wilson disease and can also be found in cholestatic liver diseases, such as primary biliary cirrhosis or intrahepatic cholestasis, associated with prolonged parenteral nutrition.

10.1.11 Serum Ceruloplasmin

Serum ceruloplasmin is typically decreased below 20 mg/dL in patients with Wilson disease.

Table 10.3 Diagnostic criteria for Wilson disease: Leipzig score [20]

Kayser–Fleischer ring (slit lamp examination)	
Present	2
Absent	0
Neurological symptoms and/or typical signs in cMRI	
Severe	2
Mild	1
Absent	0
Serum ceruloplasmin	
Normal (>0.2 g/L)	0
0.1–0.2 g/L	1
<0.1 g/L	2
Coombs-negative hemolytic anemia	
Present	1
Absent	0
Total liver copper content	
>250 μg/g dry weight	2
>50 ≤ 250 μg/g dry weight	1
Normal (<50 μg/g dry weight)	−1
If no copper quantification available: positive rhodanine staining	1
24 h-urinary copper excretion	
Normal	0
1–2x the upper limit of normal (ULN)	1
>2x ULN	2
Normal but positive D-penicillamine provocation test	2
ATP7B mutation analysis	
Present on both chromosomes	4
Present on one chromosome	1
None	0

Total score	Evaluation
4 or more	Diagnosis established
3	Diagnosis possible, more tests needed
2 or less	Diagnosis very unlikely

However, serum ceruloplasmin concentration has its limitations, as about 20% of Wilson disease patients with hepatic symptoms have serum ceruloplasmin levels in the normal range [23]. The diagnostic accuracy of serum ceruloplasmin depends on the selected cutoff values [24]. Serum ceruloplasmin concentrations below 20, 14, and 10 mg/dl showed positive predictive values of 48.3%, 100%, and 100%, respectively, and negative predictive values of 98.7%, 97.1%, and 91.9%. In line with this finding, in the Leipzig score [20], the informative cutoff is 10 mg/dL. Hormonal and inflammatory stimuli can increase the levels of the acute-phase-reactant ceruloplasmin above the lower limit of normal. For example, ceruloplasmin may be elevated in inflammatory stages, during pregnancy, and in response to exogenous administration of estrogens. Conversely, a reduced serum ceruloplasmin concentration can be seen in about 20% of ATP7B heterozygotes, in hypoproteinemia due to renal or enteric protein loss, in severe end-stage liver disease of any etiology, and in the rare condition of aceruloplasminemia. Decreased serum ceruloplasmin is, in addition, reported in patients with metabolic-associated steatotic liver disease (MASLD). In a recent study in MASLD patients (without diabetes mellitus), a decreased ceruloplasmin ratio (ceruloplasmin value divided by the lower limit of normal) was associated with a more severe histological activity, a diagnosis of metabolic-associated steatohepatitis, and hepatic iron deposition among patients with MASLD [25].

10.1.12 Total Serum Copper and Relative Exchangeable Serum Copper

In contrast to what would seem intuitive for a disorder of copper overload, total serum copper is often reduced (<70 μg/dL) in Wilson disease patients due to low serum ceruloplasmin. The copper that is not bound to ceruloplasmin is known as the serum non-ceruloplasmin-bound copper concentration and is elevated in most untreated patients.

The non-ceruloplasmin-bound "free" copper concentration can be calculated using the estimation that approximately 0.3 μg of copper is associated per mg ceruloplasmin:

$$\text{Serum copper}(\mu g/\text{dL}) - 3 \times \text{serum ceruloplasmin}(\text{mg}/\text{dL}) = \text{non} - \text{ceruloplasmin bound copper}(\mu g/\text{dL})$$

Recently, a direct exchangeable copper assay has been suggested as a robust and feasible diagnostic tool for Wilson disease. Exchangeable copper corresponds to the labile fraction of copper complexed to albumin and other peptides but not complexed within ceruloplasmin. This exchangeable copper fraction is easily exchanged in the presence of high-affinity copper-chelating agents such as EDTA and can be measured afterward—and has been proposed as a method for estimating bioavailable non-ceruloplasmin-bound copper in the circulation. For diagnostic purposes, the ratio of exchangeable copper to total serum copper, called the "relative exchangeable copper" (REC), with the cutoff set at 18.5%, distinguishes patients with Wilson disease from simple heterozygotes and normal individuals and also from adults and children with various chronic liver diseases [26–29].

10.1.13 Urinary Copper Excretion

Urinary copper excretion reflects the amount of non-ceruloplasmin copper in the circulation and is commonly increased in patients with Wilson disease. The conventional level taken as a diagnostic of Wilson disease is 100 μg/24 h (1.6 μmol/24 h)—with an upper limit of normal for daily urinary copper excretion of 40 μg/24 h (0.6 μmol/24 h). Of note, urinary copper excretion can also be increased in any disease with extensive hepatocellular necrosis, cirrhosis with cholestasis, and nephrotic syndrome.

Urinary copper excretion after provocation with D-penicillamine has only been standardized in children [30] but may be utilized as an adjunctive diagnostic test to establish the diagnosis of Wilson disease. For this test, 500 mg of D-penicillamine is administered to untreated patients orally at time zero and 12 h later during a 24-h urine collection, and an increase of urinary copper excretion to >1600 μg/24 h is considered a diagnostic for Wilson disease.

10.1.14 Liver Biopsy

Liver biopsy with the determination of hepatic copper content remains the gold standard for diagnosing Wilson disease. Normal hepatic copper content is less than 40 μg/g dry weight, and that of Wilson disease patients typically exceeds 250 μg/g dry weight. Two main studies have been published on alternate diagnostic thresholds: (1) Ferenci et al. could show that lowering the threshold value to 75 μg/g increases test sensitivity with still-acceptable specificity [31], and (2) in a large Chinese study, a threshold of 209 μg/g dry weight was proposed as the optimal threshold value (with a sensitivity of 99% and a specificity of 96%) [32].

A slightly elevated hepatic copper content can also be associated with cholestatic liver diseases, such as progressive familial intrahepatic cholestasis type 3 (PFIC 3), primary biliary cirrhosis, and primary sclerosing cholangitis [33–35].

The major problem with hepatic parenchymal copper concentration is that, in the later stages of Wilson disease, the distribution of copper within the liver is often not homogenous. Thus, the concentration can be underestimated due to sampling errors. As the accuracy of measurement is improved with an adequate specimen size, at least 1–2 cm of biopsy core length should be submitted for copper dry weight analysis [36].

Regarding liver histology, there is no single feature pathognomonic for the diagnosis of Wilson disease. Intracellular fat accumulations, hepatitis-like features, Mallory bodies, focal necrosis, fibrosis, and cirrhosis can often be found. The pathology can be similar to an ethanol-induced steatohepatitis, while other patients may show histological signs resembling autoimmune hepatitis. Although histological findings are often not helpful for the diagnosis of Wilson disease, the exclusion of other etiologies by liver biopsy may be equally important. The detection of the presence of copper staining in histological sections by rhodanine or by other means can provide supportive evidence for Wilson disease. However, especially in the early stages of Wilson disease, a negative histochemical staining for copper does not rule out increased hepatic copper content and should not be considered sufficient for the exclusion of Wilson disease. Indeed, hepatic copper concentration can be particularly high under this condition.

10.1.15 Genetic Studies

De novo diagnosis by molecular studies remains difficult due to the large number of disease-specific mutations scattered across the coding region of ATP7B. Depending on the population tested, specific mutations can be prevalent and can facilitate the otherwise cumbersome diagnostic mutation analysis [37]; in northern Europeans, the H1069Q mutation accounts for 60%–70% of the disease alleles [4, 38–40], and in Asians, the A778L mutation occurs in 30% of affected individuals.

Genetic analyses should be done in every patient with a suspicion or a confirmed diagnosis of Wilson disease. Genetic diagnosis of Wilson disease should always be corroborated with clinical and biochemical findings. The absence of two pathogenic mutations does not exclude a diagnosis of Wilson disease.

10.1.16 Other Diagnostic Tests

By ultrasound imaging, signs of liver steatosis or cirrhosis, as well as hepato- and splenomegaly, can help establish the diagnosis of Wilson disease.

Magnetic resonance imaging (MRI) of the brain may show increased density on T2-weighted images in the region of the basal ganglia and other regions, as well as cortical atrophy. MRI changes are most often seen in Wilson disease patients with neurological manifestations but may also be found in Wilson disease patients without neurological symptoms or completely asymptomatic patients.

As bone density is frequently decreased in Wilson disease patients, performing an osteodensitometry is recommended.

10.1.17 Family Screening

Screening should be performed in every first-degree relative of any Wilson disease patient. The probability of finding a homozygote in siblings is 25% and in parents or children is 0.5%. There is no single biochemical test that accurately discriminates between homozygous patients and heterozygous carriers. Kayser–Fleischer rings may be absent in the early stages of the disease. The determination of ceruloplasmin levels and 24-h urinary copper excretion can be misleading because heterozygotes can have borderline pathological values. Serum ceruloplasmin concentration as a screening tool has poor diagnostic strength due to an inadequate predictive value as a single test. Thus, individuals without Kayser–Fleischer rings who have subnormal ceruloplasmin and abnormal liver functions should undergo a liver biopsy for quantitative copper determination.

Relative exchangeable copper is useful for family screening, as it can discriminate between homozygous patients and heterozygous carriers.

In first-degree relatives of a patient with two detected mutations, targeted mutational analysis is straightforward as family screening of first-degree relatives. Mutation analysis for screening the family of an index patient with known mutations is, therefore, a very reliable tool.

10.1.18 Prognosis

Early start of lifelong anti-copper therapy and compliance are crucial for a good prognosis in Wilson disease. This is reflected in studies analyzing long-term prognosis: In Wison disease patients diagnosed early and treated correctly and with good compliance, long-term survival seems to be very similar to that of the general population [41]. However, Wilson disease patients with liver cirrhosis or primarily neurological patients diagnosed late or with insufficient treatment compliance show higher mortality compared to healthy controls [42, 43].

If therapy is started in presymptomatic patients, the development of symptoms is only rarely seen, and the prognosis is very good [44]. Symptomatic patients, in general, stabilize or improve with adequate long-term treatment. This is especially true for hepatic symptoms, while neurological symptoms can persist and, sometimes, even worsen despite treatment.

10.1.19 Treatment

Once the diagnosis of Wilson disease is established, lifelong medical treatment is recommended because copper accumulation is progressive and, ultimately, fatal without specific therapy.

As drug treatment, copper-chelating agents and zinc salts are used. Under treatment, most Wilson disease patients improve their liver function within 6–12 months of treatment. Under sufficient therapy, asymptomatic patients (e.g., diagnosed through family screening) should stay asymptomatic. Therapy should be taken lifelong. Discontinuation of medical therapy (e.g., due to noncompliance) typically leads to a progression of liver disease or of neurological symptoms.

D-penicillamine and triethylenetetramine (trientine) are chelating agents that remove copper by enhancing its urinary excretion. Therefore, chelators require adequate renal function to be effective. The mode of action of zinc therapy differs from chelators, as zinc inhibits the intestinal uptake of copper by inducing enterocyte metallothionein. Ingested copper is bound to metallothionein in enterocytes and is lost via feces due to enterocyte shedding.

In patients with symptomatic liver disease, the initial therapy should be chelating therapy, as it is more effective than zinc therapy. Although a larger body of published evidence exists for penicillamine, trientine seems to have a more favorable safety profile, especially in patients with neurological symptoms. Treatment of presymptomatic patients and lifelong maintenance therapy of successfully treated symptomatic patients can be accomplished with zinc salts or chelating agents in a reduced "maintenance" dosage. Nevertheless, definitive recommendations are difficult, as randomized head-to-head studies are missing.

In addition to medical de-coppering therapy, patients with Wilson disease should avoid the intake of copper-rich food and water.

For routine monitoring, serum copper and ceruloplasmin, liver enzymes and international normalized ratio, functional parameters, complete blood count, and urine analysis, as well as physical and neurological examinations, should be performed regularly, at least twice annually [9]. More frequent monitoring is required in the initial phase after diagnosis and initiation of treatment, if symptoms worsen, and if nonadherence to treatment is suspected.

10.1.20 Liver Transplantation

Liver transplantation corrects the underlying metabolic defect and, thereby, cures the disease. However, the great shortage of donor organs and the need for immunosuppression post- transplantation render liver transplantation only an option in fulminant Wilson disease or in patients specifically with decompensated liver disease unresponsive to medical therapy. The outcome of liver transplantation is excellent, with a 1-year survival rate of 80%–90%. Neurological symptoms can improve after liver transplantation [45], but the outcome of patients with neurological symptoms is inferior to patients without them.

10.2 Hemochromatosis

10.2.1 Introduction

Classic hemochromatosis is an autosomal recessive iron storage disease in which intestinal iron absorption is pathologically increased. If left untreated, progressive iron overload occurs, with damage to the liver, pancreatic B cells, heart, endocrine organs, and joints.

10.2.2 Genetics and Penetrance of Hemochromatosis

Hemochromatosis is a congenital iron storage disease.

In addition to the by far most common form, the classic high Fe (HFE)-associated hemochromatosis, there are other, much rarer forms of hereditary hemochromatosis that are based on mutations in other genes involved in iron metabolism.

These very rare types of hemochromatosis are referred to as non-HFE hemochromatoses to distinguish them from HFE-associated hemochromatosis. The various non-HFE hemochromatoses differ in the causally affected iron metabolism gene and in the age of manifestation resulting from the defect. In the case of severe, juvenile non-HFE hemochromatoses, the age of manifestation is even in adolescence.

By far, the most common form of hemochromatosis is autosomal recessive HFE-associated hemochromatosis. In patients with elevated transferrin saturation (defined as >50% in males and >45% in females) and elevated serum ferritin, hemochromatosis should be considered a differential diagnosis, and HFE genotyping for C282Y should be performed. In Western countries, the homozygous C282Y mutation of the HFE gene has a prevalence of approximately 1:200, with a geographical accumulation in the northern regions of Europe [46, 47]. Due to the conspicuous geographical accumulation, it is assumed that the C282Y mutation arose as a spontaneous mutation in a Celtic ancestor and caused a selective advantage through reduced iron requirements.

People who are homozygous for the C282Y variant in the HFE gene do not have manifest HFE-associated hemochromatosis per se but only a genetic predisposition. The diagnosis of HFE-associated hemochromatosis is made when a homozygous HFE-C282Y mutation is detected in connection with pathologically elevated iron metabolism parameters.

The penetrance of hemochromatosis is age- and sex-dependent. Due to the physiological blood loss in women, men are affected much more frequently and, above all, at a younger age than women. The biochemical penetrance with regard to increased serum ferritin concentrations is approximately 80% in men and 55% in women [48]. The clinical penetrance is significantly lower, at 1%–28%, and varies significantly [49]. It probably depends significantly on hitherto unknown genetic factors and exogenous influences. Regular blood loss (e.g., in premenopausal women), eating habits, and, in particular, excessive alcohol consumption play a role in the exogenous influences. Due to their physiological iron losses during menstruation, pregnancy, and lactation, women develop clinical consequences of hemochromatosis less frequently and only at an advanced age. The clinical age of onset in men is around 45 years of age. Women get the disease about 10 years later, usually in postmenopause.

Another genotype is the "compound" heterozygous C282Y and H63D carrier status, which can be detected in about 5% of hemochromatosis patients. This is—in comparison with the homozygous C282Y mutation—of significantly lower penetrance and usually only associated with a mild iron overload. When HFE was first identified as a hemochromatosis gene, C282Y and H63D were identified as disease-associated variants [47]. However, compound heterozygosity for C282Y and H63D is typically associated with, at most, a mild iron overload. Therefore, the clinical value of genetic testing for H63D that is currently discussed is increasingly controversial. In the clinical manifestation of the compound heterozygous HFE C282Y/H63D mutation, other influences (such as alcohol consumption, obesity, or metabolic syndrome) play a major role. Today, the importance of compound heterozygosity in terms of the risk of developing iron overload is estimated to be significantly lower than that of C282Y homozygosity (and a homozygous H63D mutation has an even lower risk) [46].

10.2.3 Pathogenesis of Hemochromatosis

In healthy people, iron absorption and iron loss are about the same. Depending on the iron requirement, only about 10% (1–2 mg/d) of the dietary iron is absorbed. Iron absorption is controlled by the peptide hormone hepcidin, which is primarily synthesized in the liver. This is increasingly synthesized when iron levels are high and blocks iron absorption in the intestine via its interaction partner ferroportin. In the case of iron deficiency and anemia, hepcidin levels are lower, and this leads to increased iron absorption.

In HFE-associated hemochromatosis, hepcidin is formed in inadequately low amounts. This leads to about 2–3 mg of excess iron being ingested daily. As a result, slow, progressive iron overload develops over the long term.

The excess iron is absorbed into the parenchymal cells of the liver and other organs. Iron deposition in the form of hemosiderin in pancreatic B cells, myocardium, and pituitary gonadotropic cells explains the impaired function of these organs. The joints can also be affected in the form of degenerative arthropathy.

10.2.4 Clinical Symptoms

Symptoms and clinical findings depend on the stage of iron overload at which the diagnosis is made. Without therapy, the increasing iron overload of the affected organs leads to progressive clinical symptoms, which usually begin in the 40th–50th year of life. Initially, nonspecific general symptoms appear as an expression of the liver disease. Arthralgia can develop at any point in the disease. Liver disease slowly progresses through fibrosis to cirrhosis. The risk of developing hepatocellular carcinoma is significantly increased in the presence of liver cirrhosis.

In addition to the primarily affected liver, the pancreas (diabetes mellitus), the heart (cardiomyopathy), the pituitary gland and gonads (hypofunction), the skin (pigmentation and "bronze diabetes"), and the joints (arthropathy) can also be affected as end organs. Arthropathy is typically symmetrical and frequently involves the metacarpophalangeal joints II and III.

10.2.5 Diagnosis

If iron overload is suspected, transferrin saturation and serum ferritin should first be determined. Even in the early stages of hemochromatosis, there is usually a significant increase in transferrin saturation (typically >90%). In the advanced stage, there is also a significant increase in serum ferritin, with the ferritin level usually correlating with the extent of iron overload.

Significantly more frequently, an increase in ferritin is not an expression of manifest iron overload but an epiphenomenon of other causes, such as increased alcohol consumption, metabolic syndrome, nonalcoholic or alcoholic fatty liver disease, or chronic inflammatory processes. In addition to these nonspecific increases in ferritin, which are not associated with iron overload, hemolytic and dyserythropoietic anemias can lead to secondary hemochromatosis with significant iron overload.

The transferrin saturation is helpful in distinguishing the inflammation-related ferritin increase from the "true" hemochromatosis-associated iron overload since, in contrast to iron overload, it is typically reduced or within the normal range in inflammatory states. It should be noted that increased alcohol consumption can also be the cause of increased transferrin saturation. In general, transferrin saturation should be determined in the morning. Interestingly, fasting does not increase the diagnostic value [50].

Transferrin saturation is helpful in differentiating the inflammation-related, nonspecific increase in ferritin from the "true" hemochromatosis-associated iron overload since this is usually, at most, slightly-to-moderately increased in the case of a nonspecific increase in ferritin.

If ferritin and transferrin saturation are elevated, a diagnostic HFE genetic test should be performed. The diagnosis of HFE-associated hemochromatosis is made when a homozygous HFE-C282Y mutation is detected in connection with pathologically elevated iron metabolism parameters. In patients with elevated ferritin, in combination with elevated transferrin saturation, who are not homozygous for C282Y, noninvasive quantification of liver iron using MRI is recommended in accordance with the guidelines [51]. When available, supplemental quantification of splenic iron by MRI can provide additional relevant diagnostic information since splenic iron is typically low or normal in primary hemochromatosis.

The search for mutations in the other genes associated with hemochromatosis (transferrin receptor 2, ferroportin, hepcidin, and hemojuvelin) is only indicated in exceptional cases. It can be considered in HFE-negative patients who show marked iron overload and in whom other hepatic or hematological causes have been ruled out.

Compound heterozygosity for C282Y and H63D is typically associated with only a mild iron overload. Clinical manifestation of the compound heterozygous HFE C282Y/H63D mutation is relevantly influenced by other factors such as alcohol consumption, obesity, or metabolic syndrome. A homozygous H63D mutation has an even lower risk of relevant iron overload than the compound heterozygous C282Y/H63D mutation.

It should be noted that due to the low penetrance, not all C282Y homozygous patients develop iron overload and disease symptoms, so the detection of the HFE mutation is not identical to the diagnosis of hemochromatosis. Rather, the gene carrier can only be classified as predisposed. The diagnosis of hemochromatosis, on the other hand, is always based on the combination of elevated iron metabolism parameters and genotyping.

Once the diagnosis has been made, an assessment should be made for liver fibrosis/cirrhosis and other end organ damage. In a typical constellation (elevated ferritin, in combination with homozygous HFE C282Y mutation), a liver biopsy is not necessary for diagnosis. Liver biopsy plays a certain role in HFE-associated hemochromatosis to assess the presence of liver fibrosis/cirrhosis. Advanced liver fibrosis in hemochromatosis patients can be ruled out noninvasively using transient elastography with measured stiffness values ≤6.4 kPa [46]. It is also important to note that liver fibrosis/cirrhosis is very unlikely if the initial serum ferritin value (before the start of therapy) is <1000 μg/l, normal transaminases are present, and there is no hepatomegaly (negative predictive value of approx. 95%) [52].

After the diagnosis of HFE-associated hemochromatosis, lifelong phlebotomy therapy should be carried out with the aim of de-storing the iron depots. The most effective method of removing iron from the body is phlebotomy. With a phlebotomy of 500 ml of blood, 250 mg of iron is removed from the body. The normalization of body iron levels is reflected in the reduction in serum ferritin levels. This should be checked every 2–3 months during therapy. The ferritin value should first be lowered to <50 μg/l by means of, for example, weekly bloodletting of 500 ml. In the long term, the serum ferritin value should then be between 50 and 100 μg/l by means of less frequent bloodletting.

It can also make sense to keep the transferrin saturation <50% in order to keep the damage caused by "free iron" as low as possible [53]. However, this recommendation to also regularly monitor transferrin saturation and keep it low (<50%) has not yet been included in the European Association for the Study of the Liver (EASL) guidelines [46].

Prognosis is largely determined by the degree of organ involvement at the start of therapy. In several studies of patients with homozygous HFE-C282Y hemochromatosis, the reversibility of liver fibrosis present before the initiation of phlebotomy therapy and the onset of cirrhosis could be shown. Contrary to previous assumptions, a current study was able to show that the long-term risk of HCC is significantly reduced in patients with biopsy-proven fibrosis regression [54].

It is unclear whether C282Y/H63D compound heterozygous or H63D homozygous patients with mild signs of iron overload (elevated serum ferritin) will benefit from phlebotomy, as treatment of patients with iron overload who are not C282Y homozygotes has not yet been targeted in specific studies. However, manifest iron overload should be treated by phlebotomy, regardless of genotype.

Elevated ferritin levels that occur as part of a metabolic syndrome or fatty liver disease and are not due to iron overload/hemochromatosis should not be treated with bloodletting therapy, as studies do not suggest a beneficial effect of bloodletting treatment in these patients [55].

The overall prevalence of HCC in hemochromatosis patients is around 10%–30%, and it occurs almost exclusively in patients with liver cirrhosis [56]. Rarely, HCC is also described in hemochromatosis patients with only advanced fibrosis and, in isolated cases, also in patients with mild or even no fibrosis [56]. According to the guidelines, HCC surveillance is indicated for patients with hemochromatosis and cirrhosis but is also recommended for patients with second-degree fibrosis. It should be noted here that the HCC screening should be continued in the long term, regardless of any fibrosis/cirrhosis that may have subsided under phlebotomy therapy.

Under phlebotomy therapy, there is a significant improvement in the clinical symptoms. If phlebotomy therapy begins before end organ damage occurs, the prognosis for hemochromatosis is excellent. However, the later the disease is detected, the more severe the complications, and reversibility is not guaranteed.

10.2.6 Summary

The clinical picture of the genetic copper storage disease, Wilson disease, is extremely diverse and includes hepatic and neuropsychiatric symptoms. Wilson disease should be considered in any individual with liver abnormalities or neuropsychiatric symptoms of uncertain cause. The diagnostic gold standard is hepatic copper content (measured in dry weight). Initial treatment for patients with symptomatic liver disease should include a chelating agent (D-penicillamine or trientine). Treatment is lifelong and should not be discontinued unless liver transplantation is performed.

The genetic iron storage disease, hemochromatosis, is caused by chronically increased iron absorption with subsequent iron overload. If there are elevated iron metabolism parameters in the serum (ferritin and transferrin saturation), in combination with a homozygous HFE C282Y mutation, HFE-associated hemochromatosis can be diagnosed, and therapy with phlebotomy can directly be initiated. HFE-associated hemochromatosis has a high risk of development of hepatocellular carcinoma. Therefore, HCC surveillance is indicated not only for patients with hemochromatosis and cirrhosis but is also recommended for patients with second-degree fibrosis.

References

1. Bull PC, Thomas GR, Rommens JM, Forbes JR, Cox DW. The Wilson disease gene is a putative copper transporting P-type ATPase similar to the Menkes gene. Nat Genet. 1993;5:327–37. https://doi.org/10.1038/ng1293-327.
2. Tanzi RE, et al. The Wilson disease gene is a copper transporting ATPase with homology to the Menkes disease gene. Nat Genet. 1993;5:344–50. https://doi.org/10.1038/ng1293-344.
3. Czlonkowska A, et al. Wilson disease. Nat Rev Dis Primers. 2018;4:21. https://doi.org/10.1038/s41572-018-0018-3.
4. Ferenci P, et al. Age and sex but not ATP7B genotype effectively influence the clinical phenotype of Wilson disease. Hepatology. 2019;69:1464–76. https://doi.org/10.1002/hep.30280.
5. Wiernicka A, et al. Early onset of Wilson disease: diagnostic challenges. J Pediatr Gastroenterol Nutr. 2017;65:555–60. https://doi.org/10.1097/MPG.0000000000001700.
6. Wilson DC, Phillips MJ, Cox DW, Roberts EA. Severe hepatic Wilson's disease in preschool-aged children. J Pediatr. 2000;137:719–22. https://doi.org/10.1067/mpd.2000.108569.
7. Ferenci P, et al. Late-onset Wilson's disease. Gastroenterology. 2007;132:1294–8. https://doi.org/10.1053/j.gastro.2007.02.057.
8. Merle U, Schaefer M, Ferenci P, Stremmel W. Clinical presentation, diagnosis and long-term outcome of Wilson's disease: a cohort study. Gut. 2007;56:115–20. https://doi.org/10.1136/gut.2005.087262.
9. European Association for the Study of the Liver. EASL clinical practice guidelines: Wilson's disease. J Hepatol. 2012;56:671–85. https://doi.org/10.1016/j.jhep.2011.11.007.
10. Schilsky ML, et al. A multidisciplinary approach to the diagnosis and management of Wilson disease: 2022 practice guidance on Wilson disease from the American Association for the Study of Liver Diseases. Hepatology. 2025;82(3):E41–90. https://doi.org/10.1002/hep.32801.
11. Dhawan A, et al. Wilson's disease in children: 37-year experience and revised King's score for liver transplantation. Liver Transpl. 2005;11:441–8. https://doi.org/10.1002/lt.20352.
12. Petrasek J, et al. Revised King's College score for liver transplantation in adult patients with Wilson's disease. Liver Transpl. 2007;13:55–61. https://doi.org/10.1002/lt.20920.
13. Akil M, Schwartz JA, Dutchak D, Yuzbasiyan-Gurkan V, Brewer GJ. The psychiatric presentations of Wilson's disease. J Neuropsychiatry Clin Neurosci. 1991;3:377–82. https://doi.org/10.1176/jnp.3.4.377.
14. Mura G, Zimbrean PC, Demelia L, Carta MG. Psychiatric comorbidity in Wilson's disease. Int Rev Psychiatry. 2017;29:445–62. https://doi.org/10.1080/09540261.2017.1311845.
15. Pfeiffenberger J, et al. Hepatobiliary malignancies in Wilson disease. Liver Int. 2015;35:1615–22. https://doi.org/10.1111/liv.12727.
16. van Meer S, et al. No increased risk of hepatocellular carcinoma in cirrhosis due to Wilson disease dur-

ing long-term follow-up. J Gastroenterol Hepatol. 2015;30:535–9. https://doi.org/10.1111/jgh.12716.
17. Iwadate H, et al. Hepatocellular carcinoma associated with Wilson's disease. Intern Med. 2004;43:1042–5. https://doi.org/10.2169/internalmedicine.43.1042.
18. Reyes CV. Hepatocellular carcinoma in Wilson disease-related liver cirrhosis. Gastroenterol Hepatol. 2008;4:435–7.
19. Thattil R, Dufour JF. Hepatocellular carcinoma in a non-cirrhotic patient with Wilson's disease. World J Gastroenterol. 2013;19:2110–3. https://doi.org/10.3748/wjg.v19.i13.2110.
20. Ferenci P, et al. Diagnosis and phenotypic classification of Wilson disease. Liver Int. 2003;23:139–42. https://doi.org/10.1034/j.1600-0676.2003.00824.x.
21. Nicastro E, Ranucci G, Vajro P, Vegnente A, Iorio R. Re-evaluation of the diagnostic criteria for Wilson disease in children with mild liver disease. Hepatology. 2010;52:1948–56. https://doi.org/10.1002/hep.23910.
22. Medici V, et al. Diagnosis and management of Wilson's disease: results of a single center experience. J Clin Gastroenterol. 2006;40:936–41. https://doi.org/10.1097/01.mcg.0000225670.91722.59.
23. Steindl P, et al. Wilson's disease in patients presenting with liver disease: a diagnostic challenge. Gastroenterology. 1997;113:212–8. https://doi.org/10.1016/s0016-5085(97)70097-0.
24. Mak CM, Lam CW, Tam S. Diagnostic accuracy of serum ceruloplasmin in Wilson disease: determination of sensitivity and specificity by ROC curve analysis among ATP7B-genotyped subjects. Clin Chem. 2008;54:1356–62. https://doi.org/10.1373/clinchem.2008.103432.
25. Wang Q, et al. A novel non-invasive approach based on serum ceruloplasmin for identifying non-alcoholic Steatohepatitis patients in the non-diabetic population. Front Med. 2022;9:900794. https://doi.org/10.3389/fmed.2022.900794.
26. El Balkhi S, et al. Relative exchangeable copper: a new highly sensitive and highly specific biomarker for Wilson's disease diagnosis. Clin Chim Acta. 2011;412:2254–60. https://doi.org/10.1016/j.cca.2011.08.019.
27. Guillaud O, et al. Relative exchangeable copper: a valuable tool for the diagnosis of Wilson disease. Liver Int. 2018;38:350–7. https://doi.org/10.1111/liv.13520.
28. Poujois A, et al. Exchangeable copper: a reflection of the neurological severity in Wilson's disease. Eur J Neurol. 2017;24:154–60. https://doi.org/10.1111/ene.13171.
29. Trocello JM, et al. Relative exchangeable copper: a promising tool for family screening in Wilson disease. Mov Disord. 2014;29:558–62. https://doi.org/10.1002/mds.25763.
30. Martins da Costa C, et al. Value of urinary copper excretion after penicillamine challenge in the diagnosis of Wilson's disease. Hepatology. 1992;15:609–15. https://doi.org/10.1002/hep.1840150410.
31. Ferenci P, et al. Diagnostic value of quantitative hepatic copper determination in patients with Wilson's disease. Clin Gastroenterol Hepatol. 2005;3:811–8. https://doi.org/10.1016/s1542-3565(05)00181-3.
32. Yang X, et al. Prospective evaluation of the diagnostic accuracy of hepatic copper content, as determined using the entire core of a liver biopsy sample. Hepatology. 2015;62:1731–41. https://doi.org/10.1002/hep.27932.
33. Anheim M, et al. Unexpected combination of inherited chorea-acanthocytosis with MDR3 (ABCB4) defect mimicking Wilson's disease. Clin Genet. 2010;78:294–5. https://doi.org/10.1111/j.1399-0004.2010.01386.x.
34. Shneider BL. ABCB4 disease presenting with cirrhosis and copper overload-potential confusion with Wilson disease. J Clin Exp Hepatol. 2011;1:115–7. https://doi.org/10.1016/S0973-6883(11)60131-X.
35. Sood V, Rawat D, Khanna R, Alam S. Cholestatic liver disease masquerading as Wilson disease. Indian J Gastroenterol. 2015;34:174–7. https://doi.org/10.1007/s12664-015-0552-9.
36. Liggi M, et al. Uneven distribution of hepatic copper concentration and diagnostic value of double-sample biopsy in Wilson's disease. Scand J Gastroenterol. 2013;48:1452–8. https://doi.org/10.3109/00365521.2013.845904.
37. Ferenci P. Regional distribution of mutations of the ATP7B gene in patients with Wilson disease: impact on genetic testing. Hum Genet. 2006;120:151–9. https://doi.org/10.1007/s00439-006-0202-5.
38. Caca K, et al. High prevalence of the H1069Q mutation in east German patients with Wilson disease: rapid detection of mutations by limited sequencing and phenotype-genotype analysis. J Hepatol. 2001;35:575–81. https://doi.org/10.1016/s0168-8278(01)00219-7.
39. Firneisz G, et al. Common mutations of ATP7B in Wilson disease patients from Hungary. Am J Med Genet. 2002;108:23–8. https://doi.org/10.1002/ajmg.10220.
40. Margarit E, et al. Mutation analysis of Wilson disease in the Spanish population – identification of a prevalent substitution and eight novel mutations in the ATP7B gene. Clin Genet. 2005;68:61–8. https://doi.org/10.1111/j.1399-0004.2005.00439.x.
41. Bruha R, et al. Long-term follow-up of Wilson disease: natural history, treatment, mutations analysis and phenotypic correlation. Liver Int. 2011;31:83–91. https://doi.org/10.1111/j.1478-3231.2010.02354.x.
42. Beinhardt S, et al. Long-term outcomes of patients with Wilson disease in a large Austrian cohort. Clin Gastroenterol Hepatol. 2014;12:683–9. https://doi.org/10.1016/j.cgh.2013.09.025.
43. Czlonkowska A, Tarnacka B, Litwin T, Gajda J, Rodo M. Wilson's disease-cause of mortality in 164 patients during 1992–2003 observation period. J Neurol. 2005;252:698–703. https://doi.org/10.1007/s00415-005-0720-4.

44. Walshe JM. Diagnosis and treatment of presymptomatic Wilson's disease. Lancet. 1988;2:435–7. https://doi.org/10.1016/s0140-6736(88)90423-0.
45. Weiss KH, et al. Outcome and development of symptoms after orthotopic liver transplantation for Wilson disease. Clin Transpl. 2013;27:914–22. https://doi.org/10.1111/ctr.12259.
46. European Association for the Study of the Liver. EASL clinical practice guidelines on haemochromatosis. J Hepatol. 2022;77:479–502. https://doi.org/10.1016/j.jhep.2022.03.033.
47. Kowdley KV, Brown KE, Ahn J, Sundaram V. ACG clinical guideline: hereditary hemochromatosis. Am J Gastroenterol. 2019;114:1202–18. https://doi.org/10.14309/ajg.0000000000000315.
48. Olynyk JK, et al. A population-based study of the clinical expression of the hemochromatosis gene. N Engl J Med. 1999;341:718–24. https://doi.org/10.1056/NEJM199909023411002.
49. Powell LW, Seckington RC, Deugnier Y. Haemochromatosis. Lancet. 2016;388:706–16. https://doi.org/10.1016/S0140-6736(15)01315-X.
50. Adams PC, et al. Biological variability of transferrin saturation and unsaturated iron-binding capacity. Am J Med. 2007;120:999e1–97. https://doi.org/10.1016/j.amjmed.2007.02.027.
51. European Association for the Study of the Liver. EASL clinical practice guidelines for HFE hemochromatosis. J Hepatol. 2010;53:3–22. https://doi.org/10.1016/j.jhep.2010.03.001.
52. Guyader D, et al. Noninvasive prediction of fibrosis in C282Y homozygous hemochromatosis. Gastroenterology. 1998;115:929–36. https://doi.org/10.1016/s0016-5085(98)70265-3.
53. Bardou-Jacquet E, et al. Worse outcomes of patients with HFE hemochromatosis with persistent increases in transferrin saturation during maintenance therapy. Clin Gastroenterol Hepatol. 2017;15:1620–7. https://doi.org/10.1016/j.cgh.2016.12.039.
54. Bardou-Jacquet E, et al. Regression of fibrosis stage with treatment reduces long-term risk of liver cancer in patients with hemochromatosis caused by mutation in HFE. Clin Gastroenterol Hepatol. 2020;18:1851–7. https://doi.org/10.1016/j.cgh.2019.10.010.
55. Laine F, et al. Metabolic and hepatic effects of bloodletting in dysmetabolic iron overload syndrome: a randomized controlled study in 274 patients. Hepatology. 2017;65:465–74. https://doi.org/10.1002/hep.28856.
56. Nowak A, Giger RS, Krayenbuehl PA. Higher age at diagnosis of hemochromatosis is the strongest predictor of the occurrence of hepatocellular carcinoma in the Swiss hemochromatosis cohort: a prospective longitudinal observational study. Medicine (Baltimore). 2018;97:e12886. https://doi.org/10.1097/MD.0000000000012886.

Biliary Atresia

11

Megan Anderson Adams, Dor Yoeli,
and Elizabeth Anne Pomfret

Abbreviations

BA	Biliary atresia
CMV	Cytomegalovirus
CT	Computerized tomography
HPE	Hepatic portoenterostomy
NLS	Native liver survival
PELD	Pediatric end-stage liver disease
PICU	Pediatric intensive care unit
SCC	Stool color card

11.1 Introduction

Biliary atresia (BA) is the end result of a destructive, inflammatory process that affects both intra- and extrahepatic bile ducts. This leads to fibrosis and obliteration of the biliary tract and the eventual development of biliary cirrhosis [1]. Biliary atresia is the most common cause of chronic cholestasis in infants and children and also the most frequent indication for liver transplantation in the pediatric population [2]. The exact pathogenesis is still unknown despite an evolving body of literature on the subject, but it is likely multifactorial. Some of the proposed mechanisms of the development of biliary atresia include environmental toxins, viral injury, and a genetic predispo sition with dysregulation of immunity (Fig. 11.1) [3].

M. A. Adams (✉) · D. Yoeli · E. A. Pomfret
Colorado Center for Transplantation Care, Research and Education (CCTCARE), University of Colorado Anschutz Medical Campus, University of Colorado School of Medicine, Aurora, CO, USA
e-mail: Megan.a.adams@cuanschutz.edu; dor.yoeli@cuanschutz.edu; elizabeth.pomfret@cuanschutz.edu

T. Hackert, A. Gulla (eds.), *Rare Liver and Biliary Tract Diseases*,
https://doi.org/10.1007/978-3-032-15076-9_11

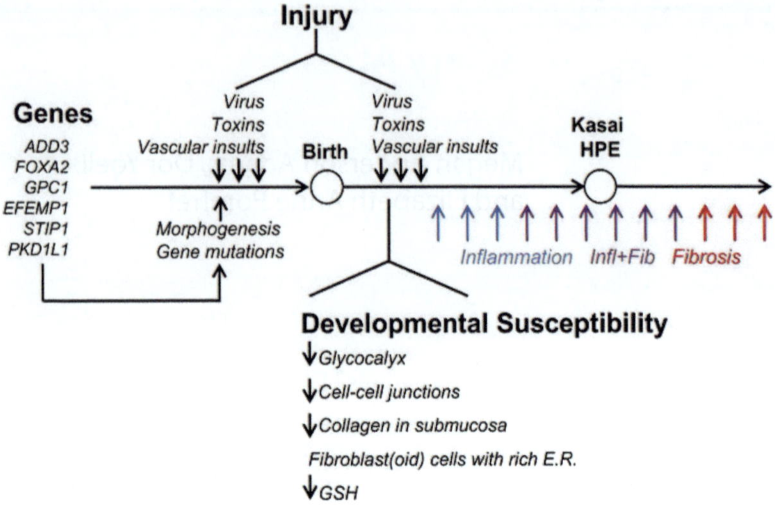

Fig. 11.1 Possible etiologies, pathogenesis, and progression of biliary atresia. (Reprinted with permission from J.A. Bezerra et al. [3]. Copyright belongs to Wolters Kluwer Health, Inc.)

11.2 Incidence

Biliary atresia is a rare disorder, with the most accurate estimates of national prevalence from the UK and France ranging from 1 in 17,000–19,000 livebirths. It is most common in East Asian countries, with a reported frequency in Taiwan of about 1 in 5000. Other estimates are 1 in 15,000 in the southeast region of the USA and 1 in 19,000 in the Netherlands [1]. There is a slight female predominance in most published series [2]. The underlying reason for the increased incidence in eastern countries is largely unknown but postulated to be related to differences in genetic makeup and environmental factors [4]. At least four phenotypes of BA are recognized: isolated BA, BA associated with laterality defects (asplenia, polysplenia, abdominal situs inversus, and intestinal malrotation), BA associated with other major congenital malformations, and BA associated with a bile duct cyst (cystic BA) [5]. Cytomegalovirus (CMV)-associated BA has also been suggested as a variant and has been demonstrated to have inferior native liver survival (NLS) in comparison to CMV-negative BA patients [6].

11.3 Clinical Presentation

Infants with BA present with jaundice (conjugated hyperbilirubinemia) and acholic stools. The presence or absence of hepatomegaly, failure to thrive, pruritus, and coagulopathy depend on the degree of disease severity at the time of presentation [2]. Ascites and muscle wasting are usually late findings after biliary cirrhosis has developed.

Timely diagnosis is important to optimize the response to a Kasai hepatic portoenterostomy (HPE) aimed at reestablishing bile flow. If the HPE is performed within the first 60 days of life, ~70% of patients will establish bile flow; after 90 days of life, <25% of patients will have bile flow [7]. Late diagnosis of BA remains a problem worldwide. Several countries have introduced use of a stool color card (SCC) to identify infants with pale stools. Japan and Taiwan were able to improve jaundice-free survival with the native liver with the use of the stool color card (SCC). Native liver survival (NLS) at 5, 10, and 15 years was 87.6%, 76.9%, and 48.5%, respectively, compared to 68.0%, 60.0%, and 51.0%, respectively, in Sendai, Japan, without the SCC [8]. In Taiwan, screening was also associated with an improved 3-year jaundice-free survival rate with native liver (56.9% with the SCC vs. 31.5% in historical controls) [8]. Because of these successes, Germany, Canada, Switzerland, and Brazil have developed variations of the stool color card program. In the USA, newborn screening with direct bilirubin has also demonstrated success, having high sensitivity and specificity for diagnosing BA, and achieving decreased time to HPE [9].

11.4 Diagnosis

The differential diagnosis of a cholestatic infant remains broad. Prompt evaluation of conjugated hyperbilirubinemia is of utmost importance to avoid delays in definitive treatment. Other causes of cholestasis such as sepsis, endocrine disorders, nutritional hepatotoxicity attributable to metabolic disease (e.g., galactosemia) and "idiopathic" neonatal intrahepatic cholestasis must be ruled out.

Early signs of BA include jaundice and/or acholic stools in a neonate. These findings in a neonate and/or laboratory findings of conjugated hyperbilirubinemia warrant further investigation for this diagnosis. Initial imaging modality of choice is abdominal ultrasound. The absence of a gallbladder and presence of the "triangular cord" sign are supportive of BA [10, 11]. The "triangular cord" sign refers to a triangular echogenicity that can be visualized near the portal vein and has a positive predictive value for BA greater than 95% (Fig. 11.2) [10, 12]. Nuclear medicine or magnetic resonance imaging can be considered adjunct imaging modalities. In children with suspected BA, a percutaneous liver biopsy is recommended, as this can help differentiate BA from other causes of neonatal cholestasis and has been reported to have a 92% accuracy, 91% sensitivity,

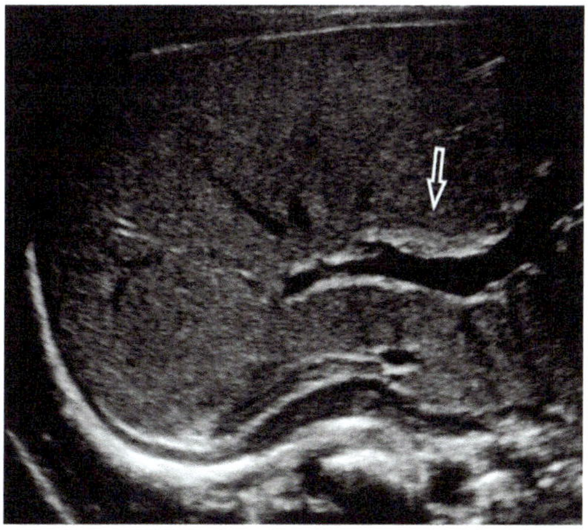

Fig. 11.2 Sonographic triangular cord sign. A 3–4-mm thickening nearing the bifurcation of the main portal vein is thought to be the fibrous remnant of the obliterated biliary duct and is highly specific for BA. (Reprinted with permission from D.D. Brahee et al. [12]. Copyright belongs to Springer Nature)

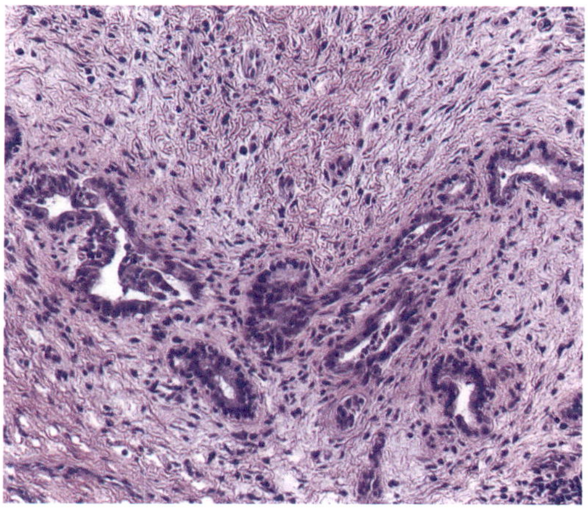

Fig. 11.3 Liver biopsy of a child with BA at the time of Kasai demonstrating histological hallmarks of BA including bile duct plugs, hepatocyte giant cell transformation, prominent bile duct proliferation, periductal inflammation, and bridging fibrosis

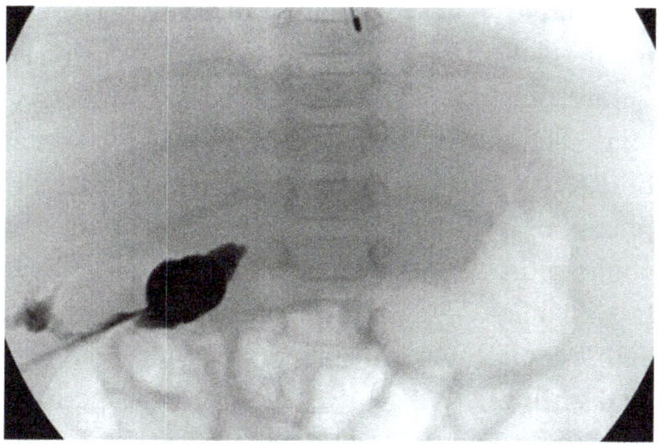

Fig. 11.4 Intraoperative cholangiogram in a child with biliary atresia demonstrates lack of proximal intrahepatic biliary filling or distal filling of the small bowel

and 93% specificity [13]. Classical histological hallmarks of BA on liver biopsy include ductular proliferation, bile plugs, and portal fibrosis (Fig. 11.3).

If the diagnosis of BA is still suspected after the above workup, an exploratory laparotomy with intraoperative cholangiogram is required to confirm the diagnosis. Obstruction of the biliary system, either to the proximal intrahepatic system or to the distal extrahepatic duct with failure to empty into the intestine, is indicative of BA (Fig. 11.4). If BA is confirmed on intraoperative cholangiogram and there is no clear evidence of cirrhosis, then the surgeon should proceed with a Kasai HPE during the same operation.

11.5 Treatment, Surgical Planning, and Management

11.5.1 Kasai Hepatoportoenterostomy

The goal of a Kasai HPE is to restore biliary-enteric drainage from the liver by excising the fibrotic biliary remnant and anastomosing a Roux limb of the small bowel to the cut edge of the portal plate at the porta hepatis (Fig. 11.5) [14, 15]. The theory behind this operation is that microscopic bile ductules at the cystic plate can then drain directly into the small bowel. NLS rates with Kasai HPE are 30–55% at 5 years [3–9] and 20–40% at 10 years (Fig. 11.6) [5, 16–21]. The benchmark for successful biliary drainage after Kasai HPE is typically considered to be total bilirubin level < 2 mg/dL at 3 months post-surgery [22, 23]. Failure of a Kasai is commonly categorized as early, referring to primary failure of biliary drainage as marked by persistently elevated bilirubin levels, and late, in which biliary drainage is successful, but long-term complications of BA, such as progressive fibrosis or cholangitis, result in death or require liver transplantation. Children with early failure typically require liver transplantation within the first year of life [24]. Age at time of HPE has perhaps been the strongest clinical prognostic factor associated with NLS, with children undergoing surgery at 30 days of age or younger achieving the best outcomes [25]. However, older age alone in the absence of evidence of end-stage liver disease does not preclude children with delayed diagnosis from undergoing an attempt at HPE, as successful biliary drainage has been reported in 25–35% of children with BA who were 90 days or older [19, 26]. Greater surgeon and center case volumes have also been associated with superior post-Kasai outcomes, with improved NLS rates achieved with the centralization of these operations in Europe [27]. Several adjuvant therapies following Kasai HPE have been proposed to prolong NLS, including steroids, immunoglobulins, antibiotics, ganciclovir, and N-acetylcysteine; though a few series have demonstrated some success at improving NLS with adjuvant treatment, the majority of trials have shown no significant difference with the currently available therapies [28–38].

11.5.2 Liver Transplantation

Indications for liver transplantation in children with biliary atresia include early HPE failure, cirrhosis due to late HPE failure or delayed diagnosis, complications of HPE (e.g., cholangitis), complications of portal hypertension, and failure to thrive, among others (Table 11.1) [5]. Children transplanted at 1 year of age or younger, typically due to early HPE failure or primary liver transplant due to delayed diagnosis, are at higher risk for both waiting list and post-transplant mortality in comparison to older candidates/recipients [24, 39].

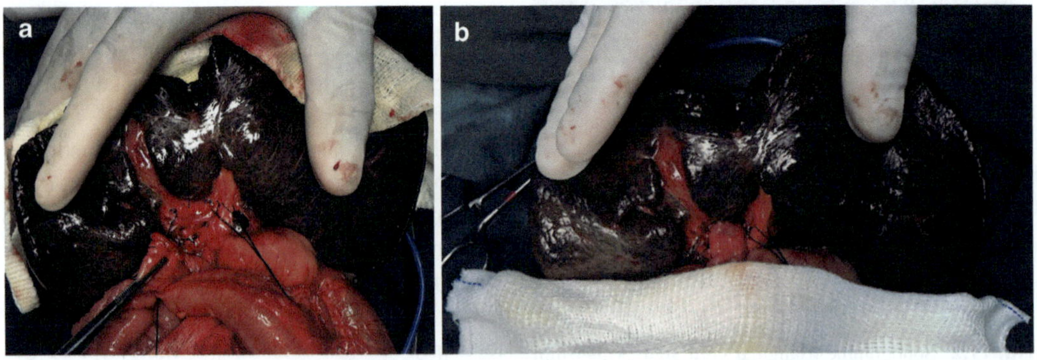

Fig. 11.5 Completed dissection of the portal hepatis (A) after excision of the fibrous biliary remnant before (**a**) and after (**b**) the entero-biliary anastomosis with Roux limb of small bowel (B). (Reprinted with permission from N.M.N de Carvalho et al. [14]. Copyright belongs to Elsevier)

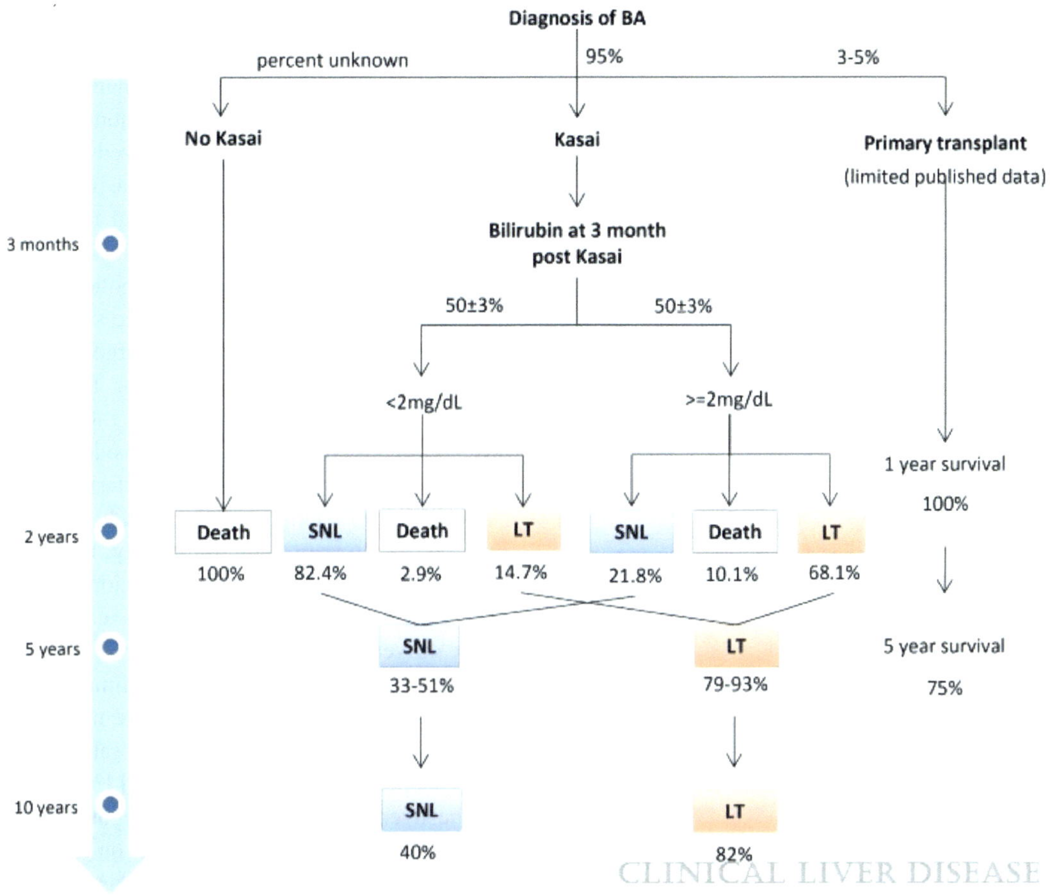

Fig. 11.6 Outcomes of children with biliary atresia. BA, biliary atresia; LT, liver transplant; SNL, survival with native liver. (Reprinted with permission from Y. Li and J.A. Bezerra [16]. Copyright belongs to Wolters Kluwer Health, Inc.)

Of those listed for liver transplant, approximately 5% of candidates with BA die while waiting for a transplant; risk factors for waiting list mortality in this patient population include rising bilirubin, portal vein thrombosis, mechanical ventilation, and ascites at time of listing [40]. The majority of BA transplant candidates experience worsening complications of cirrhosis, such as increasing ascites, need for albumin or blood transfusion, nutritional support, or hospitalizations [41]. For these reasons, early referral to a transplant center is critical.

Transplant evaluation requires a multidisciplinary approach incorporating specialists from hepatology, transplant surgery, anesthesia, transplant nurse coordinators, social work, psychology, and pharmacy, in addition to other specialists, as indicated on a case-by-case basis. During the surgery consultation, it is important to review an overview of the transplant operation, deceased vs. living donation, and the expected perioperative course. Families should be encouraged to consider living donation and reach out to potential interested living donors as early as possible. Abdominal ultrasound or computerized tomography (CT) should be obtained as part of the evaluation to document the patency of the portal vein, as the presence of a portal vein thrombosis alters peri- and intraoperative management. At our institution, we obtain a CT venogram to evaluate the portal vein and calculate liver volumes to help with donor size matching, as well as to identify other potential anatomical variations that are common in BA (i.e., presence of large portosys-

Table 11.1 Indications for liver transplantation in biliary atresia

Failed Kasai portoenterostomy
Early absence of bile flow
Late development of cirrhosis despite good bile flow
Late diagnosis: primary liver transplant
Severe nutritional compromise
Failure to thrive requiring aggressive nutritional support
Metabolic bone disease resulting in fractures
Bacterial cholangitis
Recurrent despite appropriate antibiotic therapy
Multidrug-resistant organisms
Life-threatening sepsis
Recurrent hospitalizations impairing quality of life
Complications of portal hypertension
Refractory variceal bleeding
Significant ascites and episodes of spontaneous bacterial peritonitis
Symptomatic thrombocytopenia
Severe pruritus
Pulmonary vascular disorders
Hepatopulmonary syndrome
Portopulmonary hypertension
Hepatorenal syndrome
Hepatic malignancy
Hepatocellular carcinoma
Cholangiocarcinoma

Reprinted with permission from S.S. Sundaram et al. [5]. Copyright belongs to Wolters Kluwer Health, Inc

temic shunts, situs inversus, and interrupted inferior vena cava).

Liver graft types used for transplantation of children with BA include deceased donor whole livers, deceased donor reduced sized or split grafts, and living donor grafts. The decision-making regarding graft selection and recipient-donor matching is threefold: physiologic issues, anatomic issues, and degree of metabolic disease (Fig. 11.7) [42]. While small for size syndrome (SFSS) is rare in small children, large for size (GW/RW > 3%) is not uncommon. The ideal graft vs. recipient's weight (GW/RW) ratio is ideally 1–2%, but GW/RW ≤ 3% is considered reasonable [42]. Deceased donor criteria for a "splitable" liver continue to be a subject of debate in the pediatric transplant community. Ideally, a donor that fits the following inclusion criteria would be considered as a split candidate: age < 40 years, weight 50–90 kg, liver function test not beyond 2–3 times the upper limit of normal, intensive care unit stay <5 days, no sepsis, low dose to no vasopressors, and satisfactory macroscopic appearance of the graft [43].

The liver transplant operation begins with a careful preparation of the liver graft on the back table. Identification of anatomical variations and procurement injuries, if present; preparation of

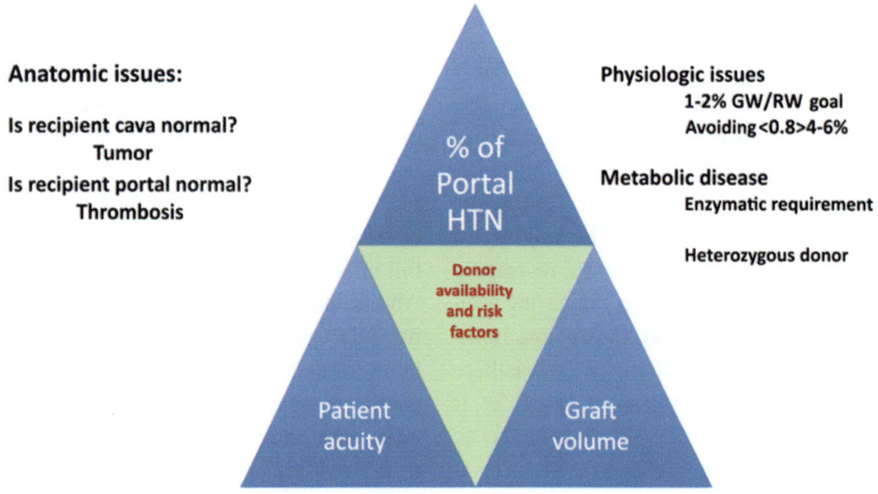

Fig. 11.7 Patient factors in graft selection decision-making for pediatric liver transplant recipients. (Reprinted with permission from G.V. Mazariegos [42]. Copyright belongs to Wolters Kluwer Health, Inc.)

vessels for implant and vascular reconstruction, if needed; and removal of excess tissue are critical aspects of the back table operation. This can often be done in conjunction with the recipient hepatectomy, though no major recipient structure should be ligated until there has been adequate verification of graft quality if completed on the back table. During the recipient hepatectomy, the liver should be mobilized and the porta hepatis dissected to gain control of the hepatic artery, portal vein, and vena cava in preparation for explant. Careful attention to the presence of large portosystemic collaterals is necessary to avoid excess blood loss. If the recipient had a prior Kasai HPE, intra-abdominal adhesions, especially around the portal plate, should be anticipated and may require additional dissection time. The Roux limb should be ligated and separated from the portal plate as part of the explant operation. Caval reconstruction can be performed with either bicaval or piggyback techniques if the recipient is receiving a whole graft, but a piggyback caval reconstruction is the only option in the case of a deceased donor partial/split or living donor graft. The portal vein and hepatic artery are anastomosed in standard fashion. Unlike in most other liver transplant recipients, duct-to-duct biliary reconstruction is not an option in BA due to the absence of a recipient extrahepatic bile duct. If a prior Kasai HPE was performed, the bile duct can be anastomosed to the recipient prior Roux limb, though the Roux limb small bowel should be excised back to fresh, healthy tissue. In the case of a primary liver transplant when a prior Kasai has not been performed, a Roux limb can be brought up for biliary reconstruction, or the donor bile duct can often be connected directly to the recipient duodenum (choledochoduodenostomy) [44]. In partial liver grafts, multiple bile ducts may be present requiring multiple biliary anastomoses.

The postoperative management of a BA liver transplant recipient varies by institution. At our institution, all pediatric liver transplant recipients are taken to the pediatric intensive care unit (PICU) for the immediate postoperative period. The majority of recipients can be extubated in the operating room prior to transfer to the PICU; young age, preoperative mechanical ventilation, and intra-operative vasopressor requirements are risk factors against early extubation in this patient population [45]. Early postoperative ultrasounds with Doppler assessment are useful to monitor for vessel patency and peri-hepatic hematomas. In small recipients or recipients of technical variant grafts, empiric anticoagulation with a heparin drip and/or aspirin is recommended to decrease the risk of hepatic artery thrombosis. Blood transfusion should be guided by assessments of hemodynamics, drain output, and frequent laboratory testing, including thromboelastography (TEG) [46, 47]. Early return to the operating room after pediatric liver transplantation is not uncommon for bleeding, bowel, vascular, or biliary complications. We encourage a low threshold for return to the operating room if there is any concern for vascular complication on labs or imaging, as hepatic artery thrombosis and other vascular complications can be devastating to the survival of the graft if not treated early, while reoperation is not a risk factor for death or graft loss [48].

Survival following pediatric liver transplantation for children with BA in the modern era is excellent, with 97% recipient survival and 90% graft survival at 5 years; these outcomes have significantly improved since the introduction of the Pediatric End-Stage Liver Disease (PELD) scoring allocation system [49, 50]. Liver transplantation is curative for BA, which does not recur in the transplanted liver. Risk factors for mortality after pediatric liver transplantation include retransplantation, small recipient size, very young donor age, and pre-transplant renal insufficiency and/or life support [49, 51]. Living donor pediatric liver transplant recipients demonstrate greater recipient and graft survival in comparison with deceased whole liver recipients [52–55]. Studies on outcomes with deceased donor split grafts have been conflicting, with some showing inferior survival and others showing equivalent survival with these grafts in comparison to deceased whole grafts [49, 51, 55, 56]. A transplant center's overall pediatric liver transplant case volume as well as deceased donor split and living donor liver transplant volumes are signifi-

Table 11.2 Complications following pediatric liver transplantation (post-2002)

Complication	Frequency (%)
Death	3
Retransplant	7
Hepatic artery thrombosis	9
Portal vein thrombosis	7
Biliary complication	13
Reoperation	37
Infection	40
Rejection	40
Post-transplant lymphoproliferative disorder	2

Data derived from Taylor et al. [49] and Elisofon et al. [50]

cantly associated with improved waiting list and post-transplant outcomes, indicating that versatility and comfort with transplanting all types of liver grafts for children is key to successfully caring for this complex patient population [57, 58]. The most common post-pediatric liver transplant complications and their reported frequencies are summarized in Table 11.2.

11.5.3 Unique Considerations

It is well known that children with BA develop an atretic portal vein which can make transplantation very difficult [59]. Often the main portal vein must be dissected back to the confluence of the splenic vein and the superior mesenteric vein in order to achieve adequate flow to the graft. Children with BA commonly develop extensive portosystemic collaterals, which need to be ligated, most commonly the left renal vein, which alleviates portal blood steal via a splenorenal shunt [59]. Because of these factors, portal vein thrombosis is a serious concern post-transplant, occurring in up to 8% of pediatric liver transplant recipients [60]. Portal vein thrombosis after Kasai is another challenge that can present at the time of transplant.

As mentioned above, BA can have many different phenotypes [1]. Biliary atresia splenic malformation syndrome (BASM) is reported in about 10% of BA patients. The estimated frequency of these clinical features in BASM is as follows: splenic malformation (100%), absent inferior vena cava (70%), intestinal malrotation (60%), cardiac anomalies (45%), preduodenal portal vein (40%), situs inversus (37%), and pancreatic anomalies (11%) [1]. These disease phenotypes are often discovered during the transplant evaluation phase. From a surgical standpoint, it is imperative to have a clear understanding of the recipient anatomy prior to selecting a graft for liver transplant.

Surgeons have long debated the utility in primary transplant for patients with BA given the high failure rate of Kasai. A recent analysis showed that candidates listed for liver transplantation after Kasai had lower bilirubin levels, and a lower MELD/PELD score and had higher waiting list and graft survival [24]. Although in children who present with cirrhosis and complications of end stage liver disease, primary liver transplantation is often the better choice. Regardless, surgery (whether it be Kasai HPE or liver transplantation) remains the backbone of treatment of biliary atresia.

11.6 Follow-Up and Recommendations

In summary, biliary atresia is a surgically treated liver disease. Early diagnosis and early Kasai are critical for improving the outcome of patients with BA [5]. If a Kasai is "non-flowing" (serum total bilirubin ≥2 mg/dL) at 90 days of life, referral for liver transplantation is recommended [5]. It is important to keep in mind that of those who still have their native liver at 2 years of age, at least 75% of those patients will develop ongoing fibrosis, portal hypertension, and cirrhosis, with the need for liver transplant later in childhood or young adulthood [3].

There are several new agents being studied in adult cholestatic and fibrotic liver disease [3]. Some of these mechanisms are by inhibiting bile acid synthesis, by inhibiting ileal reabsorption of bile acids, by inhibiting hepatocyte basolateral bile acid uptake proteins, and by using bile acid sequestrants [3]. There are also several agents that address inflammation and fibrosis of the liver [3, 61]. Future clinical trials should focus on investigating the potential of these new therapeutic agents as adjuncts to Kasai HPE to improve NLS.

Much continues to be unknown in the etiology and pathogenesis of biliary atresia. Early diagnosis and intervention continue to be the mainstay of treatment of BA. Continued efforts in prolonging native liver survival are widely described. Organ shortages continue to be present in the USA and worldwide impacting the overall survival of children after a failed Kasai. Living donor liver transplant allows children to be transplanted earlier prior to decompensation that might result in death on the waiting list for a deceased donor transplant. Despite advances in the fields of hepatology and transplantation, much work has yet to be done to elucidate the etiology for developing biliary atresia and novel therapies to treat this disease without the need for liver transplantation.

References

1. Hartley JL, Davenport M, Kelly DA. Biliary atresia. Lancet. 2009;374(9702):1704–13.
2. Bezerra JA, Mack CL, Schneider BL. Biliary atresia and other disorders of the extrahepatic bile ducts. In: Suchy F, Sokol RJ, Balistreri WF, editors. Liver disease in children. 5th ed. Cambridge: Cambridge University Press; 2021. p. 162–81.
3. Bezerra JA, Wells RG, Mack CL, Karpen SJ, Hoofnagle JH, Doo E, et al. Biliary atresia: clinical and research challenges for the twenty-first century. Hepatology. 2018;68(3):1163–73.
4. Chung PHY, Zheng S, Tam PKH. Biliary atresia: east versus west. Semin Pediatr Surg. 2020;29(4):150950.
5. Sundaram SS, Mack CL, Feldman AG, Sokol RJ. Biliary atresia: indications and timing of liver transplantation and optimization of pretransplant care. Liver Transpl. 2017;23(1):96–109.
6. Fischler B, Czubkowski P, Dezsofi A, Liliemark U, Socha P, Sokol RJ, et al. Incidence, impact and treatment of ongoing CMV infection in patients with biliary atresia in four European centres. J Clin Med. 2022;11(4):945.
7. Fawaz R, Baumann U, Ekong U, Fischler B, Hadzic N, Mack CL, et al. Guideline for the evaluation of cholestatic jaundice in infants: joint recommendations of the North American Society for Pediatric Gastroenterology, Hepatology, and Nutrition and the European Society for Pediatric Gastroenterology, Hepatology, and Nutrition. J Pediatr Gastroenterol Nutr. 2017;64(1):154–68.
8. Rabbani T, Guthery SL, Himes R, Shneider BL, Harpavat S. Newborn screening for biliary atresia: a review of current methods. Curr Gastroenterol Rep. 2021;23(12):28.
9. Harpavat S, Garcia-Prats JA, Anaya C, Brandt ML, Lupo PJ, Finegold MJ, et al. Diagnostic yield of newborn screening for biliary atresia using direct or conjugated bilirubin measurements. JAMA. 2020;323(12):1141–50.
10. Park WH, Choi SO, Lee HJ. Technical innovation for noninvasive and early diagnosis of biliary atresia: the ultrasonographic "triangular cord" sign. J Hepatobiliary Pancreat Surg. 2001;8(4):337–41.
11. Park WH, Choi SO, Lee HJ, Kim SP, Zeon SK, Lee SL. A new diagnostic approach to biliary atresia with emphasis on the ultrasonographic triangular cord sign: comparison of ultrasonography, hepatobiliary scintigraphy, and liver needle biopsy in the evaluation of infantile cholestasis. J Pediatr Surg. 1997;32(11):1555–9.
12. Brahee DD, Lampl BS. Neonatal diagnosis of biliary atresia: a practical review and update. Pediatr Radiol. 2022;52(4):685–92.
13. Lee JY, Sullivan K, El Demellawy D, Nasr A. The value of preoperative liver biopsy in the diagnosis of extrahepatic biliary atresia: a systematic review and meta-analysis. J Pediatr Surg. 2016;51(5):753–61.
14. de Carvalho NMN, Torres SM, Cavalcante JCB, Ximenes ACM, Junior JAL, da Silveira Moreira SO. Hepatoportoenterostomy surgery technique. J Pediatr Surg. 2019;54(8):1715–8.
15. Wildhaber BE. Biliary atresia: 50 years after the first kasai. ISRN Surg. 2012;2012:132089.
16. Li Y, Bezerra JA. Novel approaches to the treatment of biliary atresia. Clin Liver Dis (Hoboken). 2016;8(6):145–9.
17. Chardot C, Buet C, Serinet MO, Golmard JL, Lachaux A, Roquelaure B, et al. Improving outcomes of biliary atresia: French national series 1986-2009. J Hepatol. 2013;58(6):1209–17.
18. Serinet MO, Wildhaber BE, Broue P, Lachaux A, Sarles J, Jacquemin E, et al. Impact of age at Kasai operation on its results in late childhood and adolescence: a rational basis for biliary atresia screening. Pediatrics. 2009;123(5):1280–6.
19. Davenport M, Puricelli V, Farrant P, Hadzic N, Mieli-Vergani G, Portmann B, et al. The outcome of the older (> or = 100 days) infant with biliary atresia. J Pediatr Surg. 2004;39(4):575–81.
20. Karrer FM, Price MR, Bensard DD, Sokol RJ, Narkewicz MR, Smith DJ, et al. Long-term results with the Kasai operation for biliary atresia. Arch Surg. 1996;131(5):493–6.
21. Lykavieris P, Chardot C, Sokhn M, Gauthier F, Valayer J, Bernard O. Outcome in adulthood of biliary atresia: a study of 63 patients who survived for

over 20 years with their native liver. Hepatology. 2005;41(2):366–71.
22. Shneider BL, Brown MB, Haber B, Whitington PF, Schwarz K, Squires R, et al. A multicenter study of the outcome of biliary atresia in the United States, 1997 to 2000. J Pediatr. 2006;148(4):467–74.
23. Shneider BL, Magee JC, Karpen SJ, Rand EB, Narkewicz MR, Bass LM, et al. Total serum bilirubin within 3 months of hepatoportoenterostomy predicts short-term outcomes in biliary atresia. J Pediatr. 2016;170:211–7.e1–2.
24. Yoeli D, Choudhury RA, Sundaram SS, Mack CL, Roach JP, Karrer FM, et al. Primary vs. salvage liver transplantation for biliary atresia: a retrospective cohort study. J Pediatr Surg. 2022;57(10):407–13.
25. Hoshino E, Muto Y, Sakai K, Shimohata N, Urayama KY, Suzuki M. Age at surgery and native liver survival in biliary atresia: a systematic review and meta-analysis. Eur J Pediatr. 2023;182:2693.
26. Chardot C, Carton M, Spire-Bendelac N, Le Pommelet C, Golmard J, Reding R, et al. Is the Kasai operation still indicated in children older than 3 months diagnosed with biliary atresia? J Pediatr. 2001;138(2):224–8.
27. Stringer MD. Biliary atresia: service delivery and outcomes. Semin Pediatr Surg. 2008;17(2):116–22.
28. Meyers RL, Book LS, O'Gorman MA, Jackson WD, Black RE, Johnson DG, et al. High-dose steroids, ursodeoxycholic acid, and chronic intravenous antibiotics improve bile flow after Kasai procedure in infants with biliary atresia. J Pediatr Surg. 2003;38(3):406–11.
29. Parolini F, Hadzic N, Davenport M. Adjuvant therapy of cytomegalovirus IgM + ve associated biliary atresia: prima facie evidence of effect. J Pediatr Surg. 2019;54(9):1941–5.
30. Kuebler JF, Madadi-Sanjani O, Pfister ED, Baumann U, Fortmann D, Leonhardt J, et al. Adjuvant therapy with budesonide post-Kasai reduces the need for liver transplantation in biliary atresia. J Clin Med. 2021;10(24):5758.
31. Tessier MEM, Shneider BL, Brandt ML, Cerminara DN, Harpavat S. A phase 2 trial of N-acetylcysteine in biliary atresia after Kasai portoenterostomy. Contemp Clin Trials Commun. 2019;15:100370.
32. Mack CL, Spino C, Alonso EM, Bezerra JA, Moore J, Goodhue C, et al. A phase I/IIa trial of intravenous immunoglobulin following portoenterostomy in biliary atresia. J Pediatr Gastroenterol Nutr. 2019;68(4):495–501.
33. Zhang D, Yang HY, Jia J, Zhao G, Yue M, Wang JX. Postoperative steroids after Kasai portoenterostomy for biliary atresia: a meta-analysis. Int J Surg. 2014;12(11):1203–9.
34. Sarkhy A, Schreiber RA, Milner RA, Barker CC. Does adjuvant steroid therapy post-Kasai portoenterostomy improve outcome of biliary atresia? Systematic review and meta-analysis. Can J Gastroenterol. 2011;25(8):440–4.
35. Goh L, Phua KB, Low Y, Chiang LW, Yong C, Chiou FK. Analysis of cholangitis rates with extended perioperative antibiotics and adjuvant corticosteroids in biliary atresia. Pediatr Gastroenterol Hepatol Nutr. 2021;24(4):366–76.
36. Petersen C, Harder D, Melter M, Becker T, Wasielewski RV, Leonhardt J, et al. Postoperative high-dose steroids do not improve mid-term survival with native liver in biliary atresia. Am J Gastroenterol. 2008;103(3):712–9.
37. Bezerra JA, Spino C, Magee JC, Shneider BL, Rosenthal P, Wang KS, et al. Use of corticosteroids after hepatoportoenterostomy for bile drainage in infants with biliary atresia: the START randomized clinical trial. JAMA. 2014;311(17):1750–9.
38. Pietrobattista A, Mosca A, Liccardo D, Alterio T, Grimaldi C, Basso M, et al. Does the treatment after Kasai procedure influence biliary atresia outcome and native liver survival? J Pediatr Gastroenterol Nutr. 2020;71(4):446–51.
39. Kwong AJ, Ebel NH, Kim WR, Lake JR, Smith JM, Schladt DP, et al. OPTN/SRTR 2020 annual data report: liver. Am J Transplant. 2022;22(Suppl 2):204–309.
40. Ziogas IA, Ye F, Zhao Z, Cao S, Rauf MA, Izzy M, et al. Mortality determinants in children with biliary atresia awaiting liver transplantation. J Pediatr. 2021;228:177–82.
41. de Ville de Goyet J, Illhardt T, Chardot C, Dike PN, Baumann U, Brandt K, et al. Variability of care and access to transplantation for children with biliary atresia who need a liver replacement. J Clin Med. 2022;11(8):2142.
42. Mazariegos GV. Critical elements in pediatric allograft selection. Liver Transpl. 2017;23(S1):S56–S8.
43. Battula NR, Platto M, Anbarasan R, Perera MT, Ong E, Roll GR, et al. Intention to split policy: a successful strategy in a combined pediatric and adult liver transplant center. Ann Surg. 2017;265(5):1009–15.
44. Campsen J, Zimmerman MA, Narkewicz MR, Sokol RJ, Mandell MS, Kam I, et al. Choledochoduodenostomy in pediatric liver transplantation. Pediatr Transplant. 2011;15(3):237–9.
45. Yoeli D, Nguyen T, Wilder M, Huang J, Pahlavan S, Brigham D, et al. Immediate extubation following pediatric liver transplantation. Pediatr Transplant. 2022;26(8):e14352.
46. Sujka J, Gonzalez KW, Curiel KL, Daniel J, Fischer RT, Andrews WS, et al. The impact of thromboelastography on resuscitation in pediatric liver transplantation. Pediatr Transplant. 2018;22(4):e13176.
47. Cho JK, Moon YJ, Song IK, Kang EJ, Shin WJ, Hwang GS. A look into hemostatic characteristics during pediatric liver transplantation using the thromboelastometry (ROTEM((R))) test. Liver Transpl. 2022;28(10):1628–39.
48. Yoeli D, Ackah RL, Sigireddi RR, Kueht ML, Galvan NTN, Cotton RT, et al. Reoperative complications following pediatric liver transplantation. J Pediatr Surg. 2018;53(11):2240–4.
49. Taylor SA, Venkat V, Arnon R, Gopalareddy VV, Rosenthal P, Erinjeri J, et al. Improved out-

comes for liver transplantation in patients with biliary atresia since pediatric end-stage liver disease implementation: analysis of the Society of Pediatric Liver Transplantation registry. J Pediatr. 2020;219:89–97.
50. Elisofon SA, Magee JC, Ng VL, Horslen SP, Fioravanti V, Economides J, et al. Society of pediatric liver transplantation: current registry status 2011-2018. Pediatr Transplant. 2020;24(1):e13605.
51. Rana A, Pallister ZS, Guiteau JJ, Cotton RT, Halazun K, Nalty CC, et al. Survival outcomes following pediatric liver transplantation (Pedi-SOFT) score: a novel predictive index. Am J Transplant. 2015;15(7):1855–63.
52. Barbetta A, Butler C, Barhouma S, Hogen R, Rocque B, Goldbeck C, et al. Living donor versus deceased donor pediatric liver transplantation: a systematic review and meta-analysis. Transplant Direct. 2021;7(10):e767.
53. Shingina A, Vutien P, Uleryk E, Shah PS, Renner E, Bhat M, et al. Long-term outcomes of pediatric living versus deceased donor liver transplantation recipients: a systematic review and meta-analysis. Liver Transpl. 2022;28(3):437–53.
54. Montenovo MI, Bambha K, Reyes J, Dick A, Perkins J, Healey P. Living liver donation improves patient and graft survival in the pediatric population. Pediatr Transplant. 2019;23(1):e13318.
55. Mogul DB, Luo X, Bowring MG, Chow EK, Massie AB, Schwarz KB, et al. Fifteen-year trends in pediatric liver transplants: split, whole deceased, and living donor grafts. J Pediatr. 2018;196:148–53.e2.
56. McElroy LM, Martin AE, Feldman AG, Ng VL, Kato T, Reichman T, et al. An appraisal of technical variant grafts compared to whole liver grafts in pediatric liver transplant recipients: multicenter analysis from the SPLIT registry. Pediatr Transplant. 2023;27(1):e14415.
57. Mazariegos GV, Perito ER, Squires JE, Soltys KA, Griesemer AD, Taylor SA, et al. Center use of technical variant grafts varies widely and impacts pediatric liver transplant waitlist and recipient outcomes in the United States. Liver Transpl. 2023;29:671.
58. Yoeli D, Choudhury RA, Moore HB, Jackson WE, Nydam TL, Wachs ME, et al. Living donor liver transplant center volume influences waiting list survival among children listed for liver transplantation. Transplantation. 2022;106(9):1807–13.
59. Englesbe MJ, Mathur AK, Waits SA, Magee JC. Wow, that portal vein is small: preventing portal vein thrombosis in liver transplantation for small children. Liver Transpl. 2014;20(6):742–3.
60. Ou HY, Concejero AM, Huang TL, Chen TY, Tsang LL, Chen CL, et al. Portal vein thrombosis in biliary atresia patients after living donor liver transplantation. Surgery. 2011;149(1):40–7.
61. Yoeli D, Mack CL, Navarro-Alvarez N. Role of galectin-3 in the pathogenesis and progression of biliary atresia. Clin Liver Dis (Hoboken). 2022;20(5):170–4.

Alpha-1 Antitrypsin Deficiency

12

Andrea Briem-Richter, Uta Herden,
and Sebastian Schulz-Jürgense

12.1 Incidence

Alpha-1 antitrypsin deficiency (AATD), first reported in 1963 [23], is a genetic disorder with autosomal recessive inheritance and mutations in the SERPINA1 gene.

Clinically, AATD has an estimated incidence of around 3.4 million affected individuals worldwide. This incidence is spread across different age groups and affects the liver and lungs, either alone or together (see clinical presentation).

The calculated prevalence of patients at risk (PiZZ) from AATD in Europe varies from 1 in 1368 in Denmark to 1 in 58,319 in Poland, possibly following migration patterns [3].

More than 116 million carriers of heterozygous mutations are expected [11]. These carriers are very unevenly distributed worldwide, with a predominance of the more severe PiZ phenotypes in Northern Europe and North America. The rates of PiZ there range between 4.1 and 45/1000, while in North Africa, Central and South Africa, Eastern Europe, Asia, South America, and the Caribbean, the incidence of PiZ ranges between 0 and (rarely) 15.3/1000. A different picture is the case for PiSS, which is much more common in Southern Africa, South West Europe, and South America, reaching up to 188/1000 in Angola. A very interesting finding is the very different prevalence often existing between neighboring countries ([11], see also [4]).

Initially diagnosed based on electrophoretic patterns, the changes in the protein are attributed to different phenotypes that can occur in homozygous or heterozygous forms: PiZZ, PiSZ, PiSS, PiMZ, PiMS, and PiMM (wild type), in >99% of the affected, as well as more than 100 further sub-alleles; see Table 12.1 for the most common [17].

Of those clinically affected, 96% have a PiZZ phenotype, and 4% have a PiSZ phenotype [6]. These two phenotypes show the greatest reduction of A1AT in the bloodstream: PiZZ 10–15% of normal and PiSZ 20–30% of normal [5].

The mutations in the SERPINA1 gene can be distinguished into (1) those with defective folding and accumulation in the Endoplasmatic Reticulum (ER) of hepatocytes, leading to ER stress, hepatocellular injury, inflammation, and eventual fibrosis [30] and (2) null mutations, accounting for about 1.5%, resulting in no protein production, will leave the liver unaffected while still causing lung injury [29].

A. Briem-Richter · S. Schulz-Jürgensen (✉)
Pediatric Gastroenterology and Hepatology, University Hospital Hamburg Eppendorf, UKE, Hamburg, Germany
e-mail: a.richter@uke.de; s.schulz-juergensen@uke.de

U. Herden
Pediatric Gastroenterology and Hepatology, University Hospital Hamburg Eppendorf, UKE, Hamburg, Germany

Transplant Surgery, University Hospital Hamburg Eppendorf, UKE, Hamburg, Germany
e-mail: u.herden@uke.de

T. Hackert, A. Gulla (eds.), *Rare Liver and Biliary Tract Diseases*,
https://doi.org/10.1007/978-3-032-15076-9_12

Table 12.1 Overview of the most common alpha-1 antitrypsin deficiency alleles

rs number	Deficiency alleles	*SERPINA1* variant	Characteristic genotypes and corresponding clinical features
rs28929474	Z	p.Glu342Lys	Strong (Pi*ZZ)/mild (Pi*MZ): predisposition to liver disease and lung emphysema
rs17580	S	p.Glu264Val	Pi*SZ: moderate predisposition to liver disease and lung emphysema Pi*SS: only minimal risk
	F	p.Arg223Cys	Lung emphysema in compound heterozygotes
rs28931570	I	p.Arg39Cys	No clear phenotype
rs121912713	Pittsburgh	p.Met358Arg	Bleeding disorder via inhibition of thrombin and factor XI
	Trento	p.Glu75Val	Lung emphysema in coinheritance with Pi*Z
rs775982338	M_{maiton}	p.Phe52del (M2 variant)	Lung emphysema in coinheritance with Pi*Z
rs28931568	$M_{mineral\ springs}$	p.Gly67Glu	Liver disease and lung emphysema in homozygotes
rs28931569	$M_{procida}$	p.Leu41Pro	Lung emphysema in homozygotes
rs199422211	$Q0_{bellingham}$	p.Lys217*	Lung emphysema in homozygotes and compound heterozygotes
rs267606950	$Q0_{bolton}$	p.Δ1 bpPro362	Lung emphysema in homozygotes and compound heterozygotes
	$Q0_{granitefalls}$	p.Δ1 bpTyr160	Lung emphysema in coinheritance with Pi*Z
rs1057519610	$Q0_{hongkong}$	p.Δ2 bpLeu318	Lung emphysema in homozygotes and compound heterozygotes

From Fromme et al. [17]

The most common mutation in AATD, leading to the severe PiZZ liver phenotype, is the homozygous change Glu342Lys IN 95% of patients [30].

The diagnosis of AATD is clinically underrecognized ([39]; [17]) because many patients remain clinically inapparent, while others have a late onset, and in adults, the contribution of AATD is difficult to differentiate from common diagnoses like non-alcoholic steatohepatitis (NASH), viral hepatitis, adult-onset asthma, emphysema, or chronic obstructive pulmonary disease (COPD) [40].

12.2 Clinical Presentation

The protein encoded by the SERPINA1 gene is mainly secreted by hepatocytes and protects the lung from proteolytic damage by neutrophil elastase; therefore, the particularity of AATD is the combined affection of the liver (intracellular accumulation resulting from the impaired intracellular transport of truncated or misfolded proteins) and lungs (loss of function resulting from missing enzymatic protection from neutrophil elastase activity); see Fig. 12.1. Additionally, there is a broad clinical spectrum in the presentation and progression of both liver and lung disease, reflected in the huge heterogeneity of reported parameters. An analysis of siblings of patients with AATD found that the concordance of the presence of liver disease was 72% but that of severity was only 29% [21].

In pediatrics, AATD mostly becomes clinically apparent through liver affection, with the clinical picture of neonatal cholestatic hepatitis, with conjugated hyperbilirubinemia and differentially elevated liver function tests (LFTs), or even through accidental findings of elevated LFTs without cholestasis [26]. However, the majority of genetically affected PiZZ children will not become clinically apparent, as seen in a birth screening study with 127 diagnosed patients among the 200.000 screened: 17% had cholestasis, and 42% had only elevated alanine-aminotransferase (ALT) [32].

The liver function, measured as coagulation or detoxification, in these patients is usually preserved, and abnormal parameters (cholestasis and LFTs) mostly show a spontaneous improvement. Only single infants will show early severe mani-

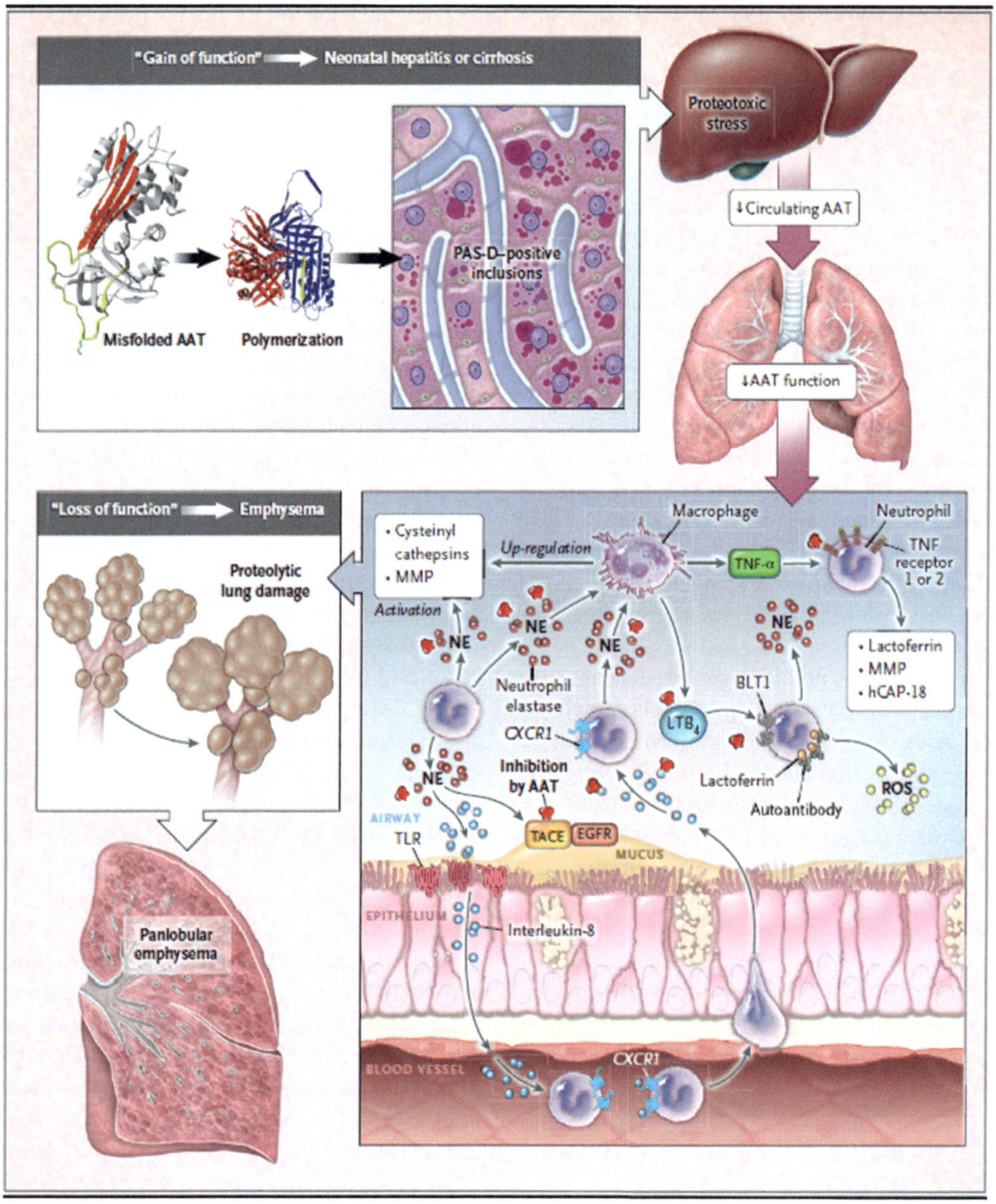

Fig. 12.1 Pathophysiology of AATD in the liver and lung. (From Strnad et al. [29])

festations like vitamin K deficiency coagulopathy, poor feeding, failure to thrive, gastrointestinal (GI) bleeding, and acute liver failure. In the pediatric and adolescent period, about 3–7% of patients develop liver changes, including fibrosis and impaired function [33, 36], but these are not limited to patients with neonatal cholestasis but are also reported in patients without neonatal cholestasis [28]. While in reported pediatric studies, cirrhosis is reported in 7.5%, portal hypertension in 6.9%, jaundice in 1.9%, and abnormal LFT/ prolonged jaundice in 9%, the incidence of liver transplantation (LTX) is reported to be 16.5%, which may be related to studies coming from tertiary transplant centers [36]. A study questioning the necessity for transplantation reported that even cirrhotic livers may show a relatively stable course and that not all pediatric patients with initial cirrhosis will need transplantation [37].

The formerly cited birth screening study later reported outcomes of the 184 identified PiZZ and PiSZ patients up to the age of 43 years. It showed 11 deaths, six of them <8 years of age and three clearly due to liver pathology. Of the five patients dying at an adult age, two deaths were clearly related to liver disease. The overall mortality was elevated compared to the statistical mean but was not statistically significant [25].

Adults mostly manifest liver disease in the fourth or fifth decade. A third of adult patients with PiZZ phenotype will show some degree of liver fibrosis [9, 20], and the lifetime risk for liver cirrhosis is present in 10–40% of AATD patients [13, 36]. In a review, cirrhosis is reported in 10.5%, portal hypertension in 3.4%, and abnormal LFTs in 3.6% of adults, with 14.7% transplantations among the reported patients. Hepatocellular carcinoma (HCC) is reported in 1.3%, which is similar to other chronic liver diseases [36].

As the majority of adult AATD patients (even with the PiZZ genotype) will show normal LFTs and gamma-glutamyl transferase (GGT), abnormal values should lead to a thorough diagnostic workup [17].

Adults' lung disease usually shows a chronic obstructive pulmonary disease (COPD) phenotype; a contribution of AATD to this diagnosis should be suspected and investigated if manifesting at <45 years or in cases of "adult-onset asthma" [40].

12.3 Workup Investigation

The basic test for AATD is the measurement of alpha-1 antitrypsin in serum with a norm of >1.1 mg/dl. In most cases of the PiZZ phenotype, this will reveal a markedly reduced level [22], while in heterozygous phenotypes, a formally normal AAT level can be found [41]. A possible confounder is the nature of AAT as an acute phase protein, leading to increased levels during inflammatory episodes [26].

The gold standard of diagnostics is the differentiation of the AAT protein phenotype (isoelectric focusing protein gel) or genotype [26].

The workup should also involve the assessment of organ affection, both liver and lung, to assess baseline values and guide therapeutic approaches. This includes liver function tests (LFTs), coagulation parameters, albumin, bilirubin, platelets, sonography of the liver and spleen (ideally with elastography), and eventual upper GI endoscopy in case of suspected varices for the liver assessment. For the lungs, initial complete lung function testing, then yearly spirometry (in children, initially at 10 years and, then, depending on results, at least from adulthood), chest x-ray, and, eventually, CT thorax in case of clinical symptoms and/or abnormal pulmonary function testing are recommended [39].

First-degree relatives of AATD patients should be offered genetic counseling and, eventually, testing, differentiating not only the AAT level but also evaluating for S and Z alleles [39].

12.4 Differential Diagnosis

Infant manifestation of AATD as cholestatic hepatitis primarily requires the exclusion of relevant differential diagnoses: (viral) hepatitis; cholestatic liver diseases, such as biliary atresia, Alagille syndrome, and progressive familial intrahepatic cholestasis (PFIC); metabolic conditions like Niemann Pick C, hereditary fructose intolerance, tyrosinemia, and Gaucher disease; and others.

In older pediatric patients with incidental findings of elevated LFTs, the differential diagnoses include viral hepatitis but, most relevantly, autoimmune hepatitis and Wilson disease.

In adults, many liver and lung diseases can be aggravated through AATD, so AATD should be considered an additional diagnosis and disease modifier. The COPD foundation recommends testing all individuals with COPD, asthma, unexplained bronchiectasis, or unexplained chronic liver disease for AATD.

12.5 Monitoring and Prognostic Markers

In pediatrics, the main focus is on the evolution of liver disease. This includes the evolution of laboratory parameters, as well as sonography and elastography, recommended in yearly intervals. In the case of progressive liver disease, the indication for liver transplant listing should be evaluated. With an increased risk of HCC in cirrhosed AATD livers, alpha-fetoprotein (AFP) should be measured in case of suspicion [31].

The deterioration of liver function, as well as the development of portal hypertension and esophageal varices, was a prognostic marker for the need for transplantation in a pediatric series [1]. In this series, only patients with the PiZZ phenotype needed transplantation, not patients with the PiMZ phenotype, although this needs further evaluation. In the analysis of the US ChiLDReN Network (consisting of tertiary referral centers), neonatal cholestasis was statistically significantly more common in patients with a severe phenotype (76%) compared to a mild phenotype (57%, $p = 0.0024$) but with a huge overlap, therefore not representing a reliable prognostic marker. Ascites, peritonitis, coagulopathy, and GI bleeding at presentation or during the course were indicative of a severe course, while other factors like age at diagnosis, AATD subtype, LFT elevation, vitamin deficiency, gender, and race were not significantly different [34]. No single longitudinal measurement was identified with the statistical power to predict the development of portal hypertension, but increasing total bilirubin, aspartate Aminotransferase (AST), GGT, and AST/platelet ratio, as well as decreasing platelet count, were associated with an increased risk of portal hypertension. Neonatal cholestasis showed an increased hazard ratio for the development of portal hypertension of 3.7 (95% CI, 1.06–12.87; $p = 0.04$) but did not reach statistical significance predicting transplantation/death with 1.93 (95% CI, 0.89–4.17; $p = 0.09$) [35].

Pulmonary monitoring is recommended from the age of 10 years with a first lung function test and, then, depending on the result, continuation or further tests from adult age. Relevant pulmonary disease is not expected before adult age, but lifestyle recommendations should already be given during adolescence (e.g., smoking, passive smoking, pressure diving, and occupational lung exposure) [31].

In adults, the focus of AATD is not only on the inherent AATD liver and lung disease but also on the modifiers that influence these affections or, from the opposite perspective, the influence of AATD on chronic liver and lung diseases, which then include not only the PiZZ phenotype but also PiSZ and PiMZ with higher prevalences. This is reflected, for example, in the contribution to liver fibrosis, liver tumors, and liver transplantation; see Fig. 12.2 (from Fromme et al. [17]).

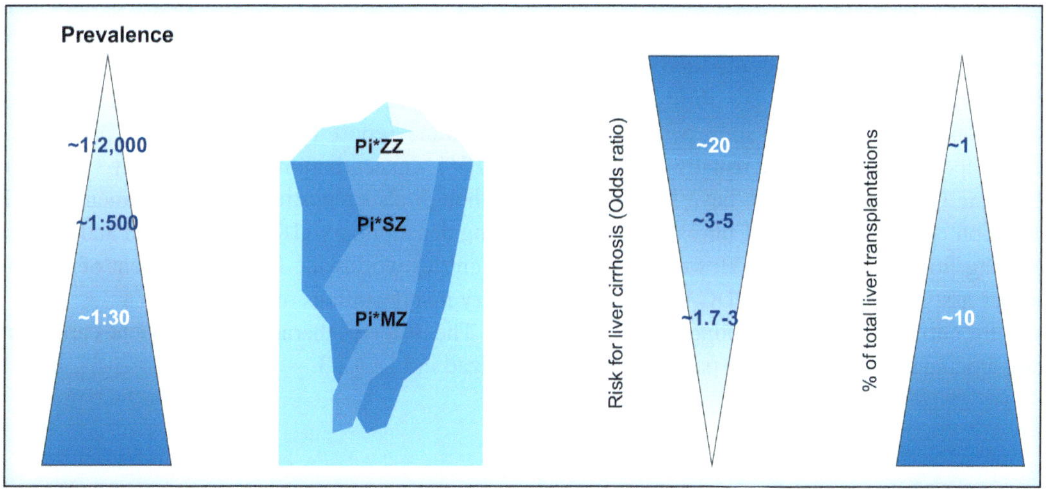

Fig. 12.2 Visualization of correlations of the prevalence, clinical visibility, risk of liver cirrhosis, and the percentage of liver transplantations. (From Fromme et al. [17])

As the majority of adult AATD patients (even with the Pi*ZZ genotype) will show normal LFTs and GGT, abnormal values should lead to a thorough diagnostic workup. In addition, liver stiffness is not directly correlated to LFT elevation; therefore, it should be investigated with elastography. Even elastography can underestimate fibrosis, thereby requiring biopsies for certain diagnoses [17].

The modifier effect of AATD makes the knowledge about AATD status, even in the heterozygote form, important in assessing other liver conditions like NASH, cystic fibrosis, or viral hepatitis.

12.6 Treatment

Being a genetic disorder with the pathophysiological mechanism involving alpha-1 antitrypsin synthesis and transport mostly in the liver, liver transplantation is a curative (gene therapy like) approach. However, considering its invasiveness and the wide phenotypic variability, this is an indication only in the context of liver failure.

Basic approaches start with lifestyle interventions: no smoking, no air-pressure diving, limiting liver toxicity through the reduction or avoidance of alcohol, preventing additional liver disease through vaccinations (hepatitis A and B), and preventing NASH [31].

In pediatrics, treatment with ursodeoxycholic acid (UDCA) has been described as successful in normalizing or improving elevated LFTs and bilirubin in 78%, with the possibility of discontinuation without relapse in some patients. Those not responding to UDCA, usually with higher baseline GGT and bilirubin, have shown a progression of liver disease and fibrosis, eventually leading to transplantation. However, while a direct association between UDCA and LFTs in the discontinuation and reintroduction of therapy was documented in individual patients, the contribution of UDCA vs. natural course cannot be fully differentiated [24].

With the aim of reducing misfolded Z-alpha-1 antitrypsin accumulation in the liver, different approaches have been tried to improve protein folding through chaperones that increase secretion of misfolded AAT medications (carbamazepine, sirolimus, and rapamycin) or block polymerization through small peptides or intrabodies (reviewed in [17, 31]). RNA interference of AAT synthesis (fazirsiran) was developed and was shown to significantly reduce Z-AAT concentration in the liver and serum, to reduce PAS-D globules and inflammation in liver histology, with a reduction of LFTs and fibrosis in a pilot trial [30]. The medication has been investigated in a phase III trial since January 2023.

Lung disease in COPD from A1ATD shows a similar pattern to that in other COPD, so the symptomatic treatment follows the same principles. However, the efficacy of these approaches comparing AATD-COPD vs. COPD without AATD is only poorly investigated [12]. Limited evidence suggested that AATD-COPD patients benefited from lung volume reduction surgery (LVRS) in terms of pulmonary testing and dyspnea but with a possibly higher mortality rate and shorter duration of benefits compared to non-AATD-COPD patients [12].

A more specific treatment is alpha-1 antitrypsin augmentation supplementation to prevent lung injury, approved by the FDA in 1987. While it is positively reviewed in the parameter CT lung densitometry (representing emphysema) and the reduction of Forced Expiratory Volume 1 (FEV1) decline [12], its efficiency is questioned in a Cochrane report focusing on other parameters (FEV1, exacerbations, and quality of life), although also reporting an improvement on CT lung densitometry [18]. It is licensed and used in countries worldwide for the treatment of pulmonary manifestations of AATD.

The different therapeutic approaches are visualized in Fig. 12.3.

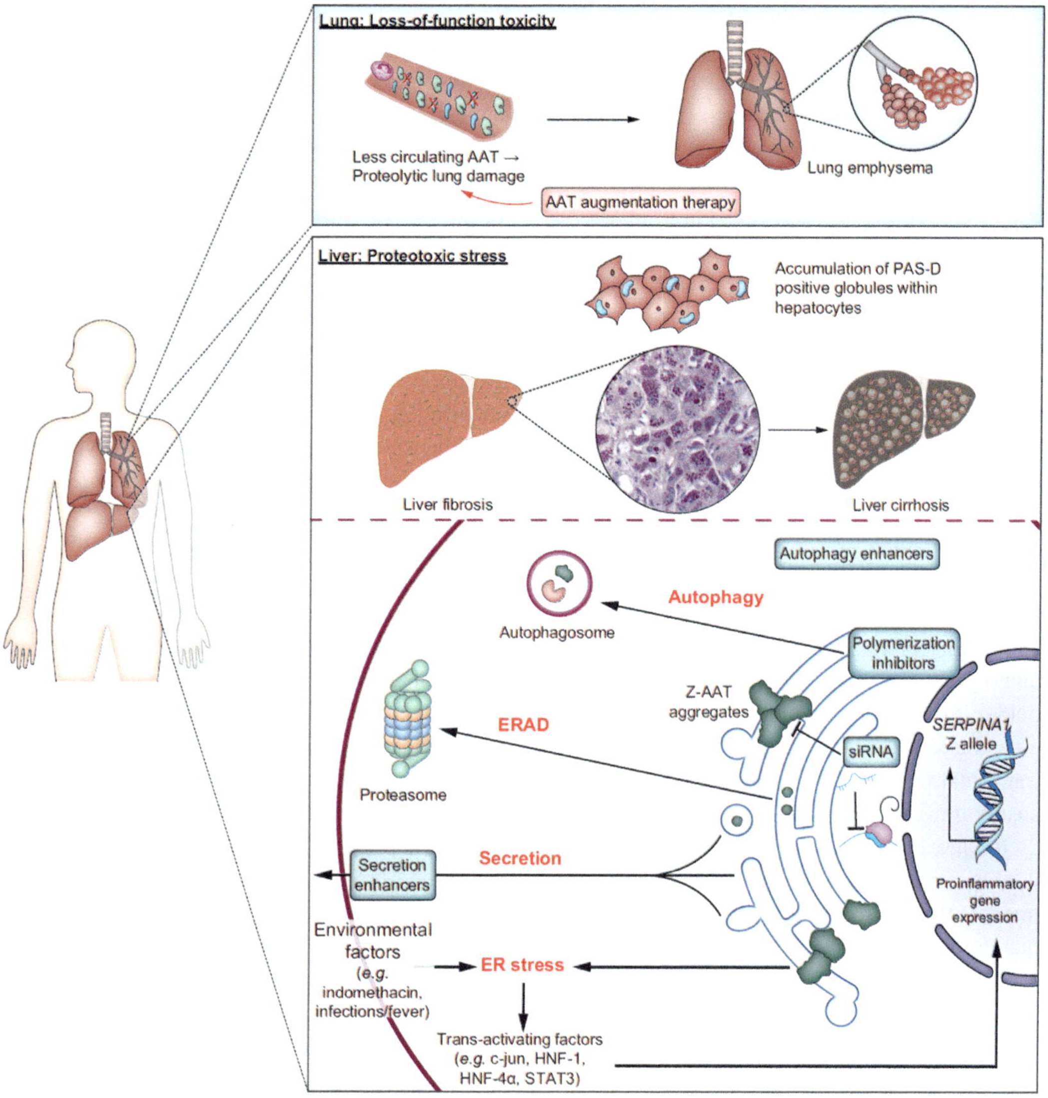

Fig. 12.3 Overview of pathomechanisms and their therapeutic approaches. (From Fromme et al. [17])

12.7 Liver Transplantation

In AATD patients with terminal liver disease, liver transplantation (LTX) is the only therapeutic option. With the low number of AATD patients reaching this condition of liver failure, AATD remains a small proportion in the indications for liver transplantation (1% in large series) (ELTR data in [42]).

In adults, lung function needs to be assessed prior to liver transplantation, as it poses a significant risk factor [8].

With AATD resulting in liver cirrhosis, the transplant procedure itself represents a standard situation in structural liver disease transplantation.

Standard surgical access in children is via a transverse upper abdominal laparotomy, if necessary, with expansion through a short upper median laparotomy. Hepatectomy is done by cutting the ligamentous attachments of the liver and the vascular structures of the liver (hepatic artery, portal vein, and hepatic vein), with preservation of the vena cava. The implantation of the left lateral liver split begins with the venous anastomosis between the donor left hepatic vein and the recipient vena cava as an end-to-side anastomosis. Portal venous anastomosis is then performed between the left portal vein branch on the donor side and the portal vein bifurcation patch on the recipient side. After completion of the portal vein connection, portal venous reperfusion of the liver takes place. Arterial anastomosis is then performed. Finally, the bile duct ostia of the left lateral split liver are connected to an intestinal loop (biliodigestive anastomosis). Repetitive duplex ultrasound examinations after reperfusion and during abdominal wall closure ensure adequate graft perfusion. In small children, in particular, a temporary abdominal wall closure using a synthetic patch can reduce the pressure on the transplant in the event of a mismatch in size and ensure transplant perfusion.

In view of the broad phenotype spectrum and various clinical developments, the indication for transplantation, the timing of listing, and transplantation for AATD represent a particular challenge.

12.8 Pediatrics

An early review reported the natural history of 16 patients, of whom 14 had neonatal cholestasis that was resolved in 13 by 8 months. The indication for transplant listing was deduced from the reappearance of cholestasis; hepatosplenomegaly; esophageal varices, sometimes with bleeding; and liver failure with ascites, leading to a mean age at LTX of 8.6 ± 4.7 years [15].

A retrospective study from Poland investigated patients with stable disease in comparison with patients requiring transplantation or dying on the waiting list and found portal hypertension with poor response to endoscopic treatment of varices and progressive liver insufficiency as factors of the second group, urging for listing and transplantation, while cholestasis and hepatitis were not prognostic [1]. The same group later published an overview of their transplanted pediatric patients, with an age range at transplant from 0.5 to 17 years (median 12 years). While four out of 20 patients were transplanted <2 years due to progressive cholestasis with coagulopathy and ascites, the other 16 patients were transplanted at >7 years with a clinical presentation of variceal bleeding, ascites, and hypersplenism but a lower rate of cholestasis [2].

Other studies report median ages at liver transplant between 3.8 and 6 years [14, 16, 27, 43].

12.9 Adults

An analysis of the American databases organ procurement & transplantation network (OPTN), National institute of diabetes and digestive and kidney diseases liver transplantation database (NIDDK) LTD, and University of Pittsburgh Medical Pittsburgh (UPMC) database) showed that while pediatric LTXs for AATD were mostly performed <5 years involving PiZZ in 88% (indicating primary AATD liver disease), the majority of transplantations (77.2% in the total cohort, 88% in the 10 years before publication) were performed at adult age, with a peak between 50 and 64 years, with PiZZ or PiSZ in only 31.6%, indicating either an age-dependent degenerative process or the importance of comorbidities. A detailed analysis of the UPMC database showed significantly higher proportions of patients with alcohol abuse in heterozygous AATD patients but also comorbidities such as hepatitis B and C, obesity, hemochromatosis, and autoimmune hepatitis in 7–45% of all AATD patients. Another remarkable finding is the male predominance in LTX for AATD (71.9% in adults, $p < 0.001$; 58.9% in children, $p < 0.001$) [10].

Indications for adult LTX listing in AATD were not specified; therefore, the diagnosis of end-stage liver disease with terminal liver failure can be assumed.

12.10 Lung Transplantation

Although not the topic of this chapter, lung transplantation has been performed in over 2000 AATD patients and has been shown to improve the survival of the transplanted patients. In some studies, survival was better than in other COPD patients, which may be related to the younger age of the AATD-COPD patients. Other studies showed more gastrointestinal complications following lung transplant in AATD and a faster FEV1 decline in AATD patients, possibly related to the ongoing pathomechanism [12].

12.11 Combined Liver and Lung Transplantation

This option is considered in patients with both end-stage liver and lung disease, making survival with only one transplantation unlikely. Due to its complexity, it is seldom considered, and case series often include only single patients with AATD as the transplant indication [38].

12.12 Prognosis of Liver Transplantation

The prognosis of liver transplantation is excellent, both in children and in adults, not different from other indications with a good prognosis ([19]; [36]).

12.13 Follow-Up/ Recommendations

Liver transplantation is pathophysiologically curative for A1ATD, also restoring normal AAT levels in the blood. Nevertheless, individual adult patients may suffer further lung deterioration after LTX [7]; therefore, pulmonology follow-up should be continued after liver transplantation.

References

1. Bakula A. Good and bad prognosis of Alpha-1-antitrypsin deficiency in children: when to list for liver transplantation. Transplant Proc. 2007;39:3186–8.
2. Bakula A. Liver transplantation in polish children with α1-antitrypsin deficiency: a single-center experience. Transplant Proc. 2016;48:3323–7.
3. Blanco I, de Serres FJ, Fernández-Bustillo E, Lara B, Miravitlles M. Estimates of the prevalence of alpha-1 antitrypsin deficiency PI*S and PI*Z alleles and the numbers at risk in Europe countries. Eur Respir J. 2006;27:77–84.
4. Blanco I, de Serres FJ, Cárcaba V, Lara B, Fernández-Bustillo E. Alpha-1 antitrypsin deficiency PI*Z and PI*S gene frequency distribution using on maps of the world by an inverse distance weighting (IDW) multivariate interpolation method. Hepat Mon. 2012;12(10 HCC):e7434. https://doi.org/10.5812/hepatmon.7434.
5. Brantly M, Nukiwa T, Crystal RG. Molecular basis of alpha-1-antitrypsin deficiency. Am J Med. 1988;84:13–31.
6. Brantly ML, Paul LD, Miller BH, Falk RT, Wu M, Crystal RG. Clinical features and history of the destructive lung disease associated with alpha-1-antitrypsin deficiency of adults with pulmonary symptoms. Am Rev Respir Dis. 1988;138:327–36.
7. Carey EJ, Iyer VN, Nelson DR, Nguyen JH, Krowka MJ. Outcomes for recipients of liver transplantation for alpha-1-antitrypsin deficiency related cirrhosis. Liver Transpl. 2013;19:1370–6.
8. Clark VC. Liver transplantation in Alpha-1 antitrypsin deficiency. Clin Liver Dis. 2017;21:355–65.
9. Clark VC, Marek G, Liu C, Collinsworth A, Shuster J, Kurtz T, Nolte J, Brantly M. Clinical and histologic features of adults with alpha-1 antitrypsin deficiency in a non-cirrhotic cohort. J Hepatol. 2018;69:1357–64.
10. Chu AS, Chopra KB, Perlmutter DH. Is severe progressive liver disease caused by Alpha-1-antitrypsin deficiency more common in children or adults? Liver Transpl. 2016;22:886–94.
11. de Serres FJ. Wordlwide racial and ethnic distribution of alpha-1-antitrypsin deficiency: summary of an analysis of published genetic epidemiologic surveys. Chest. 2002;122:1818–29.
12. Edgar RG, Patel M, Bayliss S, Crossley D, Sapey E, Turner AM. Treatment of lung disease in alpha-1 antitrypsin deficiency: a systematic review. Int J Chron Obstruct Pulmon Dis. 2017;12:1295–308.
13. Eriksson S. Alpha-1-antitrypsin deficiency: natural course and therapeutic strategies. In: Boyer JL, Blum HE, Maier KP, et al., editors. Falk symposium 115: liver cirrhosis and its development. Dordrecht: Kluwer Academic Publishers; 2001. p. 307–15.

14. Esquivel CO, Vicente E, Van Thiel D, Gordon R, Marsh W, Makowka L, Koneru B, Iwatsuki S, Madrigal M, Delgado Millan MA. Orthotopic liver transplantation for alpha-1-antitrypsin deficiency: an experience in 29 children and ten adults. Transplant Proc. 1987;19:3798–802.
15. Filipponi F, Soubrane O, Labrousse F, Devictor D, Bernard O, Valayer J, Houssin D. Liver transplantation for end-stage liver disease associated with alpha-1-antitrypsin deficiency in children: pretransplant natural history, timing and results of transplantation. J Hepatol. 1994;20:72–8. https://doi.org/10.1016/s0168-8278(05)80469-6.
16. Francavilla R, Castellaneta SP, Hadzic N, Chambers SM, Portmann B, Tung J, Cheeseman P, Rela M, Heaton ND, Mieli-Vergani G. Prognosis of alpha-1-antitrypsin deficiency-related liver disease in the era of paediatric liver transplantation. J Hepatol. 2000;32:986–92. https://doi.org/10.1016/s0168-8278(00)80103-8.
17. Fromme M, Schneider CV, Trautwein C, Brunetti-Pierri N, Strnad P. Alpha-1 antitrypsin deficiency: a resurfacing adult liver disorder. J Hepatol. 2022;76:946–58.
18. Gøtzsche PC, Johansen HK. intravenous alpha-1 antitrypsin augmentation therapy for treating patients with alpha-1 antitrypsin deficiency and lung disease. Cochrane Database Syst Rev. 2016;9:CD007851.
19. Guillaud O, Jacquemin E, Couchonnal E, Vanlemmens C, Francoz C, Chouik Y, et al. Long term results of liver transplantation for alpha-1 antitrypsin deficiency. Dig Liver Dis. 2021;53:606–11.
20. Hamesch K, Mandorfer M, Pereira VM, Moeller LS, Pons M, Dolman GE, Reichert MC, Schneider CV, Woditsch V, Voss J, Lindhauer C, Fromme M, Spivak I, Guldiken N, Zhou B, Arslanow A, Schaefer B, Zoller H, Aigner E, Reiberger T, Wetzel M, Siegmund B, Simões C, Gaspar R, Maia L, Costa D, Bento-Miranda M, van Helden J, Yagmur E, Bzdok D, Stolk J, Gleiber W, Knipel V, Windisch W, Mahadeva R, Bals R, Koczulla R, Barrecheguren M, Miravitlles M, Janciauskiene S, Stickel F, Lammert F, Liberal R, Genesca J, Griffiths WJ, Trauner M, Krag A, Trautwein C, Strnad S, et al. Liver fibrosis and metabolic alterations in adults with alpha-1-antitrypsin deficiency caused by the Pi*ZZ mutation. Gastroenterology. 2019;157:705.
21. Hinds R, Hadchouel A, Shanmugham NP, Al-Hussaini A, Chambers S, Cheeseman P, Mieli-Vergani G, Hadzić N. Variable degree of liver involvement in siblings with PiZZ alpha-1-antitrypsin deficiency-related liver disease. J Pediatr Gastroenterol Nutr. 2006;43:136–8. https://doi.org/10.1097/01.mpg.0000226370.09085.39.
22. Katzer D, Briem-Richter A, Weigert A, Lainka E, Dammann S, Pfister ED, Wirth S, Kardorff R, Ganschow R. Update Alpha-1-antitrypsin-Mangel. Monatsschr Kinderheilkd. 2022. https://doi.org/10.1007/s00112-022-01549-x.
23. Laurell C, Eriksson S. The electrophoretic alpha1-globulin pattern of serum in alpha1-antitrypsin deficiency. Scand J Clin Lab Invest. 1963;15:132–40.
24. Lykavieris P, Ducot B, Lachaux A, Dabadie A, Broué P, Sarles J, Bernard O, Jacquemin E. Liver disease associated with ZZ alpha1-antitrypsin deficiency and ursodeoxycholic acid therapy in children. J Pediatr Gastroenterol Nutr. 2008;47:623–9. https://doi.org/10.1097/MPG.0b013e31817b6dfb.
25. Mostafavi B, Piitulainen E, Tanash HA. Survival in the Swedish cohort with alpha-1-antitrypsin deficiency, up to the age of 43-45 years. Int J Chron Obstruct Pulmon Dis. 2019;14:525–30.
26. Patel D, McAllister SL, Teckman JH. Alpha-1 antitrypsin deficiency liver disease. Transl Gastroenterol Hepatol. 2021;6:23.
27. Prachalias AA, Kalife M, Francavilla R, Muiesan P, Dhawan A, Baker A, Hdzic D, Mieli-Vergani G, Rela M, Heaton ND. Liver transplantation for alpha-1-antitrypsin deficiency in children. Transpl Int. 2000;13:207–10. https://doi.org/10.1007/s001470050688.
28. Ruiz M, Lacaille F, Berthiller J, Joly P, Jérôme Dumortier J, Madeleine Aumar M, Bridoux-Henno L, Jacquemin E, Lamireau T, Broué P, Rivet C, Belmalih A, Restier L, Chapuis-Cellier C, Marion Bouchecareilh M, Lachaux A. Liver disease related to alpha1-antitrypsin deficiency in French children - the DEFI-ALPHA cohort. Liver Int. 2019;39:1136–46. https://doi.org/10.1111/liv.14035.
29. Strnad P, McElvaney NG, Lomas DA. Alpha-1-antitrypsin deficiency. N Engl J Med. 2020;382:1443–55. https://doi.org/10.1056/NEJMra1910234.
30. Strnad P, Mandorfer M, Choudhury G, Griffiths W. Fazirsiran for liver disease associated with Alpha1-antitrypsin deficiency. N Engl J Med. 2022;387:514–24.
31. Suri A, Patel D, Teckman J. Alpha-1-antitrypsin deficiency. Clin Liver Dis. 2022;19:89–92.
32. Sveger T. Liver disease in alpha1-antitrypsin deficiency detected by screening of 200,000 infants. N Engl J Med. 1976;294:1316–21.
33. Sveger T, Eriksson S. The liver in adolescents with alpha 1-antitrypsin deficiency. Hepatology. 1995;22:514–7.
34. Teckman J. Baseline analysis of a young α-1-antitrypsin deficiency liver disease cohort reveals frequent portal hypertension. J Pediatr Gastroenterol

Nutr. 2015;61:94–101. https://doi.org/10.1097/MPG.0000000000000753.
35. Teckman J. Longitudinal outcomes in young patients with Alpha-1-antitrypsin deficiency with native liver reveal that neonatal cholestasis is a poor predictor of future portal hypertension. J Pediatr. 2020;227:81–86.e4. https://doi.org/10.1016/j.jpeds.2020.07.031.
36. Townsend SA, Edgar RG, Ellis PR, Kantas D, Newsome PN, Turner AM. Systematic review: the natural history of alpha-1 antitrypsin deficiency, and associated liver disease. Aliment Pharmacol Ther. 2018;47:877–85.
37. Volpert D, Molleston JP, Permutter DH. Alpha1-antitrypsin deficiency-associated liver disease progresses slowly in some children. J Pediatr Gastroenterol Nutr. 2000;31:258–63. https://doi.org/10.1097/00005176-200009000-00011.
38. Zamora MR, Ataya A. Lung and liver transplantation in patients with alpha-1 antitrypsin deficiency. Ther Adv Chronic Dis. 2021;12:65–76.
39. Sandhaus RA, Turino G, Brantly ML, et al. The diagnosis and management of alpha-1 antitrypsin deficiency in the adult. Chronic Obstr Pulm Dis (Miami). 2016; 3(3):668–82. http://dx.doi.org/10.15326/jcopdf.3.3.2015.0182
40. Dummer J, Dobler CC, Holmes M, Chambers D, Yang IA, Parkin L, Smith S, Wark P, Dev A, Hodge S, Dabschek E, Gooi J, Samuel S, Knowles S, Holland AE. Diagnosis and treatment of lung disease associated with alpha oneantitrypsin deficiency: A position statement from the Thoracic Society of Australia and New Zealand*Respirology 2020; 25, 321–35
41. Lang T, Mühlbauer M, Strobelt M, Weidinger S, Hadorn HB. alpha-1-antitrypsin deficiency in children: liver disease is not reflected by low serum levels of alpha-1-antitrypsin – a study on 48 pediatric patients. Eur J Med Res 2005;10: 509–14.
42. Adam R, Karam V, Delvart V, O'Grady J, Mirza D, Klempnauer J, Castaing D, Neuhaus P, Jamieson N, Salizzoni M, Pollard S, Lerut J, Paul A, Garcia-Valdecasas JC, Rodríguez FSJ, Burroughs A. Evolution of indications and results of liver transplantation in Europe. A report from the European Liver Transplant Registry (ELTR). Journal of Hepatology 2012;57: 675–88
43. Hughes MG Jr, Khan KM, Gruessner AC, Sharp H, Hill M, Jie T, Kandaswamy R, Humar A, Payne WD, Gruessner RW. Long-term outcome in 42 pediatric liver transplant patients with alpha 1-antitrypsin deficiency: a single-center experience. Clin Transplant 2011;25(5):731–66.

Cirrhosis Secondary to Prolonged Total Parenteral Nutrition

13

Mareike Külzer and Markus A. Weigand

13.1 Incidence

In case of parenteral nutrition–associated liver disease (PNALD), adults are most frequently affected by steatosis, whereas in infants and neonates, cholestasis is more common. Contrary to short-term parenteral nutrition (PN), which causes ordinarily acute and potentially reversible PNALD, PNALD secondary to prolonged total parenteral nutrition (TPN) is predominantly a chronic liver injury with potential progress to fibrosis, cirrhosis, and chronic liver failure [6].

The incidence and prevalence are difficult to define because of the difficulty in differentiating between PNALD and intestinal failure–associated liver disease (IFALD), as well as a missing consensus on the diagnostic criteria for both terms [7]. The incidence of advanced PNALD varies in the literature from 0 to 50%, with a mortality from 0 to 22% in adults and up to 40% in infants and neonates [2, 3]. The incidence increases with the duration of TPN or if the underlying disease is complicated by infections (sepsis or catheter-associated infections), small bowel disease, or multi-surgical procedures [8]. The incidence of TPN-associated cirrhosis was described in 0–25% of adults [9] and 13% of pediatric patients [10], whereas approximately 15% of adults on long-term TPN develop an end-stage liver disease (ESLD) [11]. ESLD due to prolonged TPN in infants was seen only occasionally.

M. Külzer · M. A. Weigand (✉)
University of Heidelberg, Heidelberg, Germany
e-mail: mareike.kuelzer@med.uni-heidelberg.de; markus.weigand@med.uni-heidelberg.de

13.2 Clinical Presentation

Hepatobiliary complications of PN are common but generally moderate and reversible. In case of long-term TPN, more severe complications may occur, with symptoms ranging from asymptomatic cholestasis to severe cirrhosis with hepatic decompensation. A significant relationship between the duration of TPN and liver injury is well-known [10]. The predominant complication in adults is steatosis or steatohepatitis, whereas in children, cholestasis is more common. Symptoms are nonspecific; in children, commonly, the first clinical presentation includes signs of cholestasis. But even in the case of a severe liver injury, clinical symptoms can be absent, and a nonspecific abdominal discomfort due to hepatomegaly can be the only manifestation. Biochemical signs of cholestasis (elevation of γ-glutamyl-transpeptidase (γGt) and alkaline phosphatase (AP)) may occur within the first week of PN [12]. Older studies have postulated that cirrhosis may occur within 3–5 months of TPN [13]. The risk of liver injury can be reduced by reducing patient-related and PN-related risk factors [14, 15].

T. Hackert, A. Gulla (eds.), *Rare Liver and Biliary Tract Diseases*,
https://doi.org/10.1007/978-3-032-15076-9_13

Table 13.1 Risk factors for PNALD

PN-related	Patient-related
Excess of total energy delivered/excess of macronutrients	Systemic infections
Excessive glucose supply Excessive or inadequate amino acid supply Excessive fat supply	Sepsis Catheter-related bloodstream infections Digestion-related infections
Deficiency of micronutrients	Lack of enteral intake
Deficiency of choline Deficiency of carnitine	Decreased secretion of intestinal hormones (CKK, secretin, a.m.m.) Decreased emptying of the gallbladder Intestinal stasis Bacterial overgrowth Bacterial translocation Impaired gut immunity
Toxicity of micronutrients in TPN	Intestinal failure
Manganese Aluminum Chromium Copper	Severe motility disorders Short bowel syndrome (length of the short bowel is an essential risk factor) Ileocecal valve resection
Types of i.v. lipid emulsions	Disturbance of enterohepatic bile acid cycling
Omega-6 polyunsaturated fatty acids in soybean-based lipid emulsions Phytosterol in soybean-based lipid emulsions Deficiency of essential fatty acids	Increased lithogenicity Bile duct obstruction
Continuous PN infusion	Prematurity

PN parenteral nutrition, *a.m.m.* and many more, *i.v.* intravenous, *CKK* Cholezystokinin

The pathogenesis of PNALD is multifactorial and not completely understood. Table 13.1 shows the patient-related and PN-related risk factors for developing a PNALD.

13.2.1 Steatosis

Steatosis is the most frequent complication of TPN in adults, which is caused by a hepatic accumulation of lipids. An excess of carbohydrates stimulates hepatic acetyl-CoA-carboxylase, which results, first, in an increased production of fatty acids in hepatocytes and, second, in an increased production of triglycerides, which accumulate in the hepatocytes. Furthermore, an excessive infusion of lipids leads to direct liver damage (lipid overload syndrome). The mechanism still remains unclear [12]. Likewise, an amino acid imbalance can cause steatosis. A choline deficiency results in decreased synthetization of very-low-density lipoprotein (VLDL), with consequent decreased transport of triglycerides from the liver. A deficiency of carnitine (essential for lipolysis) would also lead to steatosis.

13.2.2 Cholestasis

Intrahepatic cholestasis is the most frequent complication of TPN in infants. It is defined as an elevation of conjugated bilirubin ≥2 mg/dl, often accompanied by an increase of γGt, AP, and transaminases. The elevation of bilirubin often occurs within the first 2 weeks of TPN. For the diagnosis of parenteral nutrition-related cholestasis (PNAC), the exclusion of other causes (e.g., extrahepatic reasons) of cholestasis is essential. The higher prevalence in younger age groups such as neonates and, especially premature infants, is explained by the immaturity of the biliary tract in these patients.

Pathogenesis is multifactorial. First, a lack of enteral intake results in a decreased release of gastrointestinal hormones. A decrease in the secretion of cholecystokinin, secretin, serotonin, or peptide YY causes decreased emptying of the gallbladder as well as decreased intestinal motility. This can result in bile stasis with cholestasis, cholecystitis, and bile duct obstruction. Intestinal stasis results in enterocyte hypoplasia, bacterial overgrowth with subsequent bacterial translocation, the activation of inflammatory pathways, and impaired gut immunity.

Second, there is a direct toxicity of nutritional components such as copper, manganese, aluminum, or phytosterol, which can cause PNAC.

PNAC is an accepted indication for pediatric liver or combined liver–intestinal transplantation (LIT).

13.2.3 Fibrosis, Cirrhosis, and ESLD

All the conditions mentioned above trigger a progressive process of inflammatory pathways. Cholestasis leads to portal inflammation and periportal fibrogenesis. Steatosis can turn into steatohepatitis with necrosis and panlobular fibrogenesis [8]. The end stage of these processes is characterized by fibrosis and cirrhosis. In the case of a progression to an ESLD, the prognosis is poor.

13.3 Workup Investigation

Making the diagnosis of PNALD is challenging for a variety of reasons. First, no consistent definition of PNALD exists in the recent literature. Second, to diagnose PNALD, an exclusion of numerous non-parenteral nutrition-associated causes of liver injury in patients on TPN is necessary. And last, there is no consensus on the criteria for diagnosis.

In most cases, diagnosis is made for patients on TPN only by clinical presentation and biochemical markers after the exclusion of other/non-PN-associated reasons of liver injury—optionally in combination with radiological examinations. Liver biopsy is the only method, which can demonstrate the definitive severity of fibrosis or cirrhosis but is not mandatory for diagnosis. A combination of several noninvasive radiological diagnostic tools can be used as an alternative to liver biopsy [16, 17].

Clinical Examination Because of a lack of typical clinical signs, clinical examination shows only nonspecific manifestations, such as jaundice, nausea, abdominal pain or discomfort, and hepatomegaly. In the end stage, signs of portal hypertension (e.g., abdominal/esophageal varices, splenomegaly, and ascites) can appear. However, typical signs such as esophageal varices and ascites can be absent in the case of short bowel syndrome as the underlying disease due to a low absolute mesenteric venous blood flow as a result of massive intestinal resection.

Biochemical Markers Regular biochemical monitoring of hepatic function is required, but standard liver function tests are neither specific nor reliable. There is no consensus on the criteria for diagnosing PNALD, but some serum biomarkers act as the accepted criteria. That includes an elevation of liver enzymes (alanine transferase/aspartate aminotransferase (ALT/AST) and AP) $\geq$1.5 times the upper limit of normal, which occurs within the first weeks from the beginning of TPN [7, 18, 19]. Cholestasis is usually defined as an elevated conjugated bilirubin $\geq$2 mg/dl (34,2 umol/l), and conjugated bilirubin can be a prognostic factor for liver injury during TPN [12, 20]. Usually, the first biochemical sign is an elevation of AP/γGT, followed by hyperbilirubinemia [14]. Transaminase levels increase later, but all these findings are nonspecific [12]. Furthermore, regular signs of decreased liver synthesis function and splenomegaly can occur (e.g., hypalbuminemia, low platelets, and abnormal clotting profile) in an advanced stage. Because of the important role of inflammation in the pathogenesis of PNALD, monitoring of inflammatory markers is recommended.

Beath et al. defined three severity stages of PNALD depending on biochemical markers, ultrasound findings, and histology (see Table 13.2) [18].

To diagnose liver fibrosis, some newer tests, such as the enhanced liver fibrosis (ELF) test, methionine breath test, fibrosis-4 index, and

Table 13.2 Severity stages of PNALD by Beath et al.

Type	Biochemical findings	Ultrasound findings	Histology
Type 1: mild	AP/γGT ≥ 1.5× ULN Bilirubin <3 mg/dl	Echogenic appearance of the liver	Steatosis (up to 25%) and/or periportal fibrosis
Type 2: moderate	AP/γGT ≥ 1.5× ULN Bilirubin 3–6 mg/dl	Enlarged spleen	Fatty change >25% Fibrosis >50%
Type 3: advanced	AP/γGT ≥ 3× ULN Bilirubin >6 mg/dl Platelet count <100 × 10^9 INR <1.5	Signs of portal hypertension (clinical and/or morphological imaging or histological)	

ULN upper limit of normal, *INR* international normalized ratio

aspartate-aminotransferase-to-platelet-ratio index (APRI), which are based on biochemical markers, have been developed. The diagnostic value of these tests relating to PNALD still remains unclear [18, 20].

Medical Imaging Abdominal ultrasound is helpful and is one of the first imaging steps in diagnosing PNALD. As a well-standardized, noninvasive method, it can detect several liver abnormalities and assess the liver echogenicity. Clinical liver enlargement may appear within a few days after initiating TPN [14]. Moreover, it is a good tool for regular follow-up evaluations.

Transient elastography (TE) is a noninvasive technique that correlates well with fibrosis. But relating to PNALD, there is no standardized protocol, and it is still being evaluated as a clinical tool [20]. Magnetic resonance elastography (MRE) acts as an alternative to TE.

Computed tomography (CT), magnetic resonance imaging (MRI), and magnetic resonance spectroscopy (MRS) are other imaging techniques, which are used for diagnosing PNALD. Neither CT nor MRI is sensitive enough to reliably detect fibrosis or cirrhosis, especially in the early stages, but they can be used to define the severity of cirrhosis by determining the spleen size, ascites, or vascular collaterals [21, 22]. MRS is more precise than ultrasound or CT and offers the best correlation with the results of liver biopsy. However, it is currently not part of the clinical routine.

In conclusion, conventional imaging is not able to reliably detect PNALD or the severity of PNALD, but it is important for monitoring the progress or regression of liver injury, as well as for detecting sequelae.

Liver Biopsy Liver biopsy is the only tool that can provide detailed information on the severity and structural changes relating to PNALD. Because of its invasive character and potential risks, it is not mandatory for diagnosis, and a decision should be made on a case-by-case basis. Generally indication for liver biopsy is established restrictive, especially in infants, although none of the markers mentioned above are as precise as tissue sampling [23].

13.4 Differential Diagnosis

In the case of elevated liver enzymes (Fig. 13.1), cholestasis, or signs of fibrosis or cirrhosis in patients on TPN, several differential diagnoses have to be ruled out. In critically ill patients on TPN, multiple factors can be responsible for the elevation of liver enzymes. Especially in cases with a high elevation of transaminase levels, ischemic hepatitis, acute viral or autoimmune hepatitis, and drug-induced liver injury have to be excluded. Other possible reasons are nonalcoholic fatty liver disease (NAFLD), alcohol-induced injury, and malignant or genetic diseases (e.g., Wilson's disease and hemochromatosis). In the case of elevated conjugated bilirubin (Fig. 13.1), all obstructive and nonobstructive causes of jaundice have to be taken into account (cholecystitis, choledocholithiasis, benign postoperative jaundice, sepsis, blood transfusion, and many more).

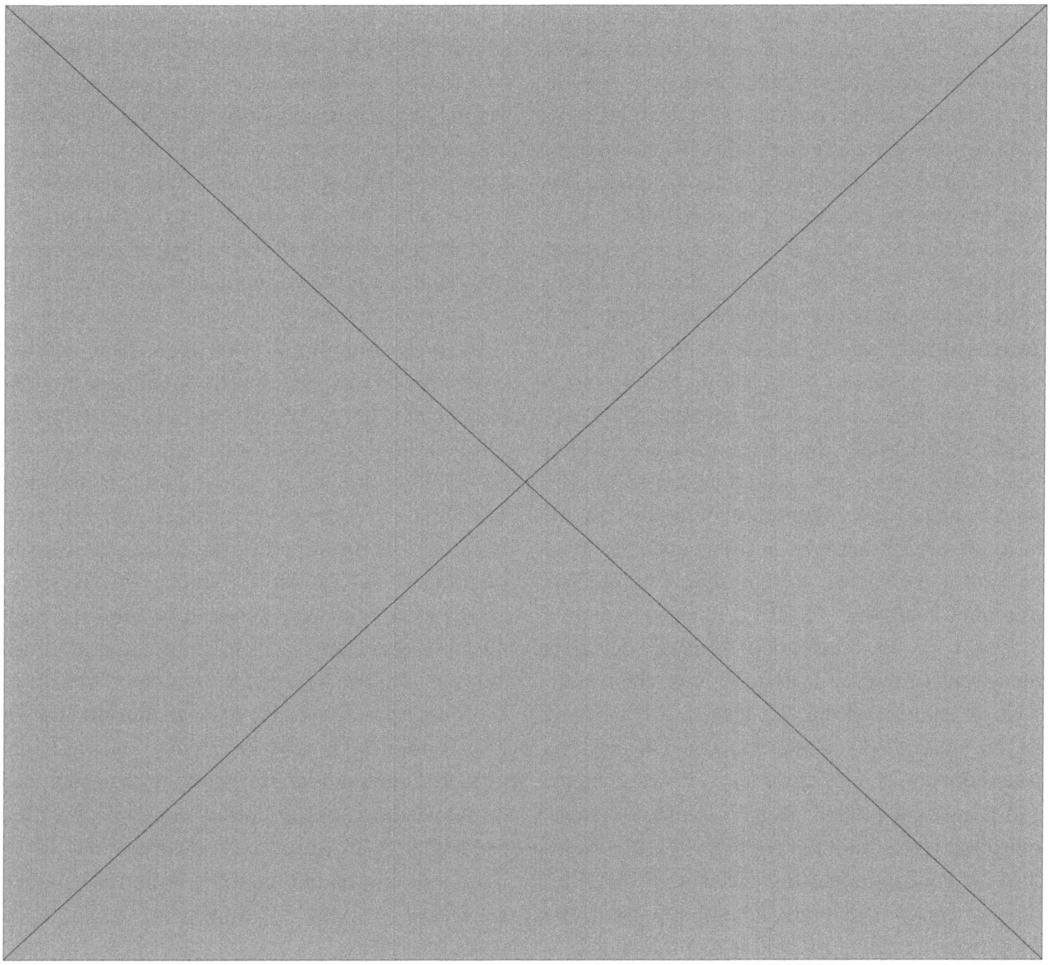

Fig. 13.1 Extract of differential diagnoses in patients on TPN with elevated liver enzymes [12, 18, 19]. NAFLD = nonalcoholic fatty liver disease

13.5 Treatment

There is no definitive treatment but intestinal transplantation (IT) or combined liver–intestinal transplantation for patients with PNALD—especially in advanced stages with cirrhosis or ESLD. Therefore, the prevention of PNALD and treatment of the underlying disease are of importance. All pathogenetic factors (mentioned in Chap. 2) have to be considered. If the underlying disease is treated or restrained carly enough, PNALD, until the stage of liver fibrosis, has the potential to regress, and even the liver architecture can revert to normal appearance [24].

The European Society for Clinical Nutrition and Metabolism (ESPEN) has enunciated several recommendations for the prevention and treatment of PNALD [2, 3, 14, 15]:

13.5.1 Prevention

First, some basic measures have to be implemented, such as common hygiene measures in the handling of central venous catheters for both clinicians/nurses and family membcrs in the case of home parenteral nutrition. Infection control plays a key role in the prevention of

PNALD. Furthermore, early enteral nutrition, if procurable, is mandatory. Enteral nutrition, even in minimal dosage, promotes bile flow and the secretion of cholecystokinin and decreases the synthesis of secondary bile acids [8]. A weaning of PN can stop further hepatic damage; therefore, special weaning protocols can be helpful.

An avoidance of overfeeding is also essential. Avoidance of an excessive glucose supply decreases insulin secretion, with consequent decreased fatty acid synthesis. Limiting intravenous lipids seems to be hepatoprotective (especially limiting the dose of soybean oil–based lipids <1 g/kg/day), but more data are needed. Potentially hepatotoxic micronutrients of PN, such as manganese, aluminum, or copper, should be removed. Furthermore, an avoidance of micronutrient deficiencies is required. Choline, for example, increases VLDL synthesis, which is essential for the transport of triglycerides from the liver. Carnitine increases long-chain fatty acid oxidation and thereby acts in a hepatoprotective manner [8]. Zalikowska and Beath proposed the addition of taurine to TPN in neonates and premature infants, which seems to decrease bilirubin levels in this population—supporting data for adults are missing [12, 18]. The ESPEN does not give a recommendation for the latter. Moreover, a cycling of TPN is recommended.

Last, several authors recommend multi-professional collaboration in expert groups, transplant centers, or specialized intestinal rehabilitation centers as a preventive measure of high importance [8, 14, 18].

13.5.2 Treatment

Some pharmaceuticals were discussed in the treatment of PNALD in the past years. Ursodeoxycholic acid was one of them, but there is still no evidence for its use. The same applies to the use of antibiotics such as metronidazole or gentamicin for the treatment of bacterial overgrowth [2, 3]. Erythromycin counteracts indirectly against bacterial overgrowth by stimulating migrating motor complexes, which results in a stimulation of intestinal motility. Evidence relating to its positive effects on PNALD is missing here as well.

Different types of lipid emulsions play a key role in the pathogenesis of PNALD—providing fish oil–based lipids may be a potential treatment [25]. Soybean oil–based lipid emulsions have a higher omega 6 ($\omega6$)/$\omega3$ polyunsaturated fatty acid (PUFA) ratio than their alternatives (olive oil–/fish oil–based lipid emulsions), a lack of long-chain PUFAs, higher amounts of phytosterol, and lower amounts of α-tocopherol (a form of vitamin E with antioxidant effects). Fish oil–based lipid emulsions have higher amounts of vitamin E, lower amounts of phytosterol, and a better $\omega6/\omega3$ ratio [15]. Composite intravenous lipid emulsions and pure fish oil–based lipid emulsions are available. In the case of PNAC in infants, $\omega3$ PUFA can be used because fish oil–based lipid emulsions seem to be protective—a sound evidence is still missing, and clinical relevance needs to be further evaluated [3]. A reduction of intravenous lipid emulsions in infants with PNAC has been shown to be controversial because of its increased risk for an essential fatty acid deficiency and potential altered development. In adults with diagnosed or suspected PNALD, intravenous lipids with a reduced $\omega6/\omega3$ ratio are recommended. More data are needed before the routine use of fish oil–based lipid emulsions can be recommended.

Ultima ratio in the case of advanced PNALD with cirrhosis or ESLD is intestinal or combined liver–intestinal transplantation. For patients with progressive liver disease, an early referral to an experienced transplantation center or intestinal failure rehabilitation center is mandatory.

13.6 Surgical Planning/Management

In the past two decades, we have seen a great improvement in surgical techniques (transplant and non-transplant surgery), as well as improvements in immunosuppressive therapies, which results in a significantly better outcome for patients with PNALD or IFALD with or without transplantation. Non-transplant surgery is targeted at improving gut function, with subsequently decreased liver injury.

13.6.1 Non-transplant Surgery

The improvements in non-transplant surgery for PNALD/IFALD effectuate an optimization of enteral food tolerance, bile acid enterohepatic circulation, and small bowel bacterial overgrowth. In the case of small bowel syndrome, lengthening strategies (i.e., serial transverse enteroplasty and longitudinal intestinal lengthening and tailoring) can result in an improvement of enteral nutrition tolerance and regression of PN-associated complications [26]. Indications for bowel-lengthening surgery include a substantial small bowel dilatation [7, 26–29]. Up to now, the optimal timing for small bowel reconstruction and lengthening strategies is undefined [7].

Other non-transplant strategies are primary anastomoses after bowel resection, whenever possible; closure of stomas as soon as possible; and prophylactic cholecystectomy during any laparotomy in case of gallstones or inspissated bile syndrome [30, 31].

13.6.2 Transplant Surgery

Because of the constant improvements in the prevention and treatment of PNALD mentioned above, the number of performed intestinal transplantations has decreased for pediatric patients since 2008 and has been relatively stable for adult patients in the past years [32]. In >60% of cases, the indication for intestinal transplantation (IT) in children and adults is a short gut. In case of an impending or overt liver failure, a listing for combined liver–intestinal transplantation (LIT) can be reasonable [5]. IT is still reserved for patients with intestinal failure who develop potentially life-threatening complications (e.g., progressive liver disease, recurring sepsis, and impending loss of central venous access) despite optimized therapies.

13.6.2.1 Indication for Transplantation

The indication criteria for pediatric IT have been published in 2001 by Kaufman et al. and were endorsed by the American Society of Transplantation. Since then, they have not been changed [33]. The criteria include an advanced liver disease (progressive IFALD/PNALD with elevated bilirubin of 3–6 mg/dl and/or signs of portal hypertension or coagulopathy), recurrent life-threatening episodes of sepsis (≥2 sepsis episodes per year), an impending loss of central venous access (loss of ≥50% of standard central venous access sites), and a high risk of death secondary to the underlying disease (i.e., ultrashort bowel syndrome).

Progressive liver injury mostly occurs in infants with very short bowel syndrome on parenteral nutrition. For a better outcome, it is of great importance to identify PNALD/IFALD in an early stage, without an irreversible liver injury.

Sepsis is a common complication in patients with PNALD or IFALD on PN. In case of two or more bacterial or fungal septic episodes or in the presence of a multi-organ failure, an intestinal transplantation should be taken into account.

The impending loss of central venous access is defined as a loss of more than 50% of the standard central venous access sites as a result of thrombosis (in infancy, two out of four: right and left jugular veins and right and left subclavian veins; in older children, three out of six: jugular veins, subclavian veins, and femoral veins).

In 2015, the indication criteria were discussed by Burghardt et al. [34]. This study showed that two of the current listing criteria had a poor predictive value (advanced liver injury defined by cholestasis and ultrashort bowel syndrome) and proposed three new criteria with a high predictive value (see Table 13.3). When two out of the three criteria are fulfilled, it predicts with 98% probability those children who are at the highest risk of death and the need for transplantation.

For adults, the recommendations for the assessment of IT are nearly the same as for pediatric patients. It is recommended that a listing for IT (with or without the liver) is required in case of impending or overt liver failure and that ideally, "patients listed for intestinal transplantation should undergo the procedure while they are in stable clinical condition" [5]. Table 13.4 shows the adult listing criteria; an assessment for IT is recommended if one of the criteria is fulfilled.

Table 13.3 Current pediatric IT listing criteria, 2001, compared to the proposed pediatric IT listing criteria, 2015

Pediatric IT listing criteria, 2001 [33]	Proposed pediatric IT listing criteria, 2015 [34]
Advanced liver disease (defined as advanced cholestasis)	Elevated conjugated bilirubin ≥75 umol/l, with no biochemical improvement following 6 weeks of lipid management strategies
≥2 sepsis episodes per year	≥2 admissions to ICU
Loss of ≥2 CVC sites related to thrombosis	Loss of ≥3 CVC sites
High risk of death secondary to the underlying disease (i.e., ultrashort bowel)	

IT intestinal transplantation, *ICU* intensive care unit, *CVC* central venous catheter

Table 13.4 Adult IT listing criteria

Adult IT listing criteria [5]	Comment
Failure of home parenteral nutrition	Defined by IFALD with one of the following:
	1. Impending or overt liver failure.
	Impending liver failure Conjugated bilirubin: 3–6 mg/dl Progressive thrombocytopenia Progressive splenomegaly Overt liver failure Portal hypertension Hepatosplenomegaly Hepatic fibrosis/cirrhosis
	2. CVC thrombosis of ≥2 central veins (jugular, subclavian, and femoral)
	3. Frequent central line sepsis
	≥2 episodes/year of systemic infection Single episode of line-related fungemia Single episode of septic shock or ARDS
	4. Frequent episodes of severe dehydration despite substitution of i.v. fluids in addition to PN
High risk of death attributable to the underlying disease	Ultrashort bowel syndrome with residual short bowel <20 cm
Intestinal failure with high morbidity or low acceptance of PN	Defined by Need for frequent hospitalization or inability to function (high-output stoma) Patients' unwillingness to accept long-term PN (i.e., young patients)

IT intestinal transplantation, *CVC* central venous catheter, *ARDS* acute respiratory distress syndrome

13.6.2.2 Transplantation Techniques

There are three possible options for transplantation in the case of severe PNALD or IFALD:

1. Isolated Intestinal Transplantation:

In the past years, there has been a significant trend toward IT without a liver component due to shorter waiting times on transplantation, with consequent lower mortality [35]. Indication is an irreversible intestinal failure without an irreversible liver disease [36]. After isolated IT, a regression of liver injury up to *restitutio ad integrum* is possible.

2. Combined Liver–Intestinal Transplantation

Combined liver–intestinal transplantation is indicated in patients with advanced IFALD/PNALD in combination with progressive/irreversible liver failure. Additionally, patients with an enteral calorie intake <50% of the estimated calories at the time of transplantation assessment should be listed for a combined graft because of a high risk of progressive liver failure due to prolonged PN. The inclusion of a liver–duodenum–pancreas graft is an option for preserving the hepatic hilus and the biliary tree. The risk of vascular and biliary complications is decreased because biliary reconstructive procedures are not necessary. That is why it is often practiced in infants. However, a transplantation of liver and intestine as individual organs without the pancreas is also prevalent [36].

3. Isolated Liver Transplantation

Isolated liver transplantation (LT) is an option for select children with PNALD and short bowel syndrome. It should be considered for children with a realistic chance of weaning from PN after transplantation. The length and functionality of the small bowel play a significant role, even though there are no definitive criteria for the assessment of isolated LT in the case of PNALD [37]. The proposed criteria are progressive liver failure with ≥50% of daily enteral energy intake for four weeks with satisfactory growth and 30 cm of functional small bowel with an ileocecal valve or 50 cm of functional small bowel in the absence of an ileocecal valve [38]. Biliary drainage may be an important technical difficulty, especially in infants.

13.6.2.3 Mortality and Complications

The graft and patient survival has significantly improved over time, while the most common cause of death still remains sepsis [32]. The mortality while waiting for IT/combined LIT is higher compared to other solid organ transplantations, which underlines the importance of an early referral to specialized intestinal transplantation centers. The recognition that performing an isolated IT before the occurrence of an irreversible liver failure resulted in a higher rate of isolated intestinal transplantations and a decreased rate of combined liver–intestinal transplantations. For children, the mortality while waiting for transplantation is higher for combined LIT than for isolated IT because of the typically longer waiting times for the former [33, 35, 36].

The main complications after transplantation are rejection and the consequences of intense immunosuppression, including infections and malignancy. The incidence of rejection is higher after IT than after other solid organ transplantations, which justifies the intense immunosuppression. Due to the latter, there is an increased incidence of infections and post-transplant lymphoproliferative syndrome (PTLD).

13.7 Follow-Up/Recommendations

One of the current problems in the prevention, diagnosis, and treatment of PNALD is the lack of a consistent definition and uniform diagnostic criteria for PNALD. For patients on TPN, the aim should be to avoid irreversible liver injury, with a potential need for intestinal or liver–intestinal transplantation. Because of the limited treatment options, preventive measures are of importance. First, a constant optimization of infection control is essential. Second, a differentiated calorie supply and an improvement in the composition of PN play a key role in the prevention of PNALD. The use of fish oil–based lipid emulsions is the current clinical practice, but valid evidence is still missing, and therefore, large randomized controlled trials are needed. Last, a multi-professional collaboration and an early referral to specialized intestinal rehabilitation centers are recommended.

In the past decades, the number of adults and children developing an advanced and irreversible type of PNALD has decreased significantly due to better monitoring, preventive measures, and differentiated management of parenteral nutrition.

References

1. Peden VH, Witzleben CL, Skelton MA. Total parenteral nutrition. J Pediatr. 1971;78(1):180–1.
2. Plauth M, Bernal W, Dasarathy S, Merli M, Plank LD, Schütz T. u. a. ESPEN guideline on clinical nutrition in liver disease. Clin Nutr. 2019;38(2):485–521.

3. Bischoff SC, Bernal W, Dasarathy S, Merli M, Plank LD, Schütz T. u. a. ESPEN practical guideline: clinical nutrition in liver disease. Clin Nutr. 2020;39(12):3533–62.
4. Lal S, Pironi L, Wanten G, Arends J, Bozzetti F, Cuerda C. u. a. Clinical approach to the management of intestinal failure associated liver disease (IFALD) in adults: a position paper from the home artificial nutrition and chronic intestinal failure special interest group of ESPEN. Clin Nutr. 2018;37(6):1794–7.
5. Pironi L, Cuerda C, Jeppesen PB, Joly F, Jonkers C, et al. ESPEN guideline on chronic intestinal failure in adults - Update 2023. Clin Nutr. 2023;42(10):1940–2021. https://doi.org/10.1016/j.clnu.2023.07.019. PMID: 37639741. Epub 2023 Jul 29.
6. Lakananurak N, Tienchai K. Incidence and risk factors of parenteral nutrition-associated liver disease in hospitalized adults: a prospective cohort study. Clin Nutr ESPEN. 2019;34:81–6.
7. Lacaille F, Gupte G, Colomb V, D'Antiga L, Hartman C, Hojsak I. u. a. Intestinal failure–associated liver disease: a position paper of the ESPGHAN Working Group of intestinal failure and intestinal transplantation. J Pediatr Gastroenterol Nutr. 2015;60(2):272–83.
8. Guglielmi FW, Boggio-Bertinet D, Federico A, Forte GB, Guglielmi A, Loguercio C. u. a. Total parenteral nutrition-related gastroenterological complications. Dig Liver Dis. 2006;38(9):623–42.
9. Shaffer JL, Bakker H, Bozzetti F, Ladefoged K, Leon-Sanz M, Messing B. u. a. P.79 a European survey on management of metaboliccomplications in home parenteral nutrition. Clin Nutr. 1997;16:43–4.
10. Zambrano E, El-Hennawy M, Ehrenkranz RA, Zelterman D, Reyes-Múgica M. Total parenteral nutrition induced liver pathology: an autopsy series of 24 newborn cases. Pediatr Dev Pathol. 2004;7(5):425–32.
11. Chan S, McCowen KC, Bistrian BR, Thibault A, Keane-Ellison M, Forse RA. u. a. Incidence, prognosis, and etiology of end-stage liver disease in patients receiving home total parenteral nutrition. Surgery. 1999;126(1):28–34.
12. Żalikowska-Gardocka M, Przybyłkowski A. Review of parenteral nutrition-associated liver disease. Clin Exp Hepatol. 2020;6(2):65–73.
13. Cohen C, Olsen MM. Pediatric total parenteral nutrition. Liver histopathology. Arch Pathol Lab Med. 1981;105(3):152–6.
14. Hartman C, Shamir R, Simchowitz V, Lohner S, Cai W, Decsi T. u. a. ESPGHAN/ESPEN/ESPR/CSPEN guidelines on pediatric parenteral nutrition: complications. Clin Nutr. 2018;37(6):2418–29.
15. Lapillonne A, Fidler Mis N, Goulet O, van den Akker CHP, Wu J, Koletzko B. u. a. ESPGHAN/ESPEN/ESPR/CSPEN guidelines on pediatric parenteral nutrition: lipids. Clin Nutr. 2018;37(6):2324–36.
16. Yoshiji H, Nagoshi S, Akahane T, Asaoka Y, Ueno Y, Ogawa K. u. a. Evidence-based clinical practice guidelines for liver cirrhosis 2020. J Gastroenterol. 2021;56(7):593–619.
17. Rockey DC, Caldwell SH, Goodman ZD, Nelson RC, Smith AD. Liver biopsy. Hepatology. 2009;49(3):1017–44.
18. Beath SV, Kelly DA. Total parenteral nutrition-induced cholestasis: prevention and management. Clin Liver Dis. 2016;20(1):159–76.
19. Mitra A, Ahn J. Liver disease in patients on Total parenteral nutrition. Clin Liver Dis. 2017;21(4):687–95.
20. Nagelkerke SCJ, Draijer LG, Benninga MA, Koot BGP, Tabbers MM. The prevalence of liver fibrosis according to non-invasive tools in a pediatric home parenteral nutrition cohort. Clin Nutr. 2021;40(2):460–6.
21. Schuppan D, Afdhal NH. Liver cirrhosis. Lancet. 2008;371(9615):838–51.
22. Popov Y, Schuppan D. Targeting liver fibrosis: strategies for development and validation of antifibrotic therapies. Hepatology. 2009;50(4):1294–306.
23. Mansoor S, Collyer E, Alkhouri N. A comprehensive review of noninvasive liver fibrosis tests in pediatric nonalcoholic fatty liver disease. Curr Gastroenterol Rep. 2015;17(6):23.
24. Fuchs BC, Wang H, Yang Y, Wei L, Polasek M, Schühle DT. u. a. Molecular MRI of collagen to diagnose and stage liver fibrosis. J Hepatol. 2013;59(5):992–8.
25. Tillman EM. Review and clinical update on parenteral nutrition–associated liver disease. Nutr Clin Pract. 2013;28(1):30–9.
26. Frongia G, Kessler M, Weih S, Nickkholgh A, Mehrabi A, Holland-Cunz S. Comparison of LILT and STEP procedures in children with short bowel syndrome — a systematic review of the literature. J Pediatr Surg. 2013;48(8):1794–805.
27. Thompson J, Sudan D. Intestinal lengthening for short bowel syndrome. Adv Surg. 2008;42:49–61.
28. D'Antiga L, Goulet O. Intestinal failure in children: the European view. J Pediatr Gastroenterol Nutr. 2013;56(2):118–26.
29. Pakarinen MP, Kurvinen A, Koivusalo AI, Iber T, Rintala RJ. Long-term controlled outcomes after autologous intestinal reconstruction surgery in treatment of severe short bowel syndrome. J Pediatr Surg. 2013;48(2):339–44.
30. Quirós-Tejeira RE, Ament ME, Reyen L, Herzog F, Merjanian M, Olivares-Serrano N. u. a. Long-term parenteral nutritional support and intestinal adaptation in children with short bowel syndrome: a 25-year experience. J Pediatr. 2004;145(2):157–63.
31. Nightingale JMD. Hepatobiliary, renal and bone complications of intestinal failure. Best Pract Res Clin Gastroenterol. 2003;17(6):907–29.
32. International Intestinal Transplant Registry Report 2019 [Internet]. [zitiert 2. November 2022]. Verfügbar unter: https://www.tts.org/irta-registries/irta-itr

33. Kaufman SS, Atkinson JB, Bianchi A, Goulet OJ, Grant D, Langnas AN. u. a. Indications for pediatric intestinal transplantation: a position paper of the American Society of Transplantation. Pediatr Transplant. 2001;5(2):80–7.
34. Burghardt KM, Wales PW, de Silva N, Stephens D, Yap J, Grant D. u. a. Pediatric intestinal transplant listing criteria – a call for a change in the new era of intestinal failure outcomes: changes in intestinal transplant criteria. Am J Transplant. 2015;15(6):1674–81.
35. Grant D, Abu-Elmagd K, Mazariegos G, Vianna R, Langnas A, Mangus R. u. a. Intestinal transplant registry report: global activity and trends: intestinal transplant registry report. Am J Transplant. 2015;15(1):210–9.
36. Martinez Rivera A, Wales PW. Intestinal transplantation in children: current status. Pediatr Surg Int. 2016;32(6):529–40.
37. Spagnuolo MI, Iorio R, Vajro P. Isolated liver transplantation in children with intestinal failure–associated liver disease: a still-debated matter. J Pediatr Gastroenterol Nutr. 2009;48(3):271–3.
38. Dell-Olio D, Beath S, de Ville de Goyet J, Clarke S, Davies P, Lloyd C. u. a. Isolated liver transplant in infants with short bowel syndrome: insights into outcomes and prognostic factors. J Pediatr Gastroenterol Nutr. 2009;48(3):334–40.

14 Echinococcosis of the Liver

Daniela Kniepeiss, Emina Talakić, and Peter Schemmer

14.1 Incidence

Echinococcosis is an important parasitic disease in humans, which is caused by *Echinococcus* (*E.*) tapeworms [1]. There is a total of four different species that can be distinguished:

- Cystic echinococcosis (CE), caused by the infection of *E. granulosus.*
- Alveolar echinococcosis (AE), caused by *E. multilocularis.*
- Polycystic echinococcosis, caused by *E. vogeli.*
- Unicystic echinococcosis, caused by *E. oligarthrus.*

E. granulosus and *E. multilocularis* are predominant in humans, representing a substantially endemic health problem in some regions of the world. The incidence of *E. granulosus* is up to 50 per 100.000 persons per year in Eastern Europe, the Middle East, China, and South America [2, 3]. In some slaughterhouses in South America, a prevalence of up to 95% is reported [4]. In contrast, *E. multilocularis* is still limited to the northern hemisphere but with a growing distribution [5]. A recent review underlined the ongoing spread of AE in humans, especially in Western, Northern, and Eastern Europe and Central Asia [6]. However, Antarctica, Tanzania, Cyprus, Malta, and New Zealand are considered echinococcosis-free regions, which is an achievement of their health policy [7].

14.2 Clinical Presentation

Cystic Echinococcosis The morbidity of CE is high, with up to 70% affection of the liver. Characteristic lesions are hydatid cysts, which can also be in the lungs, spleen, kidney, bones, and brain [8–10]. In the liver, CE is often asymptomatic for a long time. However, both biliary and vascular complications can occur and cause cholestasis, cholangitis, biliary fistula, and thrombosis or Budd–Chiari syndrome. CE in the lungs can cause clinical signs like chronic cough, chest pain, and dyspnea. In the worst cases, CE can become life-threatening, with a mortality of up to 2.2% [11].

D. Kniepeiss
Division of General, Visceral and Transplant Surgery, Department of Surgery, Medical University of Graz, Graz, Austria
e-mail: daniela.kniepeiss@medunigraz.at

E. Talakić
Division of General Radiology, Department of Radiology, Medical University of Graz, Graz, Austria
e-mail: emina.talakic@medunigraz.at

P. Schemmer (✉)
Department of Visceral Surgery, Hirslanden Hospital Beau-Site, Bern, Switzerland

General and Visceral Surgery, Schemmer-Worni Clinic, Bern, Switzerland
e-mail: peter.schemmer@hin.ch

T. Hackert, A. Gulla (eds.), *Rare Liver and Biliary Tract Diseases*,
https://doi.org/10.1007/978-3-032-15076-9_14

Alveolar Echinococcosis In 99% of cases, manifestation of the primary disease is in the liver. After an asymptomatic time of up to 10 years, the liver is slowly colonized by the parasites. The lesions grow larger and larger and often become necrotic in the center or contain calcifications. Clinically, epigastric pain, jaundice, fever, malaise, and weight loss predominate. In case of invasion of the bile ducts, cholangitis, portal hypertension, or biliary cirrhosis can occur. In 13% of the patients, the disease can affect more organs due to infiltration of the neighborhood or metastatic spread, especially into the lungs, brain, spleen, and/or bones. Without treatment, AE is progressive and life-threatening [12, 13].

14.3 Diagnostic Workup

Basically, the diagnosis of CE and AE consists of imaging and specific serology and/or molecular identification of the parasite [14].

14.3.1 Imaging

Imaging holds a central position in the accurate diagnosis of alveolar and cystic echinococcosis, providing information about parasite activity and aiding in their characterization. Specific imaging techniques are essential for the detection and understanding of these parasitic infections, while percutaneous interventions are used to treat complications arising from alveolar echinococcosis and certain cystic forms.

Alveolar Echinococcosis Alveolar echinococcosis is often discovered incidentally or due to complications such as abdominal pain or jaundice [15, 16]. The imaging manifestations of alveolar echinococcosis are largely based on the presence of infiltrative microcystic lesions, which can lead to local problems such as extrahepatic involvement and bile duct dilatation [15, 16, 17].

Ultrasound (US) and contrast-enhanced ultrasound (CEUS) are valuable tools for the diagnosis of echinococcosis. B-mode ultrasound typically shows an irregularly circumscribed, heterogeneous, echogenic mass with cystic vesicles, arising from necrotic areas and calcifications. This mass is surrounded by a hyperechogenic ring corresponding to fibrosis [18, 19].

In some cases, a rare pattern resembling a "hailstorm" with multiple hyperechogenic solid lesions may occur. This may be confused with common liver diseases such as hemangiomas, which have acoustic enhancement due to fluid content [20]. CEUS is invaluable in distinguishing alveolar echinococcosis (AE) from other diagnoses, with AE characterized by either no enhancement or limited peripheral enhancement [21].

Computed tomography (CT) plays a critical role in echinococcosis imaging. It provides a comprehensive picture of lesion characteristics, including location, quantity, and size [22, 23]. An infiltrating mass with calcifications and without contrast enhancement clearly indicates echinococcosis [24].

CT is the imaging modality of choice for the detection of calcification, a potentially crucial diagnostic feature [25]. The cystic element within the lesion varies and corresponds to necrotic regions [26]. Peripheral fibrosis may show mild enhancement on subsequent imaging [27]. In addition, intrahepatic biliary dilatation is frequently observed and occasionally manifests diffusely in cases involving the hilar region [28].

Magnetic resonance imaging (MRI) improves the characterization of the lesion and reveals an infiltrative hypovascular mass composed of a mixture of solid and cystic tissue. Among MRI sequences, T2-weighted imaging proves to be the most specific, clearly imaging metacestodal vesicles (microcysts) and areas of liquefaction necrosis (large cysts) with high signal intensity. Conversely, granuloma tissue, coagulation necrosis, and calcifications appear with low signal intensity. T2-weighted imaging can show multivesicular lesions resembling a "grape" or "honeycomb" pattern [29] (Table 14.1).

In 2003, Kodama et al. [28] introduced an MRI classification into five types (Table 14.2), with microcysts predominating in AE lesions at

Table 14.1 WHO classifications of CE and their correlation with parasitic activity

	Cystic Echinococcosis (CE)		
	OMS		Activity
CE1		Unilocular cyst with double membrane	Active
CE2		Multilocular with daughter cyst	Active
CE3a	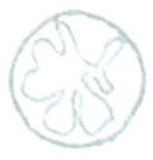	"Water-lily" sign, representing floating membranes	Transitional
CE3b	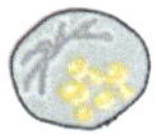	Solid daughter-cyst components	Transitional
CE4	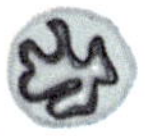	Solid component without daughters cysts	Inactive
CE5	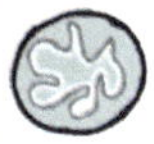	Calcified	Inactive

Table 14.2 WHO classifications of AE and their correlation with parasitic activity

	Cystic Echinococcosis (CE)		
	Kodama		Activity
1	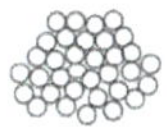	Multiple small round cysts without a solid component	Active
2	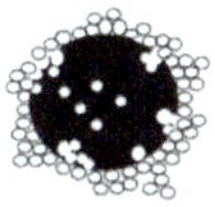	Multiple small round cysts with a solid component	Active
3	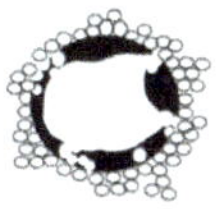	A solid component surrounding a large and/or irregular pseudo-cyst with multiple small round cysts	Active?
4	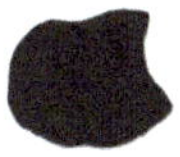	A solid component without cyst	Inactive
5	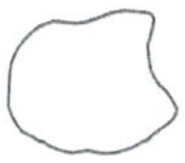	A large cyst without a solid component	Inactive

diagnosis, particularly types 2 and 3, regardless of the study (with a prevalence of 42% for type 2 and 46% for type 3) [30]. Consequently, microcysts proved to be the primary imaging feature for the positive diagnosis of alveolar echinococcosis.

MR cholangiopancreatography (MRCP) is proving to be crucial in assessing the possible invasion or compression of the bile ducts by the lesion. It serves as the basis for treatment decisions, whether curative (radical surgical resection) or palliative (percutaneous or endoscopic interventions) [31].

Radiology plays a crucial role in the diagnosis of alveolar echinococcosis (AE) and complements clinical history and serology. In areas with AE prevalence, contrast-enhanced ultrasound (CEUS) is used when an echogenic liver mass is detected; the lack of internal enhancement in AE is evident [32]. T2-weighted MRI facilitates the differentiation of AE from infiltrative masses by identifying pathognomonic microcysts [16]. In addition, diffusion-weighted MRI (DWI-MRI) helps distinguish AE from cholangiocarcinoma by increasing the Apparent Diffusion Coefficient (ADC) values [33]. Computed tomography (CT) is essential for the evaluation of infiltrative AE lesions and the detection of calcifications [34].

The increase in immunosuppressed AE cases has led to atypical imaging findings that resemble other diseases [35]. Multimodal imaging, including fluorodeoxyglucose-positron emission tomography (FDG-PET) and DWI-MRI, provides information about lesion viability [36]. Visualization of microcalcifications on CT is consistent with the hypermetabolic activity seen on FDG-PET/CT [37]. The potential of FDG-PET/MRI for AE management is currently under investigation [38].

Complications such as biliary tract involvement and vascular problems are important in AE. Biliary complications manifest as jaundice or cholangitis, while vascular complications range from sinusoidal dilatation to Budd–Chiari syndrome [39]. Extrahepatic involvement, although rare, involves areas such as the lungs and brain; therefore, chest CT and brain MRI are recommended for a thorough evaluation. Lung metastases often present as calcified nodules, with a correlation between distant extrahepatic disease and the liver lesion size [40].

Cystic Echinococcosis Cystic echinococcosis (CE) is a common endemic disease caused by the metacestode form of the tapeworm *E. granulosus*. In this introductory section, we present the global prevalence of the disease, review its clinical spectrum ranging from asymptomatic cases to severe infections, and emphasize the urgency of effective diagnostic and treatment strategies. The central role of radiological imaging in confirming the presence of CE cysts, evaluating their activity, and detecting potential complications will be highlighted.

Radiological examination begins with ultrasound (US), the most important imaging modality for preliminary CE assessment and staging. The World Health Organization Informal Working Group on Echinococcosis (WHO-IWGE) international classification is based on US imaging (Table 14.1) [41].

Magnetic resonance imaging (MRI), with its emphasis on T2-weighted sequences, is proving to be an effective tool for deciphering the inner matrix of CE cysts and the importance of contrast-enhanced T1-weighted images in the localization of biliary fistulas [4]. In addition, the role of MRI in the comprehensive evaluation of substantial cysts and the differentiation of CE from other cystic entities is focused on.

Although computed tomography (CT) is not the first diagnostic choice, it plays a critical role in the incidental detection of CE and the evaluation of complications [42, 43].

Radiologists take a lead role in CE diagnosis, especially in endemic regions. This section describes their key responsibilities in detecting signs of parasitic activity, seamlessly integrating multiple imaging modalities to confirm or clarify findings [24], and fostering a collaborative environment with clinicians to ensure accurate diagnoses and optimal treatment decisions.

Assessing parasitic activity in CE presents a relatively straightforward process when compared to its alveolar counterpart [41]. This alignment is evident through the congruence between the WHO-IWGE classification system and parasitic activity, where internal cysts or detached membranes serve as pivotal indicators [41].

Mechanical challenges such as cyst rupture and compression are potential complications. A detailed insight into intrabiliary rupture and its consequences is needed, as is a comprehensive understanding of the potential consequences of intraperitoneal rupture. The critical role of radiologists in early detection and intervention is paramount.

Given the complexity of CE, a holistic approach to treatment is essential. Collaboration between radiologists, clinicians, and surgeons is essential to develop effective treatment strategies.

14.3.2 Laboratory Tests

In most cases, routine laboratory tests are not specific for Echinococcosis. In a few cases, eosinophilia develops. Serological tests are typically performed in patients with a history of potential exposure and/or clinical presentation (i.e., imaging) of AE or CE. For the detection of antibodies against *E. granulosus*, an indirect enzyme-linked immunosorbent assay (ELISA) is used. The assay offers a semiquantitative value based on the optical density of the signal; however, in patients with hepatic CE, the indirect immunofluorescence assay (IFA) is the most sensitive test (95% sensitivity) [44]. Testing for *E. multilocularis* is a two-step procedure. First, an ELISA is performed, followed by a Western blot. In cases of an active infection, the specific immunoglobulin M and immunoglobulin G antibodies are significantly increased. Further, circulating hydatid antigen can be detected in the serum with ELISA tests and can be used for monitoring after therapy. The sensitivity of ELISA tests is up to 90% and is therefore preferred [45].

14.4 Differential Diagnosis

Possible differential diagnoses in the liver are cholangiocellular carcinoma, hepatocellular adenoma, hepatic cysts, or pyogenic hepatic abscesses. In the kidney, renal cancer and pyonephrosis must be differentiated. In the lungs, non-small cell lung cancer, small cell lung cancer, and lung metastases are possible differential diagnoses to E. In all cases, serology and imaging could provide clarity.

14.5 Treatment

Treatment of AE and CE should be multidisciplinary, comprising surgeons, gastroenterologists, infectiologists, and radiologists [14]. However, the most effective therapy against E. is surgery. Alternative treatments like chemotherapy; cyst puncture; or percutaneous aspiration, injection of chemicals, and reaspiration (PAIR) have been tried to replace surgery. These techniques are only indicated in a few cases with asymptomatic and inactive cysts, which would also disappear without any treatment.

14.5.1 Surgical Treatment

Surgery is the first-choice treatment for hepatic AE and CE. While there are some surgical treatment options for patients with CE, in cases with AE, early diagnosis and radical surgery, combined with anti-infective prophylaxis, are crucial. In cases of AE, complete resection, followed by adjuvant anthelmintic therapy, is recommended for curative treatment [46, 47]. Depending on the extent of the resection and the experience of the surgeon, an open or laparoscopic approach can be chosen. However, there are no studies that show an advantage of laparoscopic resection in AE compared to an open approach. Patients with debulking procedures have a poor prognosis compared to patients with radical surgery. Liver transplantation (LT) is performed in some cases but has no benefit compared to palliative surgery. Furthermore, immunosuppression might cause disease recurrence. However, many patients are diagnosed at an advanced stage of the disease, so no curative approach is available.

In patients with CE, a curative treatment can be achieved with various surgical approaches, including pericystectomy, liver resection, and parenchyma-sparing endocystectomy with partial cystectomy. While the latter technique can be recommended [48], the choice of the surgical technique depends on the number and size of cysts and the condition of the patient. The most important point is to avoid the spillage of cyst content and, thus, decrease the risk of recurrence [47].

In addition to liver resection, the extent of which depends on the size and number of lesions, the following surgical techniques can be offered for patients with hepatic cystic echinococcosis:

Endocystectomy with Partial Cystectomy This surgical technique is a novel parenchyma-sparing approach for CE of the liver [48]. After laparotomy and dissection of the liver from its ligaments, the location of the lesion can be verified with intraoperative ultrasound. In order to protect the surrounding tissue from contamination with hydatid fluid, a layer of cloths soaked with normal saline solution is placed in the abdomen near the liver. The first layer is covered by a second layer of cloths, which are soaked with 20% saline solution (Fig. 14.1). Subsequently, the parasite-derived cyst content is sucked out over a 12 mm trocar, which was inserted into the cyst before (Figs. 14.2 and 14.3). When the cyst is sucked empty, the trocar is removed again, and fistulas to the biliary sys-

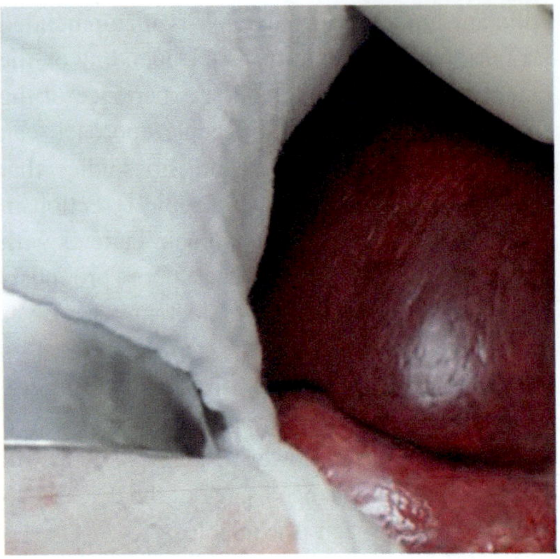

Fig. 14.1 For the protection of the surrounding tissue, a layer of cloths soaked with normal saline solution and a second layer of cloths soaked with 20% saline solution are placed around the liver

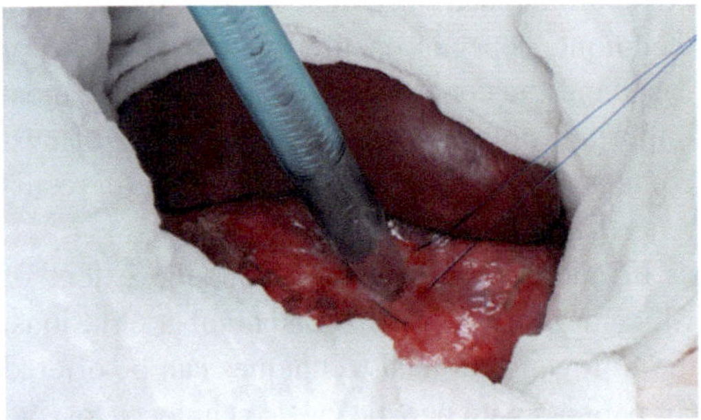

Fig. 14.2 A non-cutting 12-millimeter trocar is inserted into the cyst

tem are excluded with the white test [49]. Then, in order to devitalize remnant protoscoleces, the cyst is filled with hyperosmolar saline for 15 minutes (Fig. 14.4). Finally, the cyst is deroofed and filled with omentum.

The advantages of this procedure are an excellent view due to the open approach and good control of the parasite-derived material during surgery. Furthermore, there was no risk of recurrence of CE [50]. Rare complications could be bleeding, postoperative biloma, or fluid collection.

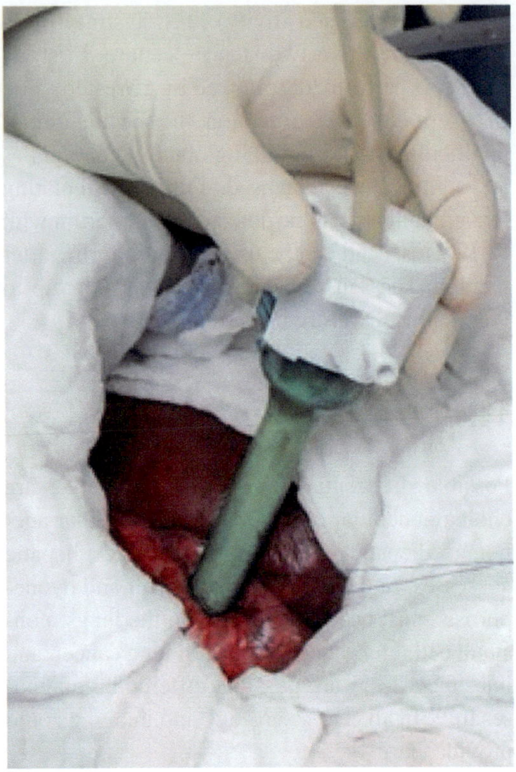

Fig. 14.3 The cyst content is evacuated through the trocar with a suction

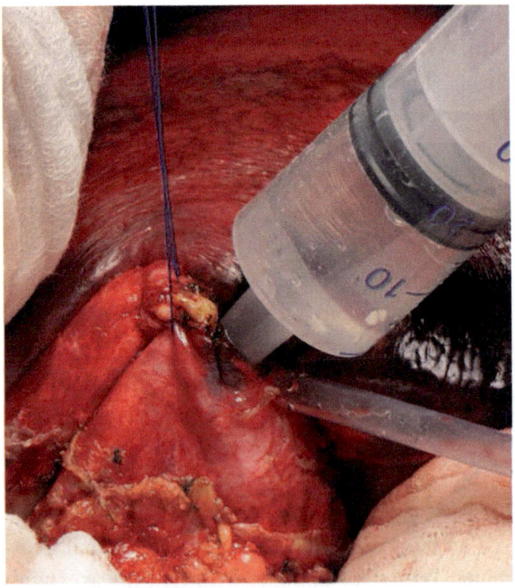

Fig. 14.4 The evacuated cyst is filled with hyperosmolar saline solution (20%)

Pericystectomy Pericystectomy comprises total cystectomy with the removal of the parasite-derived cyst components together with the entire pericyst. Pericystectomy can be performed together with the resection of the surrounding liver, which can be indicated for large, multiple, or complicated cysts. The precondition is a sufficiently large future liver remnant for good hepatic function. Pericystectomy with liver resection is a radical surgical approach that is more complex and difficult compared to less invasive techniques. There are some disadvantages, like a high risk for bile leakages, postoperative bleeding, liver failure, and wound infection or incisional hernia. Depending on the extent of the resection, the complication rate ranges from 3 to 30%, and recurrence rates of up to 4% are reported [51, 52].

Pericystectomy can also be performed without resection of the surrounding liver. The surgical technique is less radical, but the disadvantages are the risk of sclerosing cholangitis, biliary fistula, and cavity infection. There is a complication rate of up to 24% and a recurrence rate of up to 25% [53].

Laparoscopic Versus Open Approach A laparoscopic approach for the treatment of liver CE might be an option for a few patients, but there are some challenges: Cysts located in the posterior and superior segments of the liver are difficult to reach, and it is almost impossible to avoid the spilling of the cyst content [54]. Furthermore, there are some exclusion criteria for a laparoscopic technique, like intrabiliary rupture, central localization of the cyst, size of the cyst of more than 15 cm, multiple cysts, or calcified walls. Due to the higher risk of spilling the parasite-derived content of the cysts, there is a recurrence rate of up to 11% [55, 56]. Another disadvantage of the spillage is the higher risk of allergic reactions.

Liver Transplantation There are only limited data published on liver transplantation in patients with AE. However, AE can progress to severe damage of the liver, e.g., biliary stricture, recurrent cholangitis, liver abscesses, biliary cirrhosis, or Budd–Chiari syndrome [57]. In these cases, liver transplantation (LT) might be a treatment option. The first experiences with LT in patients with AE were reported in the 1980s [58]. This case series comprised a more than 11-year follow-up of patients with LT due to AE. It was cleary stated that LT should be considered very carefully due to a high risk of recurrence. The largest multicenter series consisting of 45 patients from 45 European centers [57] described a 5-year survival of 71% with a curative approach in only 50%. Based on two single-center series, LT was suggested as a reasonable treatment for AE of the liver [59]. Most patients underwent living-donor liver transplantation, with an overall survival of 80% after 16 months and no local AE recurrence. However, it was shown that the invasion of the bile duct or the portal vein was associated with higher mortality, which should be considered when choosing LT as a treatment option. In conclusion, the results of LT in AE were found to be acceptable. However, LT is indicated very rarely in patients with AE and should only be considered in cases of incurable disease or life-threatening complications.

14.5.2 Anthelmintic Drugs

Anthelmintic drugs against E. include the well-tolerated benzimidazoles (mebendazole and albendazole). Albendazole is more effective than mebendazole in patients with liver cysts [22]. Both the duration of treatment and the dosing of the medication are of importance. A therapy of at least 3 months to up to two years is highly recommended [60]. Side effects are rare and consist of liver function abnormalities, which seldom limit the treatment. Another side effect is hematologic impairment, which may be serious and could necessitate the discontinuation of the therapy. Medical therapy is usually used in addition to surgical treatment.

14.6 Surgical Planning/Management

The management of AE and CE varies worldwide and is discussed in a controversial manner. However, surgery is the most effective treatment and should be seen as the gold standard. Both forms of liver E. require a different surgical approach. Standard therapy for AE is resection. State of the art for liver CE are parenchyma-sparing approaches: partial cystectomy with removal of the pericyst components and total cystectomy or resection with removal of the parasite-derived cyst components and the entire pericyst. The modern parenchyma-sparing surgical approach comprises (i) evacuation of parasite-derived cyst content, including endocystectomy; (ii) sterilization of the cyst wall (host); and (iii) deroofing of the cyst (partial cystectomy) and can be highly recommended whenever this approach is possible [48].

Regarding the treatment of albendazole, its positive effect on recurrence is well-known, but there is no evidence on the length of treatment. It was shown that 2–3 months of albendazole preoperatively reduced the protoscolex viability to 6% to 12%. The recurrence rate following 8 weeks of preoperative albendazole was 6.25%, compared to 18% without albendazole and 0% with 8 weeks of postoperative albendazole [61]. However, a randomized controlled trial to establish the optimal length of pre- and post-procedure albendazole is still lacking.

14.7 Recommendations for Follow-Up

The follow-up of patients with echinococcosis is mainly based on imaging techniques, supported by serological tests. Visits, including an imaging examination, should be done every 3–6 months initially and once a year in patients with stable disease.

References

1. McManus DP, Thompson RC. Molecular epidemiology of cystic echinococcosis. Parasitology. 2003;127:37–51.
2. Reddy CRRM. Epidemiology of hydatic disease in Kurnool. Indian J Med Res. 1968;56(8):1205–20.
3. Bosco A, Camara Alves L, Cociancic P. Epidemiology and spatial distribution of Echinococcus granulosus in sheep and goats slaughtered in a hyperendemic European Mediterranean area. Parasites Vectors. 2021;14:421.
4. Brunetti E, Kern P, Vuitton DA. Writing panel for the WHO-IWGE expert consensus for the diagnosis and treatment of cystic and alveolar echinococcosis in humans. Acta Trop. 2010;114:1–16.
5. Torgerson PR, Budke CM. Echinococcosis—an international public health challenge. Res Vet Sci. 2003;74:191–202.
6. Baumann S, Shi R, Liu W, et al. Worldwide literature on epidemiology of human alveolar echinococcosis: a systematic review of research published in the twenty-first century. Infection. 2019;47:703–27.
7. Christofi G, Deplazes P, Christofi N, et al. Screening of dogs for Echinococcus granulosus coproantigen in a low endemic situation in Cyprus. Vet Parasitol. 2002;104(4):299–306.
8. Moro P, Schantz PM. Echinococcosis: a review. Int J Infect Dis. 2009;13(2):125–33.
9. Nunnari G, Pinzone M, Gruttadauria S, et al. Hepatic echinococcosis: clinical and therapeutic aspects. World J Gastroenterol. 2012;18(13):1448–58.
10. Khanfar N. Hydatid disease – a review update. Curr Anaesth Crit Care. 2004;15(3):173–83.
11. Brunetti E, Garlaschelli AL. Comment on "acute echinococcosis: a case report". J Clin Microbiol. 2003;41:523.
12. Eckert J, Deplazes P. Biological, epidemiological, and clinical aspects of echinococcosis, a zoonosis of increasing concern. Clin Microbiol Rev. 2004;17:107–35.
13. Kern P, Menezes da Silva A, Akhan O, et al. The Echinococcoses: diagnosis, clinical management and burden of disease. Adv Parasitol. 2017;96:259–369.
14. Brunetti E, Kern P, Vuitton DA, Autorengruppe für WHO-IWGE. Expert consensus for the diagnosis and treatment of cystic and alveolar echinococcosis in humans. Acta Trop. 2010;114(1):1–16.
15. Tamarozzi F, Akhan O, Cretu CM, et al. The global epidemiology of echinococcosis. Trop Med Int Health. 2020;25(10):1241–53.
16. Bresson-Hadni S, Delabrousse É, Blagosklonov O, et al. Imaging aspects and non-surgical interventional

treatment in human alveolar echinococcosis. Parasitol Int. 2006;55(Suppl):S267–72.
17. Zhang W, Zhang Z, Wu W, et al. Epidemiologie und Kontrolle der Echinokokkose in Zentralasien, unter besonderer Berücksichtigung der Volksrepublik China. Acta Trop. 2015;141(Pt B):235–43.
18. Brunetti E, Garcia HH, Junghanss T, et al. Cystic echinococcosis. Nat Rev Dis Primers. 2018;4:1.
19. Neumayr A, Troia G, de Bernardis C, et al. Justified concern or exaggerated fear: the risk of anaphylaxis in percutaneous treatment of cystic echinococcosis-a systematic literature review. PLoS Negl Trop Dis. 2011;5(6):e1154.
20. Dähnert I, Straub D, Völkel D, et al. Hypovaskuläre Leberläsionen auf kontrastverstärktem Ultraschall (CEUS): Unterscheidung zwischen gutartigen und bösartigen Läsionen. Clin Hemorheol Microcirc. 2012;52(2–4):179–89.
21. McManus DP, Gray DJ, Zhang W, et al. Diagnose, Behandlung und Management der Echinokokkose. BMJ. 2012;344:e3866.
22. Stojkovic M, Zwahlen M, Teggi A, et al. Treatment response of cystic echinococcosis to benzimidazoles: a systematic review. PLoS Negl Trop Dis. 2009;3(9):e524.
23. Stojkovic M, Rosenberger K, Kauczor HU, et al. Diagnosing and staging of cystic echinococcosis: how do CT and MRI perform in comparison to ultrasound? PLoS Negl Trop Dis. 2012;6(10):e1880.
24. Junghanss T, da Silva AM, Horton J, et al. Clinical management of cystic echinococcosis: state of the art, problems, and perspectives. Am J Trop Med Hyg. 2008;79(3):301–11.
25. Nunnari G, Pinzone MR, Gruttadauria S, et al. Hepatische Echinokokkose: klinische und therapeutische Aspekte. World J Gastroenterol. 2012;18(13):1448–58.
26. Rinaldi F, Brunetti E, Neumayr A, et al. Zystische Echinokokkose der Leber: klinische Merkmale und Ausgang. PLoS One. 2014;9(1):e85203.
27. Klimpel D, Römer S, Mathis A, et al. Comparative proteomic analysis of two Echinococcus multilocularis isolates. Parasitol Res. 2010;106(3):577–85.
28. Kodama Y, Fujita N, Shimizu T, et al. Alveoläre Echinokokkose: MR-Befunde in der Leber. Radiology. 2003;228:172–7.
29. Bresson-Hadni S, Spahr L, Chappuis F. Hepatische alveoläre Echinokokkose. Semin Liver Dis. 2021;41:393–408.
30. Weiner SM, Krenn V, Koelbel C, et al. Echinococcus multilocularis infection and TNF inhibitor treatment in a patient with rheumatoid arthritis. Rheumatol Int. 2011;31:1399–400.
31. Bresson-Hadni S, Vuitton DA, Bartholomot B, et al. A twenty-year history of alveolar echinococcosis: analysis of a series of 117 patients from eastern France. Eur J Gastroenterol Hepatol. 2000;12(3):327–36.
32. Gottstein B, Stojkovic M, Vuitton DA, et al. Innovationen in Diagnose, Behandlung und Vorhersage des Krankheitsverlaufs bei Echinokokkose. Trends Parasitol. 2015;31(9):407–12.
33. Kern P. Echinococcus multilocularis infection: clinical presentation, medical treatment and outcome. Langenbeck's Arch Surg. 2003;388(2):135–43.
34. Zhang W, Wang X, Liu X. Echinococcosis in China, a review of the epidemiology of Echinococcus spp. Eco Health. 2004;1(1):35–6.
35. Bulakçı M, Kartal MG, Yılmaz S, et al. Multimodality imaging in diagnosis and management of alveolar echinococcosis: an update. Diagn Interv Radiol. 2016;22(3):247–56.
36. Lötsch F, Waneck F, Groger M, et al. FDG-PET/MRI imaging for the management of alveolar echinococcosis: initial clinical experience at a reference Centre in Austria. Trop Med Int Health. 2019;24(6):663–70.
37. Rinaldi F, Brunetti E, Neumayr A, et al. Zystische Echinokokkose der Leber: eine Fibel für Hepatologen. World J Hepatol. 2014;6(5):293–305.
38. Wen H, Vuitton L, Tuxun T, et al. Echinococcosis: advances in the 21st century. Clin Microbiol Rev. 2019;32(2):e00075–18.
39. Junghanss T, Menezes da Silva A, Horton J, et al. Clinical management of cystic echinococcosis: state of the art, problems, and perspectives. Am J Trop Med Hyg. 2008;79(3):301–11.
40. Azizi A, Blagosklonov O, Lounis A, et al. Alveolar echinococcosis: correlation between hepatic MRI findings and FDG-PET/CT metabolic activity. Abdom Imaging. 2015;40(1):56–63.
41. Eckert J, Gemmell MA, Meslin, et al. WHO/OIE manual on Echinococcosis in humans and animals: a public health problem of global concern. World Health Organization.
42. Craig PS, Hegglin D, Lightowlers MW, et al. Echinococcosis: control and prevention. Adv Parasitol. 2017;96:55–158.
43. Rojas CAA, Romig T, Lightowlers MW, et al. Echinococcus granulosus sensu lato genotypes infecting humans–review of current knowledge. Int J Parasitol. 2014;44(1):9–18.
44. Manzano-Román R, Sánchez-Ovejero C, Hernández-González A, et al. Serological diagnosis and follow-up of human cystic echinococcosis: a new hope for the future? Biomed Res Int. 2015;2015:428205.
45. Brunetti E, Kern P, Vuitton DA. Expert consensus for the diagnosis and treatment of cystic and alveolar echinococcosis in humans. Acta Trop. 2010;114(1):1–16.
46. Salm LA, Lachenmayer A, Perrodin SF, et al. Surgical treatment strategies for hepatic alveolarechinococcosis. Food Waterborne Parasitol. 2019;15:e00050.
47. Siracusano A, Teggi A, Ortona E. Human cystic echinococcosis: old problems and new perspectives. Interdiscip Perspect Infect Dis. 2009;2009:474368.
48. Kniepeiss D, Talakic E, Schemmer P. Echinococcus granulosus: a novel parenchymal sparing surgical treatment. Hepatobiliary Pandreat Dis Int. 2020;19(4):390–3.

49. Nadalin S, Li J, Lang H, et al. The White test: a new dye test for intraoperative detection of bile leakage during major liver resection. Arch Surg. 2008;143(4):402–4.
50. He YB, Yao G, Tuxun T, al. Efficacy of radical and conservative surgery for hepatic cystic echinococcosis: a meta-analysis. Int J Clin Exp Med. 2015;8:7039–48.
51. Gollackner B, Längle F, Auer H, et al. Radical surgical therapy of abdominal cystic hydatid disease: factors of recurrence. World J Surg. 2000;24:717–21.
52. Dziri C, Dougaz W, Samaali I, et al. Radical surgery decreases overall morbidity and recurrence compared with conservative surgery for liver cystic echinococcosis: systematic review with meta-analysis. Ann Laparosc Endosc Surg. 2019;4:92.
53. Bostanci O, Kartal K, Yazici P, et al. Laparoscopic versus open surgery for hydatid disease of the liver. A single center experience. Ann Ital Chir. 2016;87:237–41.
54. Inaebnit EF, Molina Romero FX, Segura Sampedro JJ, et al. A review of the diagnosis and management of liver hydatid cyst. Rev Esp Enferm Dig. 2022;114(1):35–41.
55. Tuxun T, Zhang J, Zhao J, et al. World review of laparoscopic treatment of liver cystic echinococcosis—914 patients. Int J Infect Dis. 2014;24:43–5044.
56. Koch S, Bresson-Hadni S, Miguet JP, et al. Experience of liver transplantation for incurable alveolar echinococcosis: a 45-case European collaborative report. Transplantation. 2003;75:856–63.
57. Bresson-Hadni S, Koch S, Beurton I, et al. Primary disease recurrence after liver transplantation for alveolar echinococcosis: long-term evaluation in 15 patients. Hepatology. 1999;30:857–64.
58. Aydinli B, Ozturk G, Arslan S, et al. Liver transplantation for alveolar echinococcosis in an endemic region. Liver Transpl. 2015;21:1096.
59. Ozdemir F, Ince V, Barut B, et al. Living donor liver transplantation for Echinococcus alveolaris: single-center experience. Liver Transpl. 2015;21(8):1091–5.
60. Liu Y, Wang X, Wu J. Continuous long-term albendazole therapy in intraabdominal cystic echinococcosis. Chin Med J. 2000;113(9):827–32.
61. Arif SH, ul-Bari S, Wani NA, et al. Albendazole as an adjuvant to the standard surgical management of hydatid cyst liver. Int J Surg. 2008;6:448–5.

Fibrolamellar Hepatocellular Carcinoma

15

Emina Talakić, Daniela Kniepeiss, and Peter Schemmer

15.1 Incidence

Fibrolamellar hepatocellular carcinoma (FL-HCC) is a rare primary malignancy of the liver, which occurs in less than 1% of all liver malignancies [1]. In some countries, such as Mexico, the incidence is higher, with 5.8% of liver tumors [2]. Some features and clinical findings are completely different from those of conventional HCC, and patients are usually younger than patients with HCC. Mostly, patients affected with FL-HCC are in the second or third decade, and there is no gender preference. The incidence of FL-HCC is estimated to be about 0.02/100.00/year in the United States [3]. As it is a rare disease, evidence is rather limited to small retrospective, single-center studies and case series. Because of the few data, a standard of care has not been established yet. While FL-HCC is currently staged and treated similarly to conventional HCC, the survival of patients with FL-HCC is superior compared with patients with HCC.

15.2 Clinical Presentation

The etiology of FL-HCC is not understood since no underlying trigger has been identified yet. Patients with FL-HCC usually have no liver cirrhosis or chronic liver disease [4]. The clinical presentation is nonspecific, with tissue compaction, abdominal discomfort or pain, fatigue, and weight loss. Patients can also be asymptomatic, but in many cases patients present with abdominal pain from the large, aggressive tumor in the liver. At the time of diagnosis, the tumor may have an extent of about 10 centimeters, and lymphatic metastases occur in about 50% of the patients [5].

In some cases, symptoms of biliary obstruction, jaundice, male gynecomastia, fulminant liver failure, encephalopathy, ascites, or lower limb thrombophlebitis can occur. The classical HCC tumor markers (alpha-fetoprotein, AFP) are mostly normal. In imaging studies, FL-HCC presents as a unique, well-delineated mass of tissue that can sometimes be hardly differentiated from other solid lesions of the liver. At last, the biopsy confirms the diagnosis, showing well-differentiated tumor cells surrounded by thick collagen bands and a central scar [6]. The staging

E. Talakić
Division of General Radiology, Department of Radiology, Medical University of Graz, Graz, Austria
e-mail: emina.talakic@medunigraz.at

D. Kniepeiss
Division of General, Visceral and Transplant Surgery, Department of Surgery, Medical University of Graz, Graz, Austria
e-mail: daniela.kniepeiss@medunigraz.at

P. Schemmer (✉)
Department of Visceral Surgery, Hirslanden Hospital Beau-Site, Bern, Switzerland

General and Visceral Surgery, Schemmer-Worni Clinic, Bern, Switzerland
e-mail: peter.schemmer@hin.ch

T. Hackert, A. Gulla (eds.), *Rare Liver and Biliary Tract Diseases*,
https://doi.org/10.1007/978-3-032-15076-9_15

of FL-HCC is performed according to AFCC TNM staging for HCC. Many of the patients present at an advanced stage at the time of diagnosis, 37.2% with AJCC stage III and 42.3% with AJCC stage IV. The incidence of nodal positive disease is 30–40% and 33% present with distant metastases [7].

15.3 Clinical Work-Up for Diagnosis

The main goal in the work-up investigation of patients with FL-HCC is to differentiate FL-HCC from other benign or malignant liver tumors. The routine biochemical values of patients with FL-HCC are mostly normal or slightly elevated in a nonspecific way. The most important tools for the evaluation of FL-HCC are imaging and histological diagnosis. The significance of tumor markers is currently still unclear and needs to be further clarified. In recent years, progress has been made in researching the FL-HCC genome, which could make differentiation easier and enable targeted therapies in the future.

15.3.1 Imaging

In the field of liver cancer diagnosis, two tools, abdominal computed tomography (CT) and magnetic resonance imaging (MRI), have gained prominence and provide a comprehensive assessment of fibrolamellar carcinoma.

Abdominal computed tomography (CT), known for its ability to provide a holistic image of the liver and associated tumors, is the first choice for the evaluation of fibrolamellar carcinoma. To optimize the evaluation of liver tumors by CT scans, intravenous administration of an iodine-containing contrast agent is essential. However, there are practical limitations in certain patient groups, such as patients with allergies to iodine-containing contrast agents or renal insufficiency. In these cases, magnetic resonance imaging (MRI) is emerging as a preferred alternative [8–10].

In addition, ionizing radiation is not negligible with CT, making its use relatively contraindicated in certain groups such as children and women of childbearing age, and radiation exposure requires vigilant management.

Contrast-enhanced CT scans consistently show fibrolamellar hepatocellular carcinoma as a well-demarcated, 7–20 cm mass characterized by a lobular contour and heterogeneous appearance. In contrast, unenhanced CT scans often show hypoattenuation accompanied by calcifications (in 40–68% of cases) and a prominent central star-shaped scar (in 65–75% of cases) [11–14].

Magnetic resonance imaging (MRI) plays a pivotal role as a complementary modality for the detection and characterization of primary tumors. In contrast to CT, MRI has higher sensitivity in detecting multiple intrahepatic recurrent lesions. However, the sensitivity is lower in detecting extrahepatic disease. As the current research shows, fibrolamellar hepatocellular carcinoma has characteristic imaging features on MRI: hypointensity on T1-weighted images and hyperintensity on T2-weighted images. A central fibrous scar maintains its hypointensity on both T1- and T2-weighted images. Gadolinium-enhanced MRI captures the dynamic nature of fibrolamellar carcinoma, characterized by intense heterogeneous enhancement during the arterial phase and gradual attenuation during the portal venous phase [15, 16].

Despite its advantages, MRI is not without limitations. The longer duration of MRI exams compared with CT scans and ultrasound raises concerns about image quality due to motion artifacts when patients cannot remain still. MRI and a hepatocyte-specific contrast media, such as Gadovist or Primovist, are preferred.

Ultrasonography offers an alternative imaging modality, particularly for visualizing the nonspecific features of fibrolamellar hepatocellular carcinoma. These features present as well-defined masses with variable echogenicity. However, operator dependence and limitations associated with challenging patient anatomy underscore the importance of judicious application [17, 18].

In selected scenarios, the integration of radionuclide sulfur colloid scans or labeled red blood cell scans may provide a unique perspective to differentiate fibrolamellar carcinoma from other liver tumor types and further increase diagnostic specificity.

In summary, the choice of imaging modalities for the evaluation of fibrolamellar carcinoma is related to recent advances in the field. Each technique-CT, MRI, or ultrasound-brings its own strengths and limitations. A personalized approach that considers patient characteristics and requirements remains critical for optimal diagnosis and treatment in the dynamic landscape of fibrolamellar carcinoma imaging [19, 20].

15.3.2 Biopsy

The histopathological work-up is characteristic and offers the best method to differentiate between FL-HCC and HCC and confirm the diagnosis [21, 22]. Especially in cases of an uncertain imaging finding, histology is crucial. Furthermore, the biology of the tumor can be determined, and a better selection of patients who would benefit from surgical therapy can be made. The preferred technique for the biopsy is either a percutaneous core biopsy or an open biopsy via laparoscopy. Fine needle aspiration is not recommended as it has poor results, and diagnosis may be false negative due to aspiration of malignant hepatocytes without the characteristic fibrotic lamellae [23].

15.3.3 Tumor Marker

Alpha-fetoprotein (AFP) is an important marker used for the diagnosis and screening of HCC. However, FL-HCC rarely produces AFP, and therefore, patients with FL-HCC usually do not have elevated serum AFP levels [24]. Nevertheless, the significance of AFP in FL-HCC is still a matter of controversy. A few authors guess that the impact of AFP on FL-HCC has not been identified up to now because the case numbers were too low. So, it might be underreported and underappreciated [25]. Some authors suppose an association between poorly differentiated FL-HCC and the tumor size with AFP [26, 27]. A significant difference in the median overall survival for patients with FL-HCC and elevated AFP compared with patients with normal AFP was described. Associated factors were poorly differentiated tumors, increased tumor size, and older age of the patient. Furthermore, patients with elevated serum AFP levels had more aggressive tumor biology and a higher risk for recurrence after resection [28].

Further markers that have been discussed relating to FL-HCC were elevated serum vitamin B12 and serum unsaturated vitamin B12-binding capacities. Some authors described an association with FL-HCC [29, 30]. In a few cases, elevated serum neurotensin levels were thought to play a role as a biomarker, but they were not sensitive or specific enough for diagnosis [31, 32]. In general, more research is needed to evaluate the impact of AFP and other potential markers on survival and on the risk of recurrence. These markers could be used as a diagnostic and prognostic tool in patients with FL-HCC.

15.3.4 Genetic Work-Up

Historically, studies on the genomics of FL-HCC were limited due to small sample size and insufficient technology. Nevertheless, a stable genome was identified, with a lower frequency of mutations and copy number variations compared to HCC. Some abnormalities in the genome of FL-HCC were similar to those of the HCC, but a large part was different from HCC. Currently, researchers have found that at the genomic level of FL-HCC, a single 400 kB deletion in chromosome 19 exists, which leads to a functional DNAJB1-PRKACA fusion protein. This DNAJB1-PRKACA fusion transcript is supposed to be the oncogenic driver in fibrolamellar hepatocellular carcinoma [33]. Most FL-HCCs demonstrate the DNAJB1-PRKACA fusion transcript, and it is 100% specific for FL-HCC. These patterns of genomic variations can help to differentiate malignant lesions in the liver and could be used as therapeutic targets in the future [34].

15.4 Differential Diagnosis

Differential diagnosis of solitary liver lesions is sometimes very difficult or almost impossible. The most important differential diagnosis of FL-HCC is focal nodular hyperplasia (FNH), hepatocellular adenoma (HCA), and HCC. However, sometimes other lesions like giant cavernous hemangioma and metastases of neuroendocrine tumors could also be differentiated poorly. To distinguish these lesions, imaging plays a crucial role, but finally, a liver biopsy is recommended to avoid incorrect diagnosis.

15.4.1 Focal Nodular Hyperplasia

FNH is a frequent benign, hyperplastic lesion of the liver with scar-like tissue that appears in younger patients but is preferred (about 80%) in women. Sometimes it may look like FL-HCC in imaging studies, and differentiation is almost impossible [35]. Histologically, typical for FNH is characterized by functioning hepatocytes packed densely with a central scar without calcification [36]. A clear differentiation between FNH and FL-HCC is important because the clinical approach regarding both is different. FL-HCC requires surgery, whereas FNH mostly needs no treatment.

15.4.2 Hepatocellular Adenoma

HCA is a rare benign tumor of the liver that occurs preferentially in young women with a long history of estrogen-based oral contraceptive use [37]. Complications are rupture, bleeding, or malignant transformation. If lesions are bigger than 5 centimeters, resection is recommended [38]. The diagnosis of HCA comprises clinical and imaging findings. Sometimes, the differentiation between HCA and FL-HCC is challenging due to overlapping diagnostic features. In these cases, a biopsy with histological work-up should be performed.

15.4.3 Hepatocellular Carcinoma

There are a lot of differences between FL-HCC and HCC and possibilities to distinguish the two from each other. While patients are younger at diagnosis with FL-HCC, mostly they are older with HCC, and furthermore, there is a gender preference for male patients. In contrast to HCC, which is quite frequent in Africa and in Asia, there is no distinct geographic distribution in FL-HCC. Lesions of FL-HCC are mostly solitary, whereas lesions of HCC often appear multiple. The appearance of FL-HCC is not linked to chronic viral infection or liver cirrhosis, as it is in HCC. A characteristic in imaging studies of HCC is a prompt enhancement in the arterial phase with a washout of contrast in the delayed phase, which is often sufficient and clear for diagnosis. However, the most objective and accepted method to differentiate between FL-HCC and HCC is histology. The characteristic macro-finding of FL-HCC is a well-circumscribed, often lobulated mass, a central gray, and a white scar. The histological features are eosinophilic polygonal-shaped cells separated by lamellar fibrosis, a fairly uniform cell pattern, and a greater differentiation than in HCC. The macro-findings of HCC are single or massive, multifocal or nodular and mostly diffuse tumor masses. Necrosis and hemorrhage appear often. The histology shows eosinophilic thickened plates of hepatocytes with eosinophilic or clear cytoplasm. The cells are often arranged in a trabecular, pseudoglandular, or solid pattern, and the differentiation of the cells is lower than in FL-HCC [39]. The prognosis of FL-HCC is much better compared with HCC [40]. The gold standard treatment for FL-HCC is liver resection. In selected cases, liver transplantation could be performed. In patients with HCC, resection is often limited due to cirrhosis, but within defined criteria, liver transplantation offers a curative option [41].

15.5 Treatment

The best option for curative treatment in patients with resectable FL-HCC is liver resection (LR). In some cases, liver transplantation (LT) is indicated, but it is not a standard procedure for this tumor. In patients with a surgical approach, 5-year survival rates of up to 88% and 5-year disease-free survival rates of 18–50% have been described [42]. Patients with unresectable disease have a median survival of only 12 months, and the 5-year survival is 0% [43]. The role of neoadjuvant and adjuvant therapies like chemotherapy and radiotherapy is not defined and is unclear [44]. The hope of future approaches lies in targeted therapy concepts.

15.5.1 Resection

At present, surgical resection remains the best treatment option, with a reported overall survival of up to 174 months [3]. However, most patients (about 70%) need a major liver resection due to a large tumor or nodal and vascular infiltration in about 60% and 43%, respectively. In about 24% of patients, a minor hepatectomy is possible. Overall, up to 70% can be treated with a curative approach [45–47]. Results of a large monocentric study showed that less than half of the patients underwent curative resections (n = 229, 46%). In 91% of these patients, an R0 resection could be achieved, but 45% had positive lymph nodes in the final pathological findings. In this cohort of patients, worse overall survival was associated with multiple tumors, major vascular involvement, lymphovascular invasion, elevated serum AFP, regional lymph node involvement, and a microscopically positive resection margin [26]. The recurrence rate of FL-HCC after resection was described as high, with more than two-thirds of the patients [48]. The median time to recurrence ranged between 10 and 33 months and was very rare after five years. In case of a recurrent tumor, a surgical resection can be performed again [49].

15.5.2 Liver Transplantation (LT)

LT has been performed for selected cases with FL-HCC. In a systematic review [3], 14 studies including 109 patients with LT for FL-HCC were described. Survival rates after 1, 3, and 5 years ranged from 63% to 100%, 43% to 75%, and 29% to 55%, respectively. However, it is not a standard therapeutic option as it is for HCC, and the criteria for the indication are lacking. There is no priority for patients with FL-HCC on the waiting list, and regional lymph node metastases, which occur in up to 42.2% of patients with FL-HCC, are a contraindication for LT [50]. The overall published data indicate an acceptable outcome for patients undergoing liver transplantation in FL-HCC despite its advanced stage.

15.5.3 Systemic Chemotherapy

Up to now, there is no randomized controlled trial on neoadjuvant or adjuvant systemic therapy in FL-HCC showing a clear survival benefit [51]. Furthermore, it was demonstrated that FLC is not sensitive to conventional chemotherapy, but platinum-based chemotherapy regimens and combination regimens, including interferon alpha-2b, could bring some positive effects. Better results were demonstrated with multimodal concepts consisting of surgery, chemotherapy, and radiation. Patients not undergoing surgery and not receiving treatments with chemotherapy showed a mean survival of 5.9 months, significantly lower than that of patients with chemotherapy [52].

15.5.4 Radiotherapy

Only a few cases of FL-HCC are reported after treatment with radiation. It was performed in cases of unresectable primary tumors with the aim of achieving resectability or treating metastases or recurrent tumors [53].

15.6 Surgical Options

The key to successful management of patients with FL-HCC is early diagnosis with differentiation from other liver tumors and subsequently radical resection. When resection is not feasible, in some cases, LT can be considered. Although the prognosis for FL-HCC is better compared with HCC, there is a high rate of recurrence ranging from 33% to 100%. A standard of care has not been defined in FL-HCC due to the lack of data on short- and long-term outcomes related to different treatment options. Currently, experience with targeted therapies is limited to individual case reports, but it will hopefully become a promising therapy option in the future.

15.7 Follow-Up of Patients After Treatment

As recurrence rates are high, patients should be included in a careful follow-up program. In cases of recurrent disease, repeated resection might be possible and achieve a survival benefit. Most centers recommend CT or MRI scanning at 3, 6, and 12 months for the 1st year after resection/transplantation, followed by the same imaging every 6 months during the 2nd and 3rd year and once yearly until the end of the 5th year [54].

References

1. Paradis V. Histopathology of hepatocellular carcinoma. Recent Results Cancer Res. 2013;190:21–32.
2. Arista-Nasr J, Gutierrez-Villalobos L, Nuncio J, et al. Fibrolamellar hepatocellular carcinoma in Mexican patients. Pathol Oncol Res. 2002;8(2):133–7.
3. Mavros MN, Mayo SC, Hyder O, et al. A systematic review: treatment and prognosis of patients with fibrolamellar hepatocellular carcinoma. J Am Coll Surg. 2012;215(6):820–30.
4. Sobel ME. Metastasis suppressor genes. J Natl Cancer Inst. 1990;82(4):267–76.
5. Wahab MA, El Hanafy E, El Nakeeb A, et al. Clinicopathological features and surgical outcome of patients with fibrolamellar hepatocellular carcinoma (experience with 22 patients over a 15-year period). World J Gastrointest Surg. 2017;9(2):61–7.
6. Chagas AL, Kikuchi L, Herman P, et al. Clinical and pathological evaluation of fibrolamellar hepatocellular carcinomaL a single center study of 21 cases. Clinics (Sao Paulo). 2015;70(3):207–13.
7. Lee CW, Chan KM, Lee CF, et al. Hepatic resection for hepatocellular carcinoma with lymph node metastasis: clinicopathological analysis and survival outcome. Asian J Surg. 2011;34:53–62.
8. Ganeshan D, Szklaruk J, Kundra V, et al. Imaging features of fibrolamellar hepatocellular carcinoma. Am J Roentgenol. 2014;202(3):544–52.
9. Do RK, McErlean A, Ang CS, et al. CT and MRI of primary and metastatic fibrolamellar carcinoma: a case series of 37 patients. Br J Radiol. 2014;87(1040):20140024.
10. Valentino PL, Ling SC, Ng VL, et al. The role of diagnostic imaging and liver biopsy in the diagnosis of focal nodular hyperplasia in children. Liver Int. 2014;34(2):227–34.
11. Blachar A, Federle MP, Ferris JV, et al. Radiologists' performance in the diagnosis of liver tumors with central scars by using specific CT criteria. Radiology. 2002;223(2):532–9.
12. Chun YS, Zimmitti G. Fibrolamellar variant of hepatocellular carcinoma. Recent Results Cancer Res. 2013;190:101–10.
13. Ichikawa T, Federle MP, Grazioli L, et al. Fibrolamellar hepatocellular carcinoma: imaging and pathologic findings in 31 recent cases. Radiology. 1999;213(2):352–61.
14. Alexander LF, Harri P, Little B, et al. Magnetic resonance imaging of primary hepatic malignancies in patients with and without chronic liver disease: a pictorial review. Cureus. 2017;9(8):e1539.
15. Palm V, Sheng R, Mayer P, et al. Imaging features of fibrolamellar hepatocellular carcinoma in gadoxetic acid-enhanced MRI. Cancer Imaging. 2018;18(1):9.
16. Ringe KI, Husarik DB, Sirlin CB. Gadoxetate disodium-enhanced MRI of the liver. Part 1, protocol optimization and lesion appearance in the noncirrhotic liver. Am J Roentgenol. 2010;195(1):13–28.
17. Friedman AC, Lichtenstein JE, Goodman Z, et al. Fibrolamellar hepatocellular carcinoma. Radiology. 1985;157(3 Pt 1):583–7.
18. Lafaro KJ, Pawlik TM. Fibrolamellar hepatocellular carcinoma: current clinical perspectives. J Hepatocell Carcinoma. 2015;2:151–7.
19. Winston CB, Schwartz LH, Fong Y, et al. Hepatocellular carcinoma: MR imaging findings in

cirrhotic livers and noncirrhotic livers. Radiology. 1999;210(1):75–9.
20. Bartolozzi C, Battaglia V, Bozzi E. HCC diagnosis with liver-specific MRI--close to histopathology. Dig Dis. 2009;27(2):125–30.
21. Eggert T, McGlynn KA, Duffy A, et al. Fibrolamellar hepatocellular carcinoma in the USA, 2000–2010: a detailed report on frequency, treatment and outcome based on the surveillance, epidemiology, and end results database. United Eur Gastroenterol J. 2013;1(5):351–7.
22. Mitchell KA. Hepatocellular carcinoma: histologic considerations: pure, mixed, and motley. J Clin Gastroenterol. 2013;47(Suppl):S20–6. 32
23. Powers C, Ros PR, Stoupis C, et al. Primary liver neoplasms: MR imaging with pathologic correlation. Radiographics. 1994;14:459–82.
24. McLarney JK, Rucker PT, Bender GN, et al. Fibrolamellar carcinoma of the liver: radiologic-pathologic correlation. Radiographics. 1999;19:453–71.
25. Berman MA, Burnham JA, Sheahan DG. Fibrolamellar carcinoma of the liver: an immunohistochemical study of nineteen cases and review of the literature. Hum Pathol. 1988;19:784–94.
26. McDonald JD, Gupta S, Shindorf ML, et al. Elevated serum α-fetoprotein is associated with abbreviated survival for patients with Fibrolamellar hepatocellular carcinoma who undergo a curative resection. Ann Surg Oncol. 2020;27(6):1900–5.
27. Silva JP, Gorman RA, Berger NG, et al. The prognostic utility of baseline alpha-fetoprotein for hepatocellular carcinoma patients. J Surg Oncol. 2017;116(7):831–40.
28. Blank S, Wang Q, Fiel MI, et al. Assessing prognostic significance of preoperative alpha fetoprotein in hepatitis B-associated hepatocellular carcinoma: normal is not the new normal. Ann Surg Oncol. 2014;21(3):986–94.
29. Yamashita S, Vauthey JN, Kaseb AO, et al. Prognosis of fibrolamellar carcinoma compared to non-cirrhotic conventional hepatocellular carcinoma. J Gastrointest Surg. 2016;20(10):1725–31.
30. Waxman S, Gilbert HS. A tumor-related vitamin B12 binding protein in adolescent hepatoma. N Engl J Med. 1973;289:1053–6.
31. Ward SC, Waxman S. Fibrolamellar carcinoma: a review with focus on genetics and comparison to other malignant primary liver tumors. Sem Liver Disease. 2011;31:61–70.
32. Darcy DG, Malek MM, Kobos R, et al. Prognostic factors in fibrolamellar hepatocellular carcinoma in young adults. J Pediatr Surg. 2015;50:153–6.
33. Ehrenfried JA, Zhou Z, Thompson JC, et al. Expression of the neurotensin gene in fetal human liver and fibrolamellar carcinoma. Ann Surg. 1994;220:484–9.
34. Bauer J, Köhler N, Maringer Y, et al. The oncogenic fusion protein DNAJB1-PRKACA can be specifically targeted by peptide-based immunotherapy in fibrolamellar hepatocellular carcinoma. Nat Commun. 2022;13:6401.
35. Simon EP, Freije CA, Farber BA, et al. Transcriptomic characterization of fibrolamellar hepatocellular carcinoma. Proc Natl Acad Sci USA. 2015;112(44):E5916–E25.
36. Darcy DG, Chiaroni-Clarke R, Murphy JM, et al. The genomic landscape of fibrolamellar hepatocellular carcinoma: whole genome sequencing of ten patients. Oncotarget. 2015;6(2):755–70.
37. Honeyman JN, Simon EP, Robine N, et al. Detection of a recurrent DNAJB1-PRKACA chimeric transcript in fibrolamellar hepatocellular carcinoma. Science. 2014;343(6174):1010–4.
38. Hamrick-Turner JE, Shipkey FH, Cranston PE. Fibrolamellar hepatocellular carcinoma: MR appearance mimicking focal nodular hyperplasia. J Comput Assist Tomogr. 1994;18:301–4.
39. Rudolphi-Solero T, Triviño-Ibáñez EM, Medina-Benítez A, et al. Differential diagnosis of hepatic mass with central scar: focal nodular hyperplasia mimicking Fibrolamellar hepatocellular carcinoma. Diagnostics. 2022;12:44.
40. van Aalten SM, de Man RA, IJzermans JN, et al. Systematic review of haemorrhage and rupture of hepatocellular adenomas. Br J Surg. 2012;99:911–6.
41. Cho SW, Marsh JW, Steel J, et al. Surgical management of hepatocellular adenoma: take it or leave it? Ann Surg Oncol. 2008;15:2795–803.
42. Kassahun WT. Contemporary management of fibrolamellar hepatocellular carcinoma: diagnosis, treatment, outcome, prognostic factors, and recent developments. World J Surg Oncol. 2016;14:151.
43. Mazzaferro V, Citterio D, Bhoori S, et al. Liver transplantation in hepatocellular carcinoma after tumour downstaging (XXL): a randomised, controlled, phase 2b/3 trial. Lancet Oncol. 2020;21(7):947–56.
44. Stipa F, Yoon SS, Liau KH, et al. Outcome of patients with fibrolamellar hepatocellular carcinoma. Cancer. 2006;106:1331–8.
45. Kakar S, Burgart LJ, Batts KP, et al. Clinicopathologic features and survival in fibrolamellar carcinoma: comparison with conventional hepatocellular carcinoma with and without cirrhosis. Mod Pathol. 2005;18:1417–23.
46. Maniaci B, Davidson BR, Rolles K, et al. Fibrolamellar hepatocellular carcinoma—prolonged survival with multimodality therapy. EJSO. 2009;35:617–21.
47. Ang CS, Kelley RK, Choti MA, et al. Clinicopathologic characteristics and survival outcomes of patients with fibrolamellar carcinoma: data from the fibrolamellar carcinoma consortium. GCR. 2013;6(1):3–9.

48. Lafaro KJ, Eng OS, Raoof M, et al. A prognostic nomogram for patients with resected fibrolamellar hepatocellular carcinoma. Hepatobiliary Surg Nutr. 2019;8(4):338–44.
49. Mayo SC, Mavros MN, Nathan H, et al. Treatment and prognosis of patients with fibrolamellar hepatocellular carcinoma: a national perspective. J Am Coll Surg. 2014;218(2):196–205.
50. Riggle KM, Turnham R, Scott JD, et al. Fibrolamellar hepatocellular carcinoma: mechanistic distinction from adult hepatocellular carcinoma. Pediatr Blood Cancer. 2016;63:1163–7.
51. Chakrabarti S, Tella SH, Kommalapati A, et al. Clinicopathological features and outcomes of fibrolamellar hepatocellular carcinoma. J Gastrointest Oncol. 2019;10:554–61.
52. Patt YZ, Hassan MM, Lozano RD, et al. Phase II trial of systemic continuous fluorouracil and subcutaneous recombinant interferon Alfa-2b for treatment of hepatocellular carcinoma. J Clin Oncol. 2003;21:421–7.
53. Epstein BE, Pajak TF, Haulk TL, et al. Metastatic nonresectable fibrolamellar hepatoma: prognostic features and natural history. Am J Clin Oncol. 1999;22:22–8.
54. Lee M, Chang Y, Oh S, et al. Assessment of the surveillance interval at 1 year after curative treatment in hepatocellular carcinoma: risk stratification. Gut Liver. 2018;12(5):571–82.

Mesenchymal Hamartoma of the Liver

16

C. Candal-Cunha

16.1 Introduction

Mesenchymal hamartoma of the liver (MHL) is a benign liver tumor most commonly seen in children up to the age of two years (80% of cases) [1], but prenatal and adult cases have also been described [2–4]. It is the second most common benign liver tumor in children, after infantile hemangioma [5], and makes up 5–8% of all pediatric liver tumors [1, 6, 7].

It was first described by Maresch in 1903, but the term MHL was provided by Edmondson in 1956, describing a cystic mesenchymal lesion chiefly composed of connective tissue and containing much serous fluid [8].

Pediatric MHL shows a male predominance, while females are more affected in the adult population [4]. Location of the tumor in the liver also appears to be different between pediatric and adult patients: in children, about 75% of MHL is primarily located in the right lobe (the rest is found in the left lobe or involves both lobes) [9], while in adults, *Li J et al.* presented 38% of cases involving the left lobe, 49% the right lobe, and 13% extending into both lobes (all MHLs involving both lobes occurred in females). There are fewer than 50 cases of MHL in adults reported in the literature [10].

C. Candal-Cunha (✉)
Hospital Pediátrico de Coimbra, ULS Coimbra, Coimbra, Portugal
e-mail: c.cunha@ulscoimbra.min-saude.pt

16.2 Clinical Presentation

Typically, MHL presents with abdominal distension and/or an upper abdominal mass but may vary from incidental detection on physical examination or imaging of an asymptomatic mass to symptoms like abdominal pain, anorexia, and vomiting. Sometimes, the mass expands rapidly, most likely because of the accumulation of liquid within cystic spaces. (Fig. 16.1)

Other presentations of MHL differ based on the age of the patient and tumor size.

Prenatal detection of MHL usually occurs in the second and third trimesters, by ultrasound, and can be the cause of fetal demise and preterm labor due to the mass effect of the tumor, causing compression of the heart, kidneys, and umbilical veins [2]. MHL is pedunculated in 20% of cases, which can cause difficulty in determining the hepatic origin of the mass [11].

Other signs and symptoms like polyhydramnios, pericardial effusion, generalized subcutaneous edema and hydrocele (fetal hydrops), congestive heart failure (due to endocardial fibroelastosis or the enlarged hepatic mass itself), splenomegaly and secondary portal hypertension, cardiomegaly, and placentomegaly have

T. Hackert, A. Gulla (eds.), *Rare Liver and Biliary Tract Diseases*,
https://doi.org/10.1007/978-3-032-15076-9_16

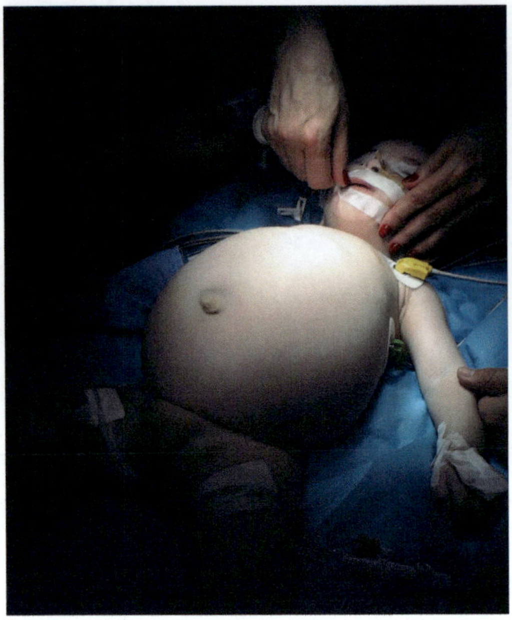

Fig. 16.1 Abdominal distension of a 7-month-old girl referred for MHL resection

also been described. Maternal α-fetoprotein (AFP) and/or β human chorionic gonadotropin (βHCG) may be elevated [12–15].

In the neonate and infant, the rapidly enlarging tumor can cause respiratory distress, cardiac failure, anorexia, vomiting, poor weight gain, vascular steal, thrombocytopenia, pulmonary hypertension, obstructive jaundice, perinatal tumor rupture with ascites, and fatal bleeding into the tumor after birth trauma. Unfortunately, the prognosis for pre- and neonatally diagnosed infants is poor, with a reported mortality of 30–35% [16, 17].

Less than 5% of MHL present after the age of five. Not so frequent presentations in older children include obstructive jaundice, disseminated intravascular coagulopathy, constipation, and abscess formation [9].

MHL is extremely rare in adults, and symptoms are usually nonspecific, but diffuse abdominal pain and distension are the most common.

16.3 Associated Anomalies

Typically, MHL is not associated with other anomalies, but associations with infantile hemangioma [18, 19], polycystic kidney disease, congenital hepatic fibrosis, biliary hamartomas [20], congenital heart disease, omphalocele, myelomeningocele, and biliary atresia have been reported. A rare case of a giant MHL in a neonate, associated with malrotation of the bowel, has been presented in the literature [17].

There are also some reports of an MHL association with Beckwith–Wiedemann syndrome [21], placental mesenchymal dysplasia [22, 23], and DICER1 syndrome [24, 25].

16.4 Investigation

16.4.1 Laboratory

Blood count and liver function tests are usually normal or mildly deranged. Serum αfetoprotein (AFP) levels are also usually normal but can be slightly elevated, and they decrease to normal after complete tumor resection [26]. It should be mentioned that the concentration of this protein in normal infants is age-specific: it is highly elevated in preterm neonates and neonates and usually declines and reaches normal concentrations at 8–12 months of age [27, 28]. AFP levels are routinely used as an important biomarker for hepatoblastoma; however, AFP is a tumor-associated, and not a tumor-specific protein, and a mild elevation can be seen in other malignant (hepatocellular carcinoma) and nonmalignant (cirrhosis, viral, and chronic active hepatitis) conditions. There are reports of some patients having received inappropriate chemotherapy for presumed hepatoblastoma based on AFP levels before the tumor was biopsied [29], or when the sample was insufficient [30], thus not correlating with imaging, histopathology, and patients' age.

16.4.2 Imaging

MHL has both cystic and solid components. The vast majority of these tumors contain cysts of varying sizes, ranging from a few mm to more than 15 cm. Rarely, the tumor may contain only the solid part, which makes it difficult to differentiate from other solid tumors (such as hepatoblastoma in children) and may be pedunculated. Typically, the tumor appears as a well-marginated, solitary mass with cystic components and internal septations. The cystic components may be either homogeneous or heterogeneous, depending on the proteinaceous content. The appearance of the lesion depends on whether it is predominantly stromal (mesenchymal) or cystic and can range from multiple small cysts in a solid mass resembling Swiss cheese to a multilocular cystic lesion with solid septa. The margin between the liver and the lesion is distinct, but a true capsule is generally not present. Beyond the outer rim of compressed liver, the hepatic architecture appears normal [31, 32].

Abdominal plain radiography may show hepatomegaly or a paucity of bowel gas in the right upper quadrant, suggesting a hepatic mass. Calcifications within the tumor are not common [33] (Fig. 16.2).

Ultrasonography (US) is usually the initial evaluation technique for suspected liver masses. It is readily accessible and can quickly delineate the cystic or solid nature of the tumor and the mass size. The presence of thin mobile septa and/or round hyperechoic parietal nodules within the cysts is highly suggestive of MHL [34] (Fig. 16.3a, b).

Color Doppler imaging shows relatively less blood flow, which is limited to solid portions and septations [35].

Computed tomography (CT) confirms sonographic findings and delineates the extent of the lesion and its relationship to other intra-abdominal organs.

At unenhanced CT, MHL has a heterogeneous appearance. The stromal elements appear hypoattenuating, whereas the cystic component is of water attenuation. In contrast-enhanced CT, the solid component, septa, and the peripheral rim may enhance, while the cystic portion does not. Hemorrhage and calcifications are rare (Fig. 16.4a, b).

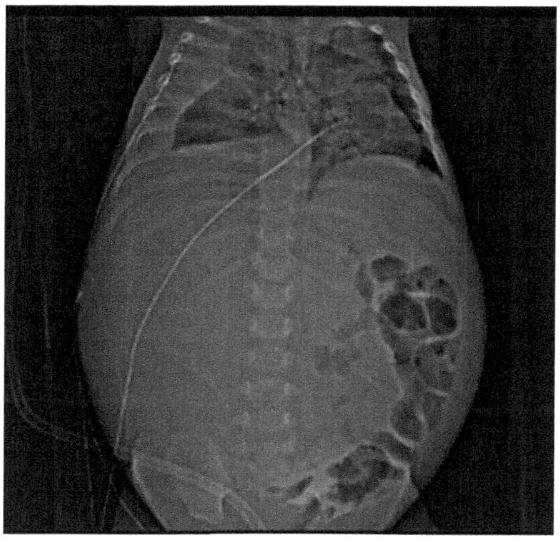

Fig. 16.2 Upright plain abdominal radiograph of a 7-month-old girl with MHL shows a large, noncalcified, soft-tissue–density abdominal mass extending through the right quadrants, epigastrium, and umbilical region; crossing the midline; displacing the bowel loops to the periphery of the abdominal cavity; and elevating the right diaphragm. There is also a right pleural effusion

CT appearance may be deceiving because cysts can mimic tumor necrosis seen in malignant hepatic neoplasms, and US and magnetic resonance imaging (MRI) are helpful to distinguish simple anechoic cysts from liquefied tissue [36, 37].

Magnetic resonance imaging (MRI) of MHL is also variable depending on the cystic versus stromal composition of the mass, as well as on the protein content of the fluid, but can confidently establish hepatic origin in cases of large, pedunculated, predominantly cystic lesions and delineate solid and cystic components, septations, and relations to surrounding structures (especially the intrahepatic vasculature and the biliary system) [36]. MRI has a low signal intensity on T1-weighted sequences and a variable signal intensity on T2-weighted sequences [38]. Mild enhancement with intravenous gadolinium contrast material is seen in the solid and stromal components [20, 35] (Fig. 16.5a, b).

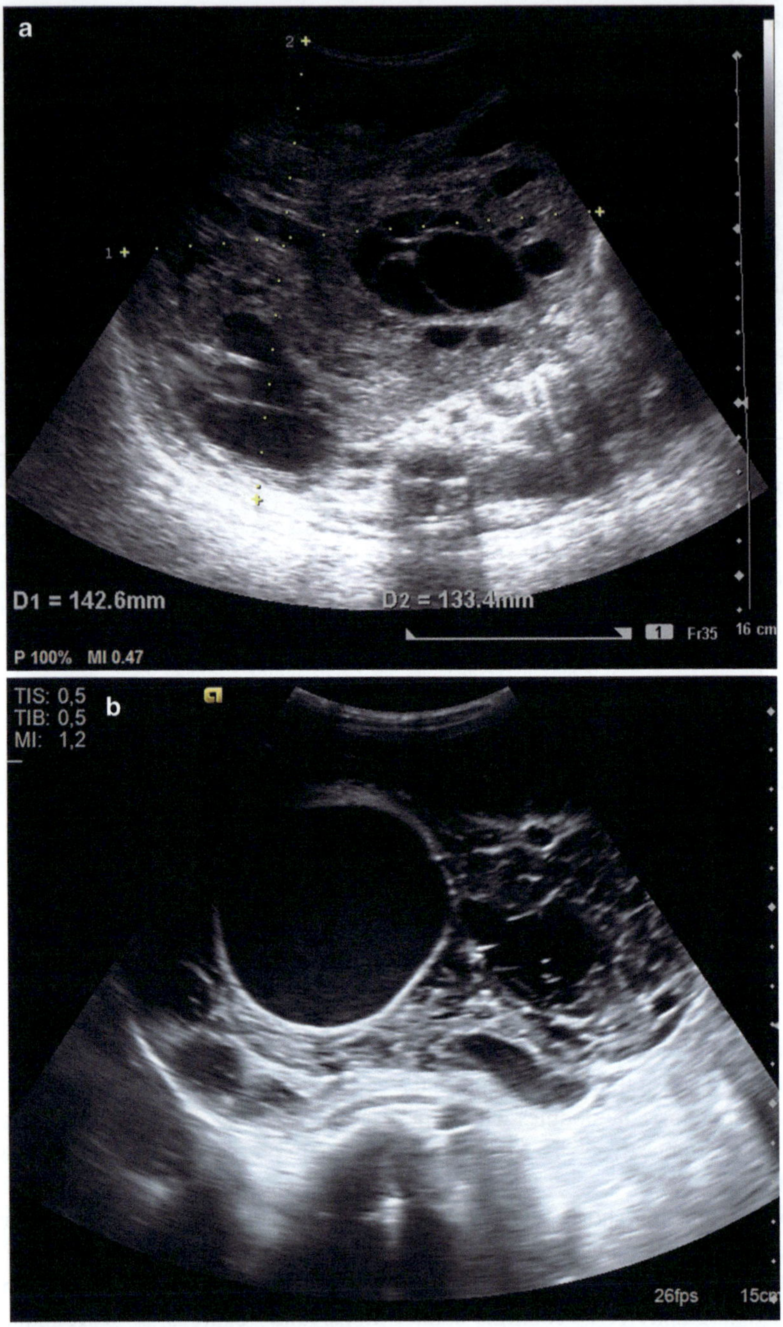

Fig. 16.3 A 7-month-old girl's abdominal ultrasound demonstrates an expansive lesion, predominantly solid but with multiple cystic areas of variable size and multiple septa, measuring about 14×13 cm, on the right lobe of the liver. (**b**) A 22-month-old boy's abdominal ultrasound shows a large, multiloculated lesion, apparently with liquid content, occupying the right lobe of the liver and measuring about 13 cm (major axis)

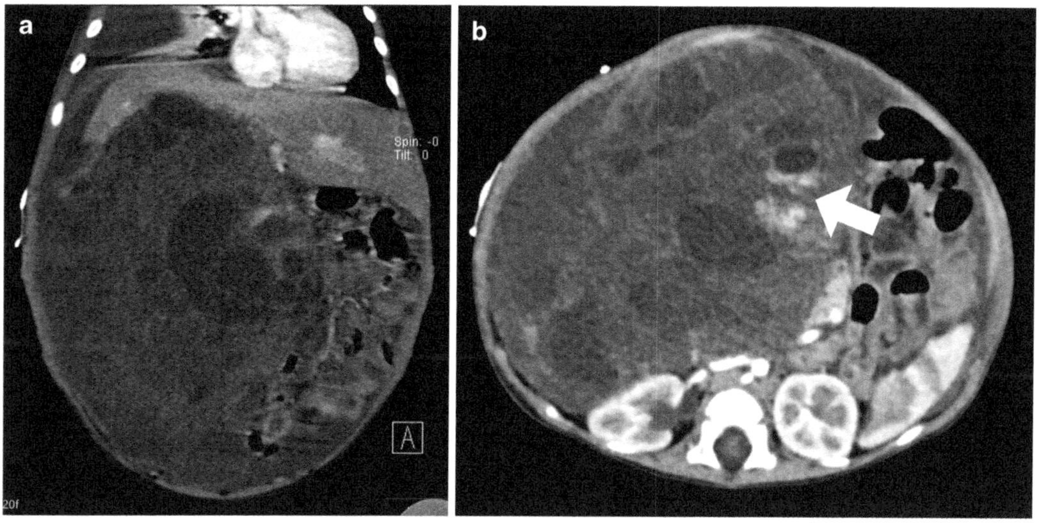

Fig. 16.4 (**a**) Contrast-enhanced CT scan. Coronal axis. (**b**) Contrast-enhanced CT scan; sagittal axis. A 7-month-old girl with MHL. There is a voluminous, multiloculated, heterogeneous cystic expansile lesion occupying almost all the right lobe of the liver, measuring 17×14×11 cm, pushing multiple abdominal organs, and showing irregular limits anteriorly because of rupture. There is also peripheral arterial enhancement from foci of intralesional bleeding (white arrow)

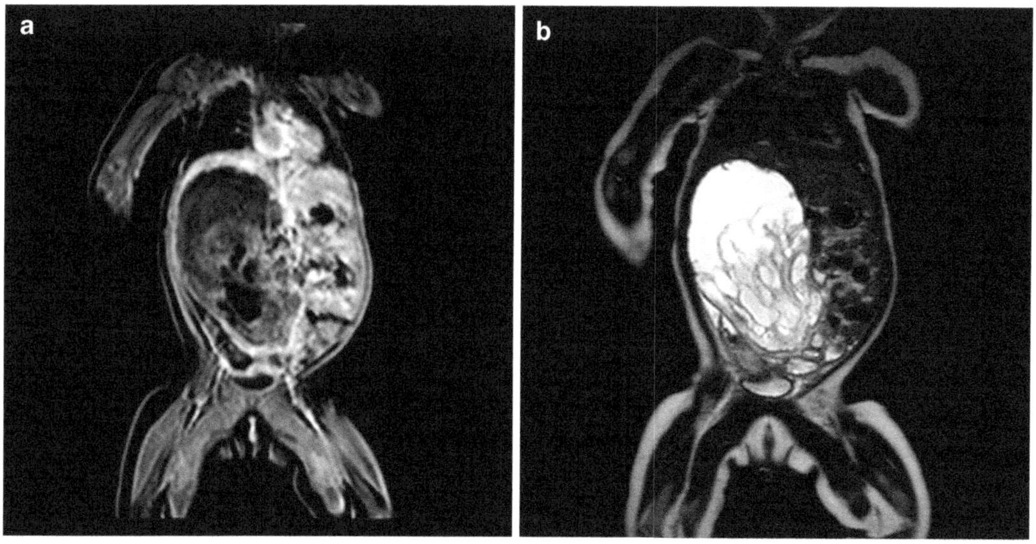

Fig. 16.5 MRI of a 5-month-old girl with MHL. (**a**) T1-weighted and (**b**) T2-weighted coronal images

Scintigraphy with technetium-labeled sulfur colloid is nonspecific and confirms the presence and position of either a solitary or multiple photopenic masses, as the MHL lacks Kupffer cells [39].

16.5 Pathology

Although MHL can be suspected by imaging, the results are nonspecific, and confirmation is obtained by histological examination. When in doubt, a tumor biopsy should be performed percutaneously or openly. Fine-needle aspiration cytology (FNAC) has been used (even in children), and findings include the presence of clusters of bile duct epithelium and hepatocytes admixed with bland mesenchymal spindle cells in a myxoid background. The presence of many long, curved, or twisted thick cords of duct epithelial cells was found to be an important clue to the cytological diagnosis [40]. However, diagnosing MHL solely on cytology is difficult and still of limited value.

MHL may be pedunculated, and its size can range from a few centimeters to 30 cm. The cut surface shows solid and cystic components. Cysts do not communicate directly with the biliary tree and are filled with clear to yellow fluid with occasional gelatinous material. Necrosis and calcifications are rare, but a thin rim of normal liver parenchyma is often seen at the periphery.

The tumor is well-circumscribed but does not have a true capsule (Fig. 16.6a–c).

Histological studies show a variable mixture of tissues from which the liver is normally formed. The predominant component is mesenchymal and consists of loose, edematous connective tissue with cyst-like collections of fluid, dilated lymphatics and blood vessels, and

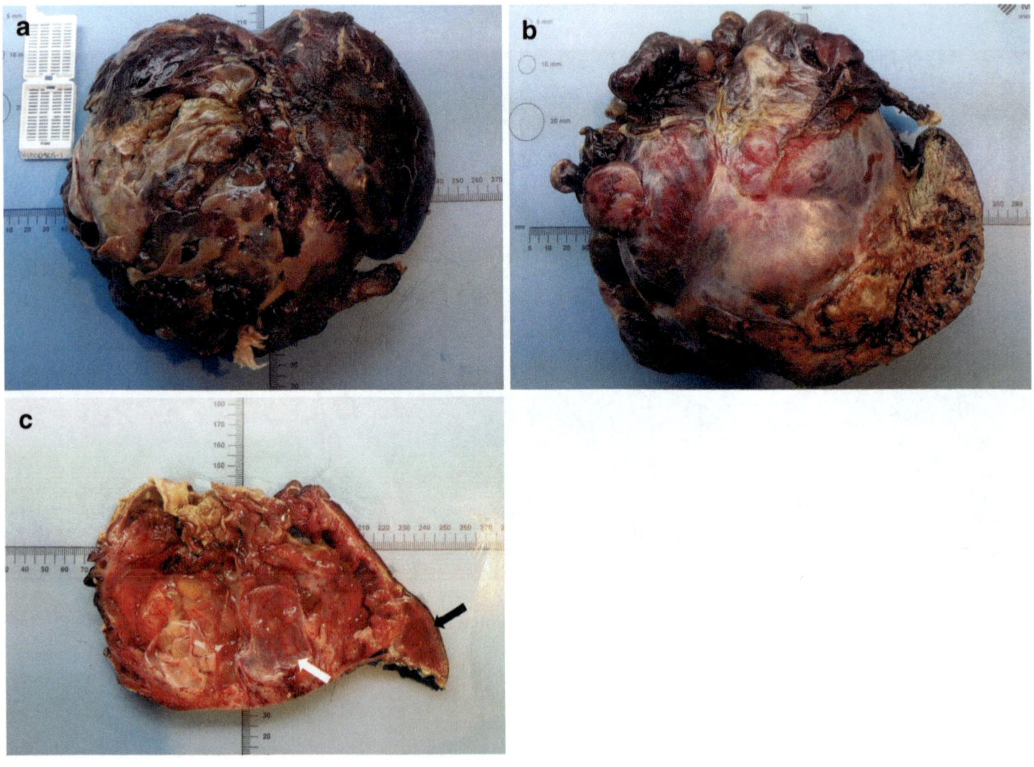

Fig. 16.6 A 7-month-old girl with MHL. Macroscopic aspect of the tumor. Weighing 1215g and measuring 15×15×6.5 cm. (**a**) Anterior view: the surface is brown and slightly bosselated with areas of rupture, hemorrhage, and necrosis. (**b**) Posterior view. (**c**) Cross section of the tumor showing multiple cysts filled with mucoid material (white arrow) and a rim of normal liver tissue (black arrow)

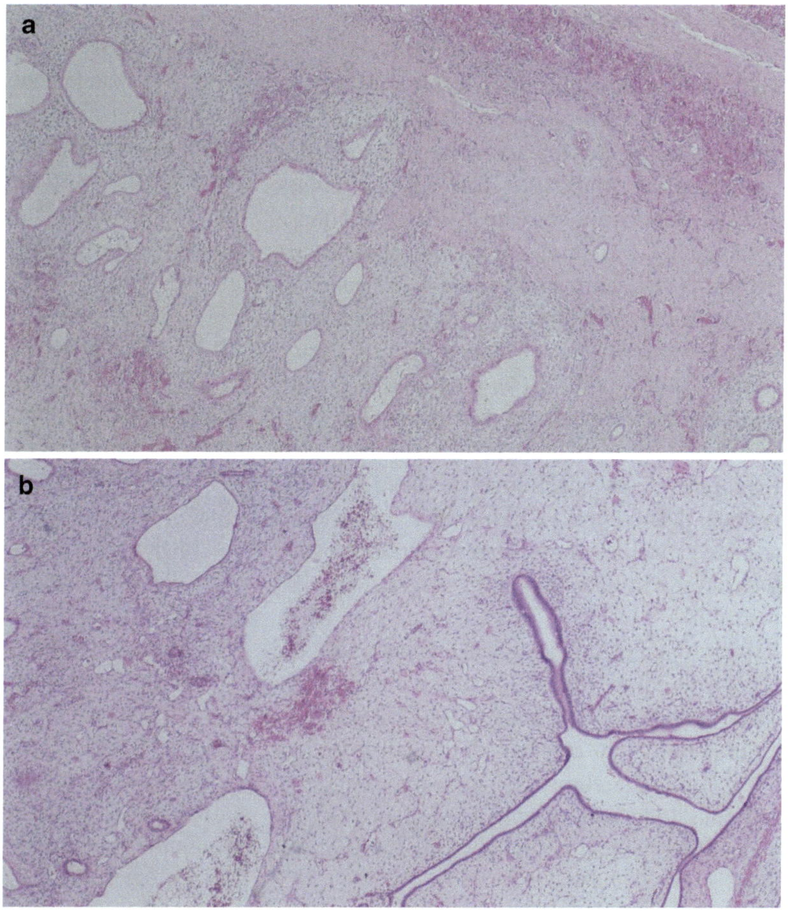

Fig. 16.7 (**a**) Pathologic findings of MHL. (**a**) Hematoxylin and eosin, 40x—small ductal structures surrounded by loose mesenchyme. (**b**) Hematoxylin and eosin, 40×—complex mixture of loose connective tissue, vessels, and bile ducts

multiple, branched, and tortuous bile ducts. Foci of extramedullary hematopoiesis are observed in 85% of cases [41] (Fig. 16.7a, b).

The cystic predominance of MHL may mimic a lymphangioma, both macroscopically and microscopically.

In adults, the stromal component is variable. In most areas, the stroma has a densely hyalinized and paucicellular appearance. Also in adults, small-caliber vessels are present within the stromal areas, and hemosiderin-laden macrophages are present focally within areas of granulation tissue associated with intralesional hemorrhage. Along most of the interface between tumor tissue and normal hepatic parenchyma, there is a proliferation of small bile ducts and thin-walled vessels. Satellite nodules may be observed in some cases, consisting of dilated and irregularly branching bile ducts in fibrous stroma [42].

16.6 Immunohistochemistry

MHL has spindle cells positive for vimentin and smooth muscle actin and negative for CD31, CD34, and S100 proteins, while the ducts stain positive for cytokeratin 7 and negative for cytokeratin 20.

There are some other markers being evaluated (HepPar1, Glypican3, CD10, CD56, CD68, arginase-1, and KI-67) with possible diagnostic and therapeutic implications, but further investigations need to be conducted [43].

16.7 Pathogenesis

MHL pathogenesis is still unknown. There are several hypotheses proposed: (1) failure of the ductal plate to develop normally in utero (this could explain similarities between the biliary ductular abnormalities seen in MHL and those observed in Caroli disease and congenital hepatic fibrosis); (2) vascular insult or reactive changes to a regional ischemic process; (3) toxic insult leading to activation of Ito cells (sinusoidal fat-storing cells) [44, 45]; (4) neoplasia [46]. Immunohistochemical and flow cytometric studies have suggested that MHL is a true neoplasm. Recurrent genetic alterations identified in MHL include androgenetic-biparental mosaicism (ABM) as well as chromosomal rearrangements, which result in activation of the chromosome 19q microRNA cluster (C19MC). Sporadic MHL lesions are frequently associated with a translocation involving the MALAT1 gene at chromosome 11q13 and the C19MC gene at 19q13.4 [47].

In addition, an atypical MHL with a tandem triplication of a chromosomal segment at chromosome 1q44 was recently described [48, 49] and a child with an inversion of chromosome 19 [50].

MHL shares a similar genetic profile with undifferentiated embryonal sarcoma (UES), a rare pediatric malignancy composed of a sarcomatous mesenchymal component, hypercellular stroma, nuclear pleomorphism, and high mitotic activity, interspersed with benign branching ductal structures. There are several reports of cases of UES developing both synchronously and metachronously with MHL, having similar genetic rearrangements in the region of 19q13.4 and histological resemblances [51–53].

There are also case reports of hepatic angiosarcoma (the most common primary sarcoma of the liver) and cholangiocarcinoma arising from an adult MHL [54–56].

16.8 Differential Diagnosis

In adults, the differential diagnosis for predominantly cystic tumors includes simple hepatic cysts, hydatid cysts, subcapsular pseudocysts, biliary cystadenocarcinoma, and cystic metastasis. In the case of a solid lesion, focal nodular hyperplasia, hepatic adenoma, cavernous hemangioma, angiomyolipoma, solitary hamartoma, and hepatocellular carcinoma are among the pathologies to consider [32].

In children, causes of intraperitoneal cystic masses should be considered, such as hydatid cysts, mesenteric cysts, gastrointestinal duplication cysts, cystic teratomas of the mesentery, and, most importantly, UES. If the lesion has a more solid appearance on imaging, then hepatoblastoma, infantile hemangioendothelioma, hepatocellular carcinoma (fibrolamellar type), and metastatic lesions should be included in the differential diagnosis [20]. There are rare, isolated cases of other entities in the literature, such as biliary mucinous cystadenomas [57] (Table 16.1).

Table 16.1 Comparison of clinical, cytological, and imagiological features of the main differential diagnoses of MHL in children [4, 40, 58–62] (hepatoblastoma (HB), undifferentiated embryonal sarcoma (UES))

	HB	UES	MHL
Age of presentation	90% within 5 years	50% in 6–10 years	80% in 2 years
Male:female ratio	1.5–2:1	-	2–3:1
Clinical presentation	Abdominal distension	Abdominal distension and pain	Abdominal distension
Serum AFP levels	90% cases elevated	Not elevated	Usually normal but can be elevated
Cytological findings	Cellular smears. Mostly epithelial cells in cohesive crowded clusters, cords, ribbons, and rosettes. Mesenchymal components and/or heterologous elements can be present. Extramedullary hematopoiesis can be seen	Hypercellular smears. Large, pleomorphic, atypical spindle cells with multinucleated tumor giant cells. PAS-positive, diastase-resistant intra- and extra-cytoplasmic globules can be seen	Scant-to-mild cellular smears. Loose myxoid mesenchymal stroma with scattered bland spindle cells, bile duct epithelium, and benign hepatocytes. Extramedullary hematopoiesis can be seen
US	Well-circumscribed solid mass that is hyperechoic relative to the adjacent liver	Shows solid-dominant mixed echogenic areas with variable anechoic cystic areas	Anechoic, multilobular mass with thin septations. Calcifications and hemorrhage are rare
CT	Well-defined heterogeneous mass, which is usually hypoattenuating compared to the adjacent liver. Frequently, there are areas of necrosis, hemorrhage, and calcifications	Well-demarcated low-attenuation mass with hyperdense septations of variable shape and thickness. A dense peripheral rim corresponds to the fibrous pseudocapsule of the tumor. Discrepancy of internal architecture on US and CT is one of the important characteristics of UES	Heterogeneous appearance. Ranges from a multilocular cystic mass with solid septa to multiple small cysts in a solid mass. Contrast administration enhances the solid component without a change in the cystic portion
MRI	Hyperintense on T2-weighted images, hypointense on T1-weighted imaging, and enhances in a heterogenous fashion. Calcification within the mass is present in 50% of cases, and hemorrhage and necrosis may also occur in variable amounts, leading to the heterogenous signal intensity	Multiloculated mass with predominantly high signal intensity on T2-weighted sequences and predominantly low signal intensity on T1-weighted sequences With gadolinium administration, there can be mild delayed heterogeneous enhancement, with a lack of enhancement of the majority of the tumor, consistent with extensive central necrosis or cystic change	The cystic component will show low signal intensity on T1-weighted images and high intensity on T2-weighted images. Solid areas are hypointense on both T1 and T2. Enhancement is mild and limited to the septa and stromal components
Angiography	Only to demonstrate normal and variant vascular anatomy	Usually hypovascular with tumoral vessels, although hypervascular and avascular patterns occur	Cystic masses appear completely avascular due to displacement of major vessels. Predominantly solid lesions are hypovascular, with small tumor vessels correlating to septa vascularization surrounding scattered cystic regions

16.9 Treatment

The recommended therapy is complete excision of the lesion, with a small margin of normal liver, because of the potential evolution or coexistent malignancy [63].

Nonetheless, multiple strategies have been used, including enucleation [64] and marsupialization into the peritoneal cavity for larger lesions, but there is a risk of recurrence of the tumor.

Intraoperative aspiration of the cysts can reduce the size of the mass and make the resection easier [65].

Fetal intervention in the form of ultrasound-guided percutaneous cyst aspiration has been reported with good outcomes [15, 66].

Surgery may be pursued by conventional "open" surgery, but some lesions are amenable to laparoscopic [67, 68] or robotic [69] resection (anatomical or non-anatomical) even in children. The method should be determined by the location of the tumor and the technical skills of surgeons in liver resection. For very large MHL, a large-scale liver resection may cause liver failure, and as for unresectable liver tumors, liver transplantation could be a good alternative [10, 38, 42, 70].

Hepatic artery embolization can be used in very sick patients for temporary clinical improvement before definitive surgery a few days later (Fig. 16.8a, b).

Complications during or after tumor excision are rare.

There are reports regarding the use of chemotherapy [30, 71, 72] and radiotherapy [73] for MHL regression, but they cannot be considered an option for definitive treatment.

Prognosis after complete resection is excellent, but long-term clinical and imagiological review is recommended [74, 75].

Spontaneous regression has been reported, questioning the need for surgical treatment, but none of the lesions disappeared completely, and the follow-up was less than 5 years.

Nonoperative management should be reserved for selected patients (e.g., tumors with a prominent vascular component) [76, 77].

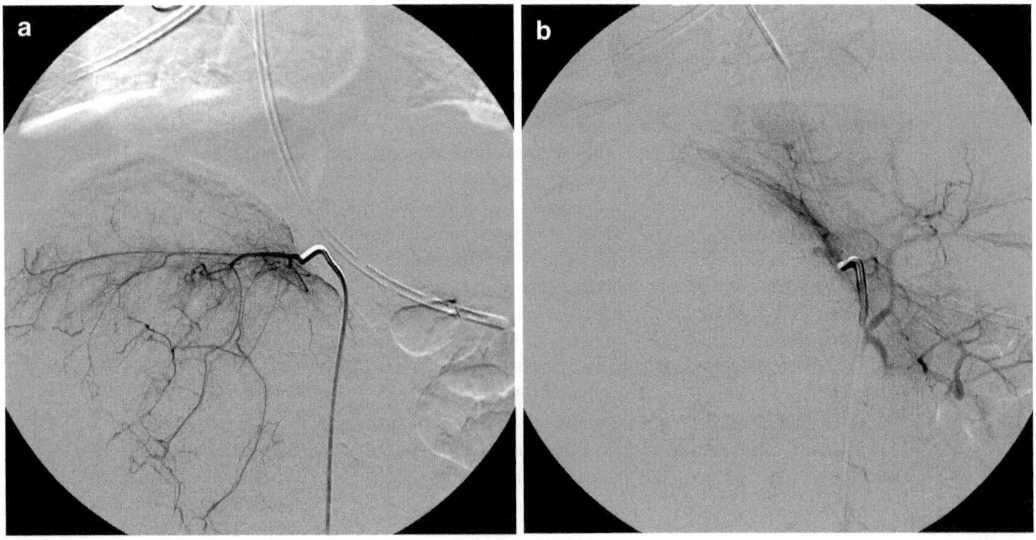

Fig. 16.8 (**a**) Angiography. (**a**) Superselective embolization of the tumor's arterial nutritive branch using 100 μ polyvinyl alcohol (PVA) particles. (**b**) Angiography after embolization

16.10 Recommendations

MHL, both in children and adults, is a rare and possibly premalignant lesion. Usually presenting as a solid and/or cystic tumor, symptoms, laboratory results, and imaging are nonspecific, variable, and inconclusive. FNAC is still of limited value, so biopsy followed by surgical excision of the mass with a margin of normal liver should be recommended. Liver transplantation can be an option for very large, unresectable tumors. Long-term follow-up is necessary.

References

1. Siddiqui MA, McKenna BJ. Hepatic mesenchymal hamartoma: a short review. Arch Pathol Lab Med. 2006;130(10):1567–9. https://doi.org/10.5858/2006-130-1567-HMHASR.
2. Laberge JM, Patenaude Y, Desilets V, Cartier L, Khalife S, Jutras L, Chen MF. Large hepatic mesenchymal hamartoma leading to mid-trimester fetal demise. Fetal Diagn Ther. 2005;20(2):141–5. https://doi.org/10.1159/000082439.
3. Mulrooney DA, Carpenter B, Georgieff M, Angel C, Hunter D, Foker J, Steiner M. Hepatic mesenchymal hamartoma in a neonate: a case report and review of the literature. J Pediatr Hematol Oncol. 2001;23(5):316–7. https://doi.org/10.1097/00043426-200106000-00017.
4. Klaassen Z, Paragi PR, Chamberlain RS. Adult Mesenchymal Hamartoma of the liver: case report and literature review. Case Rep Gastroenterol. 2010;4(1):84–92. https://doi.org/10.1159/000260183. PMID: 21103233; PMCID: PMC2988903
5. Lucas B, Ravishankar S, Pateva I. Pediatric primary hepatic tumors: diagnostic considerations. Diagnostics (Basel). 2021;11(2):333. https://doi.org/10.3390/diagnostics11020333. PMID: 33670452; PMCID: PMC7922091
6. Lack EE. Mesenchymal hamartoma of the liver. A clinical and pathologic study of nine cases. Am J Pediatr Hematol Oncol. 1986;8(2):91–8. PMID: 3740369
7. Maqbool H, Mushtaq S, Hassan U, Ahmad AH, Sarwar S, Sheikh UN. Case series of Mesenchymal Hamartoma: a rare childhood hepatic neoplasm. J Gastrointest Cancer. 2020;51(3):1030–3. https://doi.org/10.1007/s12029-020-00374-3. PMID: 32124239
8. Edmondson HA. Differential diagnosis of tumors and tumor-like lesions of liver in infancy and childhood. AMA J Dis Child. 1956;91:168–86. https://doi.org/10.1001/archpedi.1956.02060020170015. PMID: 13282629
9. Stringer MD, Alizai NK. Mesenchymal hamartoma of the liver: a systematic review. J Pediatr Surg. 2005;40(11):1681–90. https://doi.org/10.1016/j.jpedsurg.2005.07.052. PMID: 16291152
10. Li J, Cai JZ, Guo QJ, Li JJ, Sun XY, Hu ZD, Cooper DK, Shen ZY. Liver transplantation for a giant mesenchymal hamartoma of the liver in an adult: Case report and review of the literature. World J Gastroenterol. 2015;21(20):6409–16. https://doi.org/10.3748/wjg.v21.i20.6409. PMID: 26034379; PMCID: PMC4445121
11. Birkemeier KL. Imaging of solid congenital abdominal masses: a review of the literature and practical approach to image interpretation. Pediatr Radiol. 2020;50(13):1907–20. https://doi.org/10.1007/s00247-020-04678-1. Epub 2020 Nov 30. PMID: 33252758
12. Bessho T, Kubota K, Komori S, Ohtsuka Y, Uneo Y, Uematsu K, Koyama K. Prenatally detected hepatic hamartoma: another cause of non-immune hydrops. Prenat Diagn. 1996;16(4):337–41. https://doi.org/10.1002/(SICI)1097-0223(199604)16:4<337::AID-PD848>3.0.CO;2-U. PMID: 8734808
13. Tovbin J, Segal M, Tavori I, Lotan G, Maymon R. Hepatic mesenchymal hamartoma: a pediatric tumor that may be diagnosed prenatally. Ultrasound Obstet Gynecol. 1997;10(1):63–5. https://doi.org/10.1046/j.1469-0705.1997.10010063.x. PMID: 9263426
14. Dickinson JE, Knowles S, Phillips JM. Prenatal diagnosis of hepatic mesenchymal hamartoma. Prenat Diagn. 1999;19(1):81–4. PMID: 10073915
15. Kamata S, Nose K, Sawai T, Hasegawa T, Kuroda S, Sasaki T, Okada A, Tawara M. Fetal mesenchymal hamartoma of the liver: report of a case. J Pediatr Surg. 2003;38(4):639–41. https://doi.org/10.1053/jpsu.2003.50142. PMID: 12677586
16. Cignini P, Coco C, Giorlandino M, Bagolan P, Morini F, Giorlandino C. Fetal hepatic mesenchymal hamartoma: a case report. J Prenat Med. 2007;1(3):45–6. PMID: 22470828; PMCID: PMC3309338
17. Ramareddy RS, Alladi A. Neonatal mesenchymal hamartoma of liver: an unusual presentation. J Clin Neonatol. 2012;1(4):211–3. https://doi.org/10.4103/2249-4847.106001. PMID: 24027729; PMCID: PMC3762050
18. Behr GG, Fishman SJ, Caty MG, Kulungowski AM, Paltiel HJ, Alomari AI. Hepatic mesenchymal hamartoma and infantile hemangioma: a rare association. J Pediatr Surg. 2012;47(3):448–52. https://doi.org/10.1016/j.jpedsurg.2011.10.049. PMID: 22424336
19. Berte N, Filfilan A, Mainard L, Mansuy L, Lemelle JL. Co-existing infantile hepatic hemangioma and mesenchymal hamartoma in a neonate. J Surg Case Rep. 2018;2018(1):rjx260. https://doi.org/10.1093/jscr/rjx260. PMID: 29383241; PMCID: PMC5786215

20. Rosado E, Cabral P, Campo M, Tavares A. Mesenchymal hamartoma of the liver–a case report and literature review. J Radiol Case Rep. 2013;7(5):35–43. https://doi.org/10.3941/jrcr.v7i5.1334. PMID: 23705055; PMCID: PMC3661420
21. Abrahao-Machado LF, de Macedo FC, Dalence C, Stambo G, Abrahao-Machado EF, Abrahao-Machado EC, Bahrami A, Nascimento AG. Mesenchymal Hamartoma of the Liver in an Infant with Beckwith-Wiedemann Syndrome: a rare condition mimicking Hepatoblastoma. ACG Case Rep J. 2015;2(4):258–60. https://doi.org/10.14309/crj.2015.78. PMID: 26203458; PMCID: PMC4508960
22. Francis B, Hallam L, Kecskes Z, Ellwood D, Croaker D, Kent A. Placental mesenchymal dysplasia associated with hepatic mesenchymal hamartoma in the newborn. Pediatr Dev Pathol. 2007;10(1):50–4. https://doi.org/10.2350/06-03-0066.1. PMID: 17378624
23. Tortoledo M, Galindo A, Ibarrola C. Placental mesenchymal dysplasia associated with hepatic and pulmonary hamartoma. Fetal Pediatr Pathol. 2010;29(4):261–70. https://doi.org/10.3109/15513811003782474. PMID: 20594151
24. Apellaniz-Ruiz M, Segni M, Kettwig M, Glüer S, Pelletier D, Nguyen VH, Wagener R, López C, Muchantef K, Bouron-Dal Soglio D, Sabbaghian N, Wu MK, Zannella S, Fabian MR, Siebert R, Menke J, Priest JR, Foulkes WD. Mesenchymal Hamartoma of the Liver and DICER1 Syndrome. N Engl J Med. 2019;380(19):1834–42. https://doi.org/10.1056/NEJMoa1812169. PMID: 31067372
25. Vargas SO, Perez-Atayde AR. Mesenchymal Hamartoma of the Liver and DICER1 Syndrome. N Engl J Med. 2019;381(6):586–7. https://doi.org/10.1056/NEJMc1907523. PMID: 31390509
26. Le LT, Phan HT, Nguyen TS, Truong KD, Nguyen DT, Nguyen TB, Pham TTT. Infantile mesenchymal hamartoma of the liver with elevated alpha fetoprotein. BJR Case Rep. 2021;7(3):20200196. https://doi.org/10.1259/bjrcr.20200196. PMID: 34131505; PMCID: PMC8171140
27. Isaacs H Jr. Fetal and neonatal hepatic tumors. J Pediatr Surg. 2007;42(11):1797–803. https://doi.org/10.1016/j.jpedsurg.2007.07.047. PMID: 18022426
28. Wu JT, Book L, Sudar K. Serum alpha fetoprotein (AFP) levels in normal infants. Pediatr Res. 1981;15(1):50–2. https://doi.org/10.1203/00006450-198101000-00012. PMID: 6163129
29. Boman F, Bossard C, Fabre M, Diab N, Bonnevalle M, Boccon-Gibod L. Mesenchymal hamartomas of the liver may be associated with increased serum alpha foetoprotein concentrations and mimic hepatoblastomas. Eur J Pediatr Surg. 2004;14(1):63–6. https://doi.org/10.1055/s-2004-815784. PMID: 15024683
30. Unal E, Koksal Y, Akcoren Z, Tavl L, Gunel E, Kerimoglu U. Mesenchymal hamartoma of the liver mimicking hepatoblastoma. J Pediatr Hematol Oncol. 2008;30(6):458–60. https://doi.org/10.1097/MPH.0b013e318169171b. PMID: 18525464
31. Wu CH, Chiu NC, Yeh YC, Kuo Y, Yu SS, Weng CY, Liu CA, Chou YH, Chiou YY. Uncommon liver tumors: case report and literature review. Medicine (Baltimore). 2016;95(39):e4952. https://doi.org/10.1097/MD.0000000000004952. PMID: 27684838; PMCID: PMC5265931
32. Kim KA, Kim KW, Park SH, Jang SJ, Park MS, Kim PN, Lee MG, Ha HK. Unusual mesenchymal liver tumors in adults: radiologic-pathologic correlation. AJR Am J Roentgenol. 2006;187(5):W481–9. https://doi.org/10.2214/AJR.05.0659. PMID: 17056878
33. Wholey MH, Wojno KJ. Pediatric hepatic mesenchymal hamartoma demonstrated on plain film, ultrasound and MRI, and correlated with pathology. Pediatr Radiol. 1994;24(2):143–4. https://doi.org/10.1007/BF02020176. PMID: 8078720
34. Koumanidou C, Vakaki M, Papadaki M, Pitsoulakis G, Savvidou D, Kakavakis K. New sonographic appearance of hepatic mesenchymal hamartoma in childhood. J Clin Ultrasound. 1999;27(3):164–7. https://doi.org/10.1002/(sici)1097-0096(199903/04)27:3<164::aid-jcu12>3.0.co;2-j. PMID: 10064417
35. Bhargava P, Iyer RS, Moshiri M, Yeh MM, Upton MP, Foo WC, Mannelli L, Gupta RT. Radiologic-pathologic correlation of uncommon mesenchymal liver tumors. Curr Probl Diagn Radiol. 2013;42(5):183–90. https://doi.org/10.1067/j.cpradiol.2013.05.002. PMID: 24070712
36. Gray SC, Pienaar JA, Sofianos Z, Varghese J, Warnich I. Hepatic mesenchymal hamartoma: an uncommon but important paediatric diagnosis. SA J Radiol. 2020;24(1):1891. https://doi.org/10.4102/sajr.v24i1.1891. PMID: 32832122; PMCID: PMC7433248
37. Chiorean L, Cui XW, Tannapfel A, Franke D, Stenzel M, Kosiak W, Schreiber-Dietrich D, Jüngert J, Chang JM, Dietrich CF. Benign liver tumors in pediatric patients - Review with emphasis on imaging features. World J Gastroenterol. 2015;21(28):8541–61. https://doi.org/10.3748/wjg.v21.i28.8541. PMID: 26229397; PMCID: PMC4515836
38. Fernandez-Pineda I, Cabello-Laureano R. Differential diagnosis and management of liver tumors in infants. World J Hepatol. 2014;6(7):486–95. https://doi.org/10.4254/wjh.v6.i7.486. PMID: 25068000; PMCID: PMC4110540
39. Stanley P, Hall TR, Woolley MM, Diament MJ, Gilsanz V, Miller JH. Mesenchymal hamartomas of the liver in childhood: sonographic and CT findings. AJR Am J Roentgenol. 1986;147(5):1035–9. https://doi.org/10.2214/ajr.147.5.1035. PMID: 3532729
40. Thakur S, Yadav R, Agarwala S, Jana M, Jain D, Mathur SR, Iyer VK. Fine needle aspiration cytology of mesenchymal hamartoma of liver mimicking hepatoblastoma: A case report. Diagn Cytopathol. 2021;49(10):E400–4. https://doi.org/10.1002/dc.24827. Epub 2021 Jul 15. PMID: 34264026
41. Algashaamy K, Montgomery EA, Garcia-Buitrago M. Liver mesenchymal neoplasms: something old,

something new. Pathology. 2022;54(2):225–35. https://doi.org/10.1016/j.pathol.2021.09.022. Epub 2021 Dec 26. PMID: 34965900
42. Hernández JC, Alfonso C, González L, Samada M, Ramos L, Cepero-Valdez M, Antonio Abdo A, Gómez F, Castellanos R, López O, Ugarte JC, Jordán J. Solid mesenchymal hamartoma in an adult: a case report. J Clin Pathol. 2006;59(5):542–5. https://doi.org/10.1136/jcp.2004.024398. PMID: 16644886; PMCID: PMC1860273
43. Habibzadeh P, Ansari Asl M, Foroutan HR, Bahador A, Anbardar MH. Clinicopathological study of hepatic mesenchymal hamartoma and undifferentiated embryonal sarcoma of the liver: a single center study from Iran. Diagn Pathol. 2021;16(1):55. https://doi.org/10.1186/s13000-021-01117-z. PMID: 34162402; PMCID: PMC8223305
44. von Schweinitz D, Dammeier BG, Glüer S. Mesenchymal hamartoma of the liver–new insight into histogenesis. J Pediatr Surg. 1999;34(8):1269–71. https://doi.org/10.1016/s0022-3468(99)90166-5. PMID: 10466610
45. Shintaku M, Watanabe K. Mesenchymal hamartoma of the liver: a proliferative lesion of possible hepatic stellate cell (Ito cell) origin. Pathol Res Pract. 2010;206(7):532–6. https://doi.org/10.1016/j.prp.2010.02.009. PMID: 20399572
46. Otal TM, Hendricks JB, Pharis P, Donnelly WH. Mesenchymal hamartoma of the liver. DNA flow cytometric analysis of eight cases. Cancer. 1994;74(4):1237–42. https://doi.org/10.1002/1097-0142(19940815)74:4<1237::aid-cncr2820740410>3.0.co;2-5. PMID: 8055444
47. Keller RB, Demellawy DE, Quaglia A, Finegold M, Kapur RP. Methylation status of the chromosome arm 19q MicroRNA cluster in sporadic and androgenetic-Biparental mosaicism-associated hepatic mesenchymal hamartoma. Pediatr Dev Pathol. 2015;18(3):218–27. https://doi.org/10.2350/15-01-1600-OA.1. Epub 2015 Mar 9. PMID: 25751191
48. Martins-Filho SN, Putra J. Hepatic mesenchymal hamartoma and undifferentiated embryonal sarcoma of the liver: a pathologic review. Hepat Oncol. 2020;7(2):HEP19. https://doi.org/10.2217/hep-2020-0002. PMID: 32647564; PMCID: PMC7338921
49. El Demellawy D, Lee JY, McDonell L, Dyment DA, Knisely AS, McGowan-Jordan J, Ngan B, Finegold M, Kapur RP, Nasr A. Atypical hepatic Mesenchymal Hamartoma: histologic appearance, immunophenotype, and molecular findings. Pediatr Dev Pathol. 2019;22(4):365–9. https://doi.org/10.1177/1093526618806750. Epub 2018 Nov 29. PMID: 30497332
50. Shetty S, Pinto A, Roland B. Mesenchymal hamartoma of the liver with inversion of chromosome 19. Pediatr Dev Pathol. 2011;14(5):407–10. https://doi.org/10.2350/10-10-0920-CR.1. Epub 2011 Mar 22. PMID: 21426235
51. Lauwers GY, Grant LD, Donnelly WH, Meloni AM, Foss RM, Sanberg AA, Langham MR Jr. Hepatic undifferentiated (embryonal) sarcoma arising in a mesenchymal hamartoma. Am J Surg Pathol. 1997;21(10):1248–54. https://doi.org/10.1097/00000478-199710000-00018. PMID: 9331300
52. Begueret H, Trouette H, Vielh P, Laurent C, MacGrogan G, Delsol M, Belleannee G, Masson B, De Mascarel A. Hepatic undifferentiated embryonal sarcoma: malignant evolution of mesenchymal hamartoma? Study of one case with immunohistochemical and flow cytometric emphasis. J Hepatol. 2001;34(1):178–9. https://doi.org/10.1016/s0168-8278(00)00008-8. PMID: 11211901
53. Shehata BM, Gupta NA, Katzenstein HM, Steelman CK, Wulkan ML, Gow KW, Bridge JA, Kenney BD, Thompson K, de Chadarévian JP, Abramowsky CR. Undifferentiated embryonal sarcoma of the liver is associated with mesenchymal hamartoma and multiple chromosomal abnormalities: a review of eleven cases. Pediatr Dev Pathol. 2011;14(2):111–6. https://doi.org/10.2350/09-07-0681-OA.1. Epub 2010 Oct 6. PMID: 20925497
54. Li Q, Wang J, Sun Y, Cui Y, Hao X. Hepatic angiosarcoma arising in an adult mesenchymal hamartoma. Int Semin Surg Oncol. 2007;4:3. https://doi.org/10.1186/1477-7800-4-3. PMID: 17257403; PMCID: PMC1796548
55. Kulkarni MP, Agashe SR, Singh RV, Sulhyan KR. Hepatic angiosarcoma arising in an adult mesenchymal hamartoma. Indian J Pathol Microbiol. 2010;53(2):322–4. https://doi.org/10.4103/0377-4929.64311. PMID: 20551545
56. Gang S, Choi Y, Lee S, Hong SY, Suh S, Han ES, Hong SK, Yi NJ, Lee KW, Suh KS. Progression of a persisting mesenchymal hamartoma to intrahepatic cholangiocarcinoma 24 years after the initial diagnosis: a case report. Ann Hepatobiliary Pancreat Surg. 2022; https://doi.org/10.14701/ahbps.22-022. Epub ahead of print. PMID: 35995570
57. Bezabih YS, Tessema WA, Getu ME. Giant biliary mucinous cystadenoma mimicking mesenchymal hamartoma of the liver in a child: a case report. Int J Surg Case Rep. 2021;88:106523. https://doi.org/10.1016/j.ijscr.2021.106523. Epub 2021 Oct 18. PMID: 34688072; PMCID: PMC8536513
58. Shelmerdine SC, Roebuck DJ, Towbin AJ, McHugh K. MRI of paediatric liver tumours: how we review and report. Cancer Imaging. 2016;16(1):21. https://doi.org/10.1186/s40644-016-0083-3. PMID: 27526937; PMCID: PMC4986178
59. Patel RK, Pathak S. Undifferentiated embryonal sarcoma masquerading as liver abscess: a case report with typical imaging features. SA J Radiol. 2021;25(1):2179. https://doi.org/10.4102/sajr.v25i1.2179. PMID: 34522435; PMCID: PMC8424748
60. Moon WK, Kim WS, Kim IO, Yeon KM, Yu IK, Choi BI, Han MC. Undifferentiated embryonal sarcoma of the liver: US and CT findings. Pediatr

Radiol. 1994;24(7):500–3. https://doi.org/10.1007/BF02015012. PMID: 7885785

61. Psatha EA, Semelka RC, Fordham L, Firat Z, Woosley JT. Undifferentiated (embryonal) sarcoma of the liver (USL): MRI findings including dynamic gadolinium enhancement. Magn Reson Imaging. 2004;22(6):897–900. https://doi.org/10.1016/j.mri.2004.02.003. PMID: 15234460
62. Ros PR, Olmsted WW, Dachman AH, Goodman ZD, Ishak KG, Hartman DS. Undifferentiated (embryonal) sarcoma of the liver: radiologic-pathologic correlation. Radiology. 1986;161(1):141–5. https://doi.org/10.1148/radiology.161.1.3532179. PMID: 3532179
63. Sharif K, Ramani P, Lochbühler H, Grundy R, de Ville de Goyet J. Recurrent mesenchymal hamartoma associated with 19q translocation. A call for more radical surgical resection. Eur J Pediatr Surg. 2006;16(1):64–7. https://doi.org/10.1055/s--2005-873072. PMID: 16544232
64. Yen JB, Kong MS, Lin JN. Hepatic mesenchymal hamartoma. J Paediatr Child Health. 2003;39(8):632–4. https://doi.org/10.1046/j.1440-1754.2003.00250.x. PMID: 14629534
65. Anil G, Fortier M, Low Y. Cystic hepatic mesenchymal hamartoma: the role of radiology in diagnosis and perioperative management. Br J Radiol. 2011;84(1001):e91–4. https://doi.org/10.1259/bjr/41579091. PMID: 21511744; PMCID: PMC3473652
66. Tsao K, Hirose S, Sydorak R, Goldstein RB, Machin GA, Albanese CT, Farmer DL. Fetal therapy for giant hepatic cysts. J Pediatr Surg. 2002;37(10):E31. https://doi.org/10.1053/jpsu.2002.35444. PMID: 12378477
67. Dutta S, Nehra D, Woo R, Cohen I. Laparoscopic resection of a benign liver tumor in a child. J Pediatr Surg. 2007;42(6):1141–5. https://doi.org/10.1016/j.jpedsurg.2007.01.045. PMID: 17560238
68. Karpelowsky JS, Pansini A, Lazarus C, Rode H, Millar AJ. Difficulties in the management of mesenchymal hamartomas. Pediatr Surg Int. 2008;24(10):1171–5. https://doi.org/10.1007/s00383-008-2239-0. Epub 2008 Aug 28. PMID: 18751987
69. Liao W, Zhang B, Zhang W, Chen L, Zhang W, Zhang B, Chen X. A 4 and a half years old boy with mesenchymal hamartomas in the left lateral lobe of the liver: a case report and literature review. Medicine (Baltimore). 2017;96(31):e7281. https://doi.org/10.1097/MD.0000000000007281. PMID: 28767567; PMCID: PMC5626121
70. Pan ET, Yoeli D, Kueht ML, Galvan NTN, Cotton RT, O'Mahony CA, Rana A, Goss JA. Liver transplantation as definitive treatment of an unresectable mesenchymal hamartoma in a child with Beckwith-Wiedemann Syndrome. J Surg Case Rep. 2017;2017(8):rjx167. https://doi.org/10.1093/jscr/rjx167. PMID: 28928922; PMCID: PMC5597790
71. Alkalay AL, Puri AR, Pomerance JJ, Kallus M, Gans SL, Hurvitz CH, Farber SJ, Sloninsky L. Mesenchymal hamartoma of the liver responsive to cyclophosphamide therapy: therapeutic approach. J Pediatr Surg. 1985;20(2):125–8. https://doi.org/10.1016/s0022-3468(85)80283-9. PMID: 4009357
72. Kuperman AA, Kornreich L, Feinmesser M, Ash S, Yaniv I, Cohen IJ. Regression of mesenchymal hamartoma of the liver with sarcoma chemotherapy. J Pediatr Hematol Oncol. 2013;35(1):e25–6. https://doi.org/10.1097/MPH.0b013e3182667ba6. PMID: 22935658
73. Srouji MN, Chatten J, Schulman WM, Ziegler MM, Koop CE. Mesenchymal hamartoma of the liver in infants. Cancer. 1978;42(5):2483–9. https://doi.org/10.1002/1097-0142(197811)42:5<2483::aid-cncr2820420552>3.0.co;2-0. PMID: 363258
74. Ramanujam TM, Ramesh JC, Goh DW, Wong KT, Ariffin WA, Kumar G, Taib NA. Malignant transformation of mesenchymal hamartoma of the liver: case report and review of the literature. J Pediatr Surg. 1999;34(11):1684–6. https://doi.org/10.1016/s0022-3468(99)90644-9. PMID: 10591570
75. Wildhaber BE, Montaruli E, Guérin F, Branchereau S, Martelli H, Gauthier F. Mesenchymal hamartoma or embryonal sarcoma of the liver in childhood: a difficult diagnosis before complete surgical excision. J Pediatr Surg. 2014;49(9):1372–7. https://doi.org/10.1016/j.jpedsurg.2014.04.005. Epub 2014 May 15. PMID: 25148740
76. Barnhart DC, Hirschl RB, Garver KA, Geiger JD, Harmon CM, Coran AG. Conservative management of mesenchymal hamartoma of the liver. J Pediatr Surg. 1997;32(10):1495–8. https://doi.org/10.1016/s0022-3468(97)90574-1. PMID: 9349781
77. Roebuck D. Asymptomatic mesenchymal hamartoma of the liver can be treated by observation alone. J Pediatr Surg. 1998;33(10):1587. https://doi.org/10.1016/s0022-3468(98)90512-7. PMID: 9802825

Intraductal Papillary Neoplasm of the Bile Duct

17

Asmus Heumann and Thilo Hackert

17.1 Introduction

Intraductal papillary neoplasms of the bile duct (IPNB) are rare precursors of intra- and extrahepatic cholangiocarcinomas. IPNB includes the previous categories of bile duct papilloma/papillomatosis, papillary carcinoma, and mucin-secreting bile duct tumors [1]. As described by Zen et al., the low incidence and prevalence, as well as overlapping features with other precursor lesions and de novo cholangiocarcinomas, led to inconsistent findings across different studies with regard to the mentioned terminologies [2]. The WHO classification of Digestive System Tumors included IPNB as a specific tumor entity as late as 2019.

17.2 Incidence and Origin

IPNB are rare; some authors hypothesize that IPNB account for 10–15% of bile duct tumors. In fact, IPNBs are not very common, especially in Western countries, and the proportion is presumably below 5%. A recently published European multicenter survey (EUR-IPNB study) included 85 patients who underwent elective surgery for IPNB in 28 centers in 2020 [3], which underlines this. Furthermore, a current analysis of the SEER database showed a decreasing incidence of IPNB in the US over the last fifty years. The incidence of invasive IPNB decreased from 2.2 cases per 100,000 individuals in 1975 to 0.3 cases per 100,000 individuals in 2016, while, in contrast, the incidence for traditional cholangiocarcinoma increased significantly in the same time period [4].

IPNB occur predominantly in males (median age 60–66 years, male-to-female ratio 2:1 to 3:2). Risk factors include liver flukes, hepatolithiasis, primary sclerosing cholangitis (PSC), biliary malformations, and polyposis syndromes such as familial adenomatous polyposis (FAP) and Gardner syndrome [1, 5, 6].

17.3 Clinical Presentation

There are no specific early clinical signs of IPNB [7]. The symptoms are caused by bile duct occlusion due to intraductal masses/mucin or (in more advanced cases) intraductal tumor growth. In line with that, the most frequent presenting symptoms are pain and jaundice (42% and 33%, respec-

A. Heumann · T. Hackert (✉)
Department of General, Visceral and Thoracic Surgery, University Hospital Hamburg-Eppendorf, Hamburg, Germany
e-mail: a.heumann@uke.de; t.hackert@uke.de

T. Hackert, A. Gulla (eds.), *Rare Liver and Biliary Tract Diseases*,
https://doi.org/10.1007/978-3-032-15076-9_17

tively) [8]. This is accompanied by elevated alkaline phosphatase and CA 19–9 levels [6]. However, more than 10% of the patients are asymptomatic [5, 8].

17.4 Differential Diagnosis and Workup

17.4.1 Imaging

CT (Fig. 17.1) and MRI are the most relevant diagnostic tools for IPNB. Main findings are intraductal mass formation combined with biliary ductal dilatation [8]. The detection rates reach 80–89%. Ultrasound is not recommended due to its low sensitivity, low accuracy, and high user dependency, and the impossibility of adequate presurgical planning. In the European EUR-IPNB study, MRI and CT are the most commonly used preoperative diagnostic tools [3]. Endoscopic retrograde cholangiography (ERC) is used in patients with jaundice for duct decompression. In cases with involvement of the biliary bifurcation, ERC in combination with cholangioscopy helps to detect the exact tumor location and the extent of dysplasia within the bile duct system, which is a prerequisite for accurate surgical planning.

17.4.2 IPNB and Other Precursor Lesions of Biliary Carcinomas

There are three different precursor lesions of biliary carcinomas described. They bear different pathological and molecular features, but all harbor malignant potential. Biliary intraepithelial neoplasias (BilIN) arise from micropapillary lesions, while IPNB derives from macroscopically visible intraductal papillary lesions. Additionally, mucinous cystic neoplasms (MCN) give rise to invasive adenocarcinomas too [1].

The different features of BilIN, IPNB and MCN are depicted in Table 17.1.

As mentioned in the chapter by Ruff and Pawlik, it is sometimes difficult to separate MCN from IPNB. Both lesions are able to produce mucin. However, MCNs are defined as hepatic lesions without connection to the bile duct systems, whereas IPNB arises from precursor lesions within the bile duct system. MCNs are deemed to be larger than cystic IPNB and occur mainly in

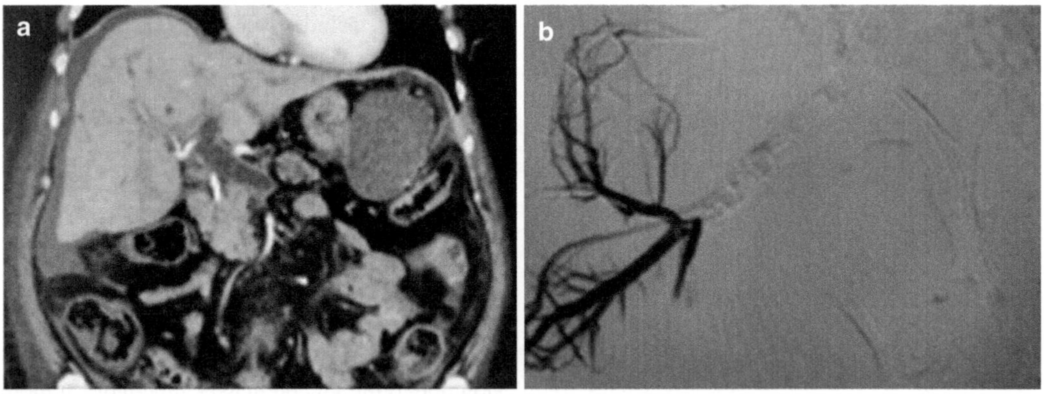

Fig. 17.1 A 65-year-old female patient with jaundice and infiltration of the main portal trunk with mucinous tumor (**a**; black arrow). Portography depicted a complete occlusion due to mucinous portal vein infiltration (**b**, black arrow—mucinous portal vein occlusion, white arrow—hepatic vein, black star—biliary stents)

Table 17.1 According to Klöppel and Lee [1, 7]

	BiIIN	IPNB	MCN
Pathology	Invasive tubular adenoca/of GNAS1 Mut.	Invasive tubular adenoca/ mucinous adenoca GNAS1 Mut	Invasive tubular adenoca /mucinous adenoca, no communication to bile duct Ovarian like stroma
Epidemiology	6–7 decades of life m = f	6–7 decades of life m: f = 2:1/3:2	5—6 decade of life m < f

middle-aged female patients. The vast majority (>90%) of MCNs are benign. Contrarily, IPNB is associated with invasive carcinoma in 40–80% of cases [3, 7].

While surgical enucleation for MCN is adequate, IPNB should be treated according to the principles of oncologic surgery.

17.4.3 Pathologic Diagnosis

Generally, IPNB includes biliary tract papilloma/papillomatosis, papillary carcinomatosis, and mucin-hypersecreting bile duct tumors. They follow the adenoma–carcinoma sequence. Consequently, they show different types of dysplasia (low-to-high grade) [1]. According to the growth pattern of the papillary components, IPNBs are classified into two different types [2]. The types have different clinicopathological features and prognosis (Table 17.2).

Type 1 IPNB is the biliary equivalent of pancreatic intraductal papillary mucinous neoplasm (IPMN) with organized papillary architecture and production of mucus [1, 2, 9]. Type 2 IPNB is less well characterized, with a more complex/irregular papillary architecture, more necrosis, and is, in most cases, associated with invasive cancer. Not surprisingly, this leads to a dismal prognosis.

The basic principle of stepwise progression from low-grade to high-grade dysplasia and finally invasive cancer is applicable to IPNB and was described in detail with its characteristic genetic alterations in a case series of 45 patients [10].

Similar to the well-described pancreatic IPMN, IPNB exhibits either a pancreatobiliary, intestinal, gastric, or oncocytic phenotype [1]. There are some geographic differences in these phenotypes, with the intestinal phenotype being more common in Asia [1, 7]. The prognostic value of these subtypes is still under debate [1]. However, epidemiologic data from the SEER database showed that non-mucin-producing tumors are associated with better overall survival (OS) and cancer-specific survival (CSS). Furthermore, the analysis showed a better prognosis for distally located tumors [4].

17.4.4 Genetic Alterations

Different genetic mutations are described in IPNB. These include APC, CTNNB1, KRAS, GNAS, P16, and TP53. Data regarding specific genetic alterations for Type 1 and Type 2 IPNB, respectively, remain conflicting, which can most likely be explained by inconsistent definitions of IPNB across the different studies [2, 11].

Table 17.2 According to Zen et al. [2]

	Type 1 IPNB	Type 2 IPNB
Prevalence Europe/Asia	<10%/33%	>90%/67%
Anatomic site	Intrahepatic/perihilar	Perihilar/distal
Gross finding	Fragile intraductal papillary tumorCystic ductal dilatation	Solid intraductal mass Upstream duct dilatation
Gross mucin	80%	10%
Histology	Regularly arranged papillae, Thin fibrovascular cores, Homogenous growth pattern; rare necrosis	Complex papillary architecture; thick fibrovascular cores, Heterogenous growth pattern; common necrosis
Histologic type	Pancreaticobiliary, intestinal, gastric, oncocytic	Pancreaticobiliary, intestinal
Grade of dysplasia	Usually high grade	Always high grade
Radiology		
Invasive cancer	50%	>95%
5 year survival	80%	40%

17.5 Treatment and Surgical Planning

The natural course of IPNB is unclear. Contrary to IPMN, no risk stratification according to "worrisome features" or "high-risk stigmata" is established. Therefore, treatment should be carefully planned after an extensive risk/benefit analysis. Age and performance status of the patient, as well as the risk of surgery, must be carefully weighed against the risk of malignancy to evaluate the potential benefits of surgery as the only curative therapeutic option.

The duration of invasive cancer development is largely unknown but probably depends on the type of IPNB. As the grade of dysplasia is generally higher in Type 2 IPNB compared to Type 1 IPNB, one can assume that the time for developing invasive cancer is significantly shorter in Type 2 cases. In Type 1 cases, Zen et al. reported 4 patients with a follow-up of more than 5 years, with microinvasion in only one case [2]. Similar to IPMN, skip lesions are described for IPNB with metachronous development of other intraductal neoplasms [12, 13].

As IPNB bear high-grade dysplasia or invasive cancer in up to 80% of cases, surgical treatment needs to be planned according to the principles of oncologic surgery [3, 6]. Even in cases without invasive carcinoma, radical surgery should be performed to eliminate the risk of malignant transformation in the future. This also includes lesions with low-grade dysplasia. Therefore, the treatment of IPNB mirrors the treatment of traditional cholangiocarcinoma [14].

The extent of IPNB within the biliary system (especially in the hilar bifurcation) can be difficult to assess, even with cholangioscopy. This is a problem for the preoperative surgical strategy because it is not clear what type of resection (e.g., left or right hemihepatectomy) is most beneficial for the patient. If the lesion is clearly located intrahepatically to the left or right side, a formal left or right hepatectomy is the standard approach, including lymphadenectomy of the hepatoduodenal ligament.

However, it is often difficult to assess the exact extent of the lesions within the biliary system intraoperatively, even when frozen sections of the cut margins are performed during the resection. This is particularly the case in patients with bile duct decompression and stent implantation prior to surgery or in patients with concomitant PSC. In these situations, it is often difficult to distinguish inflammation (e.g., caused by transpapillary stenting) from true dysplasia reflecting further intraductal growth of IPNB and requiring extension of the resection.

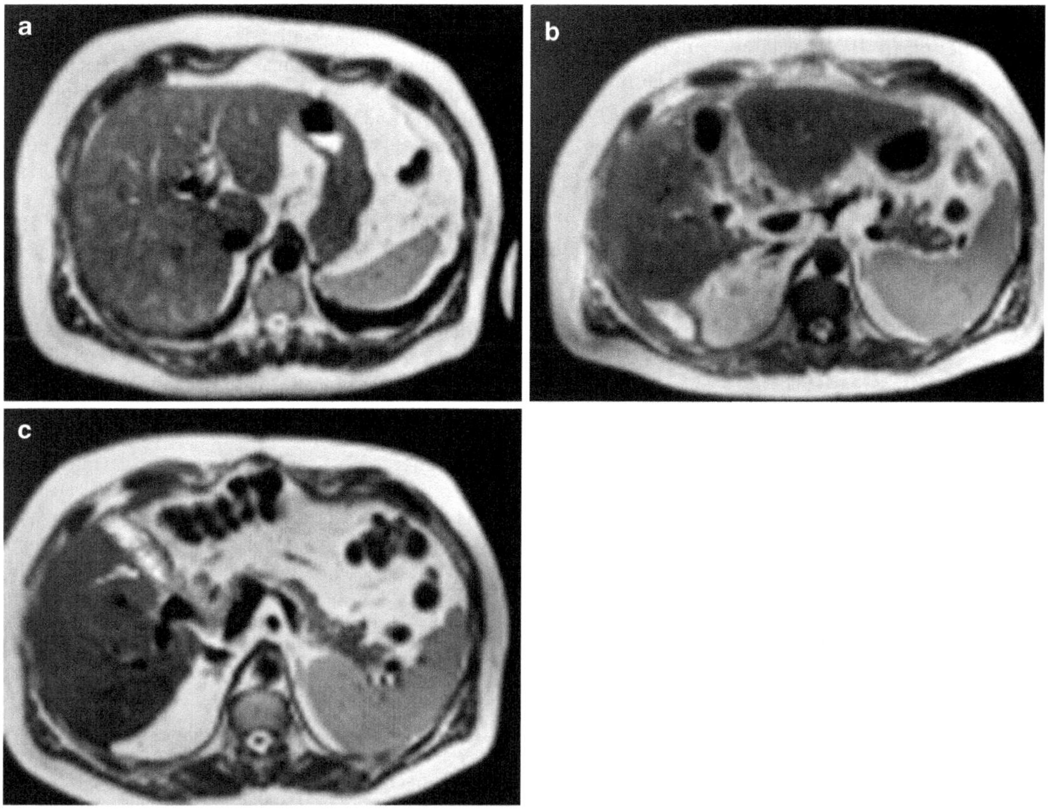

Fig. 17.2 A 51-year-old male patient with hepaticojejunostomy at the age of ten. Repeating cholangitis and jaundice due to IPNB (**a**; white arrow—dilated bile duct). Mesohepatectomy was performed with separate right- and left-sided hepaticojejunostomies (**b**; white star—jejunal loop), final histology shows left-sided high-grade dysplasia, and the resection of the left lateral sector was performed (**c**). The white arrow indicates a segmental bile duct dilatation. Histology via ERC showed dysplasia, and the patient is now scheduled for transplant

In the case of IPNB located in the hilar bifurcation (comparable to a Klatskin III/IV position), the approach of choice is the resection of the central liver segment, also known as mesohepatectomy. In this scenario, the main tumor mass is safely removed with low risk of posthepatectomy liver failure [15]. Frozen section excludes invasive carcinoma within the resection margin of the bile duct. If final pathology shows dysplasia at the resection margin, re-resection can be easily performed, resulting in completion of either extended right or extended left hepatectomy (Fig. 17.2).

In cases with technically non-resectable high-grade dysplasia, IPNB liver transplantation can be an option; however, this indication remains rare. For a patient with metastatic disease, palliative chemo–/immunotherapy is recommended, following the treatment principles of cholangiocarcinoma [14].

17.6 Follow-Up/ Recommendations

The natural outcome of IPNB is unclear, and contrary to IPMN, there is no follow-up recommendation for non-resected IPNBs. For surveillance, 6-monthly MRI examinations seem to be suitable.

In resected patients with either IPNB or associated invasive cholangiocarcinoma, postoperative surveillance and adjuvant therapy are performed according to the EASL guidelines

[14]. The OS and CSS are deemed to be significantly better in IPNB-related cancers as compared to traditional cholangiocarcinoma. The median OS in patients with invasive IPNB is 15–18 months with CSS of 24–29 months. The outcome of patients with traditional cholangiocarcinoma is significantly worse, with a median OS of 10 months and a median CSS of 16 months [4].

17.7 Conclusion

IPNB are rare precursors of cholangiocarcinoma. Their incidence is decreasing; however, they are assumed to be the underlying pathology in up to 15% of all cholangiocarcinomas. Contrary to IPMN, no morphological risk features leading to relative or absolute indications for surgery are defined. However, as up to 80% of IPNB show malignancy, radical surgery is the therapy of choice.

References

1. Klöppel G, Adsay V, Konukiewitz B, Kleeff J, Schlitter AM, Esposito I. Precancerous lesions of the biliary tree. Best Pract Res Clin Gastroenterology. 2013;27(2):285–97.
2. Zen Y, Akita M. Neoplastic progression in Intraductal papillary neoplasm of the bile duct. Arch Pathol Lab Med. 2023;148:989.
3. Lluís N, Serradilla-Martín M, Achalandabaso M, Jehaes F, Dasari BVM, Mambrilla-Herrero S, et al. Intraductal papillary neoplasms of the bile duct: a European retrospective multicenter observational study (EUR-IPNB study). Int J Surg (Lond, Engl). 2023;109(4):760–71.
4. Wu RS, Liao WJ, Ma JS, Wang JK, Wu LQ, Hou P. Epidemiology and outcome of individuals with intraductal papillary neoplasms of the bile duct. World J Gastrointest Oncol. 2023;15(5):843–58.
5. Kim JR, Jang KT, Jang JY. Intraductal papillary neoplasm of the bile duct: review of updated clinicopathological and imaging characteristics. Br J Surg. 2023;110(9):1229–40.
6. Kubota K, Nakanuma Y, Kondo F, Hachiya H, Miyazaki M, Nagino M, et al. Clinicopathological features and prognosis of mucin-producing bile duct tumor and mucinous cystic tumor of the liver: a multi-institutional study by the Japan Biliary Association. J Hepato Biliary Pancreat Sci. 2014;21(3):176–85.
7. Lee MH, Katabathina VS, Lubner MG, Shah HU, Prasad SR, Matkowskyj KA, et al. Mucin producing cystic hepatobiliary neoplasms: updated nomenclature and clinical, pathologic, and imaging features. Radiographics. 2021;41(6):1592–610.
8. Gordon-Weeks AN, Jones K, Harriss E, Smith A, Silva M. Systematic review and meta analysis of current experience in treating IPNB. Ann Surg. 2016;263(4):656–63.
9. Schlitter AM, Klöppel G, Esposito I. Intraductal papillary neoplasms of the bile duct (IPNB). Diagnostic criteria, carcinogenesis and differential diagnostics. For Pathol. 2013;34 Suppl 2(Suppl 2):235–40.
10. Schlitter AM, Born D, Bettstetter M, Specht K, Kim-Fuchs C, Riener MO, et al. Intraductal papillary neoplasms of the bile duct: stepwise progression to carcinoma involves common molecular pathways. Mod Pathol. 2014;27(1):73–86.
11. Nakanuma Y, Kakuda Y, Sugino T, Sato Y, Fukumura Y. Pathologies of precursor lesions of biliary tract carcinoma. Cancer. 2022;14(21):5358.
12. Hirono S, Shimizu Y, Ohtsuka T, Kin T, Hara K, Kanno A, et al. Recurrence patterns after surgical resection of intraductal papillary mucinous neoplasm (IPMN) of the pancreas; a multicenter, retrospective study of 1074 IPMN patients by the Japan Pancreas Society. J Gastroenterol. 2020;55(1):86–99.
13. Yokode M, Yamashita Y, Zen Y. Biliary intraductal papillary neoplasm with metachronous multiple tumors – true multicentric tumors or intrabiliary dissemination: a case report and review of the literature. Mol Clin Oncol. 2017;6(3):315–20.
14. Liver EA for the S of the, Alvaro D, Gores GJ, Walicki J, Hassan C, Sapisochin G, et al. EASL-ILCA clinical practice guidelines on the management of intrahepatic cholangiocarcinoma. J Hepatol. 2023;79(1):181–208.
15. Wang D, Sun W, Zhou S, Liu Z, Lu Z, Zhang D. Application of mesohepatectomy with caudate lobectomy for the treatment of type III–IV hilar cholangiocarcinoma: a single-center retrospective study. Eur J Méd Res. 2023;28(1):234.

Extrahepatic Biliary Atresia

18

Pratik Chandra and Christopher Wolfgang

18.1 Overview and Incidence

Biliary atresia (BA) is a rare disease unique to infancy, associated with progressive obstructive cholangiopathy. Its incidence varies according to geographic locale but can range from 1 in 8000 live births in Asia to 1 in 15,000 live births in North America [1]. It remains the number one reason for pediatric end-stage liver disease (ESLD) as well as pediatric liver transplantation in the world [2]. The underlying etiology of BA is uncertain, but the end result is epithelial injury resulting in biliary tract obstruction. The natural progression of the disease without treatment, which is primarily surgical, involves progressive cholestasis, portal fibrosis, and finally cirrhosis. The ensuing ESLD causes sequelae such as portal hypertension, coagulopathy, and encephalopathy, among others. If left untreated, death occurs by the age of 2 as a result of ESLD [2].

There are 3 different anatomical and 3 general clinical subtypes of BA (Image 18.1) [3]. The three anatomical subtypes of BA are classified according to the location of the obstruction within the extrahepatic biliary tree:

Type 1 (5%): obstruction at the level of the common bile duct, usually with proximal cystic dilatation.

Type 2 (2%): obstruction at the level of the common hepatic duct (sometimes along with the common bile duct), with patent left and right main hepatic ducts at the porta hepatis.

Type 3 (90–95%): obstruction at the level of the porta hepatis.

Clinically, BA can generally be designated into a syndromic (~20%), isolated (~70%) or CMV-associated form (~10–15%). The syndromic form of BA most commonly occurs as biliary atresia splenic malformation (BASM) syndrome, which is characterized by a variety of splenic abnormalities but also other visceral changes, including malrotation, preduodenal portal vein, complete absence of hepatic vena cava, and cardiac abnormalities [4]. Recently, CMV-associated BA has also been identified as a potentially distinct clinical phenotype of BA, which will be elaborated upon below [5].

P. Chandra · C. Wolfgang (✉)
Department of Surgery, NYU Grossman School of Medicine, New York, NY, USA
e-mail: pratik.chandra@nyulangone.org; christopher.wolfgange@nyulangone.org

T. Hackert, A. Gulla (eds.), *Rare Liver and Biliary Tract Diseases*,
https://doi.org/10.1007/978-3-032-15076-9_18

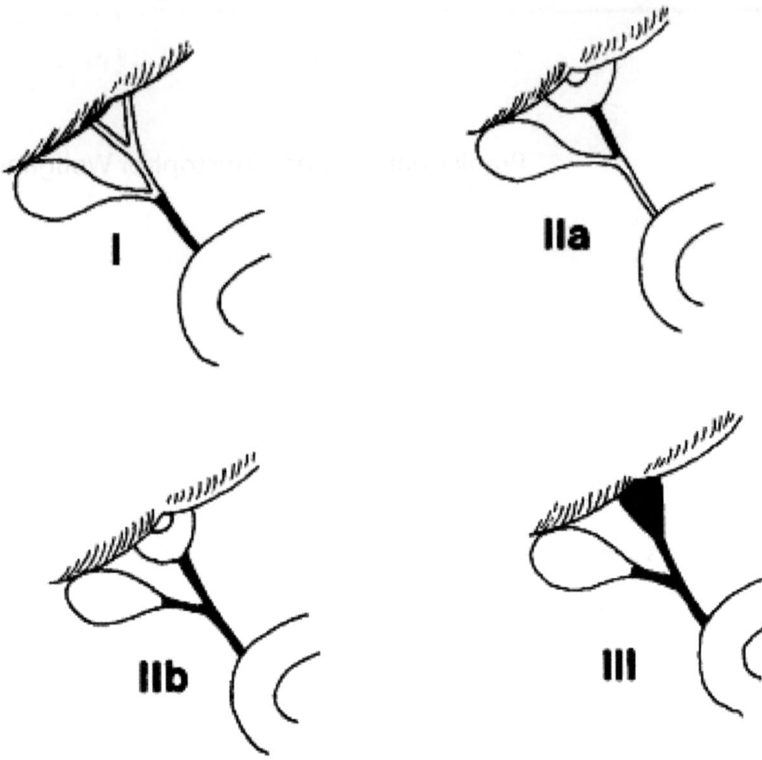

Image 18.1 Ohi classification of biliary atresia. (Reference: Lefkowitch [55])

18.2 Clinical Presentation and Differential Diagnosis

Patients with BA typically present with symptoms within the first 30–60 days of life. The hallmark symptoms of BA are similar to those of other disease processes that cause biliary obstruction: acholic stools, dark urine, and jaundice. When evaluating these patients, it is important to ascertain the temporal relationship of symptoms with birth, as it may be an indicator of disease burden. For example, an infant who has acholic stools immediately after passing meconium may have more advanced disease compared to an infant who initially has normal stools but subsequently progresses into having acholic stools.

The differential diagnosis for infantile jaundice ranges from physiologic to pathologic etiologies, with the most common cause being physiologic jaundice of the newborn [6]. Typically, the etiologies of jaundice can be categorized as benign or pathologic based on the presence of an indirect or direct hyperbilirubinemia, respectively.

A direct, or conjugated, hyperbilirubinemia has several pathologic etiologies that can be categorized broadly into either anatomic or hepatocellular causes. Anatomic causes of direct hyperbilirubinemia include BA, choledochal cysts and inspissated bile syndrome, among others. Hepatocellular causes include viral hepatitis, sepsis, Alagille syndrome, progressive familial intrahepatic cholestasis syndromes, alpha-1 antitrypsin deficiency, and certain metabolic syndromes like tyrosinemia. The differential for infantile jaundice remains broad, and the diagnosis of biliary atresia in a timely manner can be difficult [7].

18.3 Early Kasai Portoenterostomy Outcomes and Screening

Considerable work has been put into identifying the ideal timing of surgical intervention for BA. In general, it is thought that earlier surgical intervention in the form of a portoenterostomy, or Kasai procedure (KPE), is associated with improved short- and long-term outcomes. The outcomes most commonly assessed include jaundice, or bilirubin, clearance rate (JCR), and native liver survival rate (NLSR).

The Japanese Biliary Atresia Registry is a national, prospectively maintained database established in 1989, tracking the outcomes of BA patients in Japan [8]. Based on data collected from this database, previous studies have noted that the JCR was improved in patients who underwent KPE at <90 days of age when compared to >90 days of age, but there was no significant difference between those who underwent surgery at <60 days of age compared to those between 61–90 days of age [9]. Earlier age at Kasai was also noted to have improved NLSR, particularly when performed at <60 days of age, but especially when performed at <30 days of age [8].

These findings were confirmed in a recent meta-analysis evaluating early KPE outcomes. Specifically, JCR and NLSR improved when KPE was performed at <90 days of age, and the effect of performing Kasai at <60 days of age improved NLSR but had no effect on JCR [10].

There has been some conflicting data suggesting that age at Kasai is not necessarily associated with outcomes [11]. However, this may be related to a variety of factors, including the severity and timing of disease onset. If disease onset varies according to underlying etiology, which is often unknown, then age at KPE may not be a significant predictor of outcomes in BA secondary to certain etiologies. Regardless, for the majority of patients, there is still a strong correlation between outcomes and age at Kasai [9]. Thus, a significant push towards earlier diagnosis and treatment has been advocated through screening programs.

The most widely used screening protocol for BA in the world is the Stool Color Card developed in Japan (Image 18.2). Parents are provided with a card that allows them to track the color and consistency of their infants' stool. If a concerning change is identified by the parents as per the card, the infant is brought in for evaluation in the hopes of earlier referral and expedited workup. These screening programs have been shown to improve outcomes, including earlier age at KPE and significantly longer NLSR [12]. Another screening tool being assessed in the US is bilirubin fractionation. This is a two-step screen in which patients are first screened within the first 60 hours of life. If bilirubin is at or greater than the 95th percentile, then the patient is screened a second time prior to their two-week well visit with a repeat bilirubin fractionation—if the patient still has persistently elevated bilirubin >1 or a level greater than the first step, the screen is considered positive. This study demonstrated that patients had a younger age at KPE, and further analysis regarding outcomes is pending [13].

Currently, the American College of Pediatrics recommends that any neonate who has persistent jaundice beyond the first two weeks of life undergo bilirubin fractionation to identify whether there is a direct or indirect hyperbilirubinemia.

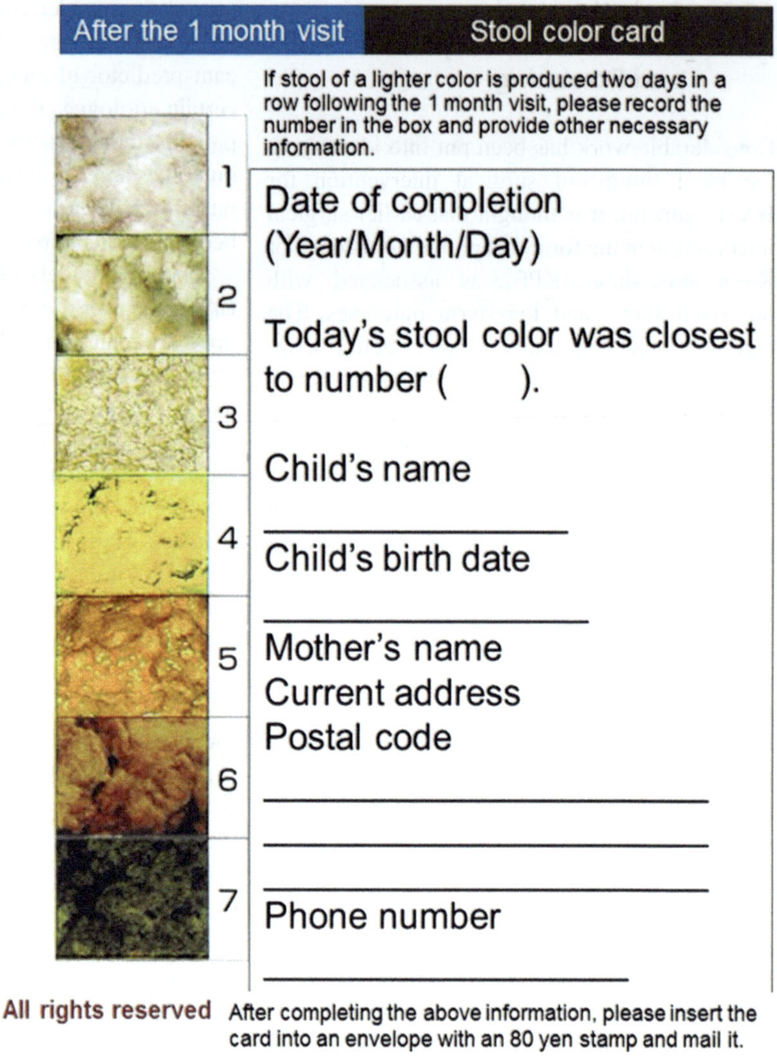

Image 18.2 Third edition stool color card used in Tochigi Prefecture from August 1994 to March 201. Images 1–3 denote abnormal stool color, whereas images 4–7 reflect normal stool color. (Reference: Gu et al. [12])

18.4 Work Up

History and physical examination are paramount in the evaluation of infantile cholestasis. With respect to BA, a focused abdominal exam may reveal hepatomegaly or sequelae of ESLD in the case of advanced presentation [7]. Alternatively, the presence of other physical exam findings, such as a heart murmur, may suggest another diagnosis, like Alagille syndrome. Additionally, direct observation of the infant's stool by the care provider is essential to establish a baseline by which the stool color can be tracked.

18.4.1 Lab Evaluation

Following history and examination, workup consists of laboratory investigation including CBC, LFTs, BMP and abdominal ultrasound (UA). Additional laboratory evaluation includes tests to assess for specific entities on the differential, as well as routine perinatal screening measures.

As mentioned earlier with respect to bilirubin fractionation, the presence of a direct (or conjugated) hyperbilirubinemia implies an obstructive or cholestatic pattern of liver injury. This is the hallmark laboratory finding of BA, but it is not specific to it. While markers of hepatocellular injury, such as an elevated transaminase, may be present, they are also not specific to BA. Gamma–glutamyl transferase (GGT), which is more specifically increased in obstructive biliary pathology, is also often elevated in BA and supports the diagnosis. However, it is also elevated in other processes, including Alagille syndrome. While alkaline phosphatase (ALP) is typically elevated in biliary or bone pathology, its levels can vary widely in infants, thus limiting its utility.

Additional pathologies that can mimic BA, such as alpha-1 antitrypsin deficiency, cystic fibrosis, and Alagille syndrome, should be assessed at this time as well [7]. This can include an immunoreactive trypsinogen for cystic fibrosis, an alpha-1 antitrypsin phenotype and molecular testing for Alagille syndrome.

18.4.2 Matrix Metalloproteinase 7

Given the relative lack of specific laboratory tests for BA and the benefit of early diagnosis/intervention in these patients, research into identifying new biomarkers to aid in diagnosis is active. One such marker is MMP-7, or matrix metalloproteinase 7. Though different studies established different cutoff values for abnormality, a recent meta-analysis evaluating biomarkers in BA found that MMP-7 had a pooled sensitivity of 96% and specificity of 91% [14]. However, other more recent papers have demonstrated lower than previously quoted sensitivity and specificity values [15]. Outside of its use in diagnosis, MMP-7 levels have not only been demonstrated to correlate with the degree of liver fibrosis in both nonalcoholic fatty liver disease in general but also in BA specifically [16, 17]. As such, it can potentially be used as a surrogate marker for post-KPE liver fibrosis [14]. Its utility as a marker in predicting the need for liver transplantation post-KPE, however, has been mixed in the literature [15–18].

18.5 Imaging

18.5.1 Ultrasound

After biochemical analysis is suggestive of an obstructive biliary pathology, further investigation takes the form of imaging. The most common first step in imaging evaluation is an abdominal ultrasound. There are several findings seen in BA, each with differing sensitivity, specificity, positive predictive value (PPV), and negative predictive value (NPV). These include gallbladder abnormalities, the triangular cord sign, hepatic artery diameter, and the ratio of hepatic artery to portal vein diameter, among others [19, 20]. A recent meta-analysis demonstrated that the combined presence of the triangular cord sign along with gallbladder abnormalities had the best diagnostic ratio and highest sensitivity/specificity when compared to any individual ultrasound finding [21]. Additional adjuncts to grayscale ultrasound include shear-wave elastography (SWE), which is used to assess liver stiffness as a surrogate for fibrosis. The use of SWE in BA has ranged from aiding in preoperative diagnosis to assessing the degree of post-KPE liver fibrosis [22]; however, it does have lower sensitivity and specificity for diagnosing BA when compared directly to grayscale ultrasonography, so its best use may be as an adjunct. However, since SWE measures liver stiffness as a surrogate for fibrosis, its clinical utility for early diagnosis may be limited when presumably the disease process is at an earlier stage with a lesser degree of fibrosis. Like grayscale ultrasonography, normal SWE findings do not exclude the diagnosis of BA.

18.5.2 Intraoperative Cholangiogram, CT and MRI

Other imaging modalities include CT and MRI, but their use is limited secondary to radiation exposure and the need for anesthesia and/or motion-artifact degradation, respectively [23]. The gold-standard imaging study for the diagnosis of biliary atresia remains an intraoperative cholangiogram. Several cholangiographic patterns exist, but the diagnosis is strongly suggested when there is non-visualization of a patent extrahepatic biliary tree [24]. However, since this requires operative intervention, the presumptive diagnosis is often made preoperatively using ultrasound.

18.5.3 Percutaneous Liver Biopsy

With suggestive imaging and biochemical findings, the next step in the workup would likely involve a percutaneous core liver biopsy. Diagnosis is achieved in up to 90% of cases with percutaneous biopsy alone [25]. Classic histopathologic findings suggestive of BA include bile duct proliferation, bile duct plugs, and portal fibrosis [3]. The development of a standardized histologic assessment system for cholestasis has resulted in high rates of successful diagnosis. However, there are still some other causes of infantile cholestasis, such as parenteral nutrition-associated cholestasis or alpha-1-antitrypsin deficiency, that can mimic BA on histology and make diagnosis difficult [3, 25]. Additionally, many of the histologic findings of BA are difficult to ascertain early in the disease process, and therefore, early biopsy may result in higher rates of false-negative findings [26]. As such, the gold standard diagnostic criterion for biliary atresia includes both pathologic assessment and imaging findings, often in the form of an intraoperative cholangiogram [7].

18.5.4 Inconclusive Biopsy and Imaging

In situations where the diagnosis remains in question despite a biopsy and imaging, some centers have advocated for the use of endoscopic retrograde cholangiopancreatography (ERCP) [27]. In a large patient cohort, Negm et al. demonstrated that ERCP matched the surgical diagnosis of BA in 95% of cases with a false-positive rate of 5% and a false-negative rate of 0%; of the false-positive patients, approximately half required expeditious surgical management anyway, while the other half required liver transplantation at follow-up. This led to a sensitivity, specificity, PPV and NPV of 100%, 79%, 89%, and 100%, respectively [28]. Despite the promising results demonstrated in this series and others, neonatal ERCP requires expert personnel as well as specialized equipment that may not be available at many centers. Additionally, it also requires that the infant be placed under general anesthesia to perform the procedure, thus reducing the extent of avoiding laparoscopic exploration [7]. For these reasons, widespread adoption of this technique has been limited.

18.5.5 Scintigraphy

Historically, a hepatobiliary scintigraphy scan was used for diagnostic purposes, but this has largely been abandoned as a result of its impact on subsequent treatment as well as its relatively low clinical utility [7]. With respect to diagnostics, scintigraphy has a very high sensitivity approaching 98% but a relatively low specificity of approximately 70% [29]. As a result, the test lends itself to being a modality to exclude BA rather than diagnose it. In order to increase the specificity of the exam, premedication with certain agents, such as phenobarbital, has been used [29]. These agents improve hepatocellular function, thereby increasing the uptake of the radiotracer into the liver. However, the premedication loading phase can take upwards of 5 days [30]. This can result in a significant delay in diagnosis that ultimately affects post-KPE outcomes [31]. Due to these limitations, scintigraphy is no longer considered to be routine practice in the workup of BA but may still have a role in excluding the diagnosis.

18.6 Treatment Paradigm

The nuance in treating BA patients lies in accurately assessing where along the natural history of the disease process each individual patient is. Prior studies have demonstrated that some patients have reasonable outcomes after KPE despite traditionally being considered advanced with respect to age [32]. This highlights the differences between each patient's natural progression of disease. As such, the decision of what to do after diagnosis is largely based on where along that spectrum each patient falls.

In general, younger patients who present before the age of 70–75 days are considered for KPE. At this age, it is hypothesized that the benefits of performing the procedure with respect to JCR and NLSR outweigh the potential operative risk associated with surgery on cirrhotic physiology. As age advances, however, the sequelae of cirrhosis may manifest, thus significantly increasing the perioperative risk associated with KPE; when coupled with the generally worse JCR and NLSR associated with late KPE, risk-benefit analysis may favor primary liver transplantation (LT) in some patients. This assessment involves the identification of any sequelae of cirrhosis and/or portal hypertension, as well as a thorough laboratory evaluation of the patient's underlying synthetic function. If the patient is presenting with more advanced liver disease, then primary LT should be considered, with evaluation by a pediatric transplant team.

18.6.1 Liver Transplant

Outcomes for LT in BA have been studied previously and have demonstrated mixed results, particularly when LT is performed after early failure (EF) of KPE, which is defined as being listed for transplant within 1 year of life, versus late failure (LF), which is defined as being listed after the age of 1. Some studies have demonstrated that patients who undergo LT for EF after KPE are associated with worse overall survival and graft survival when compared to primary transplantation (100% vs 81% and 96% vs 79%). Additionally, EF patients had an increased rate of postoperative complications, including vascular thrombosis, bile leak, and non-SSI post-transplant infections resulting in sepsis [33]. Conversely, other studies have demonstrated that KPE has no effect on LT after EF. Yoeli et al. demonstrated that there was no difference in overall survival or graft survival in patients who underwent primary LT or LT after EF of KPE. Consistent with previous literature, they found that patients who undergo LT after LF of KPE have excellent overall survival as well as graft survival rates; in general, they have higher body mass index (BMI), lower average total bilirubin levels, and lower matched MELD/PELD scores as well [34]. This leads to the conclusion that KPE has no deleterious effect on LT even in the setting of EF and leads to excellent outcomes after LF of KPE because patients are generally healthier as a result of having successful biliary drainage by the time they need transplant [34, 35].

The most common indications for requiring LT include EF of KPE, late diagnosis of BA with evidence of ESLD, failure to thrive, recurrent cholangitis, portal hypertension, pruritus, hepatopulmonary syndrome, and hepatorenal syndrome [36]. Success after the Kasai procedure is defined as a total bilirubin of <2 at 3 months postoperatively because it has been shown to significantly improve survival without transplantation compared to patients with higher bilirubin levels at that age [37]. As such, transplant evaluation should optimally begin at around that time if the patient has failure of KPE.

18.7 Kasai Portoenterostomy

The goal of the KPE operation for BA is to restore bile outflow from the liver into the intestine. The procedure is typically performed in an open fashion with a variety of differing techniques.

The first step of the operation, depending on the particular management paradigm, will typically involve a diagnostic laparoscopy. Using a small right upper quadrant transverse incision and an umbilical port, an intraoperative cholangiogram is often attempted using an angiocatheter. This provides valuable information for both diagnostic purposes, as described earlier, and also for assessing the anatomy of the biliary tree itself. Once diagnosis is confirmed and the decision is made to proceed with KPE, the right upper quadrant incision is extended transversely to the left hemiabdomen and down to the right flank. Some surgeons may elect to proceed directly into the open incision and perform an open cholangiogram, particularly in situations where the preoperative likelihood of BA is high.

The next step in the operation involves the porta hepatis dissection. This can be performed in one of two ways: by leaving the liver in situ or by exteriorization. If adequate exposure of the liver hilum is possible by leaving it in situ, then it may limit dense adhesion formation around the liver, which can otherwise complicate subsequent LT. However, this may not always be possible due to a variety of patient or technical factors. In such cases, the liver can be exteriorized by dividing the falciform and triangular ligaments, thereby allowing delivery of the liver outside the abdomen. This technique requires a generous incision because delivery of the liver can result in outflow obstruction through kinking of the hepatic veins if the incision is too small. When performed, exteriorization allows for excellent visualization of the liver hilum and permits a meticulous dissection of the porta hepatis. However, as stated previously, it can add to the technical difficulties of an ensuing LT, especially if there is a significant degree of cirrhosis present at the time of transplant, as these adhesions can become heavily vascularized.

After adequate exposure of the hilum, the gallbladder is dissected off the gallbladder fossa and can be used as a handle for retraction. Dissection is continued medially to identify the portal triad. The key landmark to identify here is the portal vein, as the remnant common bile duct may be obliterated and difficult to identify. Once the portal vein is identified, the dissection is carried cephalad toward the hilar plate, taking care to avoid injury to the hepatic arterial branches. Dissection is continued to the bifurcation of the portal vein, taking down any communicating vessels between the main right and left branches. Mobilization is carried posteriorly beyond the hilar remnant until visualization of Glisson's capsule is ensured. Dissection is then carried out laterally until the division of the second-order arterial branches. At this point, there is a characteristic triangular appearance of the hilum that is classically seen in BA. Once the fibrous mass has been dissected free, stay sutures can be placed into the mass for traction to achieve adequate retraction along with the gallbladder handle.

This retraction allows one to sharply cut across the fibrous plate, leaving Glisson's capsule intact with 1–2 mm of tissue left. The left lateral extent of the transection is determined by identifying the umbilical fissure and opening Rex's fossa to visualize the course of the main left portal vein. The right lateral extent should involve exposure of the anterior and posterior vascular pedicles. After the fibrous mass has been excised, the right upper quadrant is packed, and then attention is turned toward the creation of the Roux limb.

The Roux limb is approximately 40 cm and is typically brought to the right upper quadrant in a retrocolic fashion. The hilar plate reconstruction, or portoenterostomy, is characteristically performed in a single layer with an absorbable monofilament suture on a vascular needle.

18.7.1 Laparoscopic Kasai

The traditional and most recommended approach for performing KPE is open. While there are certainly centers offering laparoscopic KPE [38] with good results, it is not considered the standard of care for the majority of surgeons. The basis of this recommendation comes from a randomized clinical trial in which consecutive patients underwent laparoscopic KPE and were matched against open controls. The primary outcome of the study was to compare NLSR 6 months postoperatively between the laparoscopic and open groups. The study was stopped early because there was a significantly higher rate of LT, lower JCR, and lower NLSR in the laparoscopic group compared to the open controls [39].

18.8 Postoperative Management

18.8.1 Postoperative Cholangitis

Postoperative cholangitis is a dreaded and unfortunately common complication following KPE, occurring in up to 75% of patients at 1 year and 85% at 5 years in some series [40]. Postoperative cholangitis results in significant liver injury to the patient, thereby lowering their NLSR 1, 3 and 5 years post-KPE from 91.7%, 75.8% and 75.8% to 80.1%, 50.7%, and 23.3%, respectively, in some studies [41].

Given the significant morbidity associated with postoperative cholangitis, the use of prophylactic antibiotics following KPE has been the focus of much research. However, despite the ample effort that has gone into this area, results are varied. Some series have demonstrated no difference in the rates of postoperative cholangitis despite prophylactic antibiotics [42]. Others have shown improving rates of transplant-free survival, but interestingly, without a change in cholangitis rate [43]. One randomized trial demonstrated that there may be a benefit in patients who have already had a single episode of cholangitis in preventing recurrent episodes [44]. Part of the issue surrounding this topic stems from the lack of standardization with respect to therapy regimen and duration of treatment [45]. Further complicating this issue has been the considerable variation seen in the causative organisms identified in patients who develop cholangitis [40]. Regardless of this conflicting data, the use of postoperative antibiotics is widespread and serves as a testament to the morbidity associated with cholangitis following KPE.

18.8.2 Steroids

Similar to the use of postoperative antibiotics, there is some controversy and practice heterogeneity involving the postoperative use of steroids. The basis for the use of steroids is the hypothesis that significant inflammation subsequently results in the ensuing fibrosis and eventual obstruction seen in the biliary tree of BA patients. Thus, it is theorized that steroids can limit this inflammation and thus reduce the degree of fibrosis/slow disease progression.

Earlier randomized trials failed to show a difference between a low-dose steroid regimen and placebo with respect to JCR [46], while a later study from the same authors comparing low-dose and high-dose steroids to placebo did show a difference in JCR but without a change in NLSR or need for LT [47]. Some systematic reviews and meta-analyses, on the other hand, have demonstrated improved rates of JCR as well as reduced short-term need for LT [10]. The American START trial, conversely, demonstrated no statistically significant difference in JCR but did note that the steroid arm had an earlier onset of serious adverse events [48]. A follow-up study based on that trial assessed patients in the steroids arm with respect to growth parameters and demonstrated significantly lower growth parameters than the placebo group [49]. As a result of these conflicting data, there are marked differences in the use of postoperative steroids regionally across the world.

18.8.3 Other Adjuncts

Several other adjuvant therapies have been studied and are used variably across the world. These include specific postoperative nutritional supplementation in the form of fat-soluble vitamins or probiotics and medications such as ursodeoxycholic acid [50].

18.9 CMV IgM + Biliary Atresia

One of the theories surrounding BA development is a perinatal hepatobiliary virologic insult that subsequently results in the progressive cholangiopathy seen during infancy [51]. One of the proposed viruses that may play a role in this process is cytomegalovirus (CMV) [52]. It was then found that approximately 10% of BA patients have positive CMV IgM serology [53] and that they may represent a different phenotype of BA with distinct clinical factors. CMV IgM + BA patients were then found to have generally worse prognosis than non-CMV patients with respect to JCR, NLSR and overall survival (OS). Additionally, CMV IgM + BA patients had worse overall liver fibrosis, had KPE at a later age, and had worse liver function tests on presentation when compared to controls. After controlling for age, the differences in bilirubin and platelets on presentation were still significant [5]. After identifying this group as being clinically distinct, subsequent studies demonstrated that early postoperative use of antiviral therapy resulted in improved JCR and NLSR at 2 years post-KPE [54]. This growing body of literature still requires further prospective studies with larger patient populations but may at least highlight the utility of checking for CMV serology during the workup of BA.

18.10 Follow-Up and Summary

Regular and lifelong follow-up is essential in BA due to the progressive nature of the disease. Following KPE, surveillance in the form of regular laboratory work assessing bilirubin levels and trends in stool color is paramount in measuring the success of the procedure. Keeping a watchful eye for postoperative complications such as cholangitis is essential to outcomes as well. Even after successful biliary drainage is achieved by KPE, rates of LF requiring LT remain high, and so regular follow-up is necessary to assess liver health and identify the need for future interventions.

BA is a rare hepatobiliary disease of infancy, often requiring maximally invasive procedures for survival. Despite this, advances in our understanding of the disease process have led to considerable improvements in outcomes, with patients living well into adulthood. Given its rarity and complex multidisciplinary management, collaboration among institutions and even nations will be the key to future advances in the treatment of this disease.

Author Contributions P.C. wrote the initial draft; P.C. and C.W. revised and edited the manuscript—both authors read and agreed to the current version of the manuscript.

Conflicts of Interest The authors declare no conflict of interest.

Funding This received no external source of funding.

References

1. Hopkins PC, Yazigi N, Nylund CM. Incidence of biliary atresia and timing of hepatoportoenterostomy in the United States. J Pediatr. 2017;187:253–7. https://doi.org/10.1016/j.jpeds.2017.05.006.
2. Lakshminarayanan B, Davenport M. Biliary atresia: a comprehensive review. J Autoimmun. 2016;73:1–9. https://doi.org/10.1016/j.jaut.2016.06.005.
3. Morotti RA, Jain D. Pediatric cholestatic disorders: approach to pathologic diagnosis. Surg Pathol Clin. 2013;6(2):205–25. https://doi.org/10.1016/j.path.2013.03.001.
4. Davenport M, Muntean A, Hadzic N. Biliary atresia: clinical phenotypes and aetiological heterogeneity. J Clin Med. 2021;10(23) https://doi.org/10.3390/jcm10235675.
5. Zani A, Quaglia A, Hadzić N, Zuckerman M, Davenport M. Cytomegalovirus-associated biliary atresia: an aetiological and prognostic subgroup. J Pediatr Surg. 2015;50(10):1739–45. https://doi.org/10.1016/j.jpedsurg.2015.03.001.
6. Abbey P, Kandasamy D, Naranje P. Neonatal jaundice. Indian J Pediatr. 2019;86(9):830–41. https://doi.org/10.1007/s12098-019-02856-0.
7. Fawaz R, Baumann U, Ekong U, et al. Guideline for the evaluation of cholestatic jaundice in infants: joint recommendations of the north american society for pediatric gastroenterology, hepatology, and nutrition and the european society for pediatric gastroenterology, hepatology, and nutrition. J Pediatr Gastroenterol Nutr. 2017;64(1):154–68. https://doi.org/10.1097/MPG.0000000000001334.
8. Nio M. Japanese biliary atresia registry. Pediatr Surg Int. 2017;33(12):1319–25. https://doi.org/10.1007/s00383-017-4160-x.
9. Nio M, Wada M, Sasaki H, Tanaka H. Effects of age at Kasai portoenterostomy on the surgical outcome: a review of the literature. Surg Today. 2015;45(7):813–8. https://doi.org/10.1007/s00595-014-1024-z.
10. Yang C, Ke M, Zhou Y, Xu H, Diao M, Li L. Impact of early Kasai portoenterostomy on short-term outcomes of biliary atresia: a systematic review and meta-analysis. Front Surg. 2022;9:924506. https://doi.org/10.3389/fsurg.2022.924506.

11. Davenport M, De Ville de Goyet J, Stringer MD, et al. Seamless management of biliary atresia in England and Wales (1999–2002). Lancet. 2004;363(9418):1354–7. https://doi.org/10.1016/S0140-6736(04)16045-5.
12. Gu Y-H, Yokoyama K, Mizuta K, et al. Stool color card screening for early detection of biliary atresia and long-term native liver survival: a 19-year cohort study in Japan. J Pediatr. 2015;166(4):897–902.e1. https://doi.org/10.1016/j.jpeds.2014.12.063.
13. Harpavat S, Garcia-Prats JA, Anaya C, et al. Diagnostic yield of newborn screening for biliary atresia using direct or conjugated bilirubin measurements. JAMA. 2020;323(12):1141–50. https://doi.org/10.1001/jama.2020.0837.
14. He L, Ip DKM, Tam G, Lui VCH, Tam PKH, Chung PHY. Biomarkers for the diagnosis and post-Kasai portoenterostomy prognosis of biliary atresia: a systematic review and meta-analysis. Sci Rep. 2021;11(1):11692. https://doi.org/10.1038/s41598-021-91072-y.
15. Aldeiri B, Si T, Huang Z, et al. Matrix Metalloproteinase-7 and Osteopontin serum levels as biomarkers for biliary atresia. J Pediatr Gastroenterol Nutr. 2023;77(1):97–102. https://doi.org/10.1097/MPG.0000000000003792.
16. Irvine KM, Okano S, Patel PJ, et al. Serum matrix metalloproteinase 7 (MMP7) is a biomarker of fibrosis in patients with non-alcoholic fatty liver disease. Sci Rep. 2021;11(1):2858. https://doi.org/10.1038/s41598-021-82315-z.
17. Wu J-F, Jeng Y-M, Chen H-L, Ni Y-H, Hsu H-Y, Chang M-H. Quantification of serum matrix Metallopeptide 7 levels may assist in the diagnosis and predict the outcome for patients with biliary atresia. J Pediatr. 2019;208:30–37.e1. https://doi.org/10.1016/j.jpeds.2018.12.006.
18. Sakaguchi H, Konishi K-I, Yasuda R, et al. Serum matrix metalloproteinase-7 in biliary atresia: a Japanese multicenter study. Hepatol Res. 2022;52(5):479–87. https://doi.org/10.1111/hepr.13753.
19. Lee H-J, Lee S-M, Park W-H, Choi S-O. Objective criteria of triangular cord sign in biliary atresia on US scans. Radiology. 2003;229(2):395–400. https://doi.org/10.1148/radiol.292020472.
20. Kim WS, Cheon J-E, Youn BJ, et al. Hepatic arterial diameter measured with US: adjunct for US diagnosis of biliary atresia. Radiology. 2007;245(2):549–55. https://doi.org/10.1148/radiol.2452061093.
21. Napolitano M, Franchi-Abella S, Damasio MB, et al. Practical approach to imaging diagnosis of biliary atresia, part 1: prenatal ultrasound and magnetic resonance imaging, and postnatal ultrasound. Pediatr Radiol. 2021;51(2):314–31. https://doi.org/10.1007/s00247-020-04840-9.
22. Gunda ST, Chambara N, Chen XF, Pang MYC, Ying MT-C. Diagnostic efficacy of advanced ultrasonography imaging techniques in infants with biliary atresia (BA): a systematic review and meta-analysis. Children (Basel). 2022;9(11) https://doi.org/10.3390/children9111676.
23. Jain R, Gupta A, Kandasamy D, Jana M. Imaging in pediatric obstructive jaundice. Indian J Pediatr. 2022;89(9):899–907. https://doi.org/10.1007/s12098-022-04171-7.
24. Hays D, Woolley X, Snyder W. Diagnosis of 'liary atresia: relative accuracy of percutaneous liver biopsy, open liver biopJy, and operative cholangiography.
25. Russo P, Magee JC, Boitnott J, et al. Design and validation of the biliary atresia research consortium histologic assessment system for cholestasis in infancy. Clin Gastroenterol Hepatol. 2011;9(4):357–362.e2. https://doi.org/10.1016/j.cgh.2011.01.003.
26. Azar G, Beneck D, Lane B, Markowitz J, Daum F, Kahn E. Atypical morphologic presentation of biliary atresia and value of serial liver biopsies. J Pediatr Gastroenterol Nutr. 2002;34(2):212–5. https://doi.org/10.1097/00005176-200202000-00020.
27. Shteyer E, Wengrower D, Benuri-Silbiger I, Gozal D, Wilschanski M, Goldin E. Endoscopic retrograde cholangiopancreatography in neonatal cholestasis. J Pediatr Gastroenterol Nutr. 2012;55(2):142–5. https://doi.org/10.1097/MPG.0b013e318259267a.
28. Negm AA, Petersen C, Markowski A, et al. The role of endoscopic retrograde cholangiopancreatography in the diagnosis of biliary atresia: 14 years' experience. Eur J Pediatr Surg. 2018;28(3):261–7. https://doi.org/10.1055/s-0037-1602260.
29. Kianifar HR, Tehranian S, Shojaei P, et al. Accuracy of hepatobiliary scintigraphy for differentiation of neonatal hepatitis from biliary atresia: systematic review and meta-analysis of the literature. Pediatr Radiol. 2013;43(8):905–19. https://doi.org/10.1007/s00247-013-2623-3.
30. Balistreri WF. Neonatal cholestasis. J Pediatr. 1985;106(2):171–84. https://doi.org/10.1016/s0022-3476(85)80282-1.
31. Serinet M-O, Wildhaber BE, Broué P, et al. Impact of age at Kasai operation on its results in late childhood and adolescence: a rational basis for biliary atresia screening. Pediatrics. 2009;123(5):1280–6. https://doi.org/10.1542/peds.2008-1949.
32. Davenport M, Puricelli V, Farrant P, et al. The outcome of the older (> or =100 days) infant with biliary atresia. J Pediatr Surg. 2004;39(4):575–81. https://doi.org/10.1016/j.jpedsurg.2003.12.014.
33. Alexopoulos SP, Merrill M, Kin C, et al. The impact of hepatic portoenterostomy on liver transplantation for the treatment of biliary atresia: early failure adversely affects outcome. Pediatr Transplant. 2012;16(4):373–8. https://doi.org/10.1111/j.1399-3046.2012.01677.x.
34. Yoeli D, Choudhury RA, Sundaram SS, et al. Primary vs. salvage liver transplantation for biliary atresia: a retrospective cohort study. J Pediatr Surg. 2022;57(10):407–13. https://doi.org/10.1016/j.jpedsurg.2021.12.027.

35. Tambucci R, de Magnée C, Szabo M, et al. Sequential treatment of biliary atresia with Kasai hepatoportoenterostomy and liver transplantation: benefits, risks, and outcome in 393 children. Front Pediatr. 2021;9:697581. https://doi.org/10.3389/fped.2021.697581.
36. Sundaram SS, Mack CL, Feldman AG, Sokol RJ. Biliary atresia: indications and timing of liver transplantation and optimization of pretransplant care. Liver Transpl. 2017;23(1):96–109. https://doi.org/10.1002/lt.24640.
37. Shneider BL, Brown MB, Haber B, et al. A multicenter study of the outcome of biliary atresia in the United States, 1997 to 2000. J Pediatr. 2006;148(4):467–74. https://doi.org/10.1016/j.jpeds.2005.12.054.
38. Shirota C, Hinoki A, Tainaka T, et al. Laparoscopic Kasai portoenterostomy can be a standard surgical procedure for treatment of biliary atresia. World J Gastrointest Surg. 2022;14(1):56–63. https://doi.org/10.4240/wjgs.v14.i1.56.
39. Ure BM, Kuebler JF, Schukfeh N, Engelmann C, Dingemann J, Petersen C. Survival with the native liver after laparoscopic versus conventional Kasai portoenterostomy in infants with biliary atresia: a prospective trial. Ann Surg. 2011;253(4):826–30. https://doi.org/10.1097/SLA.0b013e318211d7d8.
40. Baek SH, Kang J-M, Ihn K, Han SJ, Koh H, Ahn JG. The epidemiology and etiology of cholangitis after Kasai portoenterostomy in patients with biliary atresia. J Pediatr Gastroenterol Nutr. 2020;70(2):171–7. https://doi.org/10.1097/MPG.0000000000002555.
41. Qiao G, Li L, Cheng W, Zhang Z, Ge J, Wang C. Conditional probability of survival in patients with biliary atresia after Kasai portoenterostomy: a Chinese population-based study. J Pediatr Surg. 2015;50(8):1310–5. https://doi.org/10.1016/j.jpedsurg.2015.03.062.
42. Pietrobattista A, Mosca A, Liccardo D, et al. Does the treatment after Kasai procedure influence biliary atresia outcome and native liver survival? J Pediatr Gastroenterol Nutr. 2020;71(4):446–51. https://doi.org/10.1097/MPG.0000000000002837.
43. de Vries W, de Langen ZJ, Groen H, et al. Biliary atresia in The Netherlands: outcome of patients diagnosed between 1987 and 2008. J Pediatr. 2012;160(4):638–644.e2. https://doi.org/10.1016/j.jpeds.2011.09.061.
44. Bu L-N, Chen H-L, Chang C-J, et al. Prophylactic oral antibiotics in prevention of recurrent cholangitis after the Kasai portoenterostomy. J Pediatr Surg. 2003;38(4):590–3. https://doi.org/10.1053/jpsu.2003.50128.
45. Wong ZH, Davenport M. What happens after Kasai for biliary atresia? A European multicenter survey. Eur J Pediatr Surg. 2019;29(1):1–6. https://doi.org/10.1055/s-0038-1668146.
46. Davenport M, Stringer MD, Tizzard SA, McClean P, Mieli-Vergani G, Hadzic N. Randomized, double-blind, placebo-controlled trial of corticosteroids after Kasai portoenterostomy for biliary atresia. Hepatology. 2007;46(6):1821–7. https://doi.org/10.1002/hep.21873.
47. Davenport M, Parsons C, Tizzard S, Hadzic N. Steroids in biliary atresia: single surgeon, single centre, prospective study. J Hepatol. 2013;59(5):1054–8. https://doi.org/10.1016/j.jhep.2013.06.012.
48. Bezerra JA, Spino C, Magee JC, et al. Use of corticosteroids after hepatoportoenterostomy for bile drainage in infants with biliary atresia: the START randomized clinical trial. JAMA. 2014;311(17):1750–9. https://doi.org/10.1001/jama.2014.2623.
49. Alonso EM, Ye W, Hawthorne K, et al. Impact of steroid therapy on early growth in infants with biliary atresia: the multicenter steroids in biliary atresia randomized trial. J Pediatr. 2018;202:179–185.e4. https://doi.org/10.1016/j.jpeds.2018.07.002.
50. Burns J, Davenport M. Adjuvant treatments for biliary atresia. Transl Pediatr. 2020;9(3):253–65. https://doi.org/10.21037/tp.2016.10.08.
51. Mack CL. The pathogenesis of biliary atresia: evidence for a virus-induced autoimmune disease. Semin Liver Dis. 2007;27(3):233–42. https://doi.org/10.1055/s-2007-985068.
52. Wang W, Zheng S, Shong Z, Zhao R. Development of a Guinea pig model of perinatal cytomegalovirus-induced hepatobiliary injury. Fetal Pediatr Pathol. 2011;30(5):301–11. https://doi.org/10.3109/15513815.2011.572959.
53. Rauschenfels S, Krassmann M, Al-Masri AN, et al. Incidence of hepatotropic viruses in biliary atresia. Eur J Pediatr. 2009;168(4):469–76. https://doi.org/10.1007/s00431-008-0774-2.
54. Parolini F, Hadzic N, Davenport M. Adjuvant therapy of cytomegalovirus IgM + ve associated biliary atresia: prima facie evidence of effect. J Pediatr Surg. 2019;54(9):1941–5. https://doi.org/10.1016/j.jpedsurg.2018.12.014.
55. Lefkowitch JH. Biliary atresia. Mayo Clin Proc. 1998;73(1):90–5. https://doi.org/10.1016/S0025-6196(11)63625-2.

Hepatoblastoma

19

Zachary J. Kastenberg,
Manuel I. Rodriguez-Davalos, and Talia B. Baker

19.1 Incidence

Liver malignancies account for approximately two percent of all pediatric cancers [1]. Hepatoblastoma (HB) is the most common liver malignancy of childhood, representing approximately 67 percent of pediatric liver cancers [2]. Hepatoblastoma typically occurs in infancy or toddlerhood, with the vast majority of cases presenting within the first four years of life. The incidence of HB is 1.76:1,000,000 live births and has increased significantly in recent decades (1.4–7.2 percent per year) [3, 4]. There is a strong association between prematurity and the incidence of HB, suggesting that the observed increase in overall incidence is, at least in part, due to the improved survival of contemporary preterm deliveries [5–8]. Hepatocellular carcinoma (HCC) is the second most common pediatric liver malignancy, representing 31% of pediatric liver cancers [2]. Hepatocellular carcinoma most commonly occurs in teenagers. Hepatocellular neoplasm not otherwise specified (HCN-NOS), often described as "transitional cell tumor" or "HB with HCC features," represents a much rarer malignancy that displays histologic features of both HB and HCC and tends to occur in an intermediate age group [9, 10].

19.2 Clinical Presentation

Infants and toddlers with hepatoblastoma typically present with an abdominal mass and distension. Not infrequently, the child has been treated for presumed constipation. Occasionally, tumor rupture secondary to trauma, generally fairly minor in nature, leads to the presenting symptoms of acute pain and peritonitis secondary to hemoperitoneum. By the time the patient is referred to a children's hospital or the surgical consultation is arranged, an ultrasound has often confirmed the presence of a liver mass.

Neonatal liver masses are increasingly identified by screening or directed ultrasounds performed for a variety of reasons in the neonatal intensive care unit. Incidental liver masses in this population may represent hepatoblastoma. The most common neonatal liver mass, however, is a congenital or, in some cases, infantile hemangioma. Complicating the diagnostic process in this patient population is the anticipated elevation in alpha-fetoprotein (AFP) during the neonatal period. Advanced imaging, including magnetic resonance imaging (MRI) with hepatocyte-

Z. J. Kastenberg · M. I. Rodriguez-Davalos
T. B. Baker (✉)
University of Utah School of Medicine,
Salt Lake City, UT, USA

Primary Children's Hospital, Intermountain Health,
Salt Lake City, UT, USA
e-mail: zachary.kastenburg@hsc.utah.edu;
manuel.rodriguez-davalos@hsc.utah.edu;
talia.baker@hsc.utah.edu

T. Hackert, A. Gulla (eds.), *Rare Liver and Biliary Tract Diseases*,
https://doi.org/10.1007/978-3-032-15076-9_19

specific contrast enhancement as discussed below, and AFP trends compared against age-based nomograms are helpful in formulating an initial approach to the neonate with a liver mass.

Hepatoblastoma is associated with a number of well-defined genetic conditions and, in these populations, will generally be identified in the context of routine screening. Beckwith–Wiedemann syndrome (BWS) and a variety of overgrowth syndromes are associated with the development of solid tumors, including HB. The relative risk of HB in infants and toddlers with BWS is 2280 times the risk of HB in the healthy population, with the majority of cases occurring in the first year of life [11]. While the majority of neonates and infants with Trisomy 18 succumb to cardiopulmonary complications prior to their first birthday, there is a notable increase in the development of HB in survivors and in those with Trisomy 18 mosaicism. Familial adenomatous polyposis (FAP) syndrome is also associated with an increased risk of developing HB (0.3–1.6%), with most cases occurring in the first 3 years of life [12, 13]. Screening recommendations for patients with BWS and Trisomy 18 include a complete abdominal ultrasound and AFP every three months starting at birth and continuing through the child's fourth birthday [14]. For patients with FAP, it is recommended to continue this screening through the child's seventh birthday [15].

19.3 Work-Up/Investigation

The initial diagnostic study for a child with an abdominal mass and distension is typically an ultrasound. In general, ultrasonography will help distinguish the tissue of origin and thus will give a strong indication as to the potential underlying diagnosis. Solid renal masses will most often represent Wilms tumor, suprarenal masses most often neuroblastoma, while solid tumors of the liver will be highly suspicious for hepatoblastoma.

A solid liver mass identified by ultrasonography or, in some cases, computed tomography (CT) scan, should be followed by laboratory investigation, including AFP. Alpha-fetoprotein is typically elevated in HB, often dramatically so, and is used, following diagnosis, as a marker for response to treatment and in surveillance for recurrence. While contemporary risk stratification schema (see below) describe a high-risk HB patient group for whom AFP is not elevated (less than 100 ng/mL), it is becoming increasingly recognized that this patient group likely represents, in fact, patients with rhabdoid tumor of the liver [16, 17].

Magnetic resonance imaging (MRI) of the liver with hepatocyte-specific contrast enhancement (e.g., gadoxetate disodium/Eovist® or gadopentetate dimeglumine/MultiHance®) is particularly useful in the preoperative work-up and risk stratification for patients with presumed hepatoblastoma. While the specific MRI characteristics of HB are variable, these masses are generally hypointense relative to normal liver on T1-weighted images and display decreased enhancement relative to normal liver in both the post-contrast arterial and portal venous phases, with very little retained contrast on hepatocyte-phased images [18]. Technological advances in MRI have established it as the most effective modality in the identification of macrovascular tumor involvement and in the identification of multifocal disease, two important factors in risk stratification and operative planning [19, 20].

Tissue diagnosis is recommended in cases of diagnostic uncertainty and for tumors not amenable to upfront resection. It is acceptable to biopsy these masses by open, laparoscopic, or percutaneous approach, with the key principle being that one must obtain enough tissue for both histologic and biologic evaluation. Current recommendations suggest that an operative biopsy obtain a minimum of one cubic centimeter of tumor tissue and one small wedge biopsy of normal liver, while a percutaneous biopsy should obtain a minimum of 7 cores of tumor and 2 cores of normal liver tissue with a 16-gauge core needle biopsy. It is highly recommended that the surgeon participate in the planning of the approach with the proceduralist. Specifically, the percutaneous approach should be such that the needle traverses a portion of normal liver prior to penetrating the tumor and that this section of normal liver be included in the anticipated future resection specimen. Following these guidelines will limit hemorrhage, peritoneal dissemination through capsular rupture, and morbidity related to seeding of the biopsy tract.

Importantly, percutaneous biopsy is gaining traction as the preferred tissue acquisition technique for pediatric liver tumors. A recent analysis of the Children's Oncology Group AHEP0731 study suggested the superiority of the percutaneous approach with decreased morbidity and no decrease in the rate of appropriate tissue acquisition [21]. Of the 121 children evaluated, 63 percent underwent open biopsy, 14 percent laparoscopic biopsy, and 23 percent percutaneous biopsy. All 121 procedures yielded sufficient tissue for diagnosis, while the rates of clinically significant hemorrhage were 36 percent, 24 percent, and 0 percent ($p < 0.01$) for open, laparoscopic, and percutaneous biopsy, respectively.

Upon confirming the diagnosis of HB, a complete staging work-up is necessary. Hepatoblastoma most commonly metastasizes to the lungs, necessitating a non-contrast CT scan of the chest for disease staging prior to initiating treatment. To date, there is no recognized indication for positron emission tomography or other radioisotope-based imaging in the diagnosis or staging of HB.

19.4 Differential Diagnosis

The differential diagnosis for liver masses in children is broad and age-group dependent, with not infrequent transgressions of the following generalizations. Neonates, infants, and toddlers experience hepatic hemangiomas (both congenital and infantile), mesenchymal hamartomas, rhabdoid tumor of the liver, and HB. Adolescents/teenagers experience focal nodular hyperplasia, hepatic adenomas, undifferentiated embryonal sarcoma of the liver, and HCC. Intermediate-aged children can experience any of these pathologies, while HCN-NOS occurs in this age group most commonly. Despite clues lent by the age of the patient, laboratory findings, and imaging characteristics, histologic evaluation is often required to confirm a final diagnosis.

19.5 Treatment

The current algorithm for the treatment of HB represents an international collaboration between the Children's Oncology Group (COG, North America), Societe Internationale d'Oncologie Pediatrique—Epithelia Liver Tumor Study Group (SIOPEL, Europe), and Japanese Children's Cancer Group (JCCG, Japan). The ongoing Pediatric Hepatic Malignancy International Therapeutic Trial (PHITT) employs upfront risk stratification, cisplatin-based chemotherapy, and an organized approach to operative resection. Risk stratification is based upon the imaging characteristics of the liver mass, the age of the patient, and the AFP level at presentation (Fig. 19.1) [16, 22, 23]. The radiographic components of this risk stratification are based upon the PRETEXT system created by SIOPEL in the 1990s and subsequently adopted by the COG in the 2010s (Fig. 19.2). The PRETEXT system has become an accepted international language for discussing HB and facilitating the accumulation of comparable transcontinental outcomes.

The Brisbane nomenclature (hemiliver, section, and segment) forms the basis for the PRETEXT system. A patient's PRETEXT group is defined by the number of contiguous liver sections that are tumor-free. A PRETEXT group is assigned at diagnosis, and a POST-TEXT (post-treatment extent of tumor) group is assigned following neoadjuvant therapy. A PRETEXT I mass involves one section and leaves three adjacent sections free of tumor; a PRETEXT II mass leaves two adjacent sections free of tumor; a PRETEXT III mass leaves one section free of tumor; and a PRETEXT IV mass involves all four sections. Annotation factors further describe the extent of the mass by standardizing the language surrounding vascular involvement and other important radiographic tumor characteristics. Specifically, annotation factors include involvement of the retrohepatic vena cava and hepatic veins (V), the portal vein (P), extrahe-

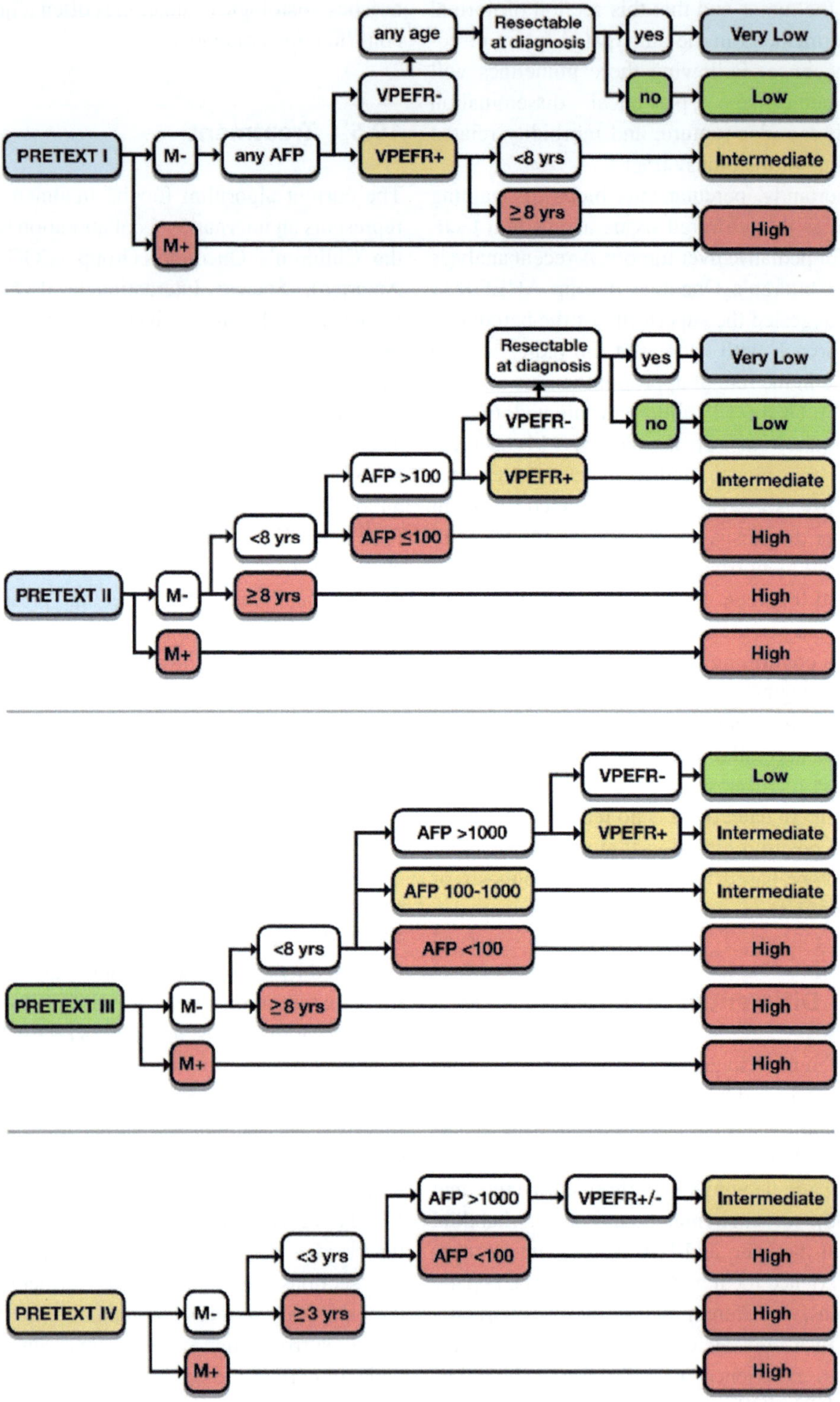

Fig. 19.1 Children's Hepatic tumor International Collaboration (CHIC) hepatoblastoma risk stratification

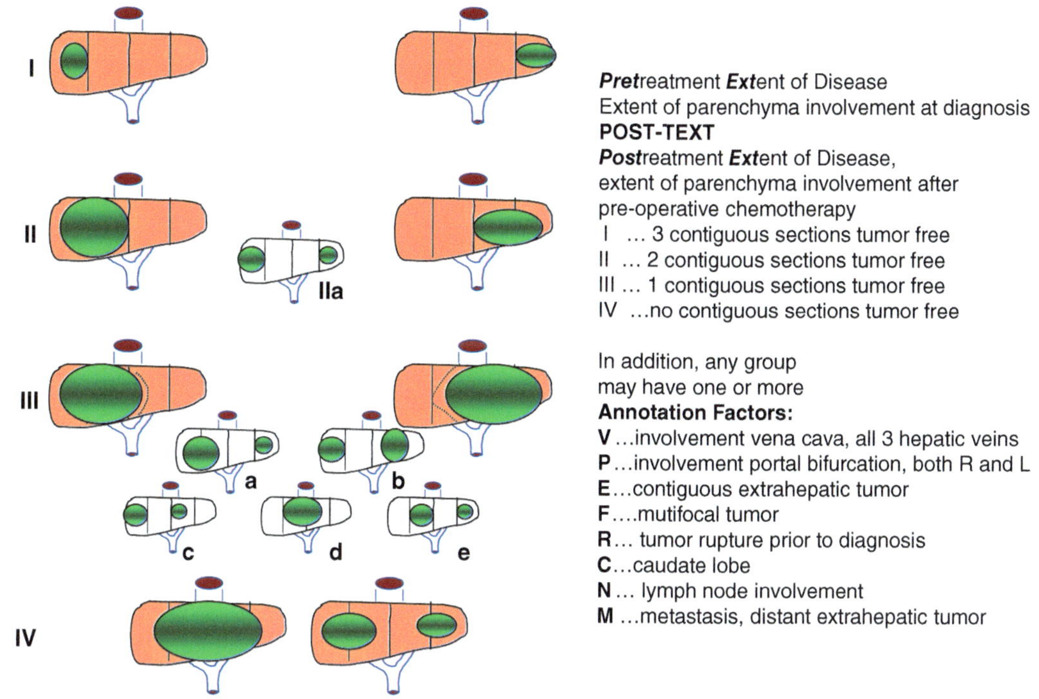

Fig. 19.2 PRETEXT and POST-TEXT groups based on extent of parenchymal involvement at diagnosis and following neo-adjuvant chemotherapy, respectively

patic contiguous disease (E), multifocal disease (F), tumor rupture (R), caudate involvement (C), lymph node involvement (N), and metastatic disease (M) [19].

Given the rarity of HB and HCC in children and adolescents, it is recommended to approach these patients from a multidisciplinary perspective and to, whenever possible, advocate for enrollment on open trial protocols through the COG, SIOPEL, JCCG, or other collaborative organizations. It is also highly recommended to engage in early consultation and referral when necessary with centers capable of advanced hepatobiliary surgery and/or liver transplantation when managing patients with liver tumors unlikely to be safely and completely resected by conventional hepatectomy.

19.6 Surgical Planning/Management

19.6.1 Resection at Diagnosis

PRETEXT I and II tumors are candidates for upfront resection if there is ≥1 cm radiographic margin at the portal vein bifurcation, the retrohepatic inferior vena cava, and the middle hepatic vein, *and* if no other annotation factors are present *and* if the mass can be resected with an anticipated negative margin by either segmentectomy, sectionectomy, or conventional hemihepatectomy [24]. Upfront resection has been championed in recent years, given the potential to reduce cumulative chemotherapy exposure and, in some cases, avoid chemotherapy altogether. Under current protocols, children undergoing upfront resection with negative margins and histopathologic confirmation of pure fetal histology require no adjuvant chemotherapy [25].

19.6.2 Resection Following Neoadjuvant Therapy

Biopsy followed by neoadjuvant chemotherapy is the standard approach for PRETEXT II tumors within 1 cm of the portal bifurcation, retrohepatic vena cava, or middle hepatic vein, or with annotation factors, and for PRETEXT III and IV tumors. Early delayed resections should be considered following two cycles of cisplatin-based chemotherapy for tumors amenable to resection by conventional sectionectomy or hemihepatectomy—POST-TEXT I or II with no annotation factors and ≥1 cm margin from the portal bifurcation, retrohepatic vena cava, and middle hepatic vein. If the patient is not a candidate for resection under these criteria, the patient is radiographically reevaluated following four cycles of chemotherapy. At this point, definitive local control should be achieved. At this juncture, it is reasonable to consider an extended hepatectomy.

It is important to acknowledge that the majority of the chemotherapy response will have been achieved following the fourth cycle of cisplatin-based chemotherapy. Further adjuvant therapy will offer little anatomic benefit and has the potential to contribute to the propagation of chemoresistant clonal populations [26–28]. In this setting, it is also important to be prepared for extreme resections with vascular reconstruction or orthotopic liver transplantation. As such, referral to a center with advanced hepatobiliary surgical expertise and liver transplant capabilities is recommended soon after diagnosis for patients with PRETEXT III, annotation-factor-positive tumors and for patients with PRETEXT IV tumors.

The decision to undertake an extreme resection with or without vascular reconstruction as opposed to proceeding directly to liver transplant is a difficult and nuanced one. Historically, rescue transplant following recurrence resulted in inferior oncologic outcomes when compared with upfront transplant, though recent studies have begun to challenge this dogma [29–31]. On the other hand, there are now many long-term survivors of extreme hepatectomy who are free of immunosuppression and the chronic issues inherent to liver transplant. The preoperative decision-making process must include interpretation of the individual anatomy, AFP response (dramatic response may make the surgical team more comfortable assuming the thrombus is bland or close margins acceptable), and the family's perspective regarding the risk/benefit discussion. In the setting where a living donor is an option, proceeding with anticipated resection while having the donor on standby provides another option in difficult cases. Certainly, when metastatic disease cannot be easily cleared, and transplant is contraindicated, one should consider resections involving vascular reconstruction, combined extended hepatectomy with nonanatomic resection, mesohepatectomy, and caudate resections as indicated.

19.6.3 Liver Transplant

Liver transplant is a well-accepted approach for patients with multifocal disease, POST-TEXT III annotation-factor-positive tumors, and POST-TEXT IV tumors when resection with negative margins and an appropriate functional liver remnant is infeasible. As noted above, there are many nuances to this decision-making process. While both the ongoing PHITT trial and the most recent past COG trial (AHEP0731) aim to identify the optimal timing of referral for transplant evaluations, it is currently a strong recommendation that the referral occur at diagnosis or after the first two cycles of chemotherapy for PRETEXT III annotation factor-positive tumors and for PRETEXT IV tumors. The goal is to minimize excessive chemotherapy while awaiting transplant, being cognizant of the fact that many of these locally advanced tumors will, in fact, become resectable following induction chemotherapy. As such, an open and ongoing dialogue should be carried out between centers to promote timely transplant when appropriate, while preventing unnecessary transplants for disease rendered amenable to conventional resection.

19.6.4 Lung Metastases

Approximately 20% of children with hepatoblastoma will present with lung metastases [32]. Response to chemotherapy is monitored by interval cross-sectional imaging and AFP trend. If metastatic disease persists following induction chemotherapy, pulmonary metastasectomy is recommended. The timing of metastasectomy can be tailored to the clinical situation and may occur prior to or after definitive local control. In the setting of liver transplant, this is a debated topic with various practice patterns. In general, pulmonary clearance (with chemotherapy or surgery) is recommended prior to proceeding with liver transplantation.

19.6.5 Lymph Nodes, Extrahepatic Extension, Tumor Rupture

Lymph nodes are rarely the site of metastatic disease for HB. Hepatocellular carcinoma is, of course, more frequently metastatic to the lymph nodes. Given that diagnostic uncertainty is not unusual at the time of resection and that HCN-NOS can be diagnosed postoperatively, portal lymph node sampling is recommended during the hilar dissection. Excision of any enlarged nodes identified at the time of exploration is also encouraged, though no formal lymphadenectomy is mandated.

Extrahepatic extension is occasionally encountered. Involved structures may include the diaphragm, abdominal wall, stomach, colon, or small bowel. Involvement of these structures or other retroperitoneal structures, such as the kidney or duodenum, should prompt consideration for possible misclassification of a more aggressive rhabdoid tumor of the liver. INI-1 retention on immunohistopathology will exclude this diagnosis. When a contiguous extrahepatic extension of the tumor is identified at exploration, if upfront resection is being attempted, a biopsy should be performed and the operation terminated in anticipation of neoadjuvant chemotherapy. If encountered following chemotherapy, *en bloc* resection without tumor transgression should be the goal.

Preoperative tumor rupture related to minor trauma is not an uncommon presenting scenario. It has been shown that neoadjuvant therapy in this setting is desirable [33]. When peritoneal fluid is identified on cross-sectional imaging, tumor rupture is confirmed when at least one of the following is present: The fluid has internal complexity or septations, density > 25 Hounsfield units, characteristics of blood degradation products by MRI, echogenic debris by US, or visible rupture of the liver capsule by imaging. Upfront resections following rupture should be limited to cases in which bleeding is refractory to less invasive maneuvers, including, if needed, transarterial embolization.

19.6.6 Adjuncts to Surgical Resection

Indocyanine green (ICG) is a fluorescent molecule that has been used as a labeling compound for decades. It has recently been described as a semi-selective tumor-labeling agent for a number of malignancies. Preoperative administration of ICG to children with hepatoblastoma has proven useful for intraoperative delineation of primary tumor margins (Fig. 19.3a), multifocal liver disease (Fig. 19.3b), and pulmonary metastasectomy (Fig. 19.3c, d), with up to 10% of patients having pulmonary metastases resected based solely upon ICG avidity [34, 35].

Transarterial radioembolization (TARE) and chemoembolization (TACE) have been used with some success in cases of unresectable HB refractory to chemotherapy [36–39]. Given the general chemosensitivity of HB, these techniques are reserved for refractory or relapsed cases. Future collaborative efforts will aim to identify radiographic and/or pathologic criteria to delineate patient subgroups who may benefit from more aggressive administration of these directed therapies.

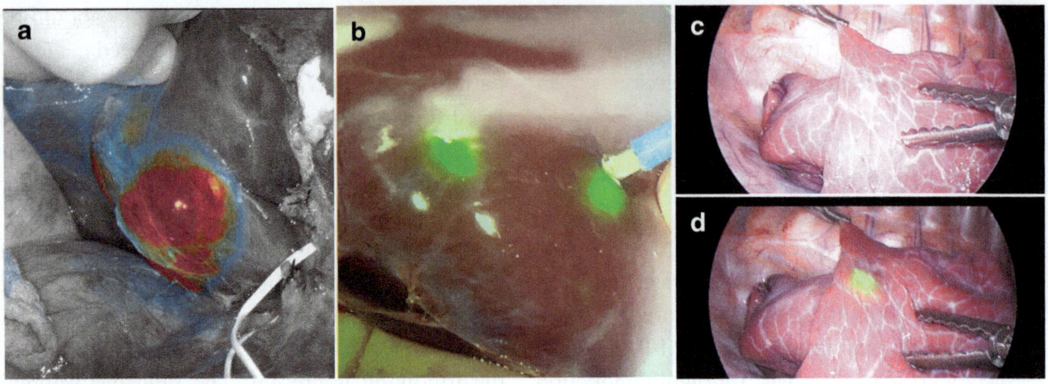

Fig. 19.3 Indocyanine green (ICG) imaging of (**a**) Segment 6 mass margin determination prior to resection; (**b**) Multifocal disease; and (**c**, **d**) Thoracoscopic identification of pulmonary metastasis

19.7 Follow-Up and Outcomes

Following resection and completion of adjuvant therapy, children will require routine physical exam, AFP monitoring, and surveillance imaging (US, CT, or MRI of the abdomen and CT of the chest) as well as routine liver function tests. Long-term implications, in addition to relapse, include the sequelae of major liver resection as well as the late effects of platinum chemotherapy. Despite these potential long-term effects, outcomes for hepatoblastoma have improved dramatically in recent years. Data from the most recent COG trial describe 100% event-free survival (EFS) and overall survival (OS) for patients in the lowest risk category, 91% EFS and 97% OS for low-risk patients, 87% EFS and 95% OS for intermediate-risk patients, and 49% EFS and 62% OS for those with metastatic disease [10]. With improved chemotherapy regimens, aggressive surgical approaches, and continued development of targeted and adjunctive therapies, it is anticipated that this trend will continue as the next generation of collaborative trials is initiated.

References

1. Siegel RL, Miller KD, Jemal A. Cancer statistics, 2020. CA Cancer J Clin. 2020;70(1):7–30. https://doi.org/10.3322/caac.21590.
2. Darbari A, Sabin KM, Shapiro CN, Schwarz KB. Epidemiology of primary hepatic malignancies in U.S. children. Hepatology. 2003;38(3):560–6. https://doi.org/10.1053/jhep.2003.50375.
3. Hubbard AK, Spector LG, Fortuna G, Marcotte EL, Poynter JN. Trends in international incidence of pediatric cancers in children under 5 years of age: 1988–2012. JNCI Cancer Spectr. 2019;3(1):pkz007. https://doi.org/10.1093/jncics/pkz007.
4. Kahla JA, Siegel DA, Dai S, et al. Incidence and 5-year survival of children and adolescents with hepatoblastoma in the United States. Pediatr Blood Cancer. 2022;69(10):e29763. https://doi.org/10.1002/pbc.29763.
5. Feusner J, Buckley J, Robison L, Ross J, Van Tornout J. Prematurity and hepatoblastoma: more than just an association? J Pediatr. 1998;133(4):585–6. https://doi.org/10.1016/s0022-3476(98)70084-8.
6. Feusner J, Plaschkes J. Hepatoblastoma and low birth weight: a trend or chance observation? Med Pediatr Oncol. 2002;39(5):508–9. https://doi.org/10.1002/mpo.10176.
7. Paquette K, Coltin H, Boivin A, Amre D, Nuyt AM, Luu TM. Cancer risk in children and young adults born preterm: a systematic review and meta-analysis. PLoS One. 2019;14(1):e0210366. https://doi.org/10.1371/journal.pone.0210366.
8. Spector LG, Johnson KJ, Soler JT, Puumala SE. Perinatal risk factors for hepatoblastoma. Br J Cancer. 2008;98(9):1570–3. https://doi.org/10.1038/sj.bjc.6604335.
9. Lopez-Terrada D, Alaggio R, de Davila MT, et al. Towards an international pediatric liver tumor consensus classification: proceedings of the Los Angeles COG liver tumors symposium. Mod Pathol. 2014;27(3):472–91. https://doi.org/10.1038/modpathol.2013.80.
10. Meyers R, Hiyama E, Czauderna P, Tiao GM. Liver tumors in pediatric patients. Surg Oncol Clin N

Am. 2021;30(2):253–74. https://doi.org/10.1016/j.soc.2020.11.006.
11. DeBaun MR, Tucker MA. Risk of cancer during the first four years of life in children from the Beckwith-Wiedemann Syndrome Registry. J Pediatr. 1998;132(3 Pt 1):398–400. https://doi.org/10.1016/s0022-3476(98)70008-3.
12. Aretz S, Koch A, Uhlhaas S, et al. Should children at risk for familial adenomatous polyposis be screened for hepatoblastoma and children with apparently sporadic hepatoblastoma be screened for APC germline mutations? Pediatr Blood Cancer. 2006;47(6):811–8. https://doi.org/10.1002/pbc.20698.
13. Giardiello FM, Offerhaus GJ, Krush AJ, et al. Risk of hepatoblastoma in familial adenomatous polyposis. J Pediatr. 1991;119(5):766–8. https://doi.org/10.1016/s0022-3476(05)80297-5.
14. Kalish JM, Doros L, Helman LJ, et al. Surveillance recommendations for children with overgrowth syndromes and predisposition to Wilms tumors and Hepatoblastoma. Clin Cancer Res. 2017;23(13):e115–22. https://doi.org/10.1158/1078-0432.CCR-17-0710.
15. Achatz MI, Porter CC, Brugieres L, et al. Cancer screening recommendations and clinical management of inherited gastrointestinal cancer syndromes in childhood. Clin Cancer Res. 2017;23(13):e107–14. https://doi.org/10.1158/1078-0432.CCR-17-0790.
16. Meyers RL, Maibach R, Hiyama E, et al. Risk-stratified staging in paediatric hepatoblastoma: a unified analysis from the Children's Hepatic tumors International Collaboration. Lancet Oncol. 2017;18(1):122–31. https://doi.org/10.1016/S1470-2045(16)30598-8.
17. Trobaugh-Lotrario AD, Tomlinson GE, Finegold MJ, Gore L, Feusner JH. Small cell undifferentiated variant of hepatoblastoma: adverse clinical and molecular features similar to rhabdoid tumors. Pediatr Blood Cancer. 2009;52(3):328–34. https://doi.org/10.1002/pbc.21834.
18. Pugmire BS, Towbin AJ. Magnetic resonance imaging of primary pediatric liver tumors. Pediatr Radiol. 2016;46(6):764–77. https://doi.org/10.1007/s00247-016-3612-0.
19. Towbin AJ, Meyers RL, Woodley H, et al. 2017 PRETEXT: radiologic staging system for primary hepatic malignancies of childhood revised for the Paediatric Hepatic International Tumour Trial (PHITT). Pediatr Radiol. 2018;48(4):536–54. https://doi.org/10.1007/s00247-018-4078-z.
20. Kolbe AB, Podberesky DJ, Zhang B, Towbin AJ. The impact of hepatocyte phase imaging from infancy to young adulthood in patients with a known or suspected liver lesion. Pediatr Radiol. 2015;45(3):354–65. https://doi.org/10.1007/s00247-014-3160-4.
21. Weldon CB, Madenci AL, Tiao GM, et al. Evaluation of the diagnostic biopsy approach for children with hepatoblastoma: a report from the children's oncology group AHEP 0731 liver tumor committee. J Pediatr Surg. 2020;55(4):655–9. https://doi.org/10.1016/j.jpedsurg.2019.05.004.
22. Czauderna P, Haeberle B, Hiyama E, et al. The Children's Hepatic tumors International Collaboration (CHIC): novel global rare tumor database yields new prognostic factors in hepatoblastoma and becomes a research model. Eur J Cancer. 2016;52:92–101. https://doi.org/10.1016/j.ejca.2015.09.023.
23. Haeberle B, Rangaswami A, Krailo M, et al. The importance of age as prognostic factor for the outcome of patients with hepatoblastoma: analysis from the Children's Hepatic tumors International Collaboration (CHIC) database. Pediatr Blood Cancer. 2020;67(8):e28350. https://doi.org/10.1002/pbc.28350.
24. Meyers RL, Tiao G, de Ville de Goyet J, Superina R, Aronson DC. Hepatoblastoma state of the art: pretreatment extent of disease, surgical resection guidelines and the role of liver transplantation. Curr Opin Pediatr. 2014;26(1):29–36. https://doi.org/10.1097/MOP.0000000000000042.
25. Malogolowkin MH, Katzenstein HM, Meyers RL, et al. Complete surgical resection is curative for children with hepatoblastoma with pure fetal histology: a report from the Children's Oncology Group. J Clin Oncol. 2011;29(24):3301–6. https://doi.org/10.1200/JCO.2010.29.3837.
26. Marin JJG, Cives-Losada C, Asensio M, Lozano E, Briz O, Macias RIR. Mechanisms of anticancer drug resistance in Hepatoblastoma. Cancers (Basel). 2019;11(3) https://doi.org/10.3390/cancers11030407.
27. Perilongo G, Maibach R, Shafford E, et al. Cisplatin versus cisplatin plus doxorubicin for standard-risk hepatoblastoma. N Engl J Med. 2009;361(17):1662–70. https://doi.org/10.1056/NEJMoa0810613.
28. Zsiros J, Brugieres L, Brock P, et al. Dose-dense cisplatin-based chemotherapy and surgery for children with high-risk hepatoblastoma (SIOPEL-4): a prospective, single-arm, feasibility study. Lancet Oncol. 2013;14(9):834–42. https://doi.org/10.1016/s1470-2045(13)70272-9.
29. Browne M, Sher D, Grant D, et al. Survival after liver transplantation for hepatoblastoma: a 2-center experience. J Pediatr Surg. 2008;43(11):1973–81. https://doi.org/10.1016/j.jpedsurg.2008.05.031.
30. Uchida H, Sakamoto S, Sasaki K, et al. Surgical treatment strategy for advanced hepatoblastoma: resection versus transplantation. Pediatr Blood Cancer. 2018;65(12):e27383. https://doi.org/10.1002/pbc.27383.
31. Umeda K, Okajima H, Kawaguchi K, et al. Prognostic and therapeutic factors influencing the clinical outcome of hepatoblastoma after liver transplantation: a single-institute experience. Pediatr Transplant. 2018;22(2) https://doi.org/10.1111/petr.13113.
32. O'Neill AF, Towbin AJ, Krailo MD, et al. Characterization of pulmonary metastases in children with Hepatoblastoma treated on children's oncology group protocol AHEP0731 (the treatment of children with all stages of Hepatoblastoma): a report from the Children's Oncology Group. J Clin Oncol.

2017;35(30):3465–73. https://doi.org/10.1200/JCO.2017.73.5654.
33. Hiyama E, Hishiki T, Watanabe K, et al. Mortality and morbidity in primarily resected hepatoblastomas in Japan: experience of the JPLT (Japanese Study Group for Pediatric Liver Tumor) trials. J Pediatr Surg. 2015;50(12):2098–101. https://doi.org/10.1016/j.jpedsurg.2015.08.035.
34. Lake CM, Bondoc AJ, Dasgupta R, et al. Indocyanine green is a sensitive adjunct in the identification and surgical management of local and metastatic hepatoblastoma. Cancer Med. 2021;10(13):4322–43. https://doi.org/10.1002/cam4.3982.
35. Whitlock RS, Patel KR, Yang T, Nguyen HN, Masand P, Vasudevan SA. Pathologic correlation with near infrared-indocyanine green guided surgery for pediatric liver cancer. J Pediatr Surg. 2022;57(4):700–10. https://doi.org/10.1016/j.jpedsurg.2021.04.019.
36. Balli HT, Aikimbaev K, Guney IB, et al. Trans-arterial Radioembolization with Yttrium-90 of Unresectable and systemic chemotherapy resistant Hepatoblastoma in three toddlers. Cardiovasc Intervent Radiol. 2022;45(3):344–8. https://doi.org/10.1007/s00270-021-03026-6.
37. Yagci-Kupeli B, Balli T. Hepatoblastoma treated successfully with drug-eluting bead transarterial chemoembolization: outcome of seven-year follow-up. Pediatr Blood Cancer. 2021;68(8):e29063. https://doi.org/10.1002/pbc.29063.
38. Hoyer M, Goli R, Barnett KK, Raabe EH, Hong K. Treatment of Hepatoblastoma with drug-eluting bead Transarterial chemoembolization in a 13-month-old infant: a case report and review of the literature. J Pediatr Hematol Oncol. 2021;43(1):e123–6. https://doi.org/10.1097/MPH.0000000000001842.
39. Aguado A, Dunn SP, Averill LW, et al. Successful use of transarterial radioembolization with yttrium-90 (TARE-Y90) in two children with hepatoblastoma. Pediatr Blood Cancer. 2020;67(9):e28421. https://doi.org/10.1002/pbc.28421.

20 Congenital Hepatic Fibrosis

Jesse Thornhill Davidson IV, Sakil S. Kulkarni, and Maria B. Majella Doyle

20.1 Incidence/Background

Congenital hepatic fibrosis (CHF) is a fibrocystic disease of the liver that typically presents within a few monogenic syndromes with varying phenotypes. The total prevalence of syndromes that include CHF is rare (1 in 10,000 to 20,000) and often accompanied by fibrocystic renal disease. These syndromes are classified as "hepatorenal ciliopathies," or disorders of primary (nonmotile) cilia, which are specialized structures that mediate signal transduction on the surface of cells. In the embryological development of the liver, primary cilia are essential for the normal formation of the ductal plate and thus the biliary system. The ductal plate forms a cylindrical layer of cells around a branch of the portal vein that then undergoes normal remodeling and involution during gestation (Fig. 20.1). CHF is one of several described ductal plate malformations (DPMs) but more specifically, it is a defect in the formation of the small peripheral interlobular bile ducts (Fig. 20.2). Such defects in the development of mature interlobular bile ducts are associated with a pro-inflammatory milieu and subsequent nearby deposition of fibrotic tissue.

The monogenic disease with the closest association to CHF is autosomal recessive polycystic kidney disease (ARPKD; OMIM# 606702), caused by a mutation of the *PKHD1* gene (polycystic kidney and hepatic disease 1), which encodes the fibrocystin/polycystin protein in primary cilia. Other diseases that may manifest with CHF include autosomal dominant polycystic kidney disease (ADPKD) as well as other rare syndromes such as Joubert syndrome (OMIM #213300), Meckel-Gruber syndrome (OMIM #249000), Bardet-Biedl syndrome (OMIM #209900), Oral-Facial-Digital 1 syndrome (OMIM #300209), Jeune syndrome (OMIM # 208500), and nephronophthisis (OMIN #256100). Congenital hepatic fibrosis in isolation, without a syndromic association, is very rare.

J. T. Davidson IV · M. B. Majella Doyle (✉)
Department of Surgery, Section of Abdominal Transplant Surgery, Washington University in St. Louis School of Medicine, St. Louis, MO, USA

Department of Surgery, Division of Organ Transplantation, Northwestern University Feinberg School of Medicine, Chicago, IL, USA
e-mail: jesse.davidson@northwestern.edu; doylem@wustl.edu

S. S. Kulkarni
Department of Pediatrics, Division of Gastroenterology, Hepatology, and Nutrition, Washington University in St. Louis School of Medicine, St. Louis, MO, USA
e-mail: kulkarni.s@wustl.edu

T. Hackert, A. Gulla (eds.), *Rare Liver and Biliary Tract Diseases*,
https://doi.org/10.1007/978-3-032-15076-9_20

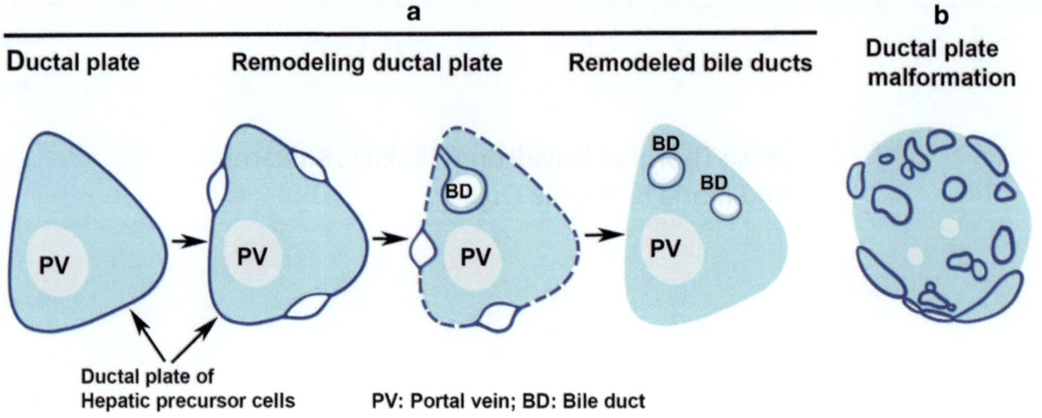

Fig. 20.1 Embryologic development of bile ducts and ductal plate malformations (DPMs). Congenital hepatic fibrosis is characterized by abnormal involution, dilation, and anastomotic networking of bile ducts with hypoplasia of portal vein radicles. (Image created by Xiaoyan Liao, MD, PhD, modified from Johnson et al. [1])

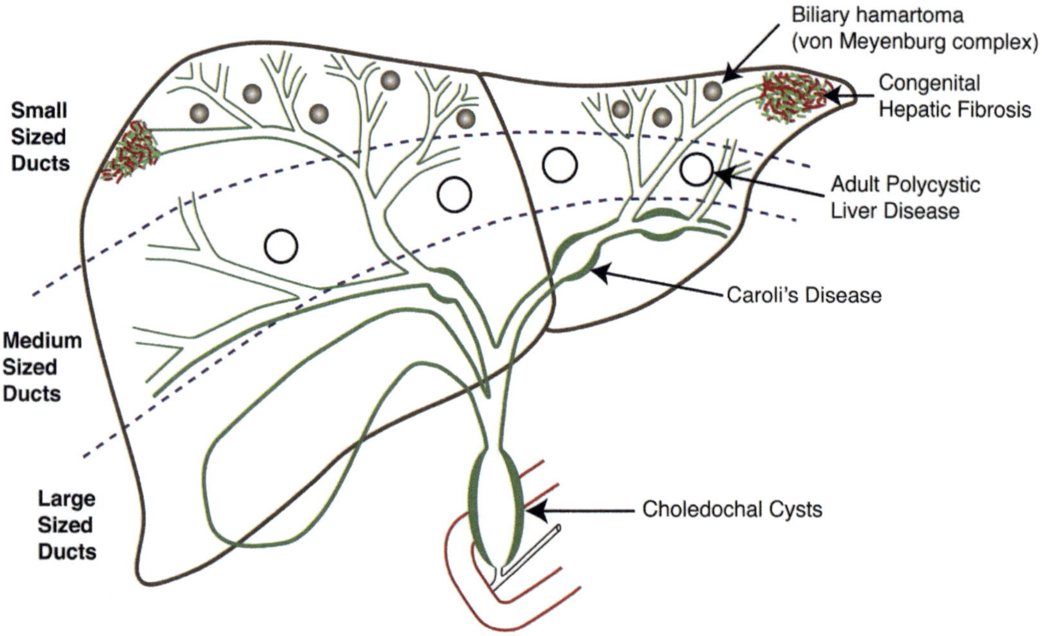

Fig. 20.2 Disease manifestations of ductal plate malformations (DPMs). Each DPM is the result of abnormal embryonic ductal plate development at various stages. (Reproduced from Venkatanarasimha et al. [3])

20.2 Clinical Presentation

Congenital hepatic fibrosis (CHF) is due to malformation of the intrahepatic bile ducts at the level of the small interlobular ducts (Fig. 20.2), leading to abnormal involution and destructive cholangiopathy with progressive biliary fibrosis. Based on the onset of symptoms, there are thought to be four subtypes of CHF: portal hypertensive, cholangitic, mixed, or latent/adult onset. CHF may present in infancy with cholestasis. As ciliopathies often manifest in multiple organs, these patients may present early in life with renal, neurologic, or ophthalmic disease and later develop hepatopathy characterized by noncirrhotic portal hypertension and/or cholangitis. The pathogenesis of portal hypertension in CHF is not precisely known, but it has been thought to be due to compression of portal vein branches in dense fibrous bands as well as anomalous hypoplastic branching of the portal vein radicles. Patients with the portal hypertensive phenotype may experience splenomegaly, thrombocytopenia, and variceal bleeding with preserved hepatic synthetic function. Development of ascites is uncommon. Acute cholangitis, usually caused by gram-negative bacteria, is a rare but serious complication of CHF, especially in patients with associated biliary dilation (Caroli syndrome). Hence, cholangitis and biliary sepsis should be considered in CHF patients with fever and abdominal pain. The progression of the disease can be extremely variable in onset and progression. The destructive cholangiopathy and subsequent fibrosis of CHF may occur at variable rates depending on the underlying etiology, and thus some cases of CHF are diagnosed in late childhood or even adulthood. Additionally, as with other ductal plate malformations, there is a low but increased risk for the development of primary liver malignancy, particularly cholangiocarcinoma.

20.3 Work-Up/Investigation

Congenital hepatic fibrosis is challenging to diagnose. As previously noted, hepatic synthetic function is usually normal, so laboratory values may not reflect underlying liver pathology. Liver biopsy is the gold standard for diagnosis, but histology requires careful interpretation alongside clinical context and cross-sectional imaging as well as adjunctive genetic testing. The classic histopathologic triad of CHF is (1) numerous small ectatic bile ducts with or without cystic dilations and inspissated bile, (2) hypoplastic or obliterated portal vein branches, and (3) portal tract expansion with dense fibrosis. Findings of cholangitis may also be present, with neutrophil or lymphocytic infiltrates along the bile duct epithelium. Distinct CT or MR imaging features of the liver have been described for CHF, with hypertrophy of the left lateral section and caudate, a normal or hypertrophied left medial section, and atrophy of the right lobe (Fig. 20.3). Biliary dilation may be seen on MR in CHF associated with Caroli's disease (Caroli's syndrome). Findings of portal hypertension, including splenomegaly, varices, and ascites, may be present. An enlarged hepatic artery has also been described. As the kidneys are the second most affected organ, renal parenchymal cysts or other architectural anomalies may be seen as well.

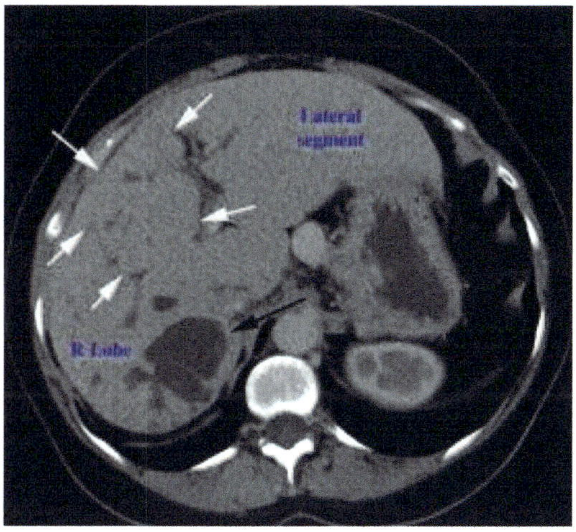

Fig. 20.3 CT findings in congenital hepatic fibrosis. The left lobe is often hypertrophied, while the right is atrophic. Hypertrophy of the left medial section is particularly characteristic of CHF (white arrows). (Reproduced from Venkatanarasimha et al. [3])

20.4 Differential Diagnosis

The differential diagnosis of congenital hepatic fibrosis includes the spectrum of other ductal plate malformations (DPMs), which differ by the level of affected ducts. Cystic dilation of large intrahepatic ducts is the hallmark of Caroli's disease, while problems with medium-sized intrahepatic ducts are seen in autosomal dominant polycystic liver/kidney disease (ADPLD/ADPKD). Abnormal development of the small peripheral interlobular ducts leads to congenital hepatic fibrosis or benign bile duct hamartomas (von Meyenburg complexes or VMCs). VMCs are usually an asymptomatic finding that requires no treatment and no further follow-up. DPMs may sometimes occur in conjunction with each other: Caroli's disease with CHF is known as Caroli's syndrome.

CHF should also be distinguished from acquired forms of portal hypertension caused by viruses, alcohol, and nonalcoholic steatohepatitis. CHF is characterized by a geographical pattern of regenerative nodularity resembling a "jigsaw" (Fig. 20.4), while in cirrhosis the nodules regenerate in a rounded, spherical shape. In addition, disorders that lead to infant cholestasis and a biliary pattern of liver fibrosis in the pediatric population (Table 20.1) may be considered in the differential diagnosis. Etiologies presenting as infant cholestasis include biliary

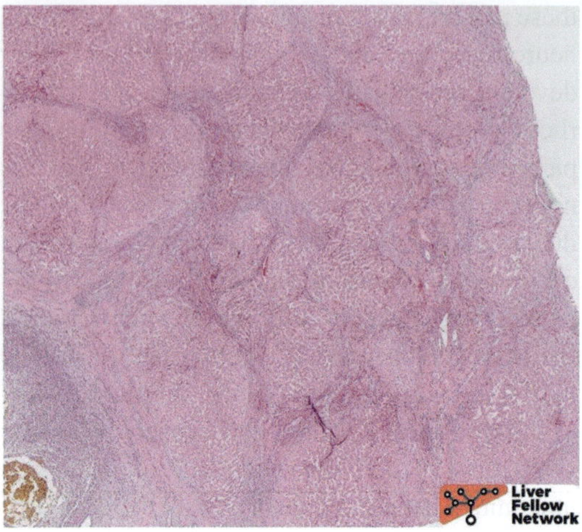

Fig. 20.4 Histopathologic findings in congenital hepatic fibrosis. Dense fibrous bands create geographic patterns of hepatocyte islands that resemble a jigsaw. (Reproduced from the American Association for the Study of Liver Disease (AASLD) Liver Fellow Network (2023))

Table 20.1 Etiologies of liver fibrosis in pediatric patients

Disease	Age of presentation	Age of fibrosis development	Risk of cirrhosis	Biopsy findings
Congenital hepatic fibrosis	Infancy, childhood	Childhood, adolescence	High (by 5–13 years old)	Triads (bile duct abnormality, portal vein hypoplasia, diffuse periportal fibrosis/ white bands encircling hepatic lobules)
Cystic fibrosis liver disease	Variable	Childhood, early adulthood	High (10% by 30 years old)	Biliary obstruction, periportal fibrosis
Biliary atresia	Neonatal	Neonatal	High	Biliary sclerosis and obliteration, loose periportal fibrosis
Primary sclerosing cholangitis	Childhood, adolescence	41% with METAVIR F3–4 fibrosis at initial biopsy (age 14 years)	High, 38% after 10 years in one study	Periductal fibrosis of extrahepatic ducts, periportal fibrosis
Alagille syndrome	Early infancy	Slower than BA; by 20 years of age, 40% developed PH	10–50%	Bile duct proliferation (early), bile duct paucity (late), lymphocyte infiltration of biliary epithelium, peribiliary fibrosis
Genetic causes of cholestasis	Early infancy	First years of life	High	Cholestasis, centrilobular and portal fibrosis, no true ductular proliferation
Autoimmune hepatitis	Puberty (type I), early childhood (type II)	Cirrhosis in 55% at diagnosis	High, 30–55% at presentation but regression at advanced fibrosis stage common	Interface hepatitis; periportal, portal-portal, portal-central fibrosis

Adapted from Ozdogan and Arikan [2]

atresia, cystic fibrosis-associated liver disease, Alagille syndrome, idiopathic (giant cell) neonatal hepatitis, and other genetic causes of intrahepatic cholestasis. Diseases that present with a biliary pattern of hepatic fibrosis include primary sclerosing cholangitis (PSC), autoimmune hepatitis, and biliary atresia.

20.5 Treatment

Mainstay medical therapy for CHF involves management of the associated complications of portal hypertension and cholangitis. Medical, endoscopic, and interventional radiology-guided management of portal hypertension follows the guidelines developed by the American Association for the Study of Liver Diseases. Complications of cholangiopathy, including bile stasis and cholangitis, can be mitigated with ursodeoxycholic acid and broad-spectrum antibiotics, respectively. There is also a low but increased risk of primary liver cancers, including cholangiocarcinoma and hepatocellular carcinoma, which require close surveillance and follow-up. When CHF is not responding to the aforementioned management strategies, the definitive treatment is liver transplant (LT). In the setting of concurrent end-stage kidney disease, patients may be good candidates for a kidney transplant (KT) as well. In an analysis by Wu et al. of the United States Scientific Registry of Transplant Recipients (SRTR), a total of 197 pediatric and adult patients with congenital hepatic fibrosis received LT from 2002 to 2018; 87 (44.2%) received LT alone, while 110 (55.8%) received a kidney transplant prior to or at the time of LT. Long-term liver allograft outcomes were excellent. Because hepatic synthetic function is preserved in CHF, most of the pediatric patients in this dataset were transplanted with MELD exception points. Interestingly, the sequence of kidney-to-liver transplant in patients did have significant implications for kidney allograft survival; KT at the time of (or subsequent to) LT was associated with superior outcomes, while KT prior to LT was associated with poorer kidney graft outcomes (Fig. 20.5). Additionally, in a study by Khan et al., the morbidity and mortality of CHF were significantly worse in pediatric patients with ARPKD that underwent isolated KT when compared with a cohort of matched KT controls without ARPKD. Therefore, a KT-first approach in patients with concurrent CHF should be avoided when possible [5].

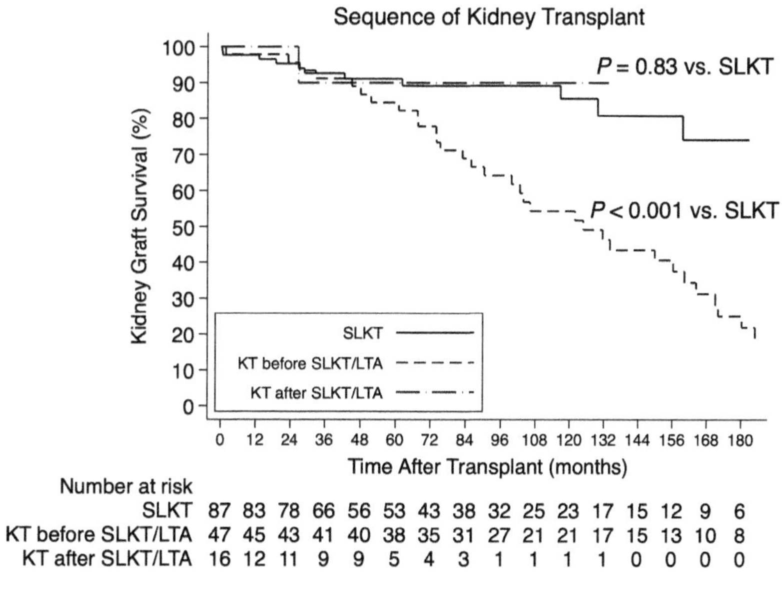

Fig. 20.5 Renal allograft survival in LT/KT patients based on the sequence of transplant. (Reproduced from Wu et al. [4])

20.6 Surgical Planning/ Management

Resective or ablative surgery does not have curative therapeutic potential in congenital hepatic fibrosis. Liver transplantation is the only definitive treatment. As stated above, in patients with combined liver and kidney disease, simultaneous liver/kidney transplant (SLK) may provide benefit over a staged approach. The organs are derived from the same donor, which reduces allosensitization and allows for immune-mediated protection of the kidney by the donor liver. The liver graft is implanted first to minimize its cold ischemia time, while the kidney is either implanted immediately to follow or up to 18–24 hours after the liver, depending on the patient's hemodynamic stability. SLK should often proceed with intraoperative continuous renal replacement therapy (CRRT) to manage metabolic acidosis, hyperkalemia, and fluid shifts, particularly in patients with end-stage renal disease.

Technical considerations in liver transplantation for CHF are not widely different from those considerations for other types of liver disease. Some authors, however, have suggested an association between CHF and cavernous transformation of the portal vein (CTPV), whereby the portal vein is obliterated or obstructed and portal flow is only present through recanalized or collateral veins. CTPV previously was an absolute contraindication to LT and now makes liver transplantation especially challenging, as there are limited options for portal inflow for the liver graft. Portal inflow can successfully be derived from a prominent collateral vein or varix, a dilated coronary vein, a jump graft from the superior mesenteric vein, portal vein arterialization, or renoportal or cavoportal anastomoses. In rare cases in which the above are not feasible, a multivisceral transplant (liver with small intestine) is a consideration as well.

20.7 Follow-Up/ Recommendations

After liver transplantation, follow-up should proceed as per institutional protocol. For patients that are not yet candidates for LT, follow-up should proceed at 6- to 12-month intervals to monitor disease progression. Regular ultrasonography +/− elastography or MRI can capture the fibrosis progression. Kidney disease should be monitored concurrently. Hepatobiliary cancers, particularly cholangiocarcinoma and hepatocellular carcinoma, occur at a slightly increased rate in patients with CHF but usually do not manifest until adulthood. There are no clear data in the literature on when to begin cancer surveillance in this population, but yearly cross-sectional imaging (CT or MRI) with tumor markers (AFP, CA19–9) would be a reasonable approach, starting in adolescence or early adulthood.

References

1. Johnson CA, Gissen P, Sergi C. Molecular pathology and genetics of congenital hepatorenal fibrocystic syndromes. J Med Genet. 2003;40(5):311–9. https://doi.org/10.1136/jmg.40.5.311.
2. Ozdogan E, Arikan C. Liver fibrosis in children: a comprehensive review of mechanisms, diagnosis, and therapy. Clin Exp Pediatr. 2023;66(3):110–24. https://doi.org/10.3345/cep.2022.00367.
3. Venkatanarasimha N, Thomas R, Armstrong EM, Shirley JF, Fox BM, Jackson SA. Imaging features of ductal plate malformations in adults. Clin Radiol. 2011;66(11):1086–93. https://doi.org/10.1016/j.crad.2011.05.008.
4. Wu WK, Ziogas IA, Izzy M, et al. Liver transplantation for congenital hepatic fibrosis. Transpl Int. 2021;34(7):1281–92. https://doi.org/10.1111/tri.13884.
5. Khan K, Schwarzenberg SJ, Sharp HL, Matas AJ, Chavers BM. Morbidity from congenital hepatic fibrosis after renal transplantation for autosomal recessive polycystic kidney disease. Am J Transplant. 2002;2(4):360–5.

21 Budd–Chiari Syndrome

Cihan Agalar and Mustafa Kerem

21.1 Introduction

Budd–Chiari syndrome (BCS) was first described in the 1800s by Hans Chiari and George Budd as a hepatic vein (HV) thrombosis and/or the presence of membranous material in the HV [1, 2].

BCS is characterized by partial or complete obstruction of hepatic venous outflow; obstructed veins may be one or more HVs and/or the inferior vena cava (IVC), and the right atrium can also be obstructed in some cases. BCS is a rare disease; the annual incidence is reported to be between 0.168 and 4.09 per million, with a prevalence of 2.40–33.10 per million [3]. It is known that advanced age is a risk factor for venous thromboembolism. However, BCS is typically diagnosed between the third and fifth decades of life [4].

21.2 Pathophysiology of BCS

When the hepatic venous outflow is obstructed, the intrahepatic sinusoidal pressure increases first in the central vein, followed by portal hypertension and congestion in the liver; hypoxia develops in the hepatocytes, and liver function begins to deteriorate. Several compensatory mechanisms are activated to limit parenchymal congestion and ischemia, the first two of which are the development of intrahepatic collaterals and increased arterial blood flow. If this clinical condition is left untreated, liver cell necrosis, fibrosis, and cirrhosis may develop [5, 6].

21.3 Classification

The classification of BCS is based on etiology, degree of obstruction, and duration of disease onset. Primary BCS causes include intravenous thrombosis, a web, and endophlebitis. Secondary BCS is caused by mechanical obstruction and may be due to primary or metastatic liver tumors, cystic liver disease, abscesses, surgery, or trauma [7, 8].

Approximately 75% of primary BCS cases result from thrombosis formation [9, 10]; predisposition to thrombosis can be acquired or hereditary. According to the literature, the most common causes of acquired prothrombotic conditions include myeloproliferative neoplasms (MPNs), essential thrombocythemia, and idiopathic myelofibrosis. Among the inherited thrombotic causes, the most common are the factor V Leiden mutation, inherited protein C and S deficiencies, and the G20210A prothrombin gene mutation.

C. Agalar
Dokuz Eylul University, Faculty of Medicine, Department of General Surgery, İzmir, Turkey

M. Kerem (✉)
Gazi University, Faculty of Medicine, Department of General Surgery, Ankara, Turkey

T. Hackert, A. Gulla (eds.), *Rare Liver and Biliary Tract Diseases*,
https://doi.org/10.1007/978-3-032-15076-9_22

Gene mutation tests can identify the cause in 90% of patients. The JAK2 V617F mutation, detected by genetic analysis, can be diagnosed in 30–50% of patients with BCS [11, 12]. These genetic tests are usually performed in the following order: if the test for JAK2 V617F is negative, then tests for JAK2 exon 12 mutations, CALR, and myeloproliferative leukemia protein (MPL) mutations are performed. In addition, next-generation sequencing techniques allow these genes to be analyzed with high sensitivity [13, 14].

Childhood BCS is a very rare condition. Polycythemia vera, paroxysmal nocturnal hemoglobinuria (PNH), and antiphospholipid antibody syndrome have been identified as risk factors in childhood BCS [15].

Around 20% of BCS patients are pregnant, are taking oral contraceptives, or have given birth within the last two months [16]. This high frequency may be due to a predisposition to coagulation; in addition, pregnancy may aggravate the predisposition to coagulation [17].

For women diagnosed with BCS during pregnancy or early postpartum, examining potential causes of hypercoagulability such as protein C and S deficiencies, factor V Leiden, paroxysmal nocturnal hemoglobinuria, and antiphospholipid syndrome is essential (Table 21.1).

Table 21.1 Prothrombotic risk factors and etiologies for Budd–Chiari syndrome

Myeloproliferative disorders	Myeloproliferative disease Polycythemia vera Essential thrombocytosis
Acquired thrombophilia	Antiphospholipid syndrome Paroxysmal nocturnal hemoglobinuria *JAK2* V617F mutation
Inherited thrombophilia	Factor V Leiden Protein C deficiency Protein S deficiency Antithrombin deficiency Prothrombin gene G20210A mutation Thalassemia
Systemic factors	Behçet disease Sarcoidosis Vasculitis
Hormonal factors	Oral contraceptive use Pregnancy Given birth within the last two months

BCS is more prevalent in women in Western countries; conversely, it is narrowly more common in men in Asia. According to research, isolated HV occlusion is more prevalent in the West, while isolated IVC or combined IVC and HV occlusion is more common in Asia [18]. Additionally, in the East, membranous occlusion of the HV and/or IVC is more prevalent [19]. The underlying cause is a bacterial infection. It has also been reported that hepatocellular carcinoma (HCC) was detected more frequently in these cases than in classical BCS cases. Due to these differences, some publications argue that the IVC membranous occlusion should be considered a disease different from BCS and define this disease as obliterative hepatocavopathy [20–22].

A retrospective study from India reported HV thrombosis in 59.1% of BCS patients [23], while a study from France investigated the thrombosis location and found 76.6% pure HV thrombosis and 37% combined HV and IVC thrombosis [24].

Portal vein (PV) thrombosis may also develop in 3.2–15% of BCS cases [7, 24].

21.4 Clinical Presentation

The clinical presentation of BCS can vary widely, from asymptomatic to fulminant liver failure. Fullness, distension, abdominal pain, jaundice, and fever are the most common presentation symptoms [4, 23, 25]; some patients may be asymptomatic due to spontaneous intrahepatic portosystemic shunts [26]. The severity of venous obstruction in the HVs and IVC determines the presentation of clinical signs and features. Patients with BCS accompanied by portal hypertension commonly present with ascites, variceal bleeding, and the caput medusae sign on the abdomen [12].

BCS should be considered a possible diagnosis when caudate lobe hypertrophy presents with new-onset ascites and hepatomegaly, particularly in young adult patients [4]. According to the severity of the clinical findings of BCS, fulminant, acute, subacute, and chronic presentations have been described [27, 28].

Acute BCS develops in less than one month and is characterized by the absence of venous collaterals, hepatic necrosis, and sudden onset of ascites. The subacute disease has an onset of 1–6 months; during this duration, collateral circulation can develop, and the subacute disease presents with less severe manifestations [4, 28]. Chronic BCS is characterized by symptoms that persist for more than six months, with cirrhosis and portal hypertension being the predominant manifestations [4, 12, 28].

Fulminant BCS, on the other hand, is characterized by the development of hepatic encephalopathy within the first eight weeks after jaundice appears. The fulminant presentation is low in incidence and occurs only when all three HVs are obstructed [12].

21.5 Work-Up Investigation

In BCS, laboratory parameters may be within normal levels, but high transaminases, high alkaline phosphatase, high bilirubin, and high international normalized ratio (INR) may be detected depending on the severity of the obstruction. The serum-ascites albumin gradient is usually calculated as 1.1 g/dL or higher [7].

Radiological examination plays a very important role in the diagnosis of BCS. Commonly used imaging modalities are Doppler ultrasound (US), computed tomography (CT), magnetic resonance imaging (MRI), and hepatic venography [29, 30].

Doppler US is the first-line imaging modality used to investigate liver dysfunction. It has several advantages, including being inexpensive, not emitting radiation, and providing information about the blood flow pattern in the splanchnic vessels. In experienced hands, Doppler US can aid in diagnosing BCS by detecting specific findings, such as failure to visualize the HV, a fibrous cord, thrombosis and stenosis, or suspicious findings, such as the presence of intrahepatic collateral circulation, caudate lobe hypertrophy, caudate vein diameter of 3 mm or more, portal thrombosis, recanalized umbilical vein, and ascites [31, 32]. USG has limitations, including its inability to identify collateral vascular structures and characterize parenchymal focal lesions [33].

However, Doppler US alone, dependent on the radiologist's experience, is often insufficient to diagnose BCS, and advanced imaging modalities such as contrast-enhanced CT and/or MRI are usually required [32].

CT imaging provides well-defined liver morphology, hepatic vascular structures, perfusion patterns, collaterals, and information about liver parenchyma and perfusion [33].

MRI can be used to differentiate between acute and chronic forms of BCS. To make this distinction, the status of collaterals, splenomegaly, ascites, HV, and IVC patency should be assessed [34, 35].

Imaging techniques can detect delayed or incomplete filling of the three main hepatic veins (right, middle, and left), narrowed or obstructed IVC, hypertrophy of the caudate lobe, and rapid clearance of contrast from the caudate lobe when the IVC is patent and the HVs are obstructed [36, 37] (Fig. 21.1). In addition to these findings, parenchymal heterogeneity, collateral structures, intravascular thrombi, or web-like structures may be observed [38].

Contrast-enhanced MRI is also helpful in diagnosing BCS [39]. The absence or reduced caliber of hepatic veins and the typical distorted "comma-shaped" intrahepatic collaterals can be easily demonstrated.

BCS with isolated hepatic vein involvement, more commonly seen in Western countries, may show a nonspecific mosaic enhancement pattern on CT and/or MRI [32].

Imaging methods can also be used to determine the classification of the disease. Acute BCS is characterized by a lack of enhancement of HVs, ascites, and hepatomegaly, whereas vascular collaterals, caudate lobe hypertrophy, and liver atrophy may characterize chronic BCS [40, 41].

Venography should be performed if there is a clinical suspicion for BCS and noninvasive tests are negative or not diagnostic. Hepatic venography can be performed percutaneously via the femoral, cephalic, or jugular vein.

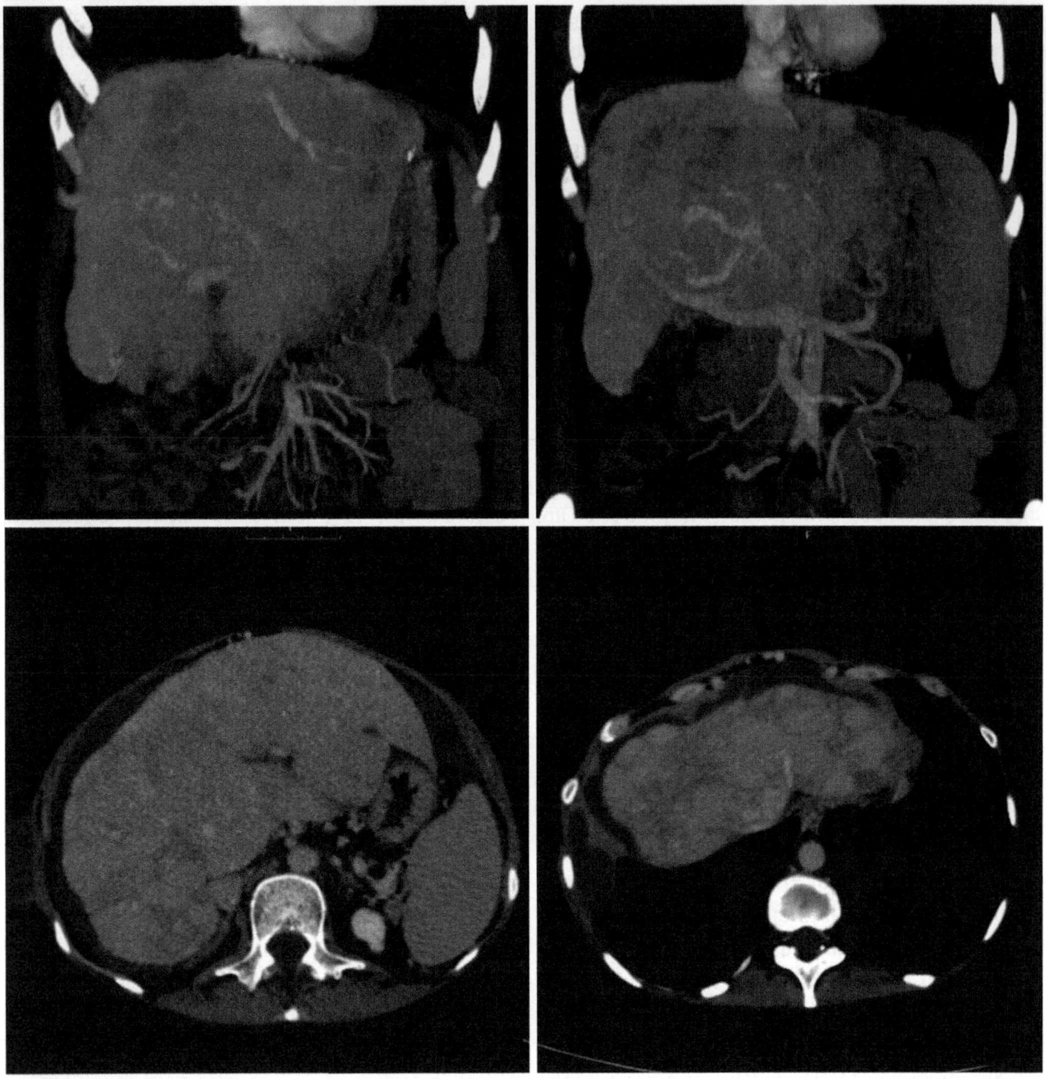

Fig. 21.1 In coronal and axial sections, Caudate lobe enlargement is observed to compress the hepatic veins in the abdominal CT

The venographic examination should include venous pressure measurements; after confirming the patency of the IVC, opacification of each hepatic vein should be attempted.

Venography of some or all hepatic veins may not be possible in many patients with Budd–Chiari syndrome. Balloon occlusion of a specific hepatic vein followed by contrast injection may facilitate visualization of the vein and show the characteristic "spider web" pattern. This model shows how the liver forms venous collaterals to bypass occluded hepatic veins [41]. Venography is critical for conducting treatment. Noninvasive studies may not fully characterize the extent or characteristics of hepatic venous flow.

Currently, there is no universal standard for diagnosing BCS. In many cases, liver histology is the only way to make a diagnosis [42, 43]. A pragmatic approach would be to consider Doppler US as the first diagnostic step, followed by CT or MRI. Liver histology should only be considered when CT and/or MRI are insufficient [32].

Liver biopsy is not routinely required for the diagnosis of BCS. Liver biopsy is not often necessary for large vessel disease. Still, it is more commonly performed in isolated small vessel involvement cases where clinical and radiologic diagnosis is more complicated.

The histologic features of BCS include centrifugal congestion, necrosis, and hemorrhage. Large regenerative nodules, obstructive portal venopathy, and fibrosis/cirrhosis may also be present [44].

The thrombotic process in Budd–Chiari syndrome may not involve all hepatic veins. Therefore, the distribution of typical pathological findings may be focal or patchy. As a result, some patients may require biopsies from both the right and left lobes of the liver. Liver biopsies are usually transjugular during hepatic venography because most patients have ascites and receive anticoagulant therapy.

It is important to note that findings on liver biopsy may not correlate with clinical outcomes. Also, it needs to be clarified whether histologic findings at diagnosis help predict survival. Tang et al. reported that histologic findings did not predict five-year survival, but survival was shorter in patients with central venous thrombosis [44].

Additionally, diagnosing hepatocellular carcinoma (HCC) in the context of BCS can be challenging. However, the radiologic criteria commonly used to diagnose HCC in cirrhosis cannot be applied to BCS. In the presence of BCS, other benign or intermediate lesions, such as regenerative nodules and adenomas, may appear hypervascular in the arterial phase. Therefore, histological confirmation by biopsy should be considered if HCC is suspected in the context of BCS [32].

21.6 Differential Diagnosis

The differential diagnosis of BCS includes alcohol-related liver disease, viral hepatitis, non-alcoholic fatty liver disease, hemochromatosis, ischemic hepatitis, metastatic liver disease, granulomatous liver disease, cystic fibrosis, right-sided heart failure, and other acute or non-alcoholic liver damage due to drug toxicity. BCS shares similar clinical features with the causes of chronic liver disease. When suspecting BCS, it is essential to consider these potential differential diagnoses and perform the necessary examinations and tests [45].

21.7 Management

Patients diagnosed with BCS require a stepwise, multidisciplinary treatment approach tailored to their individual needs based on the etiology, clinical features, and anatomical characteristics [7, 8, 46, 47].

Correct management of BCS cases is critical to survival. If BCS cases are not properly managed, up to 80% mortality can be observed over a 3-year period. However, if the syndrome is diagnosed early and managed appropriately, the risk of mortality can be significantly reduced. When BCS is properly managed, the 5-year survival rate is over 80% [14].

The European Association for the Study of the Liver (EASL) and the American Association for the Study of Liver Diseases (AASLD) have published guidelines for BCS under the category of vascular liver diseases. They suggest a stepwise approach, beginning with anticoagulation therapy and progressing to liver transplantation if minimally invasive interventions are insufficient [7, 8, 46].

The treatment objectives are to control the underlying disease if possible, prevent the spread of clots, recanalize thrombosed vessels, alleviate hepatic congestion, reduce signs and symptoms of portal hypertension, and preserve liver function [4, 32].

Anticoagulation therapy is the initial step in the treatment process; however, the possibility of coagulopathy due to liver dysfunction should be considered when initiating anticoagulant therapy.

Anticoagulant therapy is initiated with low molecular weight heparin (DMAH) for 5–7 days, followed by long-term warfarin treatment to maintain the INR level 2–3 times above normal.

The literature presents varying success rates of anticoagulant therapy. A study of 163 patients from European centers examined the effectiveness of staged treatment. In this study, 86% of patients received anticoagulant therapy, and 80 patients were treated non-invasively [10],

In another multicenter study of 157 patients 40% were treated noninvasively, and 71% of those treated noninvasively with anticoagulant therapy survived [48]. Additionally, other studies report that only a small proportion of patients (15–20%) received medical treatment alone [12, 19].

Following anticoagulation therapy, the recommended first-line treatment in the stepwise approach is thrombolysis through endovascular intervention. In cases of acute thrombus treated with endovascular intervention, locally administered thrombolytics may increase the likelihood of vessel recanalization. This treatment is applied when a well-defined clot is present [49].

Systemic thrombolysis with recombinant tissue plasminogen activator may be attempted in patients who cannot undergo selective endovascular therapy due to a high clot burden. However, systemic thrombolysis has been tried in a limited number of cases and is not expected to benefit chronic BCS [49, 50].

The next step in the stepwise approach is angioplasty/stenting in symptomatic patients with venous occlusions amenable to angiographic treatment.

Endovascular approaches such as angioplasty and stenting have become increasingly popular over the last 20 years [4]. However, it is essential to note that angioplasty/stenting may only be effective in short stenoses [32].

Approximately one-third of short HV stenosis cases are treated with recanalization by percutaneous transluminal angioplasty (PTA) with or without stenting [51, 52]. It is worth noting that recanalization is seen as a highly successful intervention in Asian centers with appropriate patient selection and high levels of experience [52, 53].

Balloon angioplasty may be appropriate for patients with combined obstruction of both the HV and IVC [54]. Angioplasty may be combined with stents, especially in cases of IVC obstruction [55, 56]. Using a stent in addition to angioplasty may provide higher success rates compared to angioplasty alone [57]. Wang et al. compared 45 BCS patients undergoing angioplasty alone with 43 patients undergoing angioplasty and routine stenting in their randomized controlled trial and reported that patients in the stent group achieved superior stenosis-free vessel patency compared to angioplasty alone at the 27-month follow-up (98% vs. 60%, respectively) [58].

For patients with acute or subacute BCS, if first-line treatments (anticoagulation, thrombolysis, and/or angioplasty (with or without stent)) fail, the following options are transjugular intrahepatic portosystemic shunt (TIPS), surgical shunts, and liver transplantation. TIPS may be applied in patients with long-segment venous occlusion who do not respond to angioplasty or in whom angioplasty is predicted to fail [4, 59].

TIPS is an intervention that involves creating a shunt between the hepatic vein and a portal vein branch through transjugular access; the aim is to reduce the portal vein pressure below 12 mmHg. TIPS has both symptomatic and therapeutic benefits, as it can alleviate hepatic congestion, which is the cause of disease progression in BCS, particularly in the early stages. Additionally, TIPS can reduce the severity of BCS syndrome. Before deciding on TIPS, it is crucial to thoroughly evaluate patients as candidates for angioplasty and stenting.

It is important to note that TIPS is not a suitable treatment option for patients with acute BCS. In a study conducted by Mancuso et al., the data of 15 BCS patients who underwent TIPS were analyzed; the study reported that although all patients with chronic BCS showed improvement in ascites and liver chemistry, half of the patients with acute BCS died shortly after TIPS placement [60].

A series of 51 patients who underwent TIPS, published from a center in China, reported 1-year, 2-year, and 3-year survival rates of 83.8%, 81.2%, and 76.9%, respectively [61]. Another series published from India reported survival rates of 93%, 89%, and 84% at one year, three years, and five years, respectively [62]. Sonavane et al. investigated the effect of TIPS and liver transplantation on survival. They found transplant-free survival rates of 86%, 81%, and

76% at one year, five years, and ten years, respectively [63].

A meta-analysis of data from 2255 patients with BCS reported a 93.7% success rate after interventional procedures (angioplasty, stenting, or TIPS), with 1-year and 5-year survival rates of 92% and 76.4%, respectively [64].

While the TIPS procedure can lead to successful outcomes in appropriate patients, it is essential to consider the potential complications. These include bile perforation, intra-abdominal bleeding, acute TIPS thrombosis, subcapsular hematoma, abnormal TIPS positioning, portal vein thrombosis, hepatic encephalopathy, and shunt dysfunction, as reported [65]. TIPS may serve as a bridge to liver transplantation, but it is crucial to consider the risk of portal vein thrombosis. If portal vein thrombosis develops, the patient's liver transplant operation may become more complicated [4].

If TIPS placement is not possible or fails, alternative treatments such as surgical shunts or liver transplantation should be considered.

21.8 Surgical Treatment

BCS surgical treatment aims to restore hepatic venous drainage and reduce liver pressure. The most common surgical method is the portocaval shunt. Surgical shunts aim to drain the portal system into the IVC or a systemic vein. If successful, shunting can lead to the acute hepatocellular regression of necrosis caused by hepatocyte compression. Before considering shunt surgery for BCS patients, it is crucial to identify and treat the underlying cause of possible thrombotic diathesis.

Various surgical shunts, including side-by-side portocaval, splenorenal, and mesocaval shunts, are available. The shunt type should be selected based on the patient's anatomical features, underlying disease, general condition, and the location of the occluded vascular structure. Before deciding on surgical shunting, it is crucial to carefully evaluate angiography and portocaval venous pressure gradients [28, 66]. If caudate lobe hypertrophy is present, a side-to-side portacaval shunt may not be technically feasible, and a mesocaval shunt may be required for this patient group. Side-by-side portocaval, splenorenal, and mesocaval shunts only show benefit if the IVC is patent [67]. In cases of IVC obstruction, a shunt can be created from the portal system to the right atrium using a combination of portocaval and cava-atrial shunts with synthetic grafts. However, it is essential to remember the risk of thrombosis associated with this shunt type [66, 68]; it is worth noting that memorial shunts have been associated with a higher rate of dysfunction [66, 69].

After shunt surgery, the two most significant factors affecting five-year survival are the maintenance of shunt patency and pre-procedural liver function status [66, 70]. Patients who underwent shunt surgery before the development of cirrhosis and whose shunts were not occluded have reported five-year survival rates of up to 90 percent [66, 70, 71].

Shunt dysfunction increases the risk of refractory ascites, portal hypertension, variceal bleeding, and death [72]. Anticoagulation therapy is recommended to reduce the risk of thrombosis after shunt surgery [73]. In addition to shunt surgery, good results have been reported in highly selected cases with posterior-superior liver resection and thrombectomy [74, 75]. The frequency of surgical shunt operations has gradually decreased, with the widespread use of TIPS in recent decades [46].

In the presence of cirrhosis, liver transplantation should be planned instead of shunt surgery.

21.9 Liver Transplantation

Liver transplantation may be considered for patients with fulminant liver failure or decompensated cirrhosis when other treatments have failed [68, 76].

In patients who develop BCS due to deficiencies in protein S, protein C, or antithrombin III, the transplanted liver will produce these enzymes in average amounts, and the clotting predisposition will be treated with liver transplantation.

Liver transplantation for BCS has shown promising outcomes. Studies have found no significant difference in survival rates between liver transplants for BCS and those for other indications of CS [77].

A multicenter study in Europe reported 5-year survival rates ranging from 65% to 71%, while more recent studies have reported 10-year survival rates between 68% and 84% [78–80]. For patients who underwent liver transplantation for BCS caused by myeloproliferative disease, there was no difference in overall survival compared to other liver transplant patients [81]. A series of 25 cases reported 92% and 88% 5-year patient and graft survival, respectively [82].

An extensive series with 510 cases found that using the Model for End-stage Liver Disease (MELD) score for cadaveric donor allocation resulted in better outcomes. Specifically, there was an improvement in 3-year graft survival (80.6% vs. 64.5%) and longer 3-year overall survival rates (84.9% vs. 72.6%) [80].

Risk factors for graft loss in patients undergoing liver transplantation for BCS include renal dysfunction, elevated bilirubin levels, history of cardiopulmonary resuscitation, advanced age, previous abdominal surgery or transplantation, advanced donor age, and prolonged duration of cold ischemia [80]; as with patients undergoing liver transplantation for other reasons, hepatic artery thrombosis, infection, and multiorgan dysfunction are among the causes of early death after transplantation [79].

Patients undergoing liver transplantation for BCS have been reported to experience more frequent vascular and thrombotic complications [77, 83]. Additionally, the JAK2 V617F mutation is associated with a higher risk of thrombosis after liver transplantation [84].

While cadaveric liver transplantation is typically the preferred method for treating BCS caused by hepatic outflow issues, there have been successful cases of living donor liver transplantation reported, particularly in countries with limited access to cadaveric donors [85–88].

21.10 Follow-Up/Recommendations

When following up with patients who have BCS, it is crucial to diagnose the underlying disease. It is also important to closely monitor for possible myelodysplastic syndrome, bleeding complications of anticoagulant therapy, and the effectiveness of appropriate anticoagulant therapy in this patient group with a predisposition to thrombosis. Additionally, patients with hepatic congestion and insufficient hepatic vein patency should be monitored carefully for rapid deterioration of liver function.

Patients in whom patency of the thrombosed vessel cannot be achieved should be closely monitored for disease progression, specifically impairment of hepatic synthesis function. It is crucial to keep in mind that Budd–Chiari Syndrome (BCS) can cause portal hypertension, which can lead to complications such as variceal bleeding; therefore, a multidisciplinary team in a center where liver transplantation can be performed should follow up and treat this patient group.

It is essential to consider that patients with BCS may face issues related to malnutrition, and therefore, their nutritional status should be assessed before they experience significant weight loss.

References

1. Chiari H. Ueber die selbstandige Phlebitis obliterans der Hauptstamme der Venae hepaticae als Todesursache. Beitr Pathol Anat. 1899;26:1–18.
2. Budd G. On diseases of the liver. 1st ed. London J: Churchill; 1845.
3. Li Y, De Stefano V, Li H, Zheng K, Bai Z, Guo X, Qi X. Epidemiology of Budd-Chiari syndrome: a systematic review and meta-analysis. Clin Res Hepatol Gastroenterol. 2019;43:468–74.

4. Haque LYK, Lim JK. Budd-Chiari syndrome: an uncommon cause of chronic liver disease that cannot be missed. Clin Liver Dis. 2020;24:453–81.
5. McCuskey RS. Morphological mechanisms for regulating blood flow through hepatic sinusoids. Liver. 2000;20:3–7.
6. Goel RM, Johnston EL, Patel KVWT. Budd-Chiari syndrome: investigation, treatment and outcomes. Postgr Med J. 2015;91:692–7.
7. DeLeve LD, Valla DC, Garcia-Tsao G. Vascular disorders of the liver. Hepatology. 2009;49:1729–64.
8. European Association for the Study of the Liver. EASL Clinical Practice Guidelines: vascular diseases of the liver. J Hepatol. 2016;64:179–202.
9. Denninger MH, Chait Y, Casadevall N, Hillaire S, Guillin MC, Bezeaud A, Erlinger S, et al. Cause of portal or hepatic venous thrombosis in adults: the role of multiple concurrent factors. Hepatology. 2000;31:587–91.
10. Murad SD, Plessier A, Hernandez-Guerra M, Fabris F, Eapen CE, Bahr MJ, Trebicka J, Morard I, Lasser L, Heller J, Hadengue A, Langlet P, Miranda H, Primignani M, Elias E, Leebeek FW, Rosendaal FR, Garcia-Pagan J-C, Valla DC, Janssen HLA, EN-Vie (European Network for Vascular Disorders of the Liver). Etiology, management, and outcome of the Budd-Chiari syndrome. Ann Intern Med. 2009;151(3):167–75.
11. Dentali F, Squizzato A, Brivio L, Appio L, Campiotti L, Crowther M, Grandi AM, et al. JAK2V617F mutation for the early diagnosis of Ph- myeloproliferative neoplasms in patients with venous thromboembolism: a meta-analysis. Blood. 2009;113:5617–23.
12. Gavriilidis P, Marangoni G, Ahmad J, Azoulay D. State of the art, current perspectives, and controversies of Budd-Chiari syndrome: a review. J Clin Med Res. 2022;14:147–57.
13. Magaz M, Alvarez-Larrán A, Colomer D, et al. Next-generation sequencing in the diagnosis of noncirrhotic splanchnic vein thrombosis. J Hepatol. 2021;74:89–95.
14. Garcia-Pagán JC, Valla D-C. Primary Budd–Chiari Syndrome. N Engl J Med. 2023;388:1307–16.
15. Nobre S, Khanna R, Bab N, et al. Primary budd-chiari syndrome in children: king's college hospital experience. J Pediatr Gastroenterol Nutr. 2017;65:93–6.
16. Khuroo MSDD. Budd-Chiari syndrome following pregnancy. Report of 16 cases, with roentgenologic, hemodynamic and histologic studies of the hepatic outflow tract. Am J Med. 1980;68:113.
17. Bissonnette J, Durand F, de Raucourt E, Ceccaldi PF, Plessier A, Valla DRP. Pregnancy and vascular liver disease. J Clin Exp Hepatol. 2015;5:41.
18. Plessier A, Valla DC. Budd-Chiari syndrome. Semin Liver Dis. 2008;28:259–69.
19. Shukla A, Shreshtha A, Mukund A, Bihari C, Eapen CE, Han G, Deshmukh H, et al. Budd-Chiari syndrome: consensus guidance of the Asian Pacific Association for the study of the liver (APASL). Hepatol Int. 2021;15:531–67.
20. Okuda K. Membranous obstruction of the inferior vena cava (obliterative hepatocavopathy, Okuda). J Gastroenterol Hepatol. 2001;16:1179–83.
21. Shrestha SM, Kage MLB. Hepatic vena cava syndrome: new concept of pathogenesis. Hepatol Res. 2017;47:603–15.
22. Shrestha SM. Liver cirrhosis and hepatocellular carcinoma in hepatic vena cava disease, a liver disease caused by obstruction of inferior vena cava. Hepatol Int. 2009;3:392–402.
23. Amarapurkar DN, Punamiya SJ, Patel ND. Changing spectrum of Budd-Chiari syndrome in India with special reference to non-surgical treatment. World J Gastroenterol. 2008;14:278–85.
24. Ollivier-Hourmand I, Allaire M, Goutte N, et al. The epidemiology of Budd-Chiari syndrome in France. Dig Liver Dis. 2018;50:931–7.
25. Dilawari JB, Bambery P, Chawla Y, et al. Hepatic outflow obstruction (Budd- Chiari syndrome). Experience with 177 patients and a review of the literature. Medicine (Baltimore). 1994;73:21–36.
26. Bhatt P, Gupta DK, Agrawal D, et al. Budd-Chiari syndrome with spontaneous intrahepatic portosystemic shunts: a case series. J Clin Exp Hepatol. 2019;9:412–5.
27. Parekh J, Matei VM, Canas-Coto A, Acute Liver Failure Study G, et al. Buddchiari syndrome causing acute liver failure: a multicenter case series. Liver Transpl. 2017;23:135–42.
28. Menon KV, Shah VKP. The Budd-Chiari syndrome. N Engl J Med. 2004;350:578–85.
29. Porrello G, Mamone G, Miraglia R. Budd-Chiari syndrome imaging diagnosis: state of the art and future perspectives. Diagnostics. 2023; https://doi.org/10.3390/diagnostics13132256.
30. Aydinli M, Bayraktar Y. Budd-Chiari syndrome: etiology, pathogenesis and diagnosis. World J Gastroenterol. 2007;13:2693–6.
31. Bargallo X, Gilabert R, Nicolau C, García-Pagán JC, Ayuso JR, Brú C. Sonography of Budd–Chiari syndrome. AJR Am J Roentgenol. 2006;197:33–41.
32. Mancuso A. Budd–Chiari syndrome management: controversies and open issues. Diagnostics. 2022; https://doi.org/10.3390/diagnostics12112670.
33. Bansal V, Gupta P, Sinha S, et al. Budd-Chiari syndrome: imaging review. Br J Radiol. 2018;91:20180441.
34. Erden A. Budd-Chiari syndrome: a review of imaging findings. Eur J Radiol. 2007;61:44–56.
35. Cheng D, Xu H, Hua R, et al. Comparative study of MRI manifestations of acute and chronic Budd-Chiari syndrome. Abdom Imaging. 2015;40:76–84.
36. Brancatelli G, Vilgrain V, Federle MP, et al. Budd-Chiari syndrome: spectrum of imaging findings. AJR Am J Roentgenol. 2007;188:168–76.
37. Bargallo X, Gilabert R, Nicolau C, et al. Sonography of the caudate vein: value in diagnosing Budd-Chiari syndrome. AJR Am J Roentgenol. 2003;181:1641–5.

38. Chaubal N, Dighe M, Hanchate V, et al. Sonography in budd-chiari syndrome. J Ultrasound Med. 2006;25(3):373–9.
39. Soyer P, Rabenandrasana A, Barge J, Laissy JP, Zeitoun G, Hay JMLM. MRI of Budd-Chiari syndrome. Abdom Imaging. 1994;19:325.
40. Lupescu IG, Dobromir C, Popa GA, et al. Spiral computed tomography and magnetic resonance angiography evaluation in Budd-Chiari syndrome. J Gastrointestin Liver Dis. 2008;17:223–6.
41. Kamath PS. Budd-Chiari syndrome: radiologic findings. Liver Transpl. 2006;12:21–2.
42. Ronot M, Kerbaol A, Rautou PE, Brancatelli G, Bedossa P, Cazals-Hatem D, Valla DC, Vilgrain V. Acute extrahepatic infectious or inflammatory diseases are a cause of transient mosaic pattern on CT and MR imaging related to sinusoidal dilatation of the liver. Eur Radiol. 2016;26:3094–101.
43. Mancuso A, Butera G, Politi F, Maringhini A. Budd Chiari syndrome presenting with hepatic transient mosaic enhancement pattern and treated with early TIPS. AME Med J. 2017;2:60.
44. Cazals-Hatem D, Vilgrain V, Genin P, Denninger MH, Durand F, Belghiti J, Valla D, Degott C. Arterial and portal circulation and parenchymal changes in Budd-Chiari syndrome: a study in 17 explanted livers. Hepatology. 2003;37:510.
45. Hitawala AA G V. Budd-Chiari Syndrome. [Updated 2023 Jan 30]. In: StatPearls [internet]. Treasure Isl. StatPearls Publ. https://www.ncbi.nlm.nih.gov/books/NBK558941/.
46. Northup PG, Garcia-Pagan JC, Garcia-Tsao G, Intagliata NM, Superina RA, Roberts LN, Lisman T, Valla DC. Vascular liver disorders, portal vein thrombosis, and procedural bleeding in patients with liver disease: 2020 practice guidance by the American Association for the Study of Liver Diseases. Hepatology. 2021;73:366–413.
47. Khan F, Armstrong MJ, Mehrzad H, et al. Review article: a multidisciplinary approach to the diagnosis and management of Budd-Chiari syndrome. Aliment Pharmacol Ther. 2019;49:840–63.
48. Seijo S, Plessier A, Hoekstra J, et al. Good long-term outcome of Budd-Chiari syndrome with a step-wise management. Hepatology. 2013;57:1962–8.
49. Sharma S, Texeira A, Texeira P, et al. Pharmacological thrombolysis in Budd Chiari syndrome: a single centre experience and review of the literature. J Hepatol. 2004;40:172–80.
50. Clark PJ, Slaughter RERD. Systemic thrombolysis for acute, severe Budd-Chiari syndrome. J Thromb Thrombolysis. 2012;34:410–5.
51. Cui YF, Fu YF, Li DCXH. Percutaneous recanalization for hepatic vein-type Budd-Chiari syndrome: long-term patency and survival. Hepatol Int. 2016;10:363–9.
52. Mukhiya G, Jiao D, Han X, Zhou X, Pokhrel G. Survival and clinical success of endovascular intervention in patients with Budd-Chiari syndrome: a systematic review. J Clin Imaging Sci. 2023;13:1–14.
53. Qi X, Han G, Guo X, et al. Review article: the aetiology of primary Budd-Chiari syndrome – differences between the West and China. Aliment Pharmacol Ther. 2016;44:1152–67.
54. Cheng DL, Xu H, Li CL, et al. Interventional treatment strategy for primary buddchiari syndrome with both inferior vena cava and hepatic vein involvement: patients from two centers in China. Cardiovasc Interv Radiol. 2019;42:1311–21.
55. Qiao T, Liu CJ, Liu C, et al. Interventional endovascular treatment for Budd- Chiari syndrome with long-term follow-up. Swiss Med Wkly. 2005;135:318–26.
56. Bi Y, Chen H, Ding P, et al. Comparison of retrievable stents and permanent stents for Budd-Chiari syndrome due to obstructive inferior vena cava. J Gastroenterol Hepatol. 2018;33:2015–21.
57. Han G, Qi X, Zhang W, et al. Percutaneous recanalization for Budd-Chiari syndrome: an 11-year retrospective study on patency and survival in 177 Chinese patients from a single center. Radiology. 2013;266:657–67.
58. Wang Q, Li K, He C, et al. Angioplasty with versus without routine stent placement for Budd-Chiari syndrome: a randomised controlled trial. Lancet Gastroenterol Hepatol. 2019;4:686–97.
59. Eapen CE, Velissaris D, Heydtmann M, et al. Favourable medium term outcome following hepatic vein recanalisation and/or transjugular intrahepatic portosystemic shunt for Budd Chiari syndrome. Gut. 2006;55:878–84.
60. Mancuso A, Fung K, Mela M, et al. TIPS for acute and chronic Budd-Chiari syndrome: a single-centre experience. J Hepatol. 2003;38:751–4.
61. Qi X, Guo W, He C, et al. Transjugular intrahepatic portosystemic shunt for Budd-Chiari syndrome: techniques, indications and results on 51 Chinese patients from a single centre. Liver Int. 2014;34:1164–75.
62. Shalimar, Gamanagatti SR, Patel AH, et al. Long-term outcomes of transjugular intrahepatic portosystemic shunt in Indian patients with Budd-Chiari syndrome. Eur J Gastroenterol Hepatol. 2017;29:1174–82.
63. Sonavane AD, Amarapurkar DN, Rathod KR, et al. Long term survival of patients undergoing TIPS in Budd-Chiari syndrome. J Clin Exp Hepatol. 2019;9:56–61.
64. Zhang F, Wang C, Li Y. The outcomes of interventional treatment for Budd-Chiari syndrome: systematic review and meta-analysis. Abdom Imaging. 2015;40:601–8.
65. Hayek G, Ronot M, Plessier A, et al. Long-term outcome and analysis of dysfunction of transjugular intrahepatic portosystemic shunt placement in chronic primary Budd-Chiari syndrome. Radiology. 2017;283:280–92.
66. Orloff MJ, Isenberg JI, Wheeler HO, et al. Budd-Chiari syndrome revisited: 38 years' experience with surgical portal decompression. J Gastrointest Surg. 2012;16(2):286–300.
67. Shill M, Henderson JMTA. The Budd-Chiari syndrome revisited. Gastroenterologist. 1994;2:27.

68. Orloff MJ, Daily PO, Orloff SL, et al. Surgical treatment of Budd-Chiari syndrome– when is liver transplant indicated? Transplant Proc. 2001;33:1435.
69. Chen H, Zhang F, Ye Y, et al. Long-term follow-up study and comparison of meso-atrial shunts and meso-cavo-atrial shunts for treatment of combined Budd-Chiari syndrome. J Surg Res. 2011;168(1):162–6.
70. Panis Y, Belghiti J, Valla D, Benhamou JPF. Portosystemic shunt in Budd-Chiari syndrome: long-term survival and factors affecting shunt patency in 25 patients in Western countries. Surgery. 1994;115:276.
71. Darwish Murad S, Valla DC, de Groen PC, Zeitoun G, Hopmans JA, Haagsma EB, van Hoek B, Hansen BE, Rosendaal FRJH. Determinants of survival and the effect of portosystemic shunting in patients with Budd-Chiari syndrome. Hepatology. 2004;39:500.
72. Bachet JB, Condat B, Hagege H, et al. long-term portosystemic shunt patency as a determinant of outcome in Budd-Chiari syndrome. J Hepatol. 2007;46:60–8.
73. Klein ASME. Surgical treatment of Budd-Chiari syndrome. Liver Transpl. 2003;9:891–6.
74. Vogt PR, Andersson LC, Jenni R, et al. Dorsocranial liver resection and direct hepatoatrial anastomosis for hepatic venous outflow obstruction: long-term outcome and functional results. Am J Gastroenterol. 1996;91:539.
75. Bansky G, Ernest C, Jenni R, et al. Treatment of Budd-Chiari syndrome by dorsocranial liver resection and direct hepatoatrial anastomosis. J Hepatol. 1986;2:101.
76. Mancuso A. Time to resize the role of liver transplant for Budd-Chiari syndrome. Liver Int. 2015;35:2339.
77. Frank U, Johann P, Ulf N, Andreas P, Gero P, Peter F, Sascha W, Sven Jonas PN. Eighteen years of liver transplantation experience in patients with advanced Budd-Chiari syndrome. Liver Transpl. 2008;14:144–50.
78. Doğrul AB, Yankol Y, Mecit N, Kanmaz T, Acarlı K, Kalayoğlu M. Orthotopic liver transplant for budd-chiari syndrome: an analysis of 14 cases. Exp Clin Transplant. 2016;14:641–5.
79. Mentha G, Giostra E, Majno PE, et al. Liver transplantation for Budd-Chiari syndrome: a European study on 248 patients from 51 centres. J Hepatol. 2006;44:520–8.
80. Dorry LS, Geoffrey CN, Jayme EL, Christopher ES, Robert AM, Warren RM, Thuluvath PJ. Twenty years of liver transplantation for Budd- Chiari syndrome: a National Registry Analysis. Liver Transpl. 2007;13:1285–94.
81. Potthoff A, Attia D, Pischke S, et al. Long-term outcome of liver transplant patients with Budd-Chiari syndrome secondary to myeloproliferative neoplasms. Liver Int. 2015;35:2042–9.
82. Chinnakotla S, Klintmalm GB, Kim P, et al. Long-term follow-up of liver transplantation for budd-chiari syndrome with antithrombotic therapy based on the etiology. Transplantation. 2011;92:341–5.
83. Cruz E, Ascher NL, Roberts JP, Bass NM, Yao FY. High incidence of recurrence and hematologic events following liver transplantation for Budd-Chiari syndrome. Clin Transpl. 2005;19:501–6.
84. Westbrook RH, Lea NC, Mohamedali AM, Smith AE, Orr DW, Roberts LN, Heaton ND, Wendon JA, O'Grady JG, Heneghan GJM MA. Prevalence and clinical outcomes of the 46/1 haplotype, Janus kinase 2 mutations, and ten-eleven translocation 2 mutations in Budd-Chiari syndrome and their impact on thrombotic complications post liver transplantation. Liver Transpl. 2012;18:819–27.
85. Yamada T, Tanaka K, Ogura Y, Ko S, Nakajima Y, Takada Y, Uemoto S. Surgical techniques and long-term outcomes of living donor liver transplantation for Budd-Chiari syndrome. Am J Transplant. 2006;6:2463–9.
86. Akamatsu N, Sugawara Y, Kokudo N. Budd-chiari syndrome and liver transplantation. Intractable Rare Dis Res. 2015;4:24–32.
87. Ara C, Akbulut S, Ince V, Karakas S, Baskiran A, Yilmaz S. Living donor liver transplantation for Budd–Chiari syndrome. Medicine (Baltimore). 2016;95:e5136.
88. Karaca C, Yilmaz C, Ferecov R, Iakobadze Z, Kilic K, Caglayan L, Aydogdu S, Kilic M. Living-donor liver transplantation for Budd-Chiari syndrome: case series. Transplant Proc. 2017;49:1841–7.

22 Urea Cycle Defects

Brian J. Shayota, Alexa Taylor,
and Andrea Gropman

Abbreviations

1HMRS	Proton magnetic resonance imaging neuroimaging
Gln	glutamine
Glu	Glutamate
HA	Hyperammonemia
OTC	Ornithine transcarbamylase deficiency
UCD	Urea cycle disorders

22.1 Introduction

The urea cycle (also known as the ornithine cycle) is the biochemical process by which nitrogen balance is maintained in ureotelic mammals. This is achieved by the conversion of nitrogen-containing compounds, primarily in the form of ammonia and various amino acids, into the non-toxic compound urea, for excretion in the urine. The entire process consists of five catalytic enzymes: (1) carbamoyl-phosphate synthase 1, CPS1; (2) ornithine transcarbamylase, OTC; (3) arginosuccinate synthase 1, ASS1; (4) arginosuccinate lyase, argininosuccinate lyase (ASL); and (5) arginase 1, ARG1. Additionally, there is an equally important cofactor-synthesizing enzyme, N-acetylglutamate synthase, NAGS, that serves as the rate-limiting step of the cycle and 2 amino acid transporters, aspartate/glutamate carrier, SLC25A13 (also known as Citrin transporter), and ornithine translocase, ORNT1. The complete urea cycle occurs only in the liver, but ASS1 and ASL are also expressed in other tissues. The pathway can be subcategorized as the proximal urea cycle, consisting of the catalytic enzymes CPS1 and OTC, as well as NAGS, which takes place in the mitochondria, and the distal urea cycle, consisting of the remaining 3 catalytic enzymes, ASS1, ASL, and ARG1, which takes place within the cytosol of the hepatocyte (Fig. 22.1).

The final product of the urea cycle is urea, which contains two nitrogen atoms derived from different steps of the cycle. Ammonia is the first nitrogen atom that enters the cycle by combining with bicarbonate, catalyzed by CPS1 and the cofactor NAGS, to form carbamoyl phosphate.

B. J. Shayota
Department of Pediatrics and Medical Genetics, University of Utah/Primary Children's Hospital, Salt Lake City, UT, USA
e-mail: brian.shayota@hsc.utah.edu

A. Taylor
Center for Experimental Neurotherapeutics, St Jude Children's Research Hospital, Memphis, TN, USA
e-mail: ataylor@childrensnational.org

A. Gropman (✉)
Department of Pediatrics, Children's National Hospital, Department of Neurology, George Washington School of Medicine and Health Sciences, Washington, DC, USA
e-mail: andrea.gropman@stjude.org

T. Hackert, A. Gulla (eds.), *Rare Liver and Biliary Tract Diseases*,
https://doi.org/10.1007/978-3-032-15076-9_22

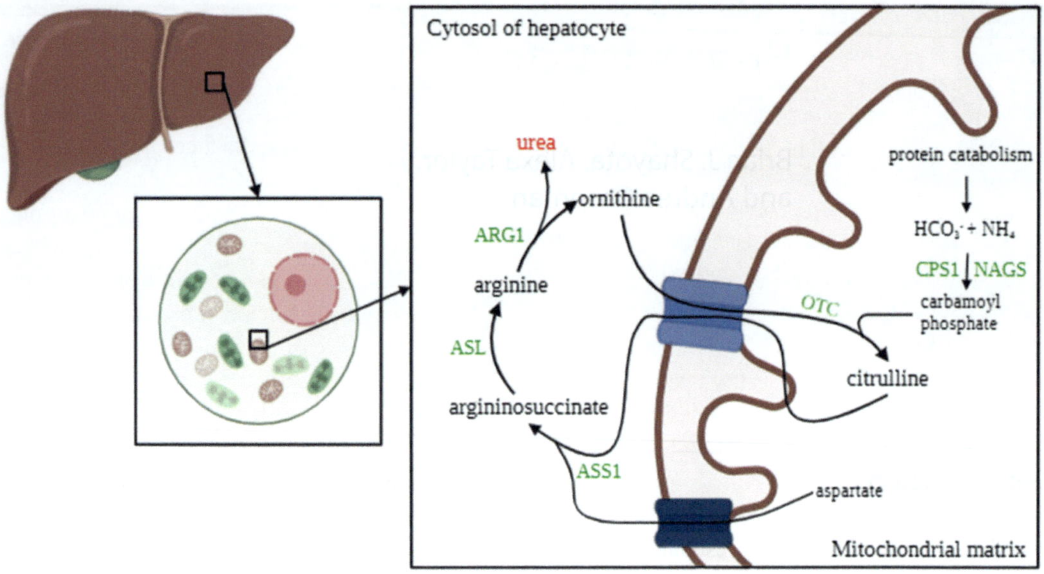

Fig. 22.1 The urea cycle takes place within the cytosol and mitochondria of hepatocytes. Proteins are broken down into amino acids, which are further catabolized into bicarbonate (HCO_3^-) and ammonia (NH_4^+). Ammonia is converted to carbamoyl phosphate via carbamoyl phosphate synthase 1 (CPS1). Carbamoyl phosphate and ornithine are catalyzed by the ornithine transcarbamylase (OTC) to form citrulline. Citrulline is transported back out to the cytosol of the hepatocyte and combined with aspartate to be catalyzed by the argininosuccinate synthetase 1 (ASS1) to form argininosuccinate. Argininosuccinate is catalyzed by the argininosuccinate lyase (ASL) to produce fumarate (not shown) and arginine. Arginine is catalyzed by arginase 1 (ARG1) to create urea and ornithine. Here, urea can enter the bloodstream and be excreted via urine by the kidneys. Ornithine can then be transported back into the mitochondrial matrix to continue the cycle

Most ammonia derives from the hydrolysis of the amide group from the amino acid glutamine, catalyzed by the enzyme glutaminase. The second nitrogen atom derives from aspartate, which is transported by the Citrin transporter out of the mitochondria and into the cytosol, where it can combine with citrulline in a reaction catalyzed by ASS1 to form arginosuccinate. Aspartate is a common byproduct of the transamination reaction of other amino acids like alanine and glutamine, which serve as a means of transporting amide groups to the liver. This is an important concept as glutamine is the most abundant amino acid in the blood and can serve as a target for diverting nitrogen away from a dysfunctional urea cycle.

Several regulatory factors ensure the proper functioning of the urea cycle. Allosteric regulation focuses on the initial catalytic step by the enzyme CPS1, which can be upregulated by deacetylation via SIRT5, typically triggered by metabolic stressors including prolonged fasting, insufficient caloric intake, and excess protein intake [19]. Furthermore, N-acetylglutamate (NAG) and carbamylglutamate serve as allosteric activators of CPS1, and as such can be targets for CPS1 and NAGS deficiency. Substrate availability can also play a vital role in normal urea cycle functioning, explaining why other inborn errors of metabolism can also present with HA. Finally, hormones like glucagon and corticosteroids play regulatory roles over the urea cycle by signaling for increased protein catabolism and suppressed urea-cycle-related gene expression [13]. As such, corticosteroid-induced HA is a well-known risk for patients with UCD and a reason to utilize caution when prescribing systemic steroids.

22.2 Incidence

UCD is rare, but the old adage "if you don't think of something, you won't diagnose it" holds true for many patients who present outside of the classic hyperammonemic crises as a neonate. Altogether, the estimated incidence of urea cycle defects is 1:35,000, with the majority (57% or 1:56,500) being OTC deficiency. ASS and ASL deficiency make up the next most common UCD (1:250,000 and 1:218,750, respectively), followed by the remaining types ≥1:1,000,000. This translates to an estimated 113 new patients born with a urea cycle disorder every year in the US [28]. Importantly, these still may be underestimates, as there is a growing appreciation for many late-onset presentations in adults that are being misdiagnosed or getting a delayed diagnosis.

22.3 Clinical Presentation

While there are common presenting features of UCD, symptoms relating to HA are the most classic finding. However, there are some notable, unique features among the different types. All UCDs pose a risk of acute HA, but the proximal defects tend to have a higher relative risk. Impaired ureagenesis intuitively results in the accumulation of free ammonia, but the mechanism by which ammonia leads to toxicity is far more complicated. The body initially tries to adapt by converting excess free ammonia into glutamine as a buffering mechanism. However, Gln then accumulates in astrocytes and disrupts their osmotic equilibrium, resulting in cerebral edema and eventual cerebellar herniation. At the same time, Gln increases mitochondrial membrane permeability, leading to free radical damage, apoptosis, and an inflammatory cascade. Additionally, excess Gln is converted to glutamate (Glu), resulting in impaired glutamatergic and GABAergic neurotransmission via altered membrane expression of Glu and GABA receptors [12].

Clinically, hyperammonemic crises can present with lethargy, nausea/vomiting, seizures, altered mental status, behavioral abnormalities, and psychosis (Table 22.1). Importantly, each UCD has the potential to manifest symptoms at any age. Additionally, the X-linked urea cycle defect, OTC deficiency, can present in females as well [25]. Female carriers may be symptomatic with deficits seen in brain Gln levels, selected dietary protein restriction, and deficits in working memory [27]. They may manifest neuropsychiatric and behavioral symptoms, and/or late HA events. Occasionally, there will be red flags in the medical history, including a family history of a male relative passing away from unknown causes during infancy in the case of OTC deficiency and early-onset aversion to high-protein foods. Preceding events to symptom onset may also provide clues to consider a urea cycle defect.

Table 22.1 Symptoms of urea cycle disorders (UCDs)

Lethargy	Nausea/vomiting
Seizures	Altered mental status
Behavioral abnormalities	Psychosis

In neonates, there will typically be a short symptom-free interval of a few days before lethargy and feeding intolerance set in. Outside of infancy, there will typically be a metabolic stressor that precipitated an episode, such as prolonged fasting, an infectious illness, excess physical exertion, or maternal recovery in the postpartum period. In adolescents and adults, episodes may mimic drug/alcohol-induced intoxication or a psychiatric disturbance and therefore will often be missed in the emergency room setting [26]. If not recognized and managed properly, encephalopathy and cerebral edema will lead to seizures, coma, and death.

HA is the defining characteristic of the proximal urea cycle defects, CPS1, OTC, and NAGS deficiency, where the frequency and severity of episodes are quite high. As one moves further down the path, the risk of HA decreases, but other phenotypic defining features can occur. For example, ASL deficiency has the additional unique findings of trichorrhexis nodosa with coarse, brittle hair, liver dysfunction leading to cirrhosis, and systemic hypertension. Additionally, neurobehavioral issues like ADHD, learning disabilities, and seizures are more common compared to other urea cycle defects, even in the absence of significant HA [1, 9]. As such, the pathophysiology of ASL deficiency differs from some of the other urea cycle defects. Notable is ASL's additional role in forming the nitrogen oxide (NO) synthesis complex. Most of the net arginine produced in the body occurs within the kidneys via ASS1 and ASL metabolism, which is then used to produce NO for vasodilation, immune response, and other signaling interactions [4, 17]. As such, NO synthesis complex-dependent NO production is at least partially responsible for the hypertension in ASL deficiency [8].

Arginase deficiency also differs phenotypically from the other urea cycle defects, with spastic paraplegia being a predominant presenting feature. While HA is rare with arginase deficiency, spasticity tends to occur regardless of HA-induced brain injury. Patients not diagnosed by newborn screening traditionally present during early childhood with developmental delays and progressive spasticity, particularly involving the lower motor neurons. The underlying biochemical mechanism of this has been hypothesized to be related to excess arginine being converted to the synthesis of guanidino compounds that interfere with neurotransmission.

Finally, the transporter defects of the urea cycle, Citrin deficiency and hyperornithinemia-hyperammonemia-homocitrullinuria (HHH) syndrome have very different presenting features than any of the catalytic enzyme deficiencies. For example, Citrin deficiency can present with different symptoms at different stages of life. Infantile symptoms include transient intrahepatic cholestasis, hepatomegaly, and parenchymal infiltration with secondary coagulopathy, hypoproteinemia, and hypoglycemia. Then, during childhood, patients develop a strong aversion to carbohydrate-rich foods and can experience failure to thrive and dyslipidemia. Finally, during adulthood, patients can have hyperammonemic crises as well as neuropsychiatric disturbances. Alternatively, ornithine translocase deficiency causes hyperornithinemia-hyperammonemia-homocitrullinuria (HHH) syndrome. A minority of HHH cases can present with neonatal HA, but the majority present in childhood or later with chronic neurocognitive deficits, slow progressive spasticity, learning disability, and seizures, as well as chronic liver dysfunction.

22.4 Work-Up/Investigation

Due to the relative simplicity of the urea cycle, diagnostic biochemical testing is rather straightforward, with measurements of plasma amino acids and urine orotic acid often being sufficient in differentiating the various types of urea cycle disorders. HA is typically the first test to raise the suspicion of a urea cycle defect in an undiagnosed patient, but it has low specificity as there are several other genetic and nongenetic causes for elevated ammonia levels. Most importantly, one should first verify the accuracy of an elevated ammonia result, as blood samples have poor stability and can easily result in a false elevation if not handled properly. A proper ammonia level should be drawn as a free-flowing sample, immediately placed on ice, and taken for direct processing within 30 minutes of the blood draw. A true elevation should be followed by plasma amino acid and urine orotic acid measurements.

The three proximal urea cycle defects (CPS1, NAGS, and OTC) have a biochemical signature that includes low plasma citrulline and elevated glutamine. OTC can then be teased out by having an elevated urine orotic acid level, which is not found in either CPS1 or NAGS deficiencies. Among the distal urea cycle defects, ASS is defined by an isolated elevation of citrulline, ASL deficiency by elevated citrulline plus the pathognomonic finding of elevated argininosuccinate, and ARG1 with elevated arginine. Currently, distal urea cycle defects are easily identified by newborn screening methods by measuring citrulline and arginine, but the detection of proximal defects is less reliable. Citrin deficiency can also be identified biochemically with plasma amino acids, but the profile is more complex with elevations in citrulline, arginine, methionine, threonine, and tyrosine, which later in life are primarily just elevated citrulline and arginine. HHH syndrome has, as its name implies, elevations of ornithine, homocitrulline, and intermittently ammonia, as well as orotic acid.

Neuroimaging may be diagnostic of UCD, particularly OTC. Common findings on a brain MRI include initial signal changes in the insula, which may progress to diffuse cerebral edema followed by atrophy, ischemic lesions in the cerebral intravascular boundary zones, and symmetric cortical involvement of the cingulate gyri, temporal lobes, and insular cortex [7, 30]. Proton magnetic resonance spectroscopy (1H MRS) can also identify a pattern of elevated Gln and reduced myoinositol and choline peaks, even in X-linked OTC carriers [10, 24, 29].

Molecular testing is common for confirmation of a diagnosis, especially when the biochemical phenotype is not as clear or when needing to differentiate CPS1 and NAGS deficiencies. Since there is a wide variety of potential causative variants in these genes, it is important to note the capabilities of the test being ordered to include sequence variants and copy number variants, as well as deep intronic and promoter region variants in the case of OTC deficiency. Newer methods to determine the pathogenicity of rare or novel variants are being developed [18].

22.5 Differential Diagnosis

One must consider all potential causes of HA when a new patient presents. This includes other inborn errors that can cause a secondary inhibition of the urea cycle. Several organic acidemias, such as propionic acidemia, methylmalonic acidemia, and isovaleric acidemia, can cause secondary inhibition of NAGS and impaired succinyl-CoA for the citric acid cycle, leading to HA [21]. Importantly, these conditions will classically present with a metabolic acidosis, whereas urea cycle disorders will have a respiratory alkalosis in the early stages. Fatty acid oxidation disorders (FAOD) can be considered as well, with carnitine acylcarnitine translocase (CACT), carnitine palmitoyltransferase II (CPT II), and multiple acyl-CoA dehydrogenase (MAD) deficiencies having a risk of HA. In this case, deficient acetyl-CoA production causes impaired NAG production and inhibition of CPS1 occurs due to fatty acylation of the active site [21]. Other rarer conditions include carbonic anhydrase VA deficiency, which can be differentiated by elevated lactic acid, and lysinuric protein intolerance, which is a rare situation in which urine amino acids are helpful to identify a pattern of increased lysine, ornithine, and arginine.

One must also consider nongenetic causes of HA, which are far more common than the genetic causes, especially when considering adult populations. Hepatic encephalopathy is a broad term and by far the most common cause of HA in adults. Liver dysfunction underlies all forms of hepatic encephalopathy, which can be caused by viral infections, autoimmune disease, toxin exposure, portosystemic bypass/shunting, and other causes of cirrhosis or portal hypertension [5]. Notably, the treatment approach is very different for hepatic encephalopathy compared to UCD, with lactulose often being effective. Less common nongenetic causes include various medications like the anticonvulsant valproic acid, chemotherapeutic drugs asparaginase hydrolysis and 5-fluorouracil, and salicylate. Finally, urinary tract infections caused by urease-producing bacteria such as *Corynebacterium, Proteus*, and *Staphylococcus* species can cause HA [14, 22].

22.6 Management

Proper management of UCD focuses on the avoidance of HA with chronic care goals in mind, as well as the acute mitigation of damage with rapid acute care during a crisis. Chronic care can be further divided into avoidance of metabolic stress, dietary modifications, and nitrogen scavenger therapies. Metabolic stress is a physiological process that occurs in response to low cellular energy levels. This results in a signaling cascade that leads to catabolism and the release of metabolites that serve as reservoirs of energy and building blocks of the cell. Metabolic stress can be caused by (1) poor caloric availability as occurs during prolonged fasting, malnutrition, and excess losses from vomiting or diarrhea, (2) increased energy demands as a result of excessive physical activity or recovery from a medical illness/surgery, (3) or a combination of the two as often occurs during infectious illnesses, particularly with those that cause nausea/vomiting and/or fevers. Therefore, it is important that patients avoid triggers of metabolic stress when reasonably possible.

Diet modifications also play a significant role in the chronic care of urea cycle defects, with a focus on protein restriction as a key component, apart from Citrin deficiency. Due to the variability of disease severity and changing rates of metabolism through different life stages, the patient's protein tolerance is a constantly moving target that requires a very specific dietary restriction as outlined by a biochemical geneticist and metabolic dietitian. Excess protein intake disrupts nitrogen homeostasis and can trigger HA even without any metabolic stressors. Some patients will also require specialized medical formulas or supplements that provide safer forms of protein by providing only essential amino acids with a low nitrogen load. Supplementation of urea cycle intermediates downstream of the enzymatic block can also be useful to ensure that specific amino acid deficiencies do not occur, while also facilitating nitrogen excretion by providing downstream metabolites to maintain residual urea cycle function.

Finally, many patients will require nitrogen scavenger therapies, which provide alternative pathways for nitrogen to be disposed of that do not require the urea cycle. The most notable of these therapies is sodium benzoate, which conjugates with glycine to form hippuric acid for urinary excretion of its single nitrogen atom, and phenylbutyrate, which conjugates with glutamine to form phenylacetylglutamine for urinary excretion of its two nitrogen atoms. Phenylbutyrate can either come attached to sodium, which has traditionally been less palatable for patients, or attached to a glycerol group that is better tolerated and has improved pharmacokinetics that allow for less frequent dosing. In the specific case of NAGS deficiency, there is the additional therapeutic carglumic acid, which serves as a structural analog to NAG and can help prevent episodes of HA.

The management of an acute crisis has a somewhat different approach, as the patient is already in a hyperammonemia crisis and requires rapid action to reduce ammonia levels as quickly as possible. With severe episodes, the fastest way to bring down ammonia levels is either dialysis or IV administration of the combined drug, sodium benzoate/sodium phenylacetate. ECMO-driven dialysis and continuous hemodialysis are the most effective forms of dialysis, whereas peritoneal dialysis has substantially less clearance and should be avoided [11]. IV sodium benzoate/sodium phenylacetate is also effective but should only be used in cases where a urea cycle diagnosis has been confirmed, since it will not be effective for some of the other causes of HA. Most protocols also call for the use of IV arginine alongside IV sodium benzoate/sodium phenylacetate, except for arginase deficiency, for the same reasons it is supplemented in chronic care.

While the above therapies will remove current endogenous ammonia, it is equally important to cease further production of ammonia. Therefore, complete protein restriction should be instituted for at least 24–48 hours and then slowly reintroduced. Avoidance of all protein intake for longer than 48 hours will trigger a catabolic state and result in endogenous release and breakdown of proteins within the body to fulfill the requirements of other processes. Calories in the form of carbohydrates and fats should be encouraged to meet the nutritional demands of the body and trigger an anabolic state. In the acutely ill patient, high-concentration dextrose IV fluids D10–20% and IV intralipids are frequently used. The body can also be rendered into anabolism by providing insulin, a hormone that is naturally released in the fed state and triggers many metabolic processes to store energy and utilize free amino acids to build proteins. Notably, when considering the risk of neurological damage following an episode, the duration of sustained HA can be as important as the magnitude of the ammonia elevation itself [7].

22.7 Surgical Planning/Management

When standard chronic care management strategies are not sufficient, liver transplantation is often the next consideration. The most common indication is recurrent episodes of HA despite optimal management. Such episodes lead to immediate risks like coma, herniation, and death but can also have a cumulative effect on neurocognitive development. Transplantation can also be considered when medical restrictions severely impact quality of life.

Liver transplantation had been avoided in the late twentieth century due to the high risks of morbidity and mortality when performed on infants. However, advances in surgical techniques and effective immunosuppressive medications have made transplantation an increasingly attractive option for patients with urea cycle disorders. Even young patients now have comparable mortality rates following liver transplantation compared to older children, so there is less benefit in delaying beyond a certain period [16]. One recent study found a survival rate of 95% of OTC patients receiving a liver transplant, but complications requiring retransplantation occurred in 10% and overall, 65% experienced at least one complication including acute rejection, hepatic artery thrombus, biliary leak, and renal dysfunction from immunosuppressive agents, so it is still not a decision to take lightly [23].

The primary benefit of liver transplantation is that it completely removes the risk of HA for all the urea cycle disorders. As such, patients may consume a normal diet without protein restriction and no longer require standard chronic care precautions. Transplantation cannot reverse any neurological damage that may have already occurred, but neurological outcomes are better in patients that have received a transplant, particularly if it was done at an early stage [6]. Different graft types may be used, with reports of grafts from living and cadaveric donors, as well as split and whole liver donors [23]. In Japan, where the availability of donors is scarce, the use of living female donors who are heterozygous for a pathogenic variant in OTC (i.e. partial donation of mother to son with OTC deficiency) has been used, though this approach is not preferred as skewed X-linked inactivation may still present a risk for HA despite a successful transplant [20]. This is less of a concern for obligate carriers of autosomal recessive urea cycle disorders serving as donors, but in rare instances, it has been reported to result in residual risk for HA during periods of metabolic stress [15].

Intraoperatively, the surgical procedure and anesthetic approach do not differ from other indications of liver transplantation. Although it is ideal to stabilize the patient from a hyperammonemia crisis prior to transplantation, there have been reports of patients undergoing transplant while requiring IV nitrogen scavengers and hemodialysis [3]. Generally, it is best to minimize preoperative fasting as much as possible and, at the very least, infuse dextrose-containing fluids and IV intralipids to maintain anabolism pre- and intraoperatively.

Postoperatively, patients are typically able to tolerate a normal diet without requiring the use of medical formulas. Nitrogen scavengers can be discontinued in most cases. It is debated whether one should supplement downstream amino acids; however, in one review of patients with CPS1 and OTC deficiency, supplementation with citrulline posttransplantation did not result in any notable difference in growth or cognitive abilities [2].

22.8 Conclusion

The outlook of UCD management is constantly shifting as improvements in existing therapies and the development of novel therapies change the medical management approach. With this progress, morbidity and mortality levels of all UCDs have improved, although significant risks and patient burdens continue to exist. Theoretically, a gene therapy approach will lead to a new paradigm in urea cycle disease care, with the added benefit of needing to target only one organ system. Human gene therapy trials are underway for some patients with proximal disorders. Until then, surgical interventions such as liver transplantation will remain a vital tool for patients with difficult-to-manage urea cycle defects.

References

1. Ah Mew N, Krivitzky L, McCarter R, Batshaw M, Tuchman M. Clinical outcomes of neonatal onset proximal versus distal urea cycle disorders do not differ. J Pediatr. 2013;162(2) https://doi.org/10.1016/j.jpeds.2012.06.065.
2. Aldrian D, Waldner B, Vogel GF, El-Gharbawy AH, McKiernan P, Vockley J, Landau YE, Al Mutairi F, Stepien KM, Kwok AMK, Yıldız Y, Honzik T, Kelifova S, Ellaway C, Lund AM, Mori M, Grünert SC, Scholl-Bürgi S, Zöggeler T, et al. Impact of citrulline substitution on clinical outcome after liver transplantation in carbamoyl phosphate synthetase 1 and ornithine transcarbamylase deficiency. J Inherit Metab Dis. 2024;47(2):220–9. https://doi.org/10.1002/jimd.12717.
3. Baba C, Yukimasa S, Yasuno R, Ichiyanagi H, Ninagawa J, Kasuya S, Kasahara M, Horikawa R, Nagasaka Y, Suzuki Y. Anesthesia management protocol for liver transplantation as treatment for ornithine transcarbamylase deficiency. Paediatr Anaesth. 2023;33(8):620–30. https://doi.org/10.1111/pan.14691.
4. Bian K, Doursout MF, Murad F. Vascular system: role of nitric oxide in cardiovascular diseases. J Clin Hypertens. 2008;10(4):304–10. https://doi.org/10.1111/j.1751-7176.2008.06632.x.
5. Butterworth RF. Hepatic encephalopathy in cirrhosis: pathology and pathophysiology. Drugs. 2019;79:17–21). Springer International Publishing. https://doi.org/10.1007/s40265-018-1017-0.
6. Campeau PM, Pivalizza PJ, Miller G, McBride K, Karpen S, Goss J, Lee BH. Early orthotopic liver transplantation in urea cycle defects: follow up of a developmental outcome study. Mol Genet Metab. 2010;100(SUPPL) https://doi.org/10.1016/j.ymgme.2010.02.012.
7. Enns GM. Neurologic damage and neurocognitive dysfunction in urea cycle disorders. Semin Pediatr Neurol. 2008;15(3):132–9. https://doi.org/10.1016/j.spen.2008.05.007.
8. Erez A, Nagamani SCS, Shchelochkov OA, Premkumar MH, Campeau PM, Chen Y, Garg HK, Li L, Mian A, Bertin TK, Black JO, Zeng H, Tang Y, Reddy AK, Summar M, O'Brien WE, Harrison DG, Mitch WE, Marini JC, et al. Requirement of argininosuccinate lyase for systemic nitric oxide production. Nat Med. 2011;17(12):1619–26. https://doi.org/10.1038/nm.2544.
9. Ficicioglu C, Mandell R, Shih VE. Argininosuccinate lyase deficiency: Longterm outcome of 13 patients detected by newborn screening. Mol Genet Metab. 2009;98(3):273–7. https://doi.org/10.1016/j.ymgme.2009.06.011.
10. Gropman AL, Fricke ST, Seltzer RR, Hailu A, Adeyemo A, Sawyer A, van Meter J, Gaillard WD, McCarter R, Tuchman M, Batshaw M. 1H MRS identifies symptomatic and asymptomatic subjects with partial ornithine transcarbamylase deficiency. Mol Genet Metab. 2008;95(1–2):21–30. https://doi.org/10.1016/j.ymgme.2008.06.003.
11. Gupta S, Fenves AZ, Hootkins R. The role of RRT in hyperammonemic patients. Clin J Am Soc Nephrol. 2016;11(10):1872–8). American Society of Nephrology. https://doi.org/10.2215/CJN.01320216.
12. Hernández-Rabaza V, Cabrera-Pastor A, Taoro-González L, Malaguarnera M, Agustí A, Llansola M, Felipo V. Hyperammonemia induces glial activation, neuroinflammation and alters neurotransmitter receptors in hippocampus, impairing spatial learning: reversal by sulforaphane. J Neuroinflammation. 2016;13(1) https://doi.org/10.1186/s12974-016-0505-y.
13. Imoto K, Tanaka M, Goya T, Aoyagi T, Takahashi M, Kurokawa M, Tashiro S, Kato M, Kohjima M, Ogawa Y. Corticosteroid suppresses urea-cycle-related gene expressions in ornithine transcarbamylase deficiency. BMC Gastroenterol. 2022;22(1) https://doi.org/10.1186/s12876-022-02213-0.
14. Inoue S, Yasuda H, Yoshida K, Mori K, Ogawa K, Yokotsuka Y, Okamoto H. A diabetic patient with prolonged Hyperammonemia due to urinary tract infection caused by urease-producing bacteria. Intern Med. 2024; https://doi.org/10.2169/internalmedicine.2817-23.
15. Kakiuchi T, Nosho T, Oka M, Tashiro K. Hyperammonemia in a carbamoyl-phosphate synthetase 1 deficiency recipient after living-donor liver transplantation from a carrier donor: a case report. Front Med. 2023;10 https://doi.org/10.3389/fmed.2023.1327854.
16. Lee B, Goss J. Long-term correction of urea cycle disorders. J Pediatr. 2001;138(1 Suppl):S62–71. https://doi.org/10.1067/mpd.2001.111838.
17. Levillain O. Expression and function of arginine-producing and consuming-enzymes in the kidney. Amino Acids. 2012;42(4):1237–52. https://doi.org/10.1007/s00726-011-0897-z.
18. Lo RS, Cromie GA, Tang M, Teng K, Owens K, Sirr A, Kutz JN, Morizono H, Caldovic L, Ah Mew N, Gropman A, Dudley AM. The functional impact of 1,570 individual amino acid substitutions in human OTC. Am J Hum Genet. 2023;110(5):863–79. https://doi.org/10.1016/j.ajhg.2023.03.019.
19. Nakagawa T, Lomb DJ, Haigis MC, Guarente L. SIRT5 deacetylates carbamoyl phosphate Synthetase 1 and regulates the urea cycle. Cell. 2009;137(3):560–70. https://doi.org/10.1016/j.cell.2009.02.026.
20. Oishi K, Arnon R, Wasserstein MP, Diaz GA. Liver transplantation for pediatric inherited metabolic disorders: considerations for indications, complications, and perioperative management. Pediatr Transplant.

2016;20(6):756–69). Blackwell Publishing Inc. https://doi.org/10.1111/petr.12741.
21. Ribas GS, Lopes FF, Deon M, Vargas CR. Hyperammonemia in inherited metabolic diseases. Cell Mol Neurobiol. 2022;42(8):2593–610. https://doi.org/10.1007/s10571-021-01156-6.
22. Roberts SC, Malik W, Ison MG. Hyperammonemia syndrome in immunosuppressed individuals. Curr Opin Infect Dis. 2022;35(3):262–8). Lippincott Williams and Wilkins. https://doi.org/10.1097/QCO.0000000000000828.
23. Seker Yilmaz B, Baruteau J, Chakrapani A, Champion M, Chronopoulou E, Claridge LC, Daly A, Davies C, Davison J, Dhawan A, Grunewald S, Gupte GL, Heaton N, Lemonde H, McKiernan P, Mills P, Morris AAM, Mundy H, Pierre G, et al. Liver transplantation in ornithine transcarbamylase deficiency: a retrospective multicentre cohort study. Mol Genet Metab Rep. 2023;37 https://doi.org/10.1016/j.ymgmr.2023.101020.
24. Sen K, Anderson AA, Whitehead MT, Gropman AL. Review of multi-modal imaging in urea cycle disorders: the old, the new, the borrowed, and the blue. Front Neurol. 2021;12). Frontiers Media S.A https://doi.org/10.3389/fneur.2021.632307.
25. Sen K, Izem R, Long Y, Jiang J, Konczal LL, McCarter RJ, Mew NA, Baumgartner MR, Berry G, Berry SA, Burgard P, Burrage LC, Cederbaum S, Coughlin C, Diaz GA, Enns G, Gallagher RC, Harding CO, Hoffmann GF, et al. Are asymptomatic carriers of OTC deficiency always asymptomatic? A multicentric retrospective study of risk using the UCDC longitudinal study database. Mol Genet Genomic Med. 2024;12(4) https://doi.org/10.1002/mgg3.2443.
26. Sloas HA, Ence TC, Mendez DR, Cruz AT. At the intersection of toxicology, psychiatry, and genetics: a diagnosis of ornithine transcarbamylase deficiency. Am J Emerg Med. 2013;31(9):1420.e5–6. https://doi.org/10.1016/j.ajem.2013.05.010.
27. Sprouse C, King J, Helman G, Pacheco-Colón I, Shattuck K, Breeden A, Seltzer R, Van Meter JW, Gropman AL. Investigating neurological deficits in carriers and affected patients with ornithine transcarbamylase deficiency. Mol Genet Metab. 2014;113(1):136–41. https://doi.org/10.1016/j.ymgme.2014.05.007.
28. Summar ML, Koelker S, Freedenberg D, Le Mons C, Haberle J, Lee HS, Kirmse B. The incidence of urea cycle disorders. Mol Genet Metab. 2013;110(1–2):179–80. https://doi.org/10.1016/j.ymgme.2013.07.008.
29. Takanashi J, Kurihara A, Tomita M, Kanazawa M, Yamamoto S, Morita F, Ikehira H, Tanada S, Kohno Y. Distinctly abnormal brain metabolism in late-onset ornithine transcarbamylase deficiency. 2002. https://www.neurology.org
30. Takanashi J-I, Barkovich AJ, Cheng SF, Weisiger K, Zlatunich CO, Mudge C, Rosenthal P, Tuchman M, Packman S. Brain MR imaging in neonatal Hyperammonemic encephalopathy resulting from proximal urea cycle disorders. AJNR Am J Neuroradiol. 2003;24(6):1184–7.

23 Mitochondrial Disease

Kimberly A. Chapman

Background The mitochondrion is the "power plant" of the cell. Primary mitochondrial disorders are a group of disorders that impact the electron transport chain, the oxidative phosphorylation regulator, mitochondrial DNA transcription, translation, and the structure of the mitochondria.

These disorders result from mitochondrial dysfunction, which impairs the energy production needed for cell function. Consequently, high-energy organs such as the brain, muscles, nervous system, eyes, heart, kidneys, pancreas, and liver are commonly affected, though symptoms can be nonspecific [1, 6].

Categorizing mitochondrial disorders is complex due to three different approaches historically used to describe them [9]. Initially, these disorders were named based on their symptoms. Later, biochemical assays, such as measuring oxidative phosphorylation activity and respiratory chain enzyme deficiencies (e.g., complex I or complex III deficiencies), were used for characterization. More recently, advances in genetic diagnostics have identified over 350 genes associated with mitochondrial disease, including 16 discovered in the past year alone [8]. Thus, the originally described disorders may not always correspond to the currently identified genetic variations and can be caused by different gene mutations. Adding to the complexity, mitochondrial disorders can arise from mutations in both mitochondrial DNA (mtDNA) and nuclear DNA (nDNA).

Mitochondrial disorders usually involve defects in energy production. According to the widely accepted "endosymbiotic hypothesis," mitochondria are relics of ancient proteobacteria that merged with early eukaryotic cells, providing them with oxidative metabolism capabilities. Mitochondria are crucial for energy production in all human tissues and not only participate in oxidative phosphorylation but also house several metabolic pathways, including the pyruvate dehydrogenase complex, amino acid catabolism, the carnitine cycle, beta-oxidation, and the tricarboxylic acid (TCA) cycle [2].

Defects in any of these pathways are considered mitochondrial diseases, but the term "mitochondrial encephalomyopathy" specifically refers to disorders caused by defects in the respiratory chain [3, 4]. The respiratory chain, located in the inner mitochondrial membrane, consists of four multi-subunit complexes (I to IV) and two small electron carriers, coenzyme Q10 (ubiquinone) and cytochrome c. The chain uses the energy from electron transfer to pump protons across the mitochondrial membrane, creating an electrochemical gradient that drives ATP produc-

K. A. Chapman (✉)
Prenatal Pediatrics Institute, Rare Disease Institute-Genetics and Metabolism, Cardiogenetics Program, Children's National Hospital, Washington, DC, USA
e-mail: kchapman@childrensnational.org

T. Hackert, A. Gulla (eds.), *Rare Liver and Biliary Tract Diseases*,
https://doi.org/10.1007/978-3-032-15076-9_23

tion via complex V (ATP synthase) in a process known as oxidative phosphorylation coupling.

A unique feature of the respiratory chain is its dual genetic control: mtDNA encodes 13 of the approximately 89 proteins required for the chain, while nDNA encodes the remaining proteins. Specifically, complex II (succinate dehydrogenase), coenzyme Q10, and cytochrome c are exclusively encoded by nDNA. In contrast, complexes I, III, IV, and V include subunits encoded by mtDNA—7 for complex I (ND1, ND2, ND3, ND4, ND4L, ND5, and ND6), 1 for complex III (cytochrome b), 3 for complex IV (COX I, COX II, and COX III), and 2 for complex V (ATPase 6 and ATPase 8) [3, 4].

Incidence Their incidence is estimated to be as high as 1 in 4300 individuals [5].

23.1 Clinical Presentation

Mitochondrial diseases, whether primary or secondary, primarily affect organs and tissues with high energy demands, including the brain, retina, cochlea, heart, pancreas, gastrointestinal tract, kidneys, and muscles. Dysfunction of genes associated with nuclear encoding usually impacts most of these organs. However, genes encoded by maternally inherited mitochondrial DNA can exhibit varying levels of heteroplasmy, meaning individuals with a higher load of dysfunctional genes may experience more severe effects.

Mitochondrial disorders can manifest at any age. When the muscle or liver is affected, lactic acidosis is often observed in the blood. Conversely, if the brain is involved, elevated lactate may be detected through magnetic resonance spectroscopy (MRS), and mitochondrial encephalopathy may occur. Gastrointestinal tract involvement is common, often leading to dysmotility, which can be aggravated by anesthesia or stress during surgery (Table 23.1).

Table 23.1 Red flags for yet-to-be-diagnosed mitochondrial disease

History	
	More than 2 high energy organs involved
	Family history of mitochondrial disease
	Family history of below signs or symptoms
Signs or symptoms (usually have more than 1)	
	Brain imaging abnormalities or encephalopathy resembling a stroke (with blood clot or bleed)
	Insulin dependent diabetes without antibodies
	Cardiomyopathy unrelated to coronary artery disease
	Cardiac arrhythmias
	Gastrointestinal dysmotility
	Lactic acidosis
	Recurrent rhabdomyolysis
	Progressive external ophthalmoplegia or ptosis
	Neurosensory hearing loss at young age or related to antibiotics
	Migraines
	Renal tubular acidosis
	Neuropathies

23.2 Workup Investigations

For individuals with known mitochondrial disease, the pre-surgical workup should focus on identifying patient-specific complications. A thorough history and physical examination will help determine if additional screening is needed. Typically, the workup may include screening blood tests such as complete blood count, comprehensive metabolic profile (which includes renal function), coagulation profiles and lactate, and possibly an electrocardiogram (EKG).

For individuals suspected of having mitochondrial disease based on history and physical examination—excluding cases requiring emergent surgery—a referral to a specialist in mitochondrial disease is recommended. The diagnostic workup typically begins with a detailed history and physical examination to identify markers of disease. This is followed by genetic testing. If no diagnosis is established but there remains a high suspicion of mitochondrial disease, a muscle or skin biopsy may be considered.

Muscle and skin biopsies for mitochondrial disorders can be analyzed using electron microscopy, oxidative phosphorylation enzyme assays, or genetic testing. Consult with a mitochondrial specialist well before the biopsy to determine the appropriate conditions for specimen collection, which specimens to collect, and where to send them for analysis.

Safety Surgery risk in individuals with mitochondrial disease is related to the organs affected. Generally, it is advisable to opt for shorter anesthesia times and less complex surgeries when possible.

Treatment Currently, therapeutic options for mitochondrial disease are limited. The most well-supported treatment is regular cardiovascular exercise. Despite common fatigue, a gradual increase in exercise has been shown to improve function.

Many patients use a "mitochondrial cocktail" consisting of various vitamins and minerals that support mitochondrial enzymes. It is important to continue these interventions without interruption.

With the growing number of clinical trials, new therapeutic options are expected to become available.

Some individuals may benefit from a ketogenic diet, although evidence supporting this is limited to specific subsets of patients. If a ketogenic diet is in use, avoid dextrose in the recommendations below and instead focus on providing intralipids as an energy source from intravenous fluids.

23.3 Surgical Planning/ Management

Preoperative planning is crucial and involves several considerations, including the selection of intravenous fluids, fasting duration, preadmission requirements, management of oral medications without intravenous alternatives, surgical duration, and post-surgical admission plans [7].

For patients with mitochondrial disease:

1. *Intravenous Fluids*: Avoid using lactated Ringer's solution, as lactate may exacerbate lactic acidosis in individuals at risk.
2. *Nutritional Support*: Prevent catabolism during surgery by providing calories, such as through 10% dextrose and electrolytes, unless the patient is on a ketogenic diet.
3. *Blood Glucose Management*: Be prepared to administer insulin if the patient is hyperglycemic.
4. *Anesthesia Considerations*: Patients with mitochondrial disease are at increased risk of anesthesia-related complications because many commonly used anesthetics are mitochondrial inhibitors [6, 7]. They may also be hypersensitive to volatile anesthetics.
   - *Respiratory Drive*: Individuals with myopathies may have decreased respiratory drive, increasing the risk of complications from muscle relaxants.
   - *Propofol*: Most mitochondrial patients do not tolerate extended use of propofol due to the risk of lactic acidosis; it should be limited to short procedures.
   - *Volatile Anesthetics*: Use these with caution, titrating slowly to avoid rapid changes in mitochondrial function.
5. *Local Anesthetics*: These are generally well tolerated in patients with mitochondrial disorders.
6. *Malignant Hyperthermia*: While there is no well-established link between malignant hyperthermia and mitochondrial disease, some myopathies associated with mitochondrial dysfunction may have a connection.

7. *Renal or Liver Medication Dosing*: Both organs can be impacted by mitochondrial disease, so screening for dysfunction prior to surgery and dosing medications appropriately is necessary.
8. *Cardiac Complications*: Individuals are at risk of cardiomyopathy and arrhythmias (especially long QTc). A thorough history and physical exam can assist with risk assessment.

Ensuring careful management in these areas can help mitigate risks and optimize outcomes for patients with mitochondrial disease undergoing surgery.

Drugs to Avoid

Valproic acid (especially in DNA polymerase subunit gamma (POLG) and those with liver disease).

Medications that cause lactic acidosis (e.g., propofol with long infusion times).

Dichloroacetate.

Aminoglycosides, if 12S rRNA encoded by mDNA (causes hearing loss); otherwise.

23.4 Medications that Can Be Used with Care (De Vries)

Analgesics/antipyretics: paracetamol, non-steroidal anti-inflammatory drugs (NSAIDs), aspirin.

Anesthetics: Articaine, bupivacaine, lidocaine, Volatile Anesthetics (see note above, including halothane, isoflurane, sevoflurane), Propofol (for induction only) (see note above), Fentanyl, Barbiturates, Ketamine, Non-depolarizing neuromuscular blocking agents with special care for those with myopathic phenotype, and Midazolam/benzodiazepines.

23.4.1 Preoperative Planning Flow Chart

1. *Diagnosis*
   (a) What is the diagnosis?
2. *Diagnosis Complications*
   (a) Does it have any specific complications?
      (i) *Yes*: Proceed to assessing complications.
      (ii) *No*: Continue to the next step.
3. *Patient Complications*
   (a) Does the patient have any complications?
4. *Surgery Details*
   (a) What is the surgery?
   (b) How long is the surgery planned?
   (c) How long is the expected nothing by mouth (NPO) (nil per os or fasting) duration?
   (d) What access will be needed (e.g., intravenous, central line)?
5. *Physical Examination, Medical History, and Family History*
   (a) Conduct a physical exam and review the patient's history.
6. *Nutritional Support*
   (a) *If on a Ketogenic Diet*:
      (i) Plan to provide electrolytes + intralipids 2–3 g/kg/d.
   (b) *If not on a Ketogenic Diet*:
      (i) Provide 10% dextrose with electrolytes at least 1.5x maintenance.
7. *Systemic Complications*
   (a) Does this patient have known systemic complications?
      (i) *Yes*: Consider additional management strategies.
      (ii) *No*: Proceed to the next step.
8. *Preoperative Screening*
   (a) Do we need to do any screening (e.g., EKG, laboratory tests, echocardiogram, etc.)?
9. *Anesthetic Approach*
   (a) Choose the anesthetic approach considering the patient's diagnosis, potential complications, and planned surgery.

This flow chart will help organize the preoperative considerations and ensure comprehensive planning for the patient.

23.5 Follow-Up and Recommendations

Individuals with mitochondrial disorders may need pre- and postoperative admissions to ensure stability. Follow-up care should be based on the type of surgery and any complications that arise.

If there are no major complications and the hospital stay is not extended, follow-up with a mitochondrial specialist can be scheduled at their discretion. Some specialists may prefer a follow-up within a few weeks, while others may opt for the usual scheduled appointments.

References

1. Barca E, Long Y, Cooley V, Schoenaker R, Emmanuele V, DiMauro S, Cohen BH, Karaa A, Vladutiu GD, Haas R, Van Hove JLK, Scaglia F, Parikh S, Bedoyan JK, DeBrosse SD, Gavrilova RH, Saneto RP, Enns GM, Stacpoole PW, Ganesh J, Larson A, Zolkipli-Cunningham Z, Falk MJ, Goldstein AC, Tarnopolsky M, Gropman A, Camp K, Krotoski D, Engelstad K, Rosales XQ, Kriger J, Grier J, Buchsbaum R, Thompson JLP, Hirano M. Mitochondrial diseases in North America: an analysis of the NAMDC registry. Neurol Genet. 2020;6(2):e402. https://doi.org/10.1212/NXG.0000000000000402. PMID: 32337332; PMCID: PMC7164977
2. Rahman J, Rahman S. Mitochondrial medicine in the omics era. Lancet. 2018;391(10139):2560–74. https://doi.org/10.1016/S0140-6736(18)30727-X. Epub 2018 Jun 18. PMID: 29903433
3. DiMauro S, Schon EA. Mitochondrial respiratory-chain diseases. N Engl J Med. 2003;348(26):2656–68. https://doi.org/10.1056/NEJMra022567. PMID: 12826641
4. DiMauro S. Mitochondrial encephalomyopathies–fifty years on: the Robert Wartenberg Lecture. Neurology. 2013;81(3):281–91. https://doi.org/10.1212/WNL.0b013e31829bfe89. PMID: 23858410; PMCID: PMC3959764
5. Gorman GS, Schaefer AM, Ng Y, Gomez N, Blakely EL, Alston CL, Feeney C, Horvath R, Yu-Wai-Man P, Chinnery PF, Taylor RW, Turnbull DM, McFarland R. Prevalence of nuclear and mitochondrial DNA mutations related to adult mitochondrial disease. Ann Neurol. 2015;77(5):753–9. https://doi.org/10.1002/ana.24362. Epub 2015 Mar 28. PMID: 25652200; PMCID: PMC4737121
6. Parikh S, Goldstein A, Karaa A, Koenig MK, Anselm I, Brunel-Guitton C, Christodoulou J, Cohen BH, Dimmock D, Enns GM, Falk MJ, Feigenbaum A, Frye RE, Ganesh J, Griesemer D, Haas R, Horvath R, Korson M, Kruer MC, Mancuso M, McCormack S, Raboisson MJ, Reimschisel T, Salvarinova R, Saneto RP, Scaglia F, Shoffner J, Stacpoole PW, Sue CM, Tarnopolsky M, Van Karnebeek C, Wolfe LA, Cunningham ZZ, Rahman S, Chinnery PF. Patient care standards for primary mitochondrial disease: a consensus statement from the Mitochondrial Medicine Society. Genet Med. 2017;19(12) https://doi.org/10.1038/gim.2017.107. Epub 2017 Jul 27. PMID: 28749475; PMCID: PMC7804217
7. Parikh S, Goldstein A, Koenig MK, Scaglia F, Enns GM, Saneto R, Anselm I, Cohen BH, Falk MJ, Greene C, Gropman AL, Haas R, Hirano M, Morgan P, Sims K, Tarnopolsky M, Van Hove JL, Wolfe L, DiMauro S. Diagnosis and management of mitochondrial disease: a consensus statement from the Mitochondrial Medicine Society. Genet Med. 2015;17(9):689–701. https://doi.org/10.1038/gim.2014.177. Epub 2014 Dec 11. PMID: 25503498; PMCID: PMC5000852
8. McCormick EM, Zolkipli-Cunningham Z, Falk MJ. Mitochondrial disease genetics update: recent insights into the molecular diagnosis and expanding phenotype of primary mitochondrial disease. Curr Opin Pediatr. 2018;30(6):714–24. https://doi.org/10.1097/MOP.0000000000000686. PMID: 30199403; PMCID: PMC6467265
9. Pavlakis SG, Hirano M. Mitochondrial diseases: a clinical and molecular history. Pediatr Neurol. 2016;63:3–5. https://doi.org/10.1016/j.pediatrneurol.2016.05.014. Epub 2016 Jun 2. PMID: 27460527; PMCID: PMC8285080

Navajo Neurohepatopathy

24

Kiley Quintana, Debra Regier, and Aiste Gulla

Overview Navajo neurohepatopathy (NNH) is a mitochondrial depletion syndrome that has been documented in the southwestern United States in Navajo families. It is an autosomal recessive disorder caused by a homozygous missense biallelic variant in the MPV17 gene, R50Q. This finding suggests it is a founder mutation. The Navajo Nation population was reduced to 8000 in 1868 [1] and has grown to approximately 400,000 in 2021 [2]. This gene is located at 2p23.3 [3]. This condition was first described in 1976 by Appenzeller et al., and was originally called Navajo neuropathy based on primarily neurological symptoms, including areflexia, weakness, and corneal ulceration secondary to corneal anesthesia [4]. Later, the name changed after the 1996 Holve et al. paper presented a large case series of affected individuals who had significant liver pathology, including liver failure[2] The incidence of this condition is estimated at 1 in 1600 live births in the Southwest Navajo population [5]. Other pathogenic variants have been described in MPV17; however, the homozygosity for the R50Q variant is almost exclusively found in Navajo families [3, 6].

Navajo neurohepatopathy is a mitochondrial DNA depletion syndrome (MDS). These disorders are characterized by a reduction in mitochondrial DNA (mtDNA) content, and the mitochondrial respiratory chain does not function correctly. The types of MDS include myopathic, encephalomyopathic, hepatocerebral, and neurogastrointestinal types. NNH falls under the MDS category of hepatocerebral, along with other genes including POLG, DGUOK, TWNK, and TFAM [7]. The MPV17 gene encodes a protein that is part of the inner mitochondrial membrane [8]. Specifically, biallelic mutations in MPV17 are also called mitochondrial DNA depletion syndrome 6 [7]. The respiratory chain complexes I, III, and IV are affected [9]. Dalla Rosa et al. found that deoxynucleotide insufficiency in the mitochondria was the cause of the DNA deletion through a study in MPV17 –/– mice [10].

Even though homozygous R50Q pathogenic variants are responsible for this condition in the Southwest Navajo population, there are three main presentations of liver involvement, even within the same family. There is an infantile form, a childhood form, and a classic form [3, 5].

K. Quintana
University of New Mexico, Washington, DC, USA
e-mail: kquintana@salud.unm.edu

D. Regier (✉)
Children's National Medical Center,
Washington, DC, USA
e-mail: dregier@childrensnational.org

A. Gulla
Department of Surgery, George Washington University, School of Medicine and Health Sciences, Washington, DC, USA

Clinic of Surgery, Gastroenterology and Nephrourology, Institute of Clinical Medicine, Faculty of Medicine, Vilnius, Lithuania
e-mail: a.gulla@gwu.edu

T. Hackert, A. Gulla (eds.), *Rare Liver and Biliary Tract Diseases*,
https://doi.org/10.1007/978-3-032-15076-9_24

The infantile form presents prior to 6 months of age with failure to thrive and jaundice, and progresses to liver failure by toddlerhood. The childhood form presents before age 5 with liver dysfunction and rapidly progresses to liver failure. The third type is the classic type, which presents at variable age, though typically from infancy to early childhood, with varying liver involvement and progressive neurological deterioration. Patients with the three forms demonstrated demyelination based on evidence of cranial imaging and nerve conduction studies [5]. The attenuated form of this condition, the classic form, is seen only with homozygous R50Q variants and not with other pathogenic variants of this gene [6].

Symptomatology Initial symptoms are often failure to thrive with growth parameters below the 5th percentile and jaundice. There is liver dysfunction, including coagulopathy, elevated AST, ALT, alkaline phosphatase, and hypoalbuminemia. Other clues in lab findings include non-anion gap metabolic acidosis and elevated lactate. Abdominal ultrasound often shows a nodular and echogenic liver [11]. The histology from a liver biopsy shows cholestatic steatohepatitis. Eventually, the child progresses to liver failure [5].

Aside from the liver symptomatology are the neurological symptoms. This is due to the degradation of myelin, causing axonal injury [5]. Symptoms include hypotonia, peripheral muscle atrophy, absent deep tendon reflexes, and sensory neuropathy. Acral mutilation and corneal anesthesia are secondary to loss of sensation, leading to injury, including corneal ulceration and poor healing [1, 5].

Histological clues on liver biopsy include cirrhosis of the liver and macrovesicular steatosis, patchy steatohepatitis, and cholestasis. Additionally, a few hepatocytes can contain megamitochondria. [11]

Diagnosis Diagnosis can be made through molecular testing showing the MPV17 homozygous R50Q missense mutation [3]. There is also a nosology, which Singleton et al. proposed in 1990 and was revised by the 1999 Holve et al. paper [1, 5]. The clinical diagnostic criteria include 4 of the 6 criteria for the new proband and 3 of the following criteria for the sibling: (1) sensory neuropathy, (2) motor neuropathy, (3) corneal anesthesia, (4) liver disease, (5) documented metabolic or infectious derangements, and (6) evidence of central nervous system demyelination on radiological imaging [5].

Differential Diagnosis Mimickers of this NNH include tyrosinemia, hepatitis B and hepatitis C, Wilson's disease, alpha-1 antitrypsin deficiency, galactosemia, Alagille syndrome, and glycogen storage diseases. For a diagnosis of tyrosinemia, succinylacetone is present. For Wilson's disease, one can evaluate for Kayser-Fleischer rings and an elevated serum copper level. Hepatitis B and C can be excluded with undetectable disease IgM markers. Alpha-1 antitrypsin deficiency has a low alpha-1-antitrypsin level. The marker for galactosemia is low galactose-1-phosphate uridyl transferase (GALT). Glycogen storage diseases have various enzyme deficiencies depending on the type.

Treatment Current treatment of NNH is largely supportive. Some treatment considerations should include a trial of vitamins and cofactors known as a "mitochondrial cocktail." There is a lack of studies showing definitive efficacy of this treatment, but it is generally low risk to try, if keeping a lookout for potential side effects of the medications and supplements. Possible medications and supplements include ubiquinol (CoQ10), B complex, L-carnitine, vitamin E, vitamin C, and alpha-lipoic acid [12].

The 2008 Parini et al. paper described avoidance of fasting as possibly slowing down progression of the disease in a small set of related patients in Italy, two siblings and a cousin, with the homozygous R50Q mutation in a consanguineous family that was not of Navajo ancestry. These children were noted to be hypoglycemic when sick with common illnesses and hospitalized for dextrose infusion. Their parents were also instructed not to let them fast beyond three hours in infancy. It was noted that when the siblings had prolonged fasting, their liver function tests worsened [6].

Surgical Treatment Options Many prior studies have been done to evaluate the outcomes of liver transplantation in these patients. Liver transplantation remains controversial as it has not been shown to improve or prevent extrahepatic manifestations of the disease [9]. A recent study from 2022 by Huang et al. presented 2 cases of infants aged 11 months and 8 months, with NNH who received liver transplantation and did not develop neurological symptoms at 3 years post-transplant and at 16 months posttransplant, respectively [13]. Their paper argued that NNH should not be a contraindication to liver transplantation.

Doctors Holve and Hu later highlighted that the follow-up of these two patients was too short to make this conclusion. Their large cohort of NNH patients, including 4 patients who underwent liver transplantation, had progression of extrahepatic symptoms after liver transplantation. They further explained that the second patient in the paper by Huang et al. developed neurological symptoms, including the inability to stand, at age 31 months [14].

The discussion of pursuing a liver transplantation for NNH should include a multidisciplinary team [11]. Families should understand the risks and benefits of the procedure and that it can cure the liver manifestations, however, not the neurological progression. Further, there is a risk of rejection and infection secondary to immunosuppression, which is a common cause of death in pediatric transplant patients.

If the decision to pursue a liver transplantation in an infant or child with NNH is made, additional testing is required. Baseline brain MRI prior to liver transplantation was performed in the patients in the above case series to monitor neurological progression after transplantation. Transplant evaluation must include an echocardiogram due to concomitant pulmonary hypertension, which has been reported as the second most common cause of mortality in these patients.

Navajo hepatopathy is a rare mitochondrial depletion disorder that is detrimental to the liver and currently does not have a cure. Liver transplantation can help mitigate the effects in the liver, but has not been shown to provide relief of neurological symptoms.

References

1. Singleton R, Helgerson SD, Snyder RD, O'Conner PJ, Nelson S, Johnsen SD, Allanson JE. Neuropathy in Navajo children: clinical and epidemiologic features. Neurology. 1990;40(2):363–7. https://doi.org/10.1212/wnl.40.2.363. PMID: 2300261
2. Becenti A. Diné enrolled population increases to 399,494, 2021-05-12 at the Wayback Machine, Navajo Times, 26 April 2021.
3. Karadimas CL, Vu TH, Holve SA, Chronopoulou P, Quinzii C, Johnsen SD, Kurth J, Eggers E, Palenzuela L, Tanji K, Bonilla E, De Vivo DC, DiMauro S, Hirano M. Navajo neurohepatopathy is caused by a mutation in the MPV17 gene. Am J Hum Genet. 2006;79(3):544–8. https://doi.org/10.1086/506913. Epub 2006 Jun 28. PMID: 16909392; PMCID: PMC1559552
4. Appenzeller O, Kornfeld M, Snyder R. Acromutilating, paralyzing neuropathy with corneal ulceration in Navajo children. Arch Neurol. 1976;24:733–8.
5. Holve S, Hu D, Shub M, Tyson RW, Sokol RJ. Liver disease in Navajo neuropathy. J Pediatr. 1999;135:482–93. https://doi.org/10.1016/S0022-3476(99)70172-1.
6. Parini R, Furlan F, Notarangelo L, Spinazzola A, Uziel G, Strisciuglio P, Concolino D, Corbetta C, Nebbia G, Menni F, Rossi G, Maggioni M, Zeviani M. Glucose metabolism and diet-based prevention of liver dysfunction in MPV17 mutant patients. J Hepatol. 2009;50(1):215–21. https://doi.org/10.1016/j.jhep.2008.08.019. Epub 2008 Oct 31. PMID: 19012992
7. Mahjoub G, Habibzadeh P, Dastsooz H, Mirzaei M, Kavosi A, Jamali L, Javanmardi H, Katibeh P, Faghihi MA, Dastgheib SA. Clinical and molecular characterization of three patients with Hepatocerebral form of mitochondrial DNA depletion syndrome: a case series. BMC Med Genet. 2019;20(1):167. https://doi.org/10.1186/s12881-019-0893-9. PMID: 31664948; PMCID: PMC6819644
8. Spinazzola A, Viscomi C, Fernandez-Vizarra E, Carrara F, D'Adamo P, Calvo S, Marsano RM, Donnini C, Weiher H, Strisciuglio P, Parini R, Sarzi E, Chan A, DiMauro S, Rötig A, Gasparini P, Ferrero I, Mootha VK, Tiranti V, Zeviani M. MPV17 encodes an inner mitochondrial membrane protein and is mutated in infantile hepatic mitochondrial DNA depletion. Nat

Genet. 2006;38(5):570–5. https://doi.org/10.1038/ng1765. Epub 2006 Apr 2. PMID: 16582910

9. Lee WS, Sokol RJ. Mitochondrial hepatopathies: advances in genetics, therapeutic approaches, and outcomes. J Pediatr. 2013;163(4):942–8. https://doi.org/10.1016/j.jpeds.2013.05.036. Epub 2013 Jun 28. PMID: 23810725; PMCID: PMC3934633
10. Dalla Rosa I, Cámara Y, Durigon R, Moss CF, Vidoni S, Akman G, Hunt L, Johnson MA, Grocott S, Wang L, Thorburn DR, Hirano M, Poulton J, Taylor RW, Elgar G, Martí R, Voshol P, Holt IJ, Spinazzola A. MPV17 loss causes deoxynucleotide insufficiency and slow DNA replication in mitochondria. PLoS Genet. 2016;12(1):e1005779. https://doi.org/10.1371/journal.pgen.1005779. PMID: 26760297; PMCID: PMC4711891
11. Bitting CP, Hanson JA. Navajo Neurohepatopathy: a case report and literature review emphasizing Clinicopathologic diagnosis. Acta Gastroenterol Belg. 2016;79(4):463–9. PMID: 28209105
12. Parikh S, Saneto R, Falk MJ, Anselm I, Cohen BH, Haas R, Medicine Society TM. A modern approach to the treatment of mitochondrial disease. Curr Treat Options Neurol. 2009;11(6):414–30. https://doi.org/10.1007/s11940-009-0046-0. PMID: 19891905; PMCID: PMC3561461
13. Huang AC, Ebel NH, Romero D, Martin B, Jhun I, Brown M, Enns GM, Esquivel C, Bonham C. Outcomes after liver transplantation in MPV17 deficiency (Navajo neurohepatopathy): a single-center case series. Pediatr Transplant. 2022;26(5):e14274. https://doi.org/10.1111/petr.14274. Epub 2022 Apr 24. PMID: 35466509
14. Holve S, Hu D. The long-term outcomes after liver transplantation in MPV-17 deficiency (Navajo Neurohepatopathy) are poor. Pediatr Transplant. 2023;27(3):e14437. https://doi.org/10.1111/petr.14437. Epub 2022 Nov 10. PMID: 36358014

25 Familial Intra-Hepatic Cholestasis (Byler disease)

Atoosa Rabiee, Roozbeh Rabiee, and Anahita Rabiee

25.1 Familial Intra-Hepatic Cholestasis

Progressive familial intrahepatic cholestasis (PFIC) is a heterogenous group of monogenic disorders characterized by impairment in bile transport and secretion. The clinical spectrum ranges from nonprogressive, intermittent cholestatic jaundice, benign recurrent intrahepatic cholestasis (BRIC), to chronic liver disease (PFIC). The most common types include PFIC 1 (deficiency of the FIC1 protein, ATP8B1 gene mutation), PFIC 2 (bile salt export pump deficiency, ABCB11 gene mutation), and PFIC 3 (multidrug resistance protein-3 deficiency, ABCB4 gene mutation). Newer variants of PFIC include PFIC 4 (loss of function of tight junction protein 2 (TJP2)), 5 (NR1H4 mutation causing Farnesoid X receptor deficiency), and 6 (MYO5B gene mutation causing microvillous inclusion disease (MVID)). Here, we discuss its incidence, clinical presentation, diagnosis, and management.

25.2 Incidence

All types of PFIC manifest in infancy or childhood, and they all have autosomal recessive inheritance. Disease variants are classified based on the specific genetic mutation resulting in bile transporter defects. The true incidence of PFIC is not known, but it is a rare disease, with an estimated incidence of 1/50,000 to 1/100,000 births. The PFIC family is responsible for 10–15% of cases of cholestasis in children and 10–15% of cases with liver transplantation in children [1]. Among the most common types of PFIC, PFIC1 and PFIC2 represent two-thirds of cases of PFIC, and PFIC3 represents the remaining third of cases [1]. Nearly two-thirds of subjects with normal gamma-glutamyltranspeptidase (GGT) do not have any mutations identified in the ATP8B1 (PFIC 1) or ABCB11 genes (PFIC2). Mutational analysis in patients with this phenotype has led to the identification of 3 more types of PFIC known as PFIC 4, 5, and 6. The exact incidence of newer variants of PFIC is not known due to the limited number of studies.

In the case of heterozygous mutations, symptoms could include transient neonatal cholestasis, intrahepatic cholestasis of pregnancy (ICP),

A. Rabiee (✉)
Department of Internal Medicine, Washington DC VA Hospital, Washington, DC, USA

R. Rabiee
Department of Gastroenterology and Hepatology, Faculty of Medicine, Azad University, Tehran, Iran

A. Rabiee
Department of Internal Medicine, West Haven VA Medical Center, Yale School of Medicine, New Haven, CT, USA
e-mail: anahita.rabiee@yale.edu

T. Hackert, A. Gulla (eds.), *Rare Liver and Biliary Tract Diseases*,
https://doi.org/10.1007/978-3-032-15076-9_25

drug-induced liver injury, cholelithiasis and choledocholithiasis [2].

25.3 Clinical Presentation

Cholestasis is a major clinical sign in all forms of PFIC. The main clinical presentation is pruritus and jaundice in the setting of cholestasis. One of the hallmarks of the disease is a low or normal GGT level, which is out of proportion to the degree of bile acid elevation in all subtypes of PFIC except PFIC 3, in which the GGT is elevated. Clinical manifestations are different based on the specific gene mutation. PFIC1 and PFIC2 usually appear in the first months of life, whereas PFIC3 can occur later in childhood or even in young adults (Table 25.1).

PFIC1 (Byler disease) is associated with an ATP8B1 gene mutation leading to FIC1 deficiency. It was first described in members of the Amish kindred, descended from Jacob Byler, in 1969, and therefore, it was called Byler disease [3]. The FIC1 membrane protein is a stabilizer of canalicular membrane lipid asymmetry, serving as a flippase for phosphatidylserine. It is characterized by recurrent episodes of jaundice, which become permanent later in the course of the disease [4]. In addition to jaundiceble, severe pruritus is usually observed. Extrahepatic features reported in PFIC1 patients include persistent short stature, sensorineural deafness, diarrhea, pancreatitis, and vitamins E and D deficiency [5]. Severe pruritus is often unresponsive to treatment with UDCA, antihistamines, or rifampicin [6].

Recurrent intrahepatic cholestasis (BRIC1) patients also have ATP8B1 mutations that rather disrupt protein function, while the mutations identified in patients with PFIC1 severely disrupt protein function. PFIC1 and BRIC1 are, in fact, two ends of a clinical spectrum. Patients with ATP8B1 deficiency, in the setting of BRIC1, usually present later in life with intermittent cholestasis and a much milder phenotype. Heterozygous ATP8B1 mutations have been identified in some cases of transient neonatal cholestasis, and intrahepatic cholestasis of pregnancy type 1 (ICP-1) [7].

PFIC2 is associated with an ABCB11 gene mutation, which encodes the ATP-dependent canalicular BSEP in the human liver. The BSEP protein is expressed at the hepatocyte canalicular membrane and is the major exporter of primary bile acids. Mutations in this protein result in decreased biliary bile salt secretion and accumulation of bile salts within the hepatocyte, resulting in severe hepatocellular damage [8]. Patients usually present with severe pruritus and cholelithiasis in the first 3 months of life. The initial presentation and the evolution are more severe, with permanent jaundice in the first months of life and rapid appearance of liver failure within the first years of life. PFIC2 patients have higher transaminase and alpha-fetoprotein serum levels at diagnosis than those with PFIC1. This group is at risk for early hepatocellular carcinoma (even in the first year of life), cholangiocarcinoma, and pancreatic adenocarcinoma.

In addition, BSEP deficiency represents a phenotypic continuum between BRIC2 and PFIC2 [9]. In BRIC2, missense mutations predominate, and mutations are seen in fewer conserved regions compared to those in PFIC1, leading to failure of protein production [10]. Heterozygosity for ABCB11 mutations has been identified in cases of ICP2 [11], drug-induced cholestasis [12], and transient neonatal cholestasis.

PFIC3 is associated with an ABCB4 gene mutation, which produces class III multidrug resistance (MDR3) of P-glycoprotein (P-gp). This is a phospholipid translocator expressed only in the canalicular membrane of hepatocytes. In the absence of biliary phospholipids, hydrophobic bile salts are not inactivated, which leads to bile canaliculi and biliary epithelial injuries. The absence of phospholipids in bile also destabilizes micelles and promotes bile lithogenicity through crystallization of cholesterol, which might result in small bile duct obstruction [1].

The most common symptoms include moderate to severe pruritus, although the onset is generally later than in other PFIC disorders. GGT is elevated, and patients are at risk of cholangiocarcinoma development. Heterozygous MDR3 defects may be involved in ICP3 [11], cholesterol gallstone disease [13], drug-induced cholestasis,

Table 25.1 Main types of PFIC and their characteristics

	PFIC1	PFIC2	PFIC3
Genetic and protein defect			
Genetic mutation	ATP8B1	ABCB11	ABCB4
Chromosome location	18q21-q22	2q24	7q21
Protein deficiency	FIC 1	BSEP	MDR 3
Functional defect	ATP-dependent aminophospholipid flippase	ATP-dependent bile acid transport in bile	ATP-dependent phosphatidylcholine floppase
Hepatocyte location	Canalicular membrane	Canalicular membrane	Canalicular membrane
Presentation			
Age at presentation	Early infancy	Early infancy	Later in childhood or young adulthood
Symptoms	Severe pruritus	Very severe pruritus	Moderate pruritus
Extra hepatic symptoms	Watery diarrhea, pancreatitis, sensorineural hearing loss	Uncommon	Uncommon
Laboratory and histology findings			
GGT	N	N	H
Bile composition	Low primary bile acid concentrations	Very low primary bile acid concentrations	Low phospholipid concentrations
Serum primary bile acid concentration	H(++) Very high	H (+++) Extremely high	H (+) High
Serum direct bilirubin	H	H	H
Serum ALP	H	H	H
Serum ALT	Mild elevation	>x5 ULN	Mild elevation
Serum AFP	N	H	N
Histology	Intracanalicular cholestasis, bile duct proliferation at the late phase	Bile duct proliferation at the late phase, lobular and portal fibrosis	Extensive bile duct proliferation, periportal fibrosis
Natural history and outcomes			
Progression to cirrhosis	Liver cirrhosis and rapid progression to end-stage liver disease	Progression even more quickly to end-stage liver disease, require liver transplantation during the first decade of life	Insidious
Risk of HCC	No	High	Mildly increased

Comparison of normal anatomy and production of bile acids, and defects seen in PFIC patients. *BSEP* Bile salt export pump, *FIC1* familial intrahepatic cholestasis, *MDR3* multidrug resistance class 3 glycoprotein, *BC* biliary canaliculus, *BA* bile acids adult idiopathic cirrhosis, and cholangiocarcinoma [14]. MDR3 deficiency could represent a clinical continuum, and a patient might experience different phenotypes during their lifetime, for example, they might initially present with cholesterol gallstones, then develop ICP during pregnancy, and later in adulthood develop biliary cirrhosis [15].

Other subtypes of normal GGT-PFIC include:

PFIC4 is associated with a TJP2 gene mutation and can present with cholestatic liver disease overlapping with FIC1; patients could also have hearing loss.

PFIC5 is a disorder with an NR1H4 gene mutation and can present with early infantile onset and rapid progression to liver failure, complicated by coagulopathy.

PFIC6 occurs with a MYO5B gene mutation; the patients can present with isolated cholestatic liver disease and could have neurologic involvement.

Lastly, PFIC7 is associated with a USP53 gene mutation, which could result in self-limited cholestasis or an episodic BRIC-like course.

25.4 Work-Up Investigation

Currently, FIC1 deficiency is typically diagnosed through a cholestasis gene panel, with a diminishing primary role for biochemical or histologic evaluations.

Serum GGT and alpha fetoprotein (AFP) are normal, ALT is only mildly elevated; normal serum cholesterol levels and very high serum bile acid concentrations are laboratory characteristics found in patients with PFIC1 [16].

In PFIC1, canalicular cholestasis and the absence of true ductular proliferation are among the early signs. As the disease progresses, periportal fibrosis and progression to biliary cirrhosis are seen. Electron microscopy shows dilatation of the canalicular lumen, filled with coarse, granular material, and focal interruption of the canalicular membrane [16, 17].

In PFIC2 patients, the same signs are seen, but the liver architecture is more perturbed, with more pronounced lobular and portal fibrosis and inflammation. Hepatocellular necrosis and giant cell transformation are also much more pronounced in PFIC2 than in PFIC1.

In PFIC3, liver histology shows portal fibrosis and true ductular proliferation with mixed inflammatory infiltrate. In a few instances, cholestasis is present in the lobule and in some ductules containing bile plugs. A slight giant cell transformation of hepatocytes can be observed. Cytokeratin immunostaining confirms the strong ductular proliferation within the portal tract. At a later stage, extensive portal fibrosis and a typical picture of biliary cirrhosis can be seen.

25.5 Differential Diagnosis

PFIC should be suspected in all children with cholestasis. Ultrasound must be done to exclude biliary tract disease and to rule out biliary atresia. Typically, ultrasonography is normal but may show a large gallbladder or gallstones. Once biliary atresia is ruled out, the most likely etiology is a monogenic defect that encompasses a large group of disorders.

The serum GGT is a good discriminant to guide initial evaluation. In a child with low or normal GGT for age and elevated serum bile acids, PFIC1 and PFIC2 are highly likely. Patients with PFIC3 have high serum GGT activity. PFIC3 patients also tend to present later in childhood or in young adulthood, as opposed to PFIC1 and PFIC2, which usually present in the first 3 months of life.

GGT value is typically higher in neonates than in older children and is generally elevated during cholestasis; therefore, the differential for normal or low GGT includes PFIC1, PFIC2, bile acid synthesis disorders (BASDs), and other subtypes of PFIC, including PFIC4 (TJP2 deficiency), PFIC5 (FXR deficiency), and PFIC6 (MYO5B deficiency). The best next step is next-generation sequencing.

In the setting when GGT is elevated, differentials could include PFIC3 and Alagille syndrome ALGS (JAG1 and NOTCH2 gene mutations). These patients have ductopenia on liver biopsy and characteristic Alagille facies, butterfly vertebrae, renal disease, and developmental cardiac defects. In cases of high serum GGT activity, sclerosing cholangitis must be excluded.

25.5.1 Liver Histology

In PFIC1 patients, liver histology is characterized by canalicular cholestasis and the absence of true ductular proliferation, with only periportal biliary metaplasia of hepatocytes.

In PFIC2 patients, in addition to the similar signs seen in PFIC1, there is usually more pronounced lobular and portal fibrosis and inflammation. Hepatocellular necrosis and giant cell transformation are also much more pronounced in PFIC2 than in PFIC1.

In PFIC3, portal fibrosis and true ductular proliferation with a mixed inflammatory infiltrate are seen. Cholestasis might be present in the lobule, and bile plugs can be seen in the ductules. Cytokeratin immunostaining usually confirms the major ductular proliferation within the portal tract. In late stages, extensive portal fibrosis and a typical picture of biliary cirrhosis can be seen. When signs of biliary obstruction appear on liver biopsy, as may be seen in PFIC3, further advanced imaging and cholangiography should be considered to exclude sclerosing cholangitis.

25.5.2 Liver Immunostaining

Commercially available MDR3 and BSEP antibodies allow liver immunostaining to be performed. Absence of canalicular or mild immunostaining favors a gene defect. However, normal staining does not rule out the disease, as a gene defect might have resulted in loss of function with only mildly decreased levels.

25.5.3 Biliary Lipid Analysis

This can be performed with gallbladder bile or with bile collected by duodenal aspiration. Biliary bile salt concentrations may be dramatically decreased in PFIC2 patients, mildly decreased in PFIC1 patients, and normal in PFIC3. However, in PFIC3 patients, the biliary phospholipid level is dramatically decreased, with a bile salt-to-phospholipid ratio fivefold higher compared to normal individuals. The percentage of biliary phospholipids appears to be directly related to the severity of the MDR3 mutation (nonsense, frameshift vs. missense).

25.5.4 Molecular Analysis and Next-Generation Sequencing

Advances in our ability to perform highly accurate next-generation sequencing have made the identification of rare diseases such as PFIC accurate and part of clinical practice. Current guidelines for the evaluation of cholestatic jaundice in infants by the North American Society for Pediatric and the European Society for Pediatric Gastroenterology, Hepatology, and Nutrition recommend the incorporation of modern, broad-based next-generation DNA sequencing technologies in the proper clinical context when working up an infant with cholestasis [18].

25.6 Medical Treatment

25.6.1 Ursodeoxycholic Acid (UDCA)

Therapy with UDCA should be considered in the initial therapeutic management of children with all types of PFIC. It is a nontoxic, hydrophilic bile acid, and is hypothesized to that it can decrease the hepatotoxicity of the accumulating endogenous bile acids. The starting dose is usually 10 mg/kg per day.

More than half of the patients with high GGT–PFIC or proven PFIC3 (especially the ones with ABCB4 alterations) responded to UDCA treatment. In one-third of PFIC3 patients, where mutations result in no expression of the MDR3 protein, patients are usually nonresponders to UDCA therapy.

In patients with low GGT–PFIC (especially PFIC 1 and 2 subtypes), UDCA therapy is usually not effective. Even in patients with a mild phenotype, such as BRIC1 and BRIC2, UDCA is not successful in preventing or aborting a cholestatic attack. Progression of disease and insufficient symptom relief may necessitate further intervention.

25.6.2 Cholestyramine

Cholestyramine is an oral, bile acid–binding resin that forms nonabsorbable micelles with the bile acids in the intestines and prevents them from entering the enterohepatic cycle. Cholestyramine should be taken at least 1 hour before or 4–6 hours after meals. However, it is rarely effective in controlling pruritus.

25.6.3 Ileal Bile Acid Transport (IBAT) Inhibitor

25.6.3.1 Bylvay

Ileal bile acid transport (IBAT) inhibitor odevixibat (Bylvay) was approved by the FDA in July 2021 for the treatment of pruritus in patients with PFIC aged 3 months and older. Odevixibat reduces reabsorption of bile acids in the terminal ileum, thereby interrupting the enterohepatic circulation by nonsurgical means. They *increase the amount of bile acids entering the colon by inhibiting their ileal absorption*. They also *interfere with ileal FXR signaling, thereby relieving the FGF19-mediated suppression of bile acid synthesis and thus augmenting bile acid production by the liver.* The recommended dose is 40 μg/kg body weight once a day in the morning, administered orally. If the response is inadequate after 3 months of continuous use, the dose may be increased up to 120 μg/kg daily, with a maximum daily dose of 6 mg in the USA.

In the phase 3 double blind trial, the percentage of patients achieving a reduction in serum bile acids by at least 70% from baseline or serum bile acids <70 μmol/L after 24 weeks of treatment was 43% in 40 μg/kg/day, 21% in 120 μg/kg/day, vs *0% in the placebo group. And a decrease in pruritus was also significantly higher in both treatment groups compared to the placebo group (58%, 52%* vs *30%, respectively). The most common adverse events were transient diarrhea (31%* vs *10% in placebo). No serious drug-related adverse event was seen* [19]. An open-label extension of the trial to evaluate long-term effects (72 weeks) is currently ongoing. Interim analysis showed sustained reductions in serum bile acids as well as pruritus up to 48 weeks. *In addition, none of the patients classified as responders after 6 months of treatment required liver transplantation for 3 years, while only 70% of nonresponders survived with their native liver for 3 years* [20].

25.6.3.2 Maralixibat

The intestine-restricted IBAT inhibitor maralixibat (LivmarliTM) was first approved for the treatment of cholestatic pruritus in patients with Alagille syndrome. In March 2024, maralixibat was also approved by the FDA for the treatment of cholestatic pruritus in PFIC patients who are at least 5 years old. The recommended starting dose for PFIC patients is 285 μg/kg body weight once daily in the morning and may be increased up to 570 μg/kg twice daily, with a maximum daily dose of 38 mg.

The effects of maralixibat in children with PFIC were studied in a number of trials. The INDIGO trial (NCT02057718), a long-term phase 2 trial, studied the efficacy and safety of maralixibat in 33 patients with FIC1 or BSEP deficiencies [21]. Seven out of 19 patients (37%) with nontruncated BSEP deficiency met the responder criteria: a reduction in serum bile acids of >75% from baseline or concentrations <102.0 μmol/L. None of the FIC1-deficient or truncated-BSEP-deficient patients met these responder criteria at any point in the study. All responding patients survived without liver transplantation after 312 weeks, compared to none of the non-responding patients. All patients experienced at least one adverse event, most commonly pyrexia (61%), diarrhea (58%), and cough (55%) [21].

Recently, the 26-week-long randomized phase 3 trial MARCH-PFIC was completed (NCT03905330) [22]. This trial included 93 PFIC patients harboring a larger range of deficiencies than in previous trials, including FIC1, non-truncated BSEP, MDR3, TJP2, and MYO5B-deficiencies. Patients received 570 μg/kg body weight maralixibat twice a day or placebo.

A significant reduction in pruritus and serum bile acids was observed after 26 weeks. In the last 10 weeks of the trial, the median proportion of days with the lowest pruritus scores was 95% in the treatment group vs. 9% in the placebo group. Least-squares mean change from baseline in total serum bile acids was −176 μmol/L (95% CI -257 to −94) for maralixibat versus 11 μmol/L (−58 to 80) for placebo ($p = 0{\cdot}0013$). Preliminary results show that the most frequent adverse effects were transient diarrhea (57.4% vs 19.6%) and abdominal pain (25.5% vs 13%) in the treatment vs. placebo group.

The ongoing open-label extension trial MARCH-ON (NCT04185363) enrolled 88 patients who had completed the MARCH-PFIC trial, studying the efficacy and safety of maralixibat up to 2 years.

25.7 Surgical Management/Planning

Partial biliary diversion (PBD) or ileal bypass (IB), are two of the non-transplant surgical interventions that can be done in patients with PFIC that interrupt the enterohepatic circulation of bile.

PBD is the therapy of choice in patients with low GGT-PFIC and should be performed as soon as possible after diagnosis to prevent liver damage [23].

Partial biliary diversion (PBD): partial diversion of bile (about 80%) while the remainder enters the duodenum; leaving the common bile duct intact reduces the accumulation of toxic bile salts by a reduction of the enterohepatic circulation. PBD may be achieved by either a jejunal conduit from the gallbladder to the abdominal wall, called partial external biliary diversion (PEBD), or one that connects the gallbladder to the colon, called partial internal biliary diversion (PIBD).

- PEBD was initially described by Withington and Withington in 1988. Reports of case series from around the world report normalization or improvement of liver function and reduced pruritus in 75–100% of patients with low GGT-PFIC. Liver biopsies post-PEBD showed resolution of hepatic morphologic abnormalities in all these patients [24–27]. Cirrhosis was proposed as the main reason for therapeutic failure, which emphasized the importance of early surgical intervention.
- PIBD: combines the advantages of external drainage and ileal bypassing by partially interrupting enterohepatic circulation without an external biliary fistula. The initial clinical and laboratory results were very promising, but long-term follow-up is needed [28].

PBD induces the loss of considerable amounts of fluids and electrolytes, and patients might become dehydrated. Adequate electrolyte and fluid supplementation is important. Other complications from intestinal surgery as stoma prolapse and intestinal obstruction.

In IB, bile salt reabsorption is diminished by bypassing the terminal ileum through an ileocolonic anastomosis.

Ileal bypass (IB) was first described by Whitington et al. in patients who were not amenable to PEBD because of a previous cholecystectomy. Additionally, this procedure does not create an external fistula. However, after a short initial response, clinical symptoms recurred in half of the treated patients with low GGT- or an undefined subtype of PFIC within a year. This is probably due to secondary adaptation of the ileum to the resection. Therefore, IB is inferior to PBD in patients with low GGT–PFIC [29–31].

25.7.1 Temporary Treatment with Recurrent Episodes of Cholestasis

Nasobiliary drainage (NBD) is a temporary treatment that can be considered in patients with BRIC1, given the intermittent nature of the disease and attack-like episodes. This can be done by endoscopically introducing a nasobiliary drain during a cholestatic episode. Because in some patients there is a transition from episodic to progressive cholestasis, PEBD should be considered when NBD fails to resolve a cholestatic episode.

25.8 Liver Transplant

Liver transplantation. Because of the high risk of complications and the lifelong need for immunosuppressive therapy, liver transplantation should be reserved for patients who have established liver cirrhosis at the time of presentation or who have progressive liver disease despite treatment.

Independent of the subtype of PFIC, the survival rate after transplantation ranges from 75–100% in more recent studies, with a median of 3 years follow-up [32–35].

The potential worsening of extrahepatic manifestations such as diarrhea has been reported, which has resulted in poor growth and severe graft steatosis/steatohepatitis. Pancreatic enzyme replacement and cholestyramine might be helpful to control diarrhea and prevent graft steatosis [36, 37].

However, a more recent study showed great graft function and only slight extrahepatic disease in the long-term follow-up with a median follow-up of more than 14 years [38].

As many of the transplant cases are done as living donor liver transplant (LDLT) from parents, one might question whether the heterozygous status of the parent donor would affect the outcomes in PFIC1 patients; however, several studies have shown similar outcomes to LDLT for non-genetic liver diseases such as biliary atresia [34, 35].

In patients transplanted for PFIC1, the liver allograft can become affected by severe steatohepatitis and cirrhosis with graft failure. This happens in patients who develop severe diarrhea, and is likely the result of the interaction between the native bowel and the liver graft by different mechanisms [37, 39]. Biliary diversion has been successfully used to treat diarrhea, resulting in improvement of graft steatofibrosis and function [40]. Biliary diversion before listing them for liver transplant (LT) or at the time of LT might be able to improve outcomes in these patients.

References

1. Davit-Spraul A, Gonzales E, Baussan C, Jacquemin E. Progressive familial intrahepatic cholestasis. Orphanet J Rare Dis. 2009;4:1.
2. Hertel PM, Hawthorne K, Kim S, Finegold MJ, Shneider BL, Squires JE, et al. Presentation and outcomes of infants with idiopathic cholestasis: a multicenter prospective study. J Pediatr Gastroenterol Nutr. 2021;73(4):478–84.
3. Clayton RJ, Iber FL, Ruebner BH, McKusick VA. Byler disease. Fatal familial intrahepatic cholestasis in an Amish kindred. Am J Dis Child. 1969;117(1):112–24.
4. Davit-Spraul A, Fabre M, Branchereau S, Baussan C, Gonzales E, Stieger B, et al. ATP8B1 and ABCB11 analysis in 62 children with normal gamma-glutamyl transferase progressive familial intrahepatic cholestasis (PFIC): phenotypic differences between PFIC1 and PFIC2 and natural history. Hepatology. 2010;51(5):1645–55.
5. Baker A, Kerkar N, Todorova L, Kamath BM, Houwen RHJ. Systematic review of progressive familial intrahepatic cholestasis. Clin Res Hepatol Gastroenterol. 2019;43(1):20–36.
6. Groen A, Romero MR, Kunne C, Hoosdally SJ, Dixon PH, Wooding C, et al. Complementary functions of the flippase ATP8B1 and the floppase ABCB4 in maintaining canalicular membrane integrity. Gastroenterology. 2011;141(5):1927–37.e1–4.
7. Klomp LW, Vargas JC, van Mil SW, Pawlikowska L, Strautnieks SS, van Eijk MJ, et al. Characterization of mutations in ATP8B1 associated with hereditary cholestasis. Hepatology. 2004;40(1):27–38.
8. Jacquemin E. Progressive familial intrahepatic cholestasis. Clin Res Hepatol Gastroenterol. 2012;36:S26–35.
9. Sohn MJ, Woo MH, Seong MW, Park SS, Kang GH, Moon JS, et al. Benign recurrent intrahepatic cholestasis type 2 in siblings with novel ABCB11 mutations. Pediatr Gastroenterol Hepatol Nutr. 2019;22(2):201–6.
10. van Mil SW, van der Woerd WL, van der Brugge G, Sturm E, Jansen PL, Bull LN, et al. Benign recurrent intrahepatic cholestasis type 2 is caused by mutations in ABCB11. Gastroenterology. 2004;127(2):379–84.
11. Pauli-Magnus C, Lang T, Meier Y, Zodan-Marin T, Jung D, Breymann C, et al. Sequence analysis of bile salt export pump (ABCB11) and multidrug resistance p-glycoprotein 3 (ABCB4, MDR3) in patients with intrahepatic cholestasis of pregnancy. Pharmacogenetics. 2004;14(2):91–102.
12. Lang C, Meier Y, Stieger B, Beuers U, Lang T, Kerb R, et al. Mutations and polymorphisms in the

bile salt export pump and the multidrug resistance protein 3 associated with drug-induced liver injury. Pharmacogenet Genomics. 2007;17(1):47–60.
13. Rosmorduc O, Poupon R. Low phospholipid associated cholelithiasis: association with mutation in the MDR3/ABCB4 gene. Orphanet J Rare Dis. 2007;2:29.
14. Wendum D, Barbu V, Rosmorduc O, Arrivé L, Fléjou JF, Poupon R. Aspects of liver pathology in adult patients with MDR3/ABCB4 gene mutations. Virchows Arch. 2012;460(3):291–8.
15. Lucena JF, Herrero JI, Quiroga J, Sangro B, Garcia-Foncillas J, Zabalegui N, et al. A multidrug resistance 3 gene mutation causing cholelithiasis, cholestasis of pregnancy, and adulthood biliary cirrhosis. Gastroenterology. 2003;124(4):1037–42.
16. Bull LN, van Eijk MJ, Pawlikowska L, DeYoung JA, Juijn JA, Liao M, et al. A gene encoding a P-type ATPase mutated in two forms of hereditary cholestasis. Nat Genet. 1998;18(3):219–24.
17. Bull LN, Carlton VE, Stricker NL, Baharloo S, DeYoung JA, Freimer NB, et al. Genetic and morphological findings in progressive familial intrahepatic cholestasis (Byler disease [PFIC-1] and Byler syndrome): evidence for heterogeneity. Hepatology. 1997;26(1):155–64.
18. Fawaz R, Baumann U, Ekong U, Fischler B, Hadzic N, Mack CL, et al. Guideline for the evaluation of Cholestatic jaundice in infants: joint recommendations of the North American Society for Pediatric Gastroenterology, Hepatology, and nutrition and the European Society for Pediatric Gastroenterology, Hepatology, and Nutrition. J Pediatr Gastroenterol Nutr. 2017;64(1):154–68.
19. Thompson RJ, Arnell H, Artan R, Baumann U, Calvo PL, Czubkowski P, et al. Odevixibat treatment in progressive familial intrahepatic cholestasis: a randomised, placebo-controlled, phase 3 trial. Lancet Gastroenterol Hepatol. 2022;7(9):830–42.
20. Thompson RJ, Artan R, Baumann U, Calvo PL, Czubkowski P, Dalgic B, et al. Interim results from an ongoing, open-label, single-arm trial of odevixibat in progressive familial intrahepatic cholestasis. JHEP Rep. 2023;5(8):100782.
21. Loomes KM, Squires RH, Kelly D, Rajwal S, Soufi N, Lachaux A, et al. Maralixibat for the treatment of PFIC: long-term, IBAT inhibition in an open-label, Phase 2 study. Hepatol Commun. 2022;6(9):2379–90.
22. Miethke AG, Moukarzel A, Porta G, Covarrubias Esquer J, Czubkowski P, Ordonez F, et al. Maralixibat in progressive familial intrahepatic cholestasis (MARCH-PFIC): a multicentre, randomised, double-blind, placebo-controlled, phase 3 trial. Lancet Gastroenterol Hepatol. 2024;9(7):620–31.
23. Stapelbroek JM, van Erpecum KJ, Klomp LW, Houwen RH. Liver disease associated with canalicular transport defects: current and future therapies. J Hepatol. 2010;52(2):258–71.
24. Kurbegov AC, Setchell KD, Haas JE, Mierau GW, Narkewicz M, Bancroft JD, et al. Biliary diversion for progressive familial intrahepatic cholestasis: improved liver morphology and bile acid profile. Gastroenterology. 2003;125(4):1227–34.
25. Whitington PF, Whitington GL. Partial external diversion of bile for the treatment of intractable pruritus associated with intrahepatic cholestasis. Gastroenterology. 1988;95(1):130–6.
26. Emond JC, Whitington PF. Selective surgical management of progressive familial intrahepatic cholestasis (Byler's disease). J Pediatr Surg. 1995;30(12):1635–41.
27. Arnell H, Bergdahl S, Papadogiannakis N, Nemeth A, Fischler B. Preoperative observations and short-term outcome after partial external biliary diversion in 13 patients with progressive familial intrahepatic cholestasis. J Pediatr Surg. 2008;43(7):1312–20.
28. Bustorff-Silva J, Sbraggia Neto L, Olímpio H, de Alcantara RV, Matsushima E, De Tommaso AM, et al. Partial internal biliary diversion through a cholecystojejunocolonic anastomosis–a novel surgical approach for patients with progressive familial intrahepatic cholestasis: a preliminary report. J Pediatr Surg. 2007;42(8):1337–40.
29. Whitington PF, Freese DK, Alonso EM, Schwarzenberg SJ, Sharp HL. Clinical and biochemical findings in progressive familial intrahepatic cholestasis. J Pediatr Gastroenterol Nutr. 1994;18(2):134–41.
30. Hollands CM, Rivera-Pedrogo FJ, Gonzalez-Vallina R, Loret-de-Mola O, Nahmad M, Burnweit CA. Ileal exclusion for Byler's disease: an alternative surgical approach with promising early results for pruritus. J Pediatr Surg. 1998;33(2):220–4.
31. Kaliciński PJ, Ismail H, Jankowska I, Kamiński A, Pawłowska J, Drewniak T, et al. Surgical treatment of progressive familial intrahepatic cholestasis: comparison of partial external biliary diversion and ileal bypass. Eur J Pediatr Surg. 2003;13(5):307–11.
32. Aydogdu S, Cakir M, Arikan C, Tumgor G, Yuksekkaya HA, Yilmaz F, et al. Liver transplantation for progressive familial intrahepatic cholestasis: clinical and histopathological findings, outcome and impact on growth. Pediatr Transplant. 2007;11(6):634–40.
33. Bassas A, Chehab M, Hebby H, Al Shahed M, Al Husseini H, Al Zahrani A, et al. Living related liver transplantation in 13 cases of progressive familial intrahepatic cholestasis. Transplant Proc. 2003;35(8):3003–5.
34. Cutillo L, Najimi M, Smets F, Janssen M, Reding R, de Ville de Goyet J, et al. Safety of living-related liver transplantation for progressive familial intrahepatic cholestasis. Pediatr Transplant. 2006;10(5):570–4.
35. Khan I, Al-Shaqrani MA, Arain ZB, Al-Hebbi HA, Wali SH, Bassas AF. One hundred and thirty-seven living donor pediatric liver transplants at Riyadh Military Hospital. Results and outlook for future. Saudi Med J. 2009;30(3):403–8.
36. Lykavieris P, van Mil S, Cresteil D, Fabre M, Hadchouel M, Klomp L, et al. Progressive familial intrahepatic cholestasis type 1 and extrahepatic features: no catch-up of stature growth, exacerbation of

diarrhea, and appearance of liver steatosis after liver transplantation. J Hepatol. 2003;39(3):447–52.
37. Miyagawa-Hayashino A, Egawa H, Yorifuji T, Hasegawa M, Haga H, Tsuruyama T, et al. Allograft steatohepatitis in progressive familial intrahepatic cholestasis type 1 after living donor liver transplantation. Liver Transpl. 2009;15(6):610–8.
38. Gül-Klein S, Öllinger R, Schmelzle M, Pratschke J, Schöning W. Long-term outcome after liver transplantation for progressive familial intrahepatic cholestasis. Medicina (Kaunas). 2021;57(8)
39. Usui M, Isaji S, Das BC, Kobayashi M, Osawa I, Iida T, et al. Liver retransplantation with external biliary diversion for progressive familial intrahepatic cholestasis type 1: a case report. Pediatr Transplant. 2009;13(5):611–4.
40. Nicastro E, Stephenne X, Smets F, Fusaro F, de Magnée C, Reding R, et al. Recovery of graft steatosis and protein-losing enteropathy after biliary diversion in a PFIC 1 liver transplanted child. Pediatr Transplant. 2012;16(5):E177–82.

26 Obstructive Biliary Tract Disease

Yusuke Kazami, Yoshikuni Kawaguchi,
and Kiyoshi Hasegawa

26.1 Introduction

Biliary strictures are encountered in daily clinical practice by clinicians specializing in hepatobiliary–pancreatic diseases. Although the diagnosis of typical cases is more accurate because of advances in imaging studies, clinical challenges remain in differentiating between benign and malignant strictures and identifying the cause of benign strictures. Therefore, elaborate pretreatment investigations using imaging studies and pathological examinations are required.

Biliary strictures are caused by benign diseases, including bile duct stones and immune-related diseases, and malignant diseases, such as biliary and pancreatic cancers. This chapter provides an overview of recent updates on biliary strictures caused by benign or malignant etiologies.

26.2 Causes of Biliary Strictures

The main causes of benign biliary strictures include common bile duct stone (CBS)-induced strictures, primary sclerosing cholangitis (PSC), IgG4-related sclerosing cholangitis (IgG4-SC), and postoperative biliary strictures, including iatrogenic biliary tract injury. Additionally, studies report other causes for secondary sclerosing cholangitis (Table 26.1). In contrast, malignant biliary strictures result from bile duct cancer, pancreatic head cancer with bile duct invasion, or lymph node metastasis from nonbiliary malignancies.

Y. Kazami · Y. Kawaguchi · K. Hasegawa (✉)
Hepato-Biliary-Pancreatic Surgery Division, and Artificial Organ and Transplantation Division, Department of Surgery, Graduate School of Medicine, The University of Tokyo, Tokyo, Japan
e-mail: hasegawa-2su@h.u-tokyo.ac.jp

T. Hackert, A. Gulla (eds.), *Rare Liver and Biliary Tract Diseases*,
https://doi.org/10.1007/978-3-032-15076-9_26

Table 26.1 Other secondary sclerosing cholagitis

Congenital	Caroli's disease
	Cystic fibrosis
Infectious	HIV-related cholangiopathy
	Recurrent pyogenic cholagitis
	Parastic infection (echinococcosis, hydatid cyst, etc.)
Iscemic	Posttraumatic sclerosing cholagitis
	Intra-arterial chemotherapy
	Transcatheter arterial embolization therapy
	Post-transplantation hepatic artery thrombosis
	Hepatic allograft rejection(acute, chronic)
Toxic	Accidental alcohol
	Formaldehyde
	Hypertonic saline
Immunologic	Eosinophilic cholangitis
	Mast cell cholangiopathy
Anatomic obstruction	Cystic fibrosis liver disease
	Portal hypertensive biliopathy
	Sickle cell cholangipathy
	Choledochal cyst
Drug-induced	Immunotherapy with immune check point inhibitor
Infiltrative disorders	Systemic vasculitis
	Amyloidosis
	Radiation injury
	Sarcoidosis
	Systemic mastocytosis
	Hypereosinophilic syndrome
	Hodgkin's disease

26.3 Biliary Obstruction Caused by Non-neoplastic Diseases

1. *Common Bile Duct Stone*

- Incidence

Primary common bile duct stones (CBDS) are newly formed intra- and extrahepatic bile duct stones. Secondary CBDSs originate in the gallbladder and migrate to the bile ducts through the cystic duct. The proportion of secondary CBDSs is reportedly high and is found in approximately 10–20% of patients with symptomatic gallstones [1].

- Clinical Presentation

One-third of patients with CBDS are asymptomatic, and the remaining experience epigastric pain, right upper abdominal pain, fever, partial or complete obstruction of the bile ducts, obstructive cholangitis, liver abscess, pancreatitis, and other severe complications. CBDS may lead to secondary biliary cirrhosis in a few patients [2]. All patients diagnosed with CBDS should be treated because of the potential for these complications.

- Work-Up Investigation

Blood chemistry data on hepatobiliary enzymes and transabdominal ultrasound scanning (USS) are recommended as initial tests. If CBDS is highly suspected based on these tests, other tests are not required to confirm the diagnosis. Enhanced computed tomography (CT) is recommended before CBDS treatment to rule out bile duct obstruction due to malignancy. Magnetic resonance cholangiopancreatography (MRCP) and endoscopic ultrasonography (EUS) are imaging studies that identify CBDS when hepatobiliary enzymes are within normal limits and when USS imaging does not visualize CBDS. The choice between these two modalities is determined by facility preferences and/or patient acceptance. Although CT is beneficial in identifying and staging malignant bile duct obstruction, it is not routinely used to detect CBDS because the accuracy of detecting CBDS with CT is not high. Endoscopic retrograde cholangiography (ERC) should only be performed in patients who require endoscopic treatment.

- Treatment

Treatment options include endoscopic therapy, surgery (open or minimally invasive surgeries), and percutaneous transhepatic treatment. Consideration should be given to either "stone extraction by ERC + cholecystectomy" or "cholecystectomy + intraoperative stone extraction," and if both are not feasible, percutaneous transhepatic treatment is performed. Despite being the least invasive, ERC is technically complicated. ERC is performed under propofol or general anesthesia. To reduce the risk of post-ERC pancreatitis (PEP), the use of diclofenac or indomethacin suppositories (100 mg) is recommended [3]. Stent placement in the pancreatic duct is recommended when multiple cannulations are performed. Endoscopic papillary balloon dilation (EPBD) is used to dilate the papilla of Vater. Endoscopic retrograde bile duct lithotripsy achieves a high rate of stone removal (73–97%) [1]. Surgical treatment is needed for secondary stones, and cholecystectomy is performed for patients with cholelithiasis with or without a history of CBDS. One-stage CBDS removal with transcystic or transductal laparoscopic bile duct exploration (LBDE) during the surgery is effective. Both LBDE and perioperative ERC are considered equally effective treatment methods [4]. One-stage LBDE during laparoscopic cholecystectomy is associated with shorter hospital stays and lower costs than the two-stage approach of ERC and laparoscopic cholecystectomy [5].

- Surgical Planning/Management

Currently, more than 95% of cholecystectomies for cholelithiasis are performed laparoscopically, and LBDE is being increasingly used. LBDE requires a flexible choledochoscope, light source, camera, and disposable instruments (basket, balloon, stent, etc.) similar to those used in ERC. Because optical magnification, direct visualization, and more delicate instruments are available during LBDE, the risk of bile duct injury is limited. Bile duct closure is often performed in a single stage. This reduces the various events associated with traditional T-tube placement and achieves similar risks of bile leakage and stone recurrence, resulting in a shorter hospital stay and lower hospital costs. The following two surgical approaches are used: the transcystic and transductal approaches [6].

- Follow-Up/Recommendations

The rate of stone recurrence is reported to range from 2% to 21%, depending on the series [7]. Risk factors for recurrence include an endoscopic sphincterotomy before cholecystectomy, stone size of 9 mm or larger, CBD diameter of 10 mm or larger, and a history of previous laparoscopic cholecystectomy [8].

2. *Primary Sclerosing Cholangitis (PSC)*

Primary sclerosing cholangitis (PSC) is a chronic fibroinflammatory disease of the bile duct. Biliary strictures are observed at all levels of the biliary tree. PSC is an autoimmune disease; however, its pathophysiology remains unclear. Approximately 70% of patients have concurrent inflammatory bowel disease (IBD), and the overlap of PSC and autoimmune hepatitis (PSC-AIH) is observed in 35% and 5% of pediatric and adult patients with PSC, respectively [9]. Some patients show a clinical presentation called "small duct PSC": namely, PSC is histologically characterized despite normal bile duct imaging.

- Incidence

To date, studies have shown that the estimated incidence and prevalence rates are approximately 1–1.5 cases per 100,000 person-years and 6–16 cases per 100,000 individuals, respectively, in North America and Western Europe [10]. No differences in sexes have been reported. The peak onset is between 25 and 45 years of age, with a median age at diagnosis of 36–39 years. PSC can develop at any age [11].

- Clinical Presentation

Signs of PSC include fatigue, abdominal pain, fever, pruritus, anxiety, and depression. Approximately 50% of adult patients with PSC exhibit persistent or intermittent symptoms, and approximately 20% develop these symptoms within 5 years of diagnosis [11]. With disease progression, PSC often leads to jaundice from obstructive cholestatic liver disease, and further complications, such as liver cirrhosis and liver failure, can occur, resulting in various associated symptoms. Additionally, PSC significantly increases the risk of cholangiocarcinoma (CCA) and colorectal cancer (CRC), leading to the development of symptoms related to these malignancies.

- Work-up Investigation

Although biochemical markers are sensitive, they are not specific for diagnosing PSC. Elevation of liver enzymes such as alkaline phosphatase (ALP) and gamma-glutamyltransferase (GGT), suggestive of cholestasis, is observed in approximately 75% of patients [12].

The primary imaging tests for patients suspected to have PSC include magnetic resonance imaging/magnetic resonance cholangiopancreatography (magnetic resonance imaging (MRI)/MRCP) with bile and pancreatic duct imaging, and 1 mm-slice T2-weighted (T2w) and three-dimensional (3D) MRCP aid in diagnosis. Contrast-enhanced MRI can be useful, especially when suspecting CCA [13].

Before the clinical use of MRI/MRCP, endoscopic retrograde cholangiography (ERC) was considered the gold standard for PSC diagnosis. Owing to the associated complications, such as post-ERC pancreatitis (PEP), and because the diagnostic accuracy of MRI/MRCP is reportedly comparable to that of ERC, routine use of MRI/MRCP is recommended. However, the role of ERC remains important, and ERC is performed in patients who show newly developed or worsening pruritus, unexplained weight loss, worsening serum liver function tests, elevated serum CA 19–9, recurrence of bacterial cholangitis, and progressive bile duct dilation [14]. Evaluation using ultrasound scanning (USS) or computed tomography (CT) alone is insufficient. Imaging findings reveal short intrahepatic strictures distributed diffusely or alternately with normal or minimally dilated segments in the early stages of the disease (Fig. 26.1) [15]. When patients progress to fibrosis, biliary strictures, or bile duct obstruction, T2W and diffusion-weighted MRI reveal localized signal abnormalities in the liver parenchyma. The progression of fibrosis manifests as liver lobe atrophy, surface lobulation, and/or an increased ratio of the caudate lobe to the right lobe.

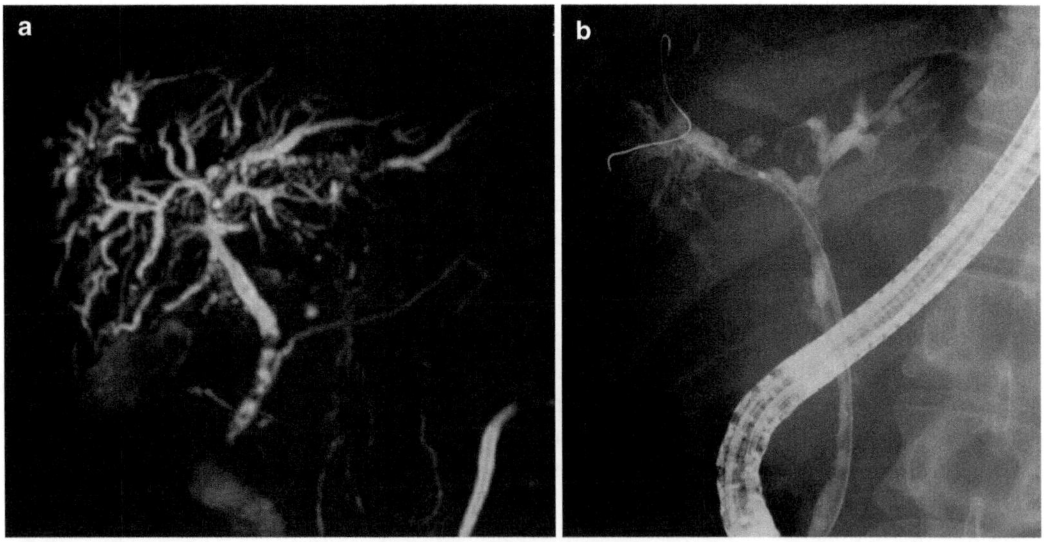

Fig. 26.1 Typical imaging findings in primary sclerosing cholangitis (PSC), (**a**) Magnetic resonance cholangiopancreatography (MRCP), (**b**) Endoscopic retrograde cholangiography (ERC)

Advancements in imaging have reduced the need for liver biopsies. However, when there are concerns about overlap with small duct PSC or AIH, which are considered to represent the early stage of the disease, a liver biopsy should be considered. Circumferential fibrosis resembling "onion-skin" fibrosis is a histological feature seen in PSC and other obstructive cholangiopathies. Typical histological features of PSC include periductal fibrosis and fibroobliterative duct lesions, and compatible features include bile duct loss, ductular reaction (also known as bile duct proliferation), interface hepatitis patterns, and chronic cholestatic changes in periportal hepatocytes [16].

- Differential Diagnosis

The prominent differential diagnosis is IgG4-related sclerosing cholangitis, for which serum IgG4 levels should be measured. A comparison between IgG4-related sclerosing cholangitis and PSC is presented in Table 26.2 and Fig. 26.2. Secondary sclerosing cholangitis should be carefully excluded, particularly in the absence of concurrent IBD.

Table 26.2 Each characteristics of PSC and IgG4-SC

	Primary sclerosing cholangitis (PSC)	IgG4-related sclerosing cholangitis (IgG4-SC)
Age on set	Younger	Elderly
Gender	Both	Male
Blood test	Not particular	IgG4↑
Coexisting disease	Inflammatory bowel disease Autoimmune hepatitis	Autoimmune pancreatitis IgG4-related dacryoadenitis/sialadenitis IgG4-related retroperitoneal fibrosis IgG4-related kidney disease
Image of bile duct	Short strictures with: Band-like stricture Beaded appearance Pruned-tree appearance Diverticulum-like outpouching	Long strictures Lower bile duct strictures Dilatation after confluent stricture
Inflammatory site in bile duct	Lumen surface	All layers
Epithelial damage	Severe	Rare
Pathological findings	Periductal onion-skin fibrosis Fibrous obliterative cholangitis	Abundant IgG4-positive plasma cell infiltration
Treatment	Drugs including UDCA Liver transplantation	Steroid

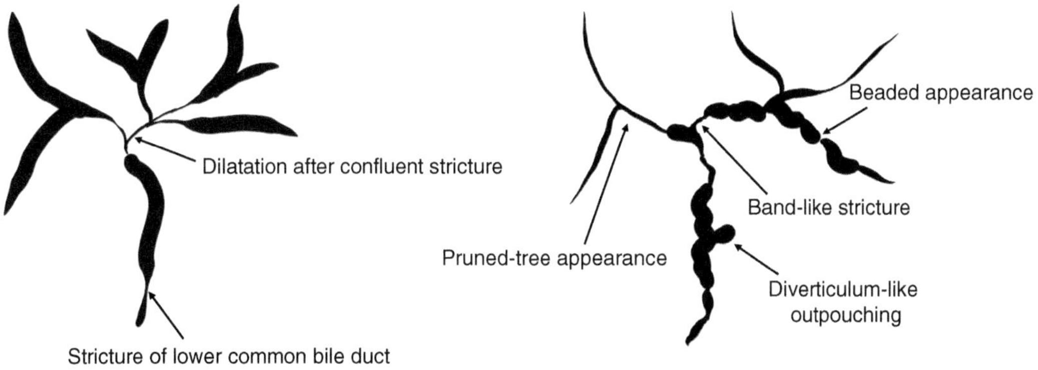

Fig. 26.2 Characteristics of the bile duct image of primary sclerosing cholangitis (PSC) and IgG4-related sclerosing cholangitis (IgG4-SC)

- Treatment

However, an effective treatment for PSC has not yet been established. Therefore, treatment mainly focuses on managing the complications associated with PSC. Liver transplantation may be performed to treat cirrhosis as the disease progresses to advanced stages. Furthermore, PSC is a risk factor for PSC-related hepatobiliary cancers, especially cholangiocarcinoma (CCA), and specific treatments are required if these malignancies occur (refer to the section on malignancies).

- Surgical Planning/Management

Excluding the treatment of malignant tumors, liver transplantation is the primary surgical treatment for PSC. Considering the risk of bile duct strictures and CCA in the remaining bile ducts, Roux-en-Y hepaticojejunostomy is preferred for bile duct reconstruction. However, some facilities perform duct-to-duct (DD) anastomosis in patients who show a normal bile duct appearance or in those who do not show high-grade dysplasia in the bile duct at the time of transplantation. DD anastomosis is associated with a lower incidence of post-transplant biliary strictures, with no impact on overall transplant outcomes [17].

Post-transplant complications in patients with PSC are generally similar to those in patients transplanted for other indications; however, they have a higher incidence of steroid-resistant allograft rejection. The post-transplant immunosuppression protocol for patients with PSC remains an unresolved issue [18].

- Follow-up/Recommendations

The disease recurrence rate after liver transplantation for PSC is approximately 15–20%. The risk factors for recurrence include male sex, extended-criteria grafts, steroid-free antithymocyte globulin induction protocols, primary immunosuppression with tacrolimus, allograft rejection, and new or poorly controlled IBD. In addition, one of the most debated and significant risk factors for PSC recurrence is the use of living-related donors. Moreover, in living donor liver transplantation (LDLT), donor age ≥45 years and monotherapy or no use of immunosuppressive agents in the first year after LT have been identified as risk factors for recurrence. In cases of recurrence, retransplantation may be considered [19].

3. *IgG4-related Sclerosing Cholangitis (IgG4-SC)*

IgG4-related sclerosing cholangitis (IgG4-SC) is characterized by elevated serum IgG4 levels, fibrotic narrowing of the bile duct walls caused by IgG4-positive plasma cells and lymphocytes, and obstructive phlebitis. IgG4-SC frequently develops in autoimmune pancreatitis (AIP) and is recognized as a biliary manifestation of systemic IgG4-related diseases. The differential diagnosis is primary sclerosing cholangitis (PSC) [20]. The characteristics of both diseases are summarized in Table 26.2 and Fig. 26.2.

- Incidence

Based on epidemiological studies, the estimated overall prevalence of IgG4-SC in Japan is 2.0 per 100,000 people, with a calculated patient count of 2500 individuals [21]. Approximately 80% of the patients are men. The average or median age at diagnosis of IgG4-SC is 60–70 years, and the incidence of IgG4-SC has not been reported in children or adolescents [22].

- Clinical presentation

Symptoms related to bile stasis (jaundice, pruritus, fever, and abdominal pain due to obstructive cholangitis) are similar to those observed in PSC. Among these, jaundice is the most frequently observed symptom at the time of diagnosis and is found in over 70% of patients [21]. When IgG4-related diseases (autoimmune pancreatitis, sclerosing sialadenitis, retroperitoneal fibrosis, etc.) coexist, symptoms related to these clinical manifestations occur. Unlike PSC, IgG4-SC does not progress to liver cirrhosis, nor does it present with symptoms of end-stage liver failure.

- Work-up investigation

The diagnosis of IgG4-SC is based on the following four criteria: (1) elevated serum IgG4 levels (2), characteristic biliary imaging findings (3), coexistence of IgG4-related diseases outside the bile duct, and (4) characteristic histological findings.

Elevated serum IgG4 levels are observed in 90% of patients with IgG4-SC. However, elevated serum IgG4 levels can be found in 8–14% of patients with cholangiocarcinoma. Therefore, the diagnosis of IgG4-SC should not be solely based on elevated serum IgG4 levels (sensitivity 64–90%, specificity 87–93%) [23].

Among the imaging studies, magnetic resonance imaging/magnetic resonance cholangiopancreatography (MRI/MRCP) is useful for evaluating bile ducts. Computed tomography (CT) is helpful in differentiating IgG4-SC from cholangiocarcinoma (CCA) when imaging findings are similar. Whole-body screening using CT may be useful for confirming the presence of other IgG4-related diseases. According to clinical guidelines, endoscopic retrograde cholangiography (ERC) is preferred over MRCP for the evaluation of bile duct images. The imaging features of IgG4-SC include: (1) concentric thickening of the bile duct wall in the longitudinal direction, (2) smooth inner and outer margins, (3) mild dilation of the upper bile ducts and visual confirmation of bile duct patency at the stenotic site, and (4) continuous thickening of the bile duct wall covering both the intrahepatic and extrahepatic bile ducts. IgG4-related SC is classified into four types based on bile duct imaging, and the characteristics are illustrated in Fig. 26.3 [24]. Endoscopic ultrasonography (EUS) and intraductal ultrasonography (IDUS) are effective in differentiating IgG4-SC from CCA, and the wall thickening at the stenotic site of the bile ducts is characterized by a concentrically symmetric, smooth outer and inner margin, and homogenous internal echogenicity. The most characteristic finding of IDUS is wall thickening of the bile ducts in nonstenotic areas, which is vital for distinguishing it from local tumor findings in CCA or pancreatic cancer [25].

Marked transmural lymphoplasmacytic infiltration and fibrosis are observed in the liver and extrahepatic bile ducts obtained by bile duct or duodenal papillary biopsy, indicating thickening of the bile duct wall. Storiform fibrosis and obliterative phlebitis are crucial histological findings for the diagnosis of IgG4-SC. Storiform fibrosis is characterized by collagen with irregu-

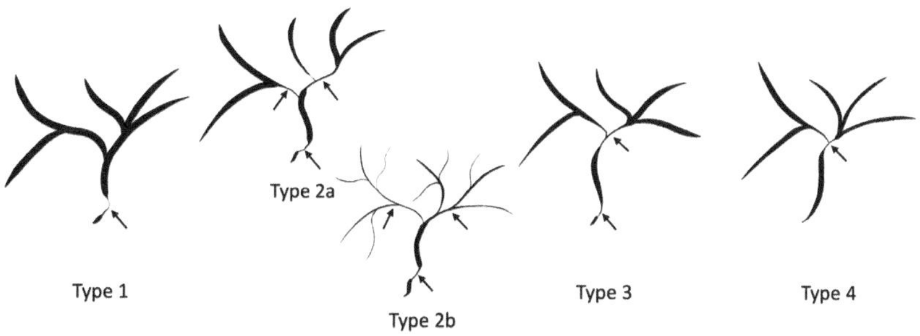

	Type 1	Type 2	Type 3	Type 4
Incidence	64%	13% (a:5%, b:8%)	10%	10%
Differential diagnosis	Cholangiocarcinoma Pancreatic cancer Chronic pancreatitis	Primary sclerosing cholagitis	Cholangiocarcinoma Gallbladder cancer	
Useful examination	EUS IDUS EUS-FNA/Biopsy	MRCP ERCP IDUS Biopsy	EUS IDUS Biopsy	

Fig. 26.3 Type of IgG4 SC, incidence, differential diagnosis, and useful examinations

larly swirling arrangements containing inflammatory cells, and obliterative phlebitis is caused by inflammation and fibrosis by inflammatory cells, resulting in occlusion of the venous lumen. IgG4-SC lesions extend not only to the bile duct wall but also to the perihilar fat tissue, peripheral nerves, and portal vein. An increase in IgG4-positive cells is characteristic but not specific [26].

- Treatment

Steroids are used for the treatment of IgG4-SC. Defining a definitive diagnosis is challenging. In patients who do not have a definitive diagnosis based on imaging findings or biopsies and in patients who show an insufficient response to steroid treatment, surgical resection may be performed because of the possibility of malignancy. Endoscopy or percutaneous biliary drainage may be required for patients with biliary stricture-related obstructive jaundice. The need for such procedures is limited to patients who do not respond well to steroid treatment.

- Surgical Planning/Management

As mentioned previously, surgical treatment is not required if the diagnosis of IgG4-SC is definitive. However, if a definitive diagnosis cannot be established, surgical resection is recommended. This procedure is similar to that used for malignant tumors at the site of bile duct stenosis.

- Follow-up/Recommendations

IgG4-SC shows a good response to steroid therapy; however, disease recurrence occurs in 30–57% of patients with IgG4-SC, especially during steroid maintenance therapy or after steroid discontinuation, particularly within the first 2–3 years [27]. Predictors of recurrence include high serum IgG4 levels at the time of diagnosis, the presence of multiple bile duct strictures, and thickening of the bile duct wall at the initial presentation [28]. Although reports on the use of other drugs (immunosuppressive agents or rituximab) are available, evidence in terms of the efficacy of the treatments is unknown.

4. *Congenital Biliary Atresia (CBA)*

Congenital biliary atresia (CBA) is a destructive inflammatory obliterative cholangiopathy that refers to destructive inflammation and obstruction of the bile ducts in newborns. A similar pathological process was not observed in older children or adults. If left untreated, the condition progresses to liver cirrhosis, leading to death by the age of 2 years. CBA is classified according to the degree of bile duct obstruction. Approximately 20% of patients have other congenital anatomical abnormalities [29]. Biliary atresia and splenic malformation syndrome are commonly observed. However, the exact cause of CBA remains unclear. Genetics, infection, inflammation, and toxic insults are associated with the incidence of CBA.

- Incidence

Epidemiological studies from the United Kingdom and France have estimated an incidence rate of approximately 1 in 17,000–1 in 19,000 births. Ethnic differences have been reported [30]. Reports from the United States suggest that children born to Black mothers have a 2–5 times higher likelihood than those born to White mothers [31].

- Clinical presentation

Newborns with normal birth weights present with persistent jaundice, acholic (pale gray/white) stools, and dark urine immediately after birth. Any full-term newborn with persistent jaundice after 14 days (and 21 days) of life requires evaluation for liver disease.

- Work-up investigation

In physiological or breast milk jaundice, the serum concentration of unconjugated bilirubin increases, whereas in jaundice secondary to most liver diseases, conjugated bilirubin levels increase. However, an increase in conjugated bilirubin can also be observed in other liver diseases, making this symptom non-specific. Serum gamma-glutamyl transferase (GGT) levels are higher in patients with biliary atresia than in those with other neonatal cholestatic diseases [30].

Endoscopic retrograde cholangiography (ERC) is required when the diagnosis is uncertain; however, ERC is technically challenging in infants. MRCP also has technical limitations due to the small bile duct size in infants; however, its importance for diagnosis may increase in the future. Identification of hepatoduodenal ligament enlargement, known as the "triangular cord sign" on ultrasound (US), is a specific finding in almost all cases; however, the success rate for visualizing this sign depends on the operator, and the sensitivity is not high [32]. Operative cholangiography performed before Kasai portoenterostomy, if CBA is suspected, remains the gold standard for diagnosis.

Histopathological diagnosis using percutaneous liver biopsy typically reveals cholestasis with varying degrees of portal fibrosis, edema, bile duct proliferation, and the presence of bile plugs, confirming extrahepatic biliary obstruction. However, liver biopsy samples obtained in the early stages of CBA (before 6 weeks of age) may not show typical histological features, necessitating multiple biopsies for diagnosis.

In some cases, after administering phenobarbital at 5 mg/kg/day for 3–5 days, a radionuclide excretion test using an N-tert-butylimino diacetic acid (TEBIDA) scan may be performed. For CBA, hepatic uptake is usually good; however, there is little to no excretion into the intestine within 24 h [30]. However, this finding is not specific to CBA. Duodenal tube tests are commonly performed in Japan and China. Transparent bile-stained intestinal secretions over 24 h strongly suggest biliary atresia [33].

- Differential diagnosis

Differentiating CBA from other cholestatic diseases, such as Alagille syndrome, is important.

- Treatment

Surgical treatment is the only available treatment option. Kasai portoenterostomy (first reported by the Japanese surgeon Morio Kasai in the 1950s) and liver transplantation remain the key treatments for CBA. Kasai portoenterostomy improves jaundice and restores excretory and synthetic liver functions, allowing healthy growth and development [34].

- Surgical planning/management

In Kasai portoenterostomy, the entire extrahepatic biliary system is excised, and the porta hepatis is transected at the height of the liver capsule, exposing any remaining (usually minute) ducts. A jejunal Roux loop is anastomosed to the cut surface to complete the reconstruction [35]. The role of minimally invasive techniques is debatable. The success of the Kasai procedure is determined by the normalization of bilirubin levels within 6 months of surgery. Several factors, such as age at surgery, severity of liver disease, and expertise and experience of the surgeons, influence the success of the surgery [36]. Performing this surgery on infants older than 100 days remains controversial, and some centers prefer to perform primary liver transplantation.

- Follow-up/Recommendations

Prevention and treatment of complications, such as cholangitis, as well as providing nutritional and family support, are essential. To prevent malnutrition, all affected infants should receive nutritional and fat-soluble vitamin supplements.

Kasai portoenterostomy is a palliative procedure and does not cure CBA. In approximately 70% of children who undergo successful surgery, the disease progresses to fibrosis, portal hypertension, and liver cirrhosis. However, more than 80% of successfully treated patients maintain their quality of life and survive for more than 10 years with their original liver.

In patients without successful bile drainage after Kasai portoenterostomy, liver transplantation is usually indicated within 6 months to 2 years. Even in patients with successful surgery, if progressive cholestasis, liver cirrhosis, or portal hypertension with uncontrollable ascites and variceal bleeding develop despite medical management, liver transplantation should be considered.

The prognosis after liver transplantation has improved over time, with early (1–3 years) survival rates ranging from 85% to 94%, 10-year graft survival rates of 73%, and patient survival rates of 86% [37].

5. *Postoperative Bile Duct Anastomotic Strictures*

Bile duct strictures are common after liver transplantation. In patients who underwent liver and bile duct resection with biliary reconstruction, hepaticojejunostomy/choledochojejunostomy show stenosis at the anastomotic sites.

- Incidence

The overall incidence of postoperative bile duct strictures after liver transplantation is 13%, accounting for 12% and 19% in patients who received deceased donor liver transplants (DDLT) and living donor liver transplants (LDLT), respectively. Most cases occur within 1 year after transplantation, with an average interval of 5–8 months post-transplant. Risk factors for bile duct stricture include LDLT, postoperative bile leakage, and the presence of a narrow bile duct diameter or multiple reconstructed bile ducts [38]. Studies from the United States indicate that the stricture rate for hepaticojejunostomy/choledochojejunostomy outside of liver transplant was 11.9%, with a lower stricture rate in individuals aged ≤65 years. Patients who underwent preoperative biliary stent placement have a higher stricture rate [39].

- Clinical Presentation

Blood investigations indicate abnormal liver function, and patients present with fever due to recurrent cholangitis.

- Work-up investigation

Elevated serum levels of bilirubin, transaminases, serum gamma-glutamyltransferase (GGT), and alkaline phosphatase (ALP) are commonly observed which aid in diagnosis.

In addition to ultrasound scanning (USS), computed tomography (CT), and magnetic resonance imaging (MRI) (including magnetic resonance cholangiopancreatography (MRCP)), the diagnosis can be confirmed using endoscopic retrograde cholangiography (ERC) or percutaneous transhepatic cholangiography.

- Differential diagnosis

Particularly in post-liver transplantation cases, differentiation from non-anastomotic strictures of the bile duct, such as due to ischemic changes, is necessary.

- Treatment, Surgical Planning/Management

The treatment of postoperative bile duct strictures after liver transplantation is primarily endoscopic balloon dilation and/or stent placement, with a success rate of 80–90% [40]. Some institutions that perform biliary reconstruction using the hepaticojejunostomy technique for LDLT may consider surgical reimplantation or a percutaneous approach as the first choice [41]. However, with the increasing use of duct-to-duct reconstruction and technical advancements in ERC for LDLT, the endoscopic approach is now the first choice in most centers.

In cases other than liver transplantation, reconstruction is often performed via hepaticojejunostomy, making endoscopic treatment more challenging. Nevertheless, considering its invasiveness, endoscopic treatment remains the first choice [42].

- Follow-up/Recommendations

Following ERC treatment for post-liver transplant anastomotic strictures, approximately 20% of patients experience stricture recurrence; however, it can be effectively treated with repeat ERC [43].

The main issues with endoscopic treatment include the need for multiple procedures over an extended period and the risk of associated complications, such as cholangitis and pancreatitis.

However, considering the risk of reoperation, this is generally acceptable [44].

6. *Iatrogenic Biliary Tract Injury*

Intraoperative iatrogenic bile duct injury is one of the causes of postoperative bile duct stricture, particularly occurring at a frequency of 0.5% during laparoscopic cholecystectomy [45]. Laparoscopic cholecystectomy is one of the most common surgeries in general surgery. However, bile duct injury can not only lead to a reduced quality of life but also life-threatening complications, making it the most crucial concern during the procedure.

In cases of major bile duct injury, reconstruction with a hepaticojejunostomy is required; however, post-reconstruction anastomotic stenosis is challenging. The risk factors for anastomotic stenosis after reconstruction include vascular injury, post-repair bile leakage, and lack of surgical expertise [42].

- Work-up Investigation, Surgical Planning/Management

Avoiding bile duct injuries is imperative. A comprehensive understanding of preoperative anatomy is essential, and safe intraoperative manipulation is crucial for avoiding such injuries. Studies have reported indocyanine green (ICG)-fluorescence imaging for intraoperative bile duct visualization to prevent intraoperative bile duct injury [46]. ICG has the property of fluorescing under near-infrared light, and after intravenous injection, it is absorbed by the liver and excreted into the bile, which enhances the ability to identify bile ducts during surgery (Fig. 26.4). While the most common protocol involves an intravenous injection of ICG (2.5 mg) immediately before surgery, the lack of fluorescence contrast between the bile ducts and background liver remains problematic, leading to decreased discriminative capability. To address this issue, injecting 0.025 mg of ICG intravenously the night before surgery reduces background liver fluorescence and improves bile duct visualization [47]. Additionally, direct injection of ICG into the bile ducts further enhances visibility.

Severe gallbladder inflammation is associated with an increased risk of bile duct injury owing to misidentification caused by inflammation and adhesions. Consequently, a drainage-based approach with conservative laparoscopic cholecystectomy after drainage is recommended based on objective criteria [48]. Percutaneous transhepatic gallbladder drainage is the standard approach for gallbladder drainage; however, the presence of an external drainage tube until cholecystectomy can cause pain and affect the quality of life. Endoscopic ultrasonography-guided gallbladder drainage (EUS-GBD) can resolve these issues. Previous reports have described laparoscopic cholecystectomy under navigation using ICG fluorescence imaging after

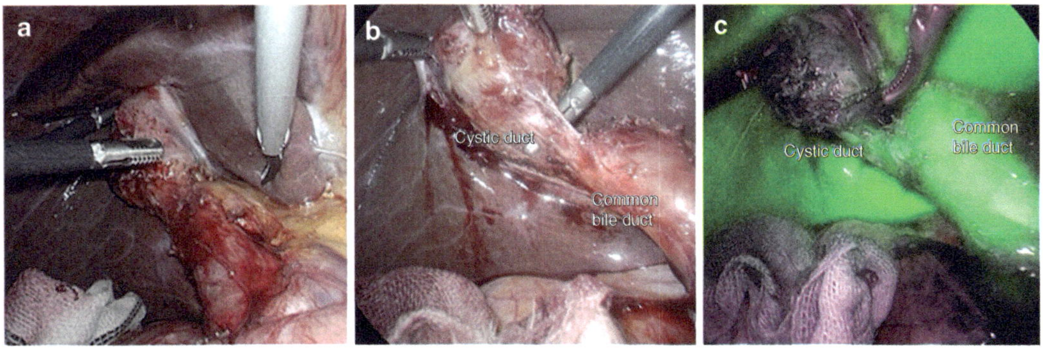

Fig. 26.4 Indocyanine green (ICG)-fluorescence imaging for intraoperative bile duct visualization in a patient. The gallbladder was atrophic due to chronic inflammation (**a**), which made it difficult to identify the cholecystic duct (**b**), but ICG fluorescence was used to safely secure the cystic duct (**c**)

EUS-GBD. In these cases, ICG is injected through the endoscopic nasobiliary tube during EUS-GBD, clearly visualizing the cystic and common bile ducts under fluorescence and allowing safe management of the bile ducts [49].

26.4 Neoplastic Diseases

Neoplasms that cause bile duct strictures are mainly pancreatic head and biliary tract cancers. Biliary tract cancers can be further classified into intrahepatic cholangiocarcinoma (CCA), hilar CCA, distal CCA, ampullary cancer, and gallbladder cancer.

- Incidence

Gallbladder cancer is the most common biliary tract cancer, with an age-standardized rate of 1.2 per 100,000 individuals. Other types of CCAs are rare worldwide, with the following reported rates per 100,000 individuals: intrahepatic CCA 1.49, hilar and distal CCA 0.96, ampullary cancer 0.45, and duplicate or other lesions in the biliary tract 0.24. Gallbladder cancer is more common in women, whereas other types of biliary tract cancer are more frequent in men [50–52].

Pancreatic cancer has an age-standardized rate of 4.9 per 100,000 individuals, comprising approximately 75% of pancreatic head cancer cases. Pancreatic cancer includes a majority of adenocarcinomas but may also consist of exocrine and neuroendocrine tumors [50, 53]. Biliary tract cancers are predominantly adenocarcinomas.

- Clinical Presentation

Except for intrahepatic CCA, bile duct obstruction can cause jaundice. Weight loss and pain are also possible symptoms of tumors.

- Work-up Investigation

Blood investigations reveal elevated tumor markers along with the presence of a bile duct stricture/obstruction. CA19–9 is commonly used as a serum biomarker for biliary tract cancer and pancreatic ductal adenocarcinoma (PDAC), with a sensitivity and specificity of 80–90% in symptomatic patients with PDAC. However, CA19–9 may not be detectable in individuals with Lewis antigen negativity (approximately 7% of the general population), which is a limitation [54].

Computed tomography (CT) and magnetic resonance imaging/magnetic resonance cholangiopancreatography (MRI/MRCP) are used to detect tumors. CT accurately evaluates tumor vascular invasion, and MRI/MRCP, especially contrast-enhanced MRI, demonstrates high diagnostic accuracy in detecting biliary invasion and liver metastases [55]. EUS can detect small tumors that might not be visible on CT or MRI and can provide a reliable tissue diagnosis via fine-needle aspiration under EUS guidance [56]. Endoscopic retrograde cholangiopancreatography (ERCP) can detect malignant biliary strictures and provide information about the horizontal extent of the tumor. Intraductal ultrasonography (IDUS) is helpful in assessing the vertical and horizontal tumor extents, and cholangioscopy allows direct visualization of the biliary mucosa to evaluate the horizontal spread. In some cases of ampullary cancer, swollen papillae can be observed under direct visualization. Positron emission tomography (PET) scans are not routinely performed but are useful in detecting distant metastases. A summary of the ERC, IDUS, and hilar CCA biopsy results is shown in Fig. 26.5.

- Differential Diagnosis

As previously mentioned for IgG4-related sclerosing cholangitis, differentiating between distal CCA and pancreatic head cancer based on IgG4-SC Type 1, and between hilar CCA and IgG4-SC Type 4 is crucial. Thickening of the gallbladder wall may increase the suspicion of gallbladder cancer; however, diffuse and homogeneous thickening might indicate benign conditions such as chronic cholecystitis or xanthogranulomatous cholecystitis.

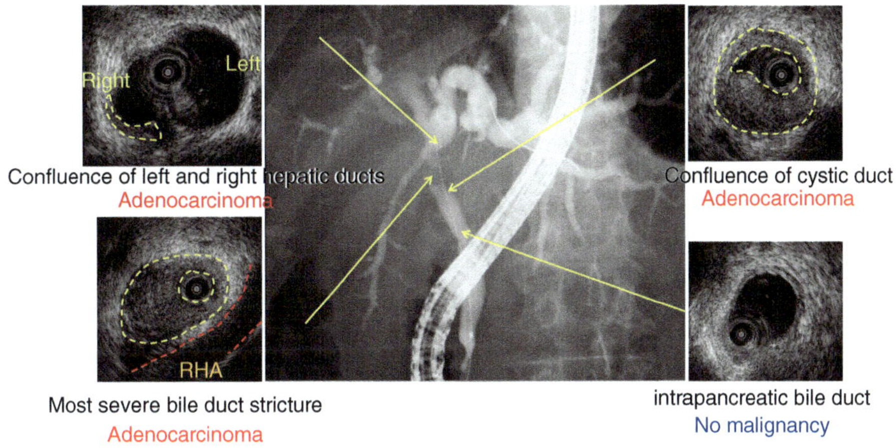

Fig. 26.5 Summary of ERC, intraductal ultrasonography (IDUS), and biopsy results in hilar cholangiocarcinoma

- Treatment

Both biliary tract and pancreatic head cancers require surgical resection with curative intent. A consensus on whether preoperative biliary drainage should be performed in all patients with obstructive jaundice caused by malignant biliary lesions is lacking. However, in resectable hilar CCA requiring major hepatectomy for radical resection, preoperative biliary drainage reduces postoperative mortality rates. Endoscopic nasobiliary drainage (ENBD) is the first choice of drainage, and transgastric drainage is also considered an option. Percutaneous transhepatic biliary drainage (PTBD) is performed only when other methods are not possible because it increases the risk of intrahepatic metastasis and seeding by puncture [57, 58].

Preoperative therapy followed by surgery is recommended for PDAC [59]; however, the existing evidence for this approach in biliary tract cancer is not well established. Postoperative adjuvant therapy is effective in both types of cancer and is recommended when applicable [60, 61]. In unresectable cases, endoscopic or percutaneous biliary drainage is performed, followed by systemic chemotherapy or radiation therapy.

- Surgical Planning/Management

For intrahepatic CCA, the extent of liver resection is determined based on tumor localization. Lymph node dissection is a debatable topic. For hilar CCA, resection is determined using the Bismuth classification, and the procedure includes extrahepatic bile duct resection, extended hepatectomy, and regional lymph node dissection. In patients requiring major hepatectomy, preoperative portal vein embolization may be performed to increase the future remnant liver volume [62]. In the presence of an underlying chronic liver disease, such as primary sclerosing cholangitis (PSC), liver transplantation after neoadjuvant therapy can provide a good prognosis [63]. Distal CCA and ampullary cancer are resected with pancreaticoduodenectomy (Whipple procedure); limited resections such as extrahepatic bile duct resection may be considered in selected cases [51]. For gallbladder cancer, the extent of resection varies depending on the degree of tumor invasion. Simple cholecystectomy is curative for early-stage gallbladder cancer without lymph node metastasis. However, in patients with serosal or liver invasion, additional liver bed resection is necessary. If the tumor invades the bile duct, extrahepatic bile duct resection is required; in extensive cases involving the surrounding vessels, extended right hepatectomy or pancreaticoduodenectomy may be performed. Lymph node dissection focuses on the hepaticoduodenal ligament for advanced cancers; however, this may not be required for early-stage cancers without lymph node metastasis

[52]. Pancreaticoduodenectomy with regional lymph node dissection is the standard procedure for pancreatic head cancer [53].

- Follow-up/Recommendations

Regular follow-ups are essential, and in cases of recurrence, systemic chemotherapy is often the first choice, considering the patient's overall condition. Targeted therapies for specific genetic mutations have been effective. Repeat surgical resection should be considered under certain conditions.

26.5 Conclusion

We outlined the diseases that can cause biliary strictures associated with non-neoplastic benign and neoplastic diseases. Even with the advancements in diagnostic imaging, a diagnosis based solely on imaging findings can be challenging, and preoperative histopathological examination fails to provide a definitive diagnosis. Treatment approaches differ between patients with malignant and benign diseases. Therefore, establishing a definitive diagnosis before treatment planning is imperative.

Financial Support None

Disclosures Nothing to disclose.

References

1. Williams E, Beckingham I, El Sayed G, Gurusamy K, Sturgess R, Webster G, Young T. Updated guideline on the management of common bile duct stones (CBDS). Gut. 2017;66(5):765–82.
2. Cox MR, Budge JP, Eslick GD. Timing and nature of presentation of unsuspected retained common bile duct stones after laparoscopic cholecystectomy: a retrospective study. Surg Endosc. 2015;29(7):2033–8.
3. Elmunzer BJ, Scheiman JM, Lehman GA, Chak A, Mosler P, Higgins PD, Hayward RA, Romagnuolo J, Elta GH, Sherman S, Waljee AK, Repaka A, Atkinson MR, Cote GA, Kwon RS, McHenry L, Piraka CR, Wamsteker EJ, Watkins JL, Korsnes SJ, Schmidt SE, Turner SM, Nicholson S, Fogel EL, Endoscopy USCfORi. A randomized trial of rectal indomethacin to prevent post-ERCP pancreatitis. N Engl J Med. 2012;366(15):1414–22.
4. Alexakis N, Connor S. Meta-analysis of one- vs. two-stage laparoscopic/endoscopic management of common bile duct stones. HPB (Oxford). 2012;14(4):254–9.
5. Rhodes M, Sussman L, Cohen L, Lewis MP. Randomised trial of laparoscopic exploration of common bile duct versus postoperative endoscopic retrograde cholangiography for common bile duct stones. Lancet. 1998;351(9097):159–61.
6. Riciardi R, Islam S, Canete JJ, Arcand PL, Stoker ME. Effectiveness and long-term results of laparoscopic common bile duct exploration. Surg Endosc. 2003;17(1):19–22.
7. Gonzalvez-Guardiola P, Paya-Llorente C, Domingo-Del Pozo C, Martinez-Perez A. Predictors for stone recurrence after a successful common bile duct surgical exploration for choledocholithiasis. Langenbeck's Arch Surg. 2022;407(4):1545–52.
8. Park SY, Hong TH, Lee SK, Park IY, Kim TH, Kim SG. Recurrence of common bile duct stones following laparoscopic common bile duct exploration: a multicenter study. J Hepatobiliary Pancreat Sci. 2019;26(12):578–82.
9. Mack CL, Adams D, Assis DN, Kerkar N, Manns MP, Mayo MJ, Vierling JM, Alsawas M, Murad MH, Czaja AJ. Diagnosis and management of autoimmune hepatitis in adults and children: 2019 practice guidance and guidelines from the American Association for the Study of Liver Diseases. Hepatology. 2020;72(2):671–722.
10. Bowlus CL, Arrive L, Bergquist A, Deneau M, Forman L, Ilyas SI, Lunsford KE, Martinez M, Sapisochin G, Shroff R, Tabibian JH, Assis DN. AASLD practice guidance on primary sclerosing cholangitis and cholangiocarcinoma. Hepatology. 2023;77(2):659–702.
11. Kuo A, Gomel R, Safer R, Lindor KD, Everson GT, Bowlus CL. Characteristics and outcomes reported by patients with primary sclerosing cholangitis through an online registry. Clin Gastroenterol Hepatol. 2019;17(7):1372–8.
12. Lunder AK, Hov JR, Borthne A, Gleditsch J, Johannesen G, Tveit K, Viktil E, Henriksen M, Hovde O, Huppertz-Hauss G, Hoie O, Hoivik ML, Monstad I, Solberg IC, Jahnsen J, Karlsen TH, Moum B, Vatn M, Negard A. Prevalence of sclerosing cholangitis detected by magnetic resonance cholangiography in patients with long-term inflammatory bowel disease. Gastroenterology. 2016;151(4):660–9. e664.
13. Schramm C, Eaton J, Ringe KI, Venkatesh S, Yamamura J, IPSCSG MRIwgot. Recommendations on the use of magnetic resonance imaging in PSC-A position statement from the International PSC Study Group. Hepatology. 2017;66(5):1675–88.
14. Aabakken L, Karlsen TH, Albert J, Arvanitakis M, Chazouilleres O, Dumonceau JM, Farkkila M, Fickert P, Hirschfield GM, Laghi A, Marzioni M, Fernandez

M, Pereira SP, Pohl J, Poley JW, Ponsioen CY, Schramm C, Swahn F, Tringali A, Hassan C. Role of endoscopy in primary sclerosing cholangitis: European Society of Gastrointestinal Endoscopy (ESGE) and European Association for the Study of the Liver (EASL) clinical guideline. Endoscopy. 2017;49(6):588–608.

15. Khoshpouri P, Habibabadi RR, Hazhirkarzar B, Ameli S, Ghadimi M, Ghasabeh MA, Menias CO, Kim A, Li Z, Kamel IR. Imaging features of primary sclerosing cholangitis: from diagnosis to liver transplant follow-up. Radiographics. 2019;39(7):1938–64.
16. Ponsioen CY, Assis DN, Boberg KM, Bowlus CL, Deneau M, Thorburn D, Aabakken L, Farkkila M, Petersen B, Rupp C, Hubscher SG, Group PSCS. Defining primary sclerosing cholangitis: results from an international primary sclerosing cholangitis study group consensus process. Gastroenterology. 2021;161(6):1764–75. e1765.
17. Prokopic M, Beuers U. Management of primary sclerosing cholangitis and its complications: an algorithmic approach. Hepatol Int. 2021;15(1):6–20.
18. Karlsen TH, Folseraas T, Thorburn D, Vesterhus M. Primary sclerosing cholangitis - a comprehensive review. J Hepatol. 2017;67(6):1298–323.
19. Akamatsu N, Hasegawa K, Egawa H, Ohdan H, Yoshizawa A, Kokudo N, Tazuma S, Tanaka A, Takikawa H. Donor age (>/=45 years) and reduced immunosuppression are associated with the recurrent primary sclerosing cholangitis after liver transplantation - a multicenter retrospective study. Transpl Int. 2021;34(5):916–29.
20. Kamisawa T, Zen Y, Pillai S, Stone JH. IgG4-related disease. Lancet. 2015;385(9976):1460–71.
21. Kamisawa T, Nakazawa T, Tazuma S, Zen Y, Tanaka A, Ohara H, Muraki T, Inui K, Inoue D, Nishino T, Naitoh I, Itoi T, Notohara K, Kanno A, Kubota K, Hirano K, Isayama H, Shimizu K, Tsuyuguchi T, Shimosegawa T, Kawa S, Chiba T, Okazaki K, Takikawa H, Kimura W, Unno M, Yoshida M. Clinical practice guidelines for IgG4-related sclerosing cholangitis. J Hepatobiliary Pancreat Sci. 2019;26(1):9–42.
22. Tanaka A, Tazuma S, Okazaki K, Nakazawa T, Inui K, Chiba T, Takikawa H. Clinical features, response to treatment, and outcomes of IgG4-related sclerosing cholangitis. Clin Gastroenterol Hepatol. 2017;15(6):920–926 e923.
23. Ohara H, Nakazawa T, Kawa S, Kamisawa T, Shimosegawa T, Uchida K, Hirano K, Nishino T, Hamano H, Kanno A, Notohara K, Hasebe O, Muraki T, Ishida E, Naitoh I, Okazaki K. Establishment of a serum IgG4 cut-off value for the differential diagnosis of IgG4-related sclerosing cholangitis: a Japanese cohort. J Gastroenterol Hepatol. 2013;28(7):1247–51.
24. Nakazawa T, Ohara H, Sano H, Ando T, Joh T. Schematic classification of sclerosing cholangitis with autoimmune pancreatitis by cholangiography. Pancreas. 2006;32(2):229.
25. Hirano K, Tada M, Isayama H, Yamamoto K, Mizuno S, Yagioka H, Yashima Y, Sasaki T, Kogure H, Togawa O, Arizumi T, Matsubara S, Nakai Y, Sasahira N, Tsujino T, Kawabe T, Omata M. Endoscopic evaluation of factors contributing to intrapancreatic biliary stricture in autoimmune pancreatitis. Gastrointest Endosc. 2010;71(1):85–90.
26. Zen Y. The pathology of IgG4-related disease in the bile duct and pancreas. Semin Liver Dis. 2016;36(3):242–56.
27. Hart PA, Kamisawa T, Brugge WR, Chung JB, Culver EL, Czako L, Frulloni L, Go VL, Gress TM, Kim MH, Kawa S, Lee KT, Lerch MM, Liao WC, Lohr M, Okazaki K, Ryu JK, Schleinitz N, Shimizu K, Shimosegawa T, Soetikno R, Webster G, Yadav D, Zen Y, Chari ST. Long-term outcomes of autoimmune pancreatitis: a multicentre, international analysis. Gut. 2013;62(12):1771–6.
28. Hart PA, Topazian MD, Witzig TE, Clain JE, Gleeson FC, Klebig RR, Levy MJ, Pearson RK, Petersen BT, Smyrk TC, Sugumar A, Takahashi N, Vege SS, Chari ST. Treatment of relapsing autoimmune pancreatitis with immunomodulators and rituximab: the Mayo Clinic experience. Gut. 2013;62(11):1607–15.
29. Davenport M, Tizzard SA, Underhill J, Mieli-Vergani G, Portmann B, Hadzic N. The biliary atresia splenic malformation syndrome: a 28-year single-center retrospective study. J Pediatr. 2006;149(3):393–400.
30. Hartley JL, Davenport M, Kelly DA. Biliary atresia. Lancet. 2009;374(9702):1704–13.
31. The NS, Honein MA, Caton AR, Moore CA, Siega-Riz AM, Druschel CM, National Birth Defects Prevention S. Risk factors for isolated biliary atresia, national birth defects prevention study, 1997–2002. Am J Med Genet A. 2007;143A(19):2274–84.
32. Roquete ML, Ferreira AR, Fagundes ED, Castro LP, Silva RA, Penna FJ. Accuracy of echogenic periportal enlargement image in ultrasonographic exams and histopathology in differential diagnosis of biliary atresia. J Pediatr. 2008;84(4):331–6.
33. Larrosa-Haro A, Caro-Lopez AM, Coello-Ramirez P, Zavala-Ocampo J, Vazquez-Camacho G. Duodenal tube test in the diagnosis of biliary atresia. J Pediatr Gastroenterol Nutr. 2001;32(3):311–5.
34. Pakarinen MP, Rintala RJ. Surgery of biliary atresia. Scand J Surg. 2011;100(1):49–53.
35. Garcia AV, Cowles RA, Kato T, Hardy MA. Morio Kasai: a remarkable impact beyond the Kasai procedure. J Pediatr Surg. 2012;47(5):1023–7.
36. McKiernan PJ, Baker AJ, Kelly DA. The frequency and outcome of biliary atresia in the UK and Ireland. Lancet. 2000;355(9197):25–9.
37. Barshes NR, Lee TC, Balkrishnan R, Karpen SJ, Carter BA, Goss JA. Orthotopic liver transplantation for biliary atresia: the U.S. experience. Liver Transpl. 2005;11(10):1193–200.
38. Akamatsu N, Sugawara Y, Hashimoto D. Biliary reconstruction, its complications and management of

biliary complications after adult liver transplantation: a systematic review of the incidence, risk factors and outcome. Transpl Int. 2011;24(4):379–92.
39. Dimou FM, Adhikari D, Mehta HB, Olino K, Riall TS, Brown KM. Incidence of hepaticojejunostomy stricture after hepaticojejunostomy. Surgery. 2016;160(3):691–8.
40. Morelli G, Fazel A, Judah J, Pan JJ, Forsmark C, Draganov P. Rapid-sequence endoscopic management of posttransplant anastomotic biliary strictures. Gastrointest Endosc. 2008;67(6):879–85.
41. Sharma S, Gurakar A, Jabbour N. Biliary strictures following liver transplantation: past, present and preventive strategies. Liver Transpl. 2008;14(6):759–69.
42. Halle-Smith JM, Hall LA, Mirza DF, Roberts KJ. Risk factors for anastomotic stricture after hepaticojejunostomy for bile duct injury-a systematic review and meta-analysis. Surgery. 2021;170(5):1310–6.
43. Alazmi WM, Fogel EL, Watkins JL, McHenry L, Tector JA, Fridell J, Mosler P, Sherman S, Lehman GA. Recurrence rate of anastomotic biliary strictures in patients who have had previous successful endoscopic therapy for anastomotic narrowing after orthotopic liver transplantation. Endoscopy. 2006;38(6):571–4.
44. Williams ED, Draganov PV. Endoscopic management of biliary strictures after liver transplantation. World J Gastroenterol. 2009;15(30):3725–33.
45. Ishizawa T, Bandai Y, Ijichi M, Kaneko J, Hasegawa K, Kokudo N. Fluorescent cholangiography illuminating the biliary tree during laparoscopic cholecystectomy. Br J Surg. 2010;97(9):1369–77.
46. Kawaguchi Y, Velayutham V, Fuks D, Christidis C, Kokudo N, Gayet B. Usefulness of indocyanine green-fluorescence imaging for visualization of the bile duct during laparoscopic liver resection. J Am Coll Surg. 2015;221(6):e113–7.
47. Matsumura M, Kawaguchi Y, Kobayashi Y, Kobayashi K, Ishizawa T, Akamatsu N, Kaneko J, Arita J, Kokudo N, Hasegawa K. Indocyanine green administration a day before surgery may increase bile duct detectability on fluorescence cholangiography during laparoscopic cholecystectomy. J Hepatobiliary Pancreat Sci. 2021;28(2):202–10.
48. Yokoe M, Hata J, Takada T, Strasberg SM, Asbun HJ, Wakabayashi G, Kozaka K, Endo I, Deziel DJ, Miura F, Okamoto K, Hwang TL, Huang WS, Ker CG, Chen MF, Han HS, Yoon YS, Choi IS, Yoon DS, Noguchi Y, Shikata S, Ukai T, Higuchi R, Gabata T, Mori Y, Iwashita Y, Hibi T, Jagannath P, Jonas E, Liau KH, Dervenis C, Gouma DJ, Cherqui D, Belli G, Garden OJ, Gimenez ME, de Santibanes E, Suzuki K, Umezawa A, Supe AN, Pitt HA, Singh H, Chan ACW, Lau WY, Teoh AYB, Honda G, Sugioka A, Asai K, Gomi H, Itoi T, Kiriyama S, Yoshida M, Mayumi T, Matsumura N, Tokumura H, Kitano S, Hirata K, Inui K, Sumiyama Y, Yamamoto M. Tokyo guidelines 2018: diagnostic criteria and severity grading of acute cholecystitis (with videos). J Hepatobiliary Pancreat Sci. 2018;25(1):41–54.
49. Okada Y, Kawaguchi Y, Matsumura M, Matsubara S, Nakai Y, Ichida A, Ishizawa T, Akamatsu N, Kaneko J, Arita J, Koike K, Hasegawa K. A safe sequential treatment approach for patients who have acute cholecystitis with severe inflammation: transmural gallbladder drainage followed by laparoscopic cholecystectomy under the guidance of fluorescence imaging. Asian J Endosc Surg. 2022;15(1):230–4.
50. World Cancer Research Fund International. https://www.wcrf.org/.
51. Rizvi S, Khan SA, Hallemeier CL, Kelley RK, Gores GJ. Cholangiocarcinoma - evolving concepts and therapeutic strategies. Nat Rev Clin Oncol. 2018;15(2):95–111.
52. Roa JC, Garcia P, Kapoor VK, Maithel SK, Javle M, Koshiol J. Gallbladder cancer. Nat Rev Dis Primers. 2022;8(1):69.
53. Wood LD, Canto MI, Jaffee EM, Simeone DM. Pancreatic cancer: pathogenesis, screening, diagnosis, and treatment. Gastroenterology. 2022;163(2):386–402 e381.
54. Nehls O, Gregor M, Klump B. Serum and bile markers for cholangiocarcinoma. Semin Liver Dis. 2004;24(2):139–54.
55. Ruys AT, van Beem BE, Engelbrecht MR, Bipat S, Stoker J, Van Gulik TM. Radiological staging in patients with hilar cholangiocarcinoma: a systematic review and meta-analysis. Br J Radiol. 2012;85(1017):1255–62.
56. Mohamadnejad M, DeWitt JM, Sherman S, LeBlanc JK, Pitt HA, House MG, Jones KJ, Fogel EL, McHenry L, Watkins JL, Cote GA, Lehman GA, Al-Haddad MA. Role of EUS for preoperative evaluation of cholangiocarcinoma: a large single-center experience. Gastrointest Endosc. 2011;73(1):71–8.
57. Moole H, Bechtold M, Puli SR. Efficacy of preoperative biliary drainage in malignant obstructive jaundice: a meta-analysis and systematic review. World J Surg Oncol. 2016;14(1):182.
58. Nagino M, Hirano S, Yoshitomi H, Aoki T, Uesaka K, Unno M, Ebata T, Konishi M, Sano K, Shimada K, Shimizu H, Higuchi R, Wakai T, Isayama H, Okusaka T, Tsuyuguchi T, Hirooka Y, Furuse J, Maguchi H, Suzuki K, Yamazaki H, Kijima H, Yanagisawa A, Yoshida M, Yokoyama Y, Mizuno T, Endo I. Clinical practice guidelines for the management of biliary tract cancers 2019: the 3rd English edition. J Hepatobiliary Pancreat Sci. 2021;28(1):26–54.
59. Versteijne E, van Dam JL, Suker M, Janssen QP, Groothuis K, Akkermans-Vogelaar JM, Besselink MG, Bonsing BA, Buijsen J, Busch OR, Creemers GM, van Dam RM, Eskens F, Festen S, de Groot JWB, Groot Koerkamp B, de Hingh IH, Homs MYV, van Hooft JE, Kerver ED, Luelmo SAC, Neelis KJ, Nuyttens J, Paardekooper G, Patijn GA, van der Sangen MJC, de Vos-Geelen J, Wilmink JW, Zwinderman AH, Punt CJ, van Tienhoven G, van Eijck CHJ, Dutch Pancreatic Cancer G. Neoadjuvant chemoradiotherapy versus upfront surgery for resectable and borderline resectable pancreatic cancer: long-

term results of the Dutch randomized PREOPANC trial. J Clin Oncol. 2022;40(11):1220–30.
60. Oettle H, Neuhaus P, Hochhaus A, Hartmann JT, Gellert K, Ridwelski K, Niedergethmann M, Zulke C, Fahlke J, Arning MB, Sinn M, Hinke A, Riess H. Adjuvant chemotherapy with gemcitabine and long-term outcomes among patients with resected pancreatic cancer: the CONKO-001 randomized trial. JAMA. 2013;310(14):1473–81.
61. Nakachi K, Ikeda M, Konishi M, Nomura S, Katayama H, Kataoka T, Todaka A, Yanagimoto H, Morinaga S, Kobayashi S, Shimada K, Takahashi Y, Nakagohri T, Gotoh K, Kamata K, Shimizu Y, Ueno M, Ishii H, Okusaka T, Furuse J, Hepatobiliary, Pancreatic Oncology Group of the Japan Clinical Oncology G. Adjuvant S-1 compared with observation in resected biliary tract cancer (JCOG1202, ASCOT): a multicentre, open-label, randomised, controlled, phase 3 trial. Lancet. 2023;401(10372):195–203.
62. Aoki T, Sakamoto Y, Kohno Y, Akamatsu N, Kaneko J, Sugawara Y, Hasegawa K, Makuuchi M, Kokudo N. Hepatopancreaticoduodenectomy for biliary cancer: strategies for near-zero operative mortality and acceptable long-term outcome. Ann Surg. 2018;267(2):332–7.
63. Rosen CB, Heimbach JK, Gores GJ. Liver transplantation for cholangiocarcinoma. Transpl Int. 2010;23(7):692–7.

Surgical Treatment of Choledochal Cysts

27

Hiroyuki Ishida, Richard D. Schulick, and Marco Del Chiaro

27.1 Introduction

Choledochal cysts (CCs), also known as congenital biliary dilation, are rare congenital cystic dilations of the extrahepatic and/or intrahepatic bile ducts. CCs are diagnosed both in children and adults, although more than half of patients present before the age of 10 years [1, 2]. It is also well known that CCs are more common in females than in males, with a female-to-male ratio of 3–4:1 [1, 3]. The incidence of CCs is reported to be higher in East Asia than in Western countries, ranging from 1 in 1000 in Japan to 1 in 50,000–150,000 in Western countries [4–7]. CCs are usually associated with pancreatobiliary maljunction and have a potential risk of biliary tract cancer. Therefore, resection of the dilated bile duct with biliary reconstruction should be considered even in asymptomatic patients [8]. This chapter reviews the pathophysiology and classification of CCs and discusses current topics in surgical treatments.

H. Ishida
Division of Surgical Oncology, Department of Surgery, University of Colorado School of Medicine, Aurora, CO, USA

Department of Hepatobiliary and Pancreatic Surgery, Institute of Science Tokyo, Tokyo, Japan
e-mail: hiroyuki.ishida@cuanschutz.edu

R. D. Schulick · M. Del Chiaro (✉)
Division of Surgical Oncology, Department of Surgery, University of Colorado School of Medicine, Aurora, CO, USA
e-mail: richard.schulick@cuanschutz.edu; marco.delchiaro@cuanschutz.edu

27.2 Etiology and Pathophysiology

CCs are mostly associated with congenital pancreatobiliary maljunction (PBM). Patients with PBM have the junction of the pancreatic and bile ducts outside the wall of the duodenum, usually showing a long common duct. The sphincter of Oddi does not regulate the function of the pancreatobiliary junction, and regurgitation can occur in both directions: pancreatic juice can regurgitate into the bile duct, and bile can regurgitate into the pancreatic duct. Since the pressure in the pancreatic duct is usually higher than in the bile duct, pancreatic juice often refluxes into the bile duct in patients with PBM.

The mixing of bile and pancreatic juice leads to the production of hazardous substances, such as lithostathine, which stagnate in the dilated biliary tree [9]. These substances irritate the epithelium, resulting in hyperplasia that can progress to carcinoma. Lithostathine is cleaved into an insoluble form by activated trypsin, which then aggregates to form an obstructive plug of protein. This condition causes abdominal pain, vomiting, and jaundice in childhood and biliary tract cancer in adulthood [10].

T. Hackert, A. Gulla (eds.), *Rare Liver and Biliary Tract Diseases*,
https://doi.org/10.1007/978-3-032-15076-9_27

27.3 Classification of Pancreatobiliary Maljunction

Various classifications of PBM have been created based on the form of the confluence between the bile duct and the pancreatic duct [11–14]. In 1977, Komi et al. [12] classified PBM into three types according to the type of pancreatobiliary junction: (a) the narrow common bile duct joins the pancreatic duct (C-P type), (b) the pancreatic duct joins the common bile duct (P-C type), and (c) complex type. This classification was later modified to classify PBM into three types, with subtypes based on the presence of common channel dilatation [13]. However, since this classification was considered complex, a new classification was proposed by the Committee on Diagnostic Criteria of the Japanese Study Group on Pancreaticobiliary Maljunction (JSGPM) in 2015 [15]. In this classification, PBM is divided into four types: (A) stenotic type, (B) non-stenotic type, (C) dilated channel type, and (D) complex type [15].

27.4 Classification of Choledocal Cysts

The existence of CCs was first described by Vater and Ezler in 1723 [16]. In 1959, CCs were first classified by Alonso-Lej into three types: (Type I) congenital cystic dilatation of the common bile duct, (Type II) congenital diverticulum of the common bile duct, and (Type III) choledochocele [17]. This classification was modified by Todani in 1977 into five types due to the recognition of intrahepatic involvement, including Caroli disease, and later revised based on the concept of PBM (Fig. 27.1) [18–20].

According to Todani's classification, Type I is divided into three subtypes: (Ia) cystic dilatation with PBM, (Ib) segmental dilatation without PBM, and (Ic) diffuse dilatation with PBM. Type II is diverticular dilatation of the bile duct without PBM. Type III is a choledochocele in the duodenal wall without PBM. Type IV is multiple cysts, at least including one in the extrahepatic bile duct, and is subdivided into two types. Type IV-A is multiple cysts in both the extrahepatic and intrahepatic bile ducts, and PBM is accompanied. Type IV-B also has multiple cysts, but confined to the extrahepatic bile duct alone. The presence of malunion is uncertain due to the lack of data. Type V, also known as Caroli disease, is a single or multiple dilatations of the intrahepatic duct without PBM. In summary, types Ia, Ic, and IV-A are accompanied by PBM, while types Ib, II, III, IV-B, and V are not accompanied by PBM. The most frequent type of CCs is Type I, followed by Type IV.

Of note, in Japan, a congenital malformation involving both local dilatation of the extrahepatic bile duct and PBM is currently defined as congenital biliary dilatation by the JSGPM. Therefore, types Ia, Ic, and IV-A in Todani's classification are included in congenital biliary dilatation [21].

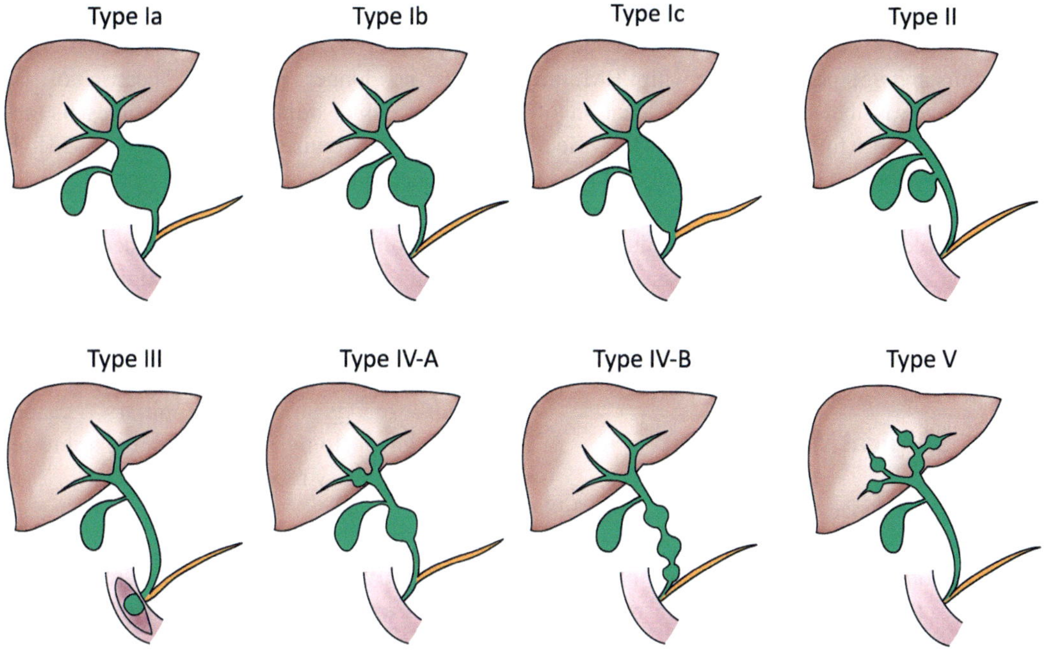

Fig. 27.1 Todani's classification of choledochal cysts

27.5 Clinical Symptoms

The classic symptom triad of patients with CCs is right upper quadrant pain, jaundice, and an abdominal mass. However, this triad is present in fewer than 20% of patients [22]. A multi-institutional study by 8 institutions in North America and Europe included 135 children and 259 adults and showed that abdominal pain was the most common presenting symptom (61.2%), followed by pancreatitis (18.8%) and jaundice (18.5%). None had the triad of symptoms. Adults were more likely to present with abdominal pain (71.8% vs. 40.7%, $p < 0.001$), and children were more likely to have jaundice (31.9% vs. 11.6%, $p < 0.001$) [22]. The Japanese nationwide survey ($n = 2561$) included 950 children and 997 adult patients between 1990 and 2007 and showed that the incidence of clinical symptoms was more frequent in children than in adult patients (94.3% vs. 74.0%, $p < 0.001$) [10]. In children, the most frequent symptom was abdominal pain, followed by vomiting and jaundice. Abdominal pain was most frequent in adult patients as well, followed by jaundice and back pain.

27.6 Incidence of Associated Biliary Tract Cancer

CCs are associated with various complications, including obstructive jaundice, choledocholithiasis, pancreatitis, cholangitis, and spontaneous rupture of the bile duct [23]. Besides these complications, CCs are known to have an increased risk of biliary tract cancer. The association of cancer with CCs was first reported by Irwin and Morison in 1944 [24]. The risk of cancer is known to increase with age. Patients diagnosed with CCs during the first decade of life had a cancer risk of 0.7%, compared to 6.8% and 14.3% for patients diagnosed with CCs at ages 11–20 years and 20 years and older, respectively [25]. The Japanese nationwide registry also reported that the incidence of biliary cancers in CCs was 21.6% in adult patients, while 0.1% in pediatric patients [10]. Moreover, the risk of cancer is associated with CC types [26–28]. Todani et al. showed that 68% of biliary tract cancers occurred in Type I, 5% in Type II, 1.6% in Type III, 21% in Type IV, and 6% in Type V [29]. Regarding the location of cancer, cancer occurs in both the bile duct and gallbladder. According to the Japanese nationwide registry, including 997 adults and 950 pediatric CCs with PBM, the gallbladder was the most common location of cancer (62.3%), followed by the bile duct (32.1%), and both the gallbladder and bile duct (4.7%) in adult patients [10]. Bile duct cancer was observed in only one of 950 children. The age of onset of bile duct cancer was reportedly younger than that of gallbladder cancer (52.0 vs. 60.1 years old, $p < 0.001$).

27.7 Surgical Management

As mentioned above, the risk of developing biliary tract cancer in patients with CCs depends on the location and distribution of the cysts. Therefore, the indication and timing of surgery and the optimal procedure should be determined according to the type of CCs. Furthermore, the principle of surgery varies depending on whether PBM exists or not.

27.8 Type I and IV

27.8.1 Surgical Indication and Standard Procedure

Types Ia, Ic, and IV-A are usually associated with PBM. There is no clear consensus on when CC patients with PBM should undergo surgical resection. However, given the higher risk of biliary tract cancer in CC patients with PBM, surgery is recommended when a definitive diagnosis is made for children and young adults. On the other hand, the timing of surgery for neonates and infants should be determined carefully. Symptomatic neonates and infants should be operated on as soon as possible, whereas elective operations at around 3–6 months of age may be considered for asymptomatic cases while their organ functions are monitored carefully [21].

The standard procedure is complete excision of the cysts with a Roux-en-Y hepaticojejunostomy. Historically, internal drainage with cholecystoenterostomy was first reported by Swain et al. in 1894, which was supported by Brun and Hartman in 1897 [30]. However, internal drainage is no longer preferred because of the increased risk of biliary stones, cholangitis, and cancer in the remnant biliary tree [31–33]. In 1970, the importance of the removal of the dilated bile duct was reported to reduce postoperative morbidity and prevent cancer [34, 35]. Regarding the biliary reconstruction, hepaticoduodenostomy was previously considered as an option. However, since it was found that hepaticoduodenostomy was associated with the development of gastric and biliary cancer, hepaticojejunostomy is currently the preferred method for biliary reconstruction [36].

27.8.2 Optimal Range of Excision: Pancreatic and Hepatic Sides and the Need for Hepatectomy

The pancreatic side of the common bile duct should be resected just above the pancreatobiliary junction to prevent postoperative complications, including cancer in the remnant bile duct, pancreatitis, and pancreatic stones [37, 38]. Identification of the narrow segment allows the complete resection of the dilated bile duct just above the pancreatobiliary junction. The extent of bile duct resection on the hepatic side should be determined by the type of CCs.

In type I CCs, the complete resection of the dilated bile duct is mandatory. When stenosis of the common hepatic duct is suspected, incision of both the right and left hepatic ducts to create a large anastomosis is essential to prevent the intrahepatic carcinoma associated with postoperative biliary stasis [39]. In Type IV-A CCs, it remains unknown to what extent the hepatic bile ducts should be resected and whether hepatectomy should be added to achieve a complete resection of the dilated duct [40]. Ando et al. showed that the orifice of the left and right hepatic ducts was the common site of stenosis in Type IV-A and that there were two types of stenosis: membranous and septal [41]. They also reported that lateral incision of the hepatic duct or dilation by resection from the divided end of the common hepatic duct should be performed to treat stenoses [42]. Regarding the need for hepatectomy, several studies showed the results of concomitant hepatectomies for Type IV-A CCs [43–47]. Generally, partial hepatectomy should be considered if the dilated bile ducts and stenosis are confined to a single lobe in adult patients. A study investigating the risk of carcinogenesis in CCs suggests that hepatectomy should be considered for Type IV-A choledochal cysts because cholangiocarcinoma can arise from the intrahepatic bile duct years after the extrahepatic cyst excision [46]. Nevertheless, the evidence of hepatectomy for Type IV-A with bilobar disease is scarce. In a retrospective study including 28 patients who underwent hepatectomy for Type IV-A with bilobar bile duct cysts, the postoperative morbidity and mortality were 57.1% and 3.6%, respectively [46]. They also reported that no malignant transformation occurred after hepatectomy during a mean follow-up of 31 months. Further studies with long-term follow-up are needed.

27.9 Type II

Type II CCs are very rare, and reports are limited. In this type, diverticula arise laterally from the wall of the extrahepatic bile duct. Ligation and excision can be performed at the neck of cysts without the need for bile duct reconstruction. However, when cysts have larger connections, closure over a T-tube after excision or en bloc cyst excision with the extrahepatic bile duct and a Roux-en-Y hepaticojejunostomy is required [48]. In a retrospective European multicenter study including 19 Type II CCs, the diverticulum occurred in the upper, middle, and lower parts of the extrahepatic bile duct in 58%, 21%, and 21% of patients, respectively [49]. Diverticulum excision was performed in all patients, and 58% of patients required the concomitant resection of the extrahepatic bile duct. The overall complication rate was 15.8%, including one severe complication of biliary fistula requiring percutaneous radiological drainage in 1 patient. The mortality rate was 0% [49].

27.10 Type III

Type III CCs, also known as choledochoceles, are abnormalities of cystic or diverticular dilatation of the terminal intramural portion of the bile duct. Although this type of CC is rare, previous studies showed that 14.3–27% of all choledochoceles harbored cancers [50, 51]. Therefore, cysts should be resected or at least should be under endoscopic surveillance. Regarding the treatment for Type III CCs, transduodenal excision and sphincteroplasty were historically performed. However, the endoscopic approach has been increasingly chosen for this type. A recent systematic review by Lobeck et al. evaluated the management of this type in both pediatric and adult patients [52]. Of the 13 pediatric patients, endoscopic sphincterotomy was the most frequent treatment ($n = 5$). Of the 58 adult patients, 21 patients (36%) underwent endoscopic therapy, including endoscopic sphincterotomy ($n = 17$), endoscopic cyst marsupialization ($n = 1$), and a combination of percutaneous and endoscopic sphincterotomy ($n = 1$). On the other hand, 30 patients (52%) underwent open surgery, including transduodenal cyst excision ($n = 12$), followed by pancreatoduodenectomy ($n = 5$). The authors also recommended cyst wall biopsy because the presence of biliary epithelium is believed to be a risk factor for malignant transformation [53, 54]. According to their proposal, cyst resection and sphincteroplasty are sufficient if intestinal mucosa is present, while pancreatoduodenectomy could be considered if biopsy shows the presence of biliary epithelium [52]. Further studies are needed to determine the optimal procedure.

27.11 Type V

Type V CCs, also known as Caroli disease, result from abnormal remodeling of the ductal plate responsive to segmental and communicating saccular or cystic dilatation of the intrahepatic bile ducts [55]. Caroli disease predisposes to biliary stasis, resulting in intrahepatic lithiasis and septic complications, including recurrent episodes of cholangitis, liver abscesses, septicemia, and ultimately secondary biliary cirrhosis. In addition, the risk of developing intrahepatic cholangiocarcinoma in patients with Caroli disease is 100 times higher than in healthy individuals [56]. The dilated hepatic ducts are connected to the common hepatic duct and are prone to infection and stone formation. Percutaneous or endoscopic drainage and stents are used, but are often not effective at preventing recurrent symptoms [57]. Recurrent cholangitis and intrahepatic lithiasis are the most common indications for hepatectomy in patients with Caroli disease. Partial hepatectomy can be an option when the intrahepatic duct dilation is localized and without congenital hepatic fibrosis [58, 59]. Liver transplantation is required, especially in patients with bilobar disease with complications including cirrhosis and portal hypertension [60, 61].

27.12 Minimally Invasive Surgery in Choledochal Cysts

In 1995, Farello et al. first described laparoscopic surgery (LS) for a 6-year-old female with Type I CCs [62]. Since then, minimally invasive surgery has replaced traditional open surgery (OS) for CCs [63]. Liem et al. reported outcomes of laparoscopic surgery for 400 patients with CCs and showed that the rate of postoperative biliary leakage and conversion to open surgery was 2% and 0.5%, respectively [64]. A systematic review including 1767 pediatric patients showed improved postoperative outcomes with LS compared to OS [65].

Additionally, in 2006, Woo et al. performed the first robotic surgery (RS) for a 5-year-old female with Type I CCs [66]. Thereafter, RS has been widely adopted [67–70]. RS can provide a clearer vision of anatomy and more precise operation movement than LS [71]. In that sense, RS is deemed more beneficial than LS, especially in the part of biliary reconstruction. In a comparative study of RS and LS in pediatric patients, the RS group showed significantly shorter operative time, shorter hepaticojejunostomy time, and earlier postoperative recovery than the LS group [72, 73]. Zhang et al. conducted a systematic review and meta-analysis to compare the efficacy of RS and LS in pediatric patients with CCs [74]. There were no differences in the postoperative comparison rates, such as intestinal obstruction or ileus, anastomotic bleeding, anastomotic or bile leakage, and anastomotic stenosis. However, the RS groups showed less intraoperative blood loss and shorter postoperative hospital stay than the LS group. Although comparative studies between RS and LS in adult patients are few, recent studies showed that RS and LS had comparable surgical outcomes [68, 75, 76].

27.13 Remnant Biliary Cancer

The long-term follow-up has revealed that cancer can occur in the remnant bile duct even after excision of CCs. The incidence of remnant biliary tree cancer after excision of CCs has been reported to be 0.3–6.5% [3, 28, 36, 38, 77–80]. Ohashi et al. reported that the cumulative incidence after 15, 20, and 25 years was 1.6%, 3.9%, and 11.3%, respectively [28]. If the primary excision of the dilated bile duct is insufficient, the remnant bile duct has a higher risk of cancer. However, even after the resection of CCs, the remnant bile duct has already been exposed by reflux of pancreatic juice in adult CC patients with PBM. Thus, the malignant potential of the remnant bile duct is deemed present. Therefore, cancer can occur in various locations of the remnant bile duct, including the anastomotic site and the intrahepatic bile duct [79]. Surgical procedures should be determined depending on the location of the cancer.

27.14 Conclusion

Choledochal cysts are rare but pose a significant risk of biliary tract cancer. Early diagnosis and surgical treatment, when appropriate, are crucial to prevent the development of cancers. Tailored surgical management is required based on Todani's classification. Long-term follow-up is necessary because of the risk of cancer development in the remnant bile duct.

References

1. Yamaguchi M. Congenital choledochal cyst: analysis of 1,433 patients in the Japanese literature. Am J Surg. 1980;140(5):653–7.
2. Todani T. Congenital choledochal dilatation: classification, clinical features, and long-term results. J Hepato-Biliary-Pancreat Surg. 1997;4:276–82.
3. Soares KC, Kim Y, Spolverato G, et al. Presentation and clinical outcomes of choledochal cysts in children and adults: a multi-institutional analysis. JAMA Surg. 2015;150(6):577–84.
4. Miyano T, Yamataka A. Choledochal cysts. Curr Opin Pediatr. 1997;9(3):283–8.
5. Olbourne NA. Choledochal cysts. A review of the cystic anomalies of the biliary tree. Ann R Coll Surg Engl. 1975;56(1):26.
6. Howell CG, Templeton JM, Weiner S, Glassman M, Betts JM, Witzleben CL. Antenatal diagnosis and early surgery for choledochal cyst. J Pediatr Surg. 1983;18(4):387–93.
7. Lenriot JP, Gigot JF, Ségol P, et al. Bile duct cysts in adults: a multi-institutional retrospective study. Ann Surg. 1998;228(2):159–66.
8. Ten Hove A, De Meijer VE, Hulscher JBF, De Kleine RHJ. Meta-analysis of risk of developing malignancy in congenital choledochal malformation. Br J Surg. 2018;105(5):482–90.
9. Kamisawa T, Kaneko K, Itoi T, Ando H. Pancreaticobiliary maljunction and congenital biliary dilatation. Lancet Gastroenterol Hepatol. 2017;2(8):610–8. https://doi.org/10.1016/S2468-1253(17)30002-X.
10. Morine Y, Shimada M, Takamatsu H, et al. Clinical features of pancreaticobiliary maljunction: update analysis of 2nd Japan-nationwide survey. J Hepatobiliary Pancreat Sci. 2013;20(5):472–80. https://doi.org/10.1007/s00534-013-0606-2.
11. Kimura K, Ohto M, Ono T, et al. Congenital cystic dilatation of the common bile duct: relationship to anomalous pancreaticobiliary ductal union. Am J Roentgenol. 1977;128(4):571–7.
12. Komi N, Udaka H, Ikeda N, Kashiwagi Y. Congenital dilatation of the biliary tract; new classification and study with particular reference to anomalous arrangement of the pancreaticobiliary ducts. Gastroenterol Jpn. 1977;12:293–304.
13. Komi N, Takehara H, Kunitomo K, Miyoshi Y, Yagi T. Does the type of anomalous arrangement of pancreaticobiliary ducts influence the surgery and prognosis of choledochal cyst? J Pediatr Surg. 1992;27(6):728–31.
14. Hara H, Morita S, Sako S, et al. Relationship between types of common channel and development of biliary tract cancer in pancreaticobiliary maljunction. Hepato-Gastroenterology. 2002;49(44):322–5.
15. Urushihara N, Hamada Y, Kamisawa T, et al. Classification of pancreaticobiliary maljunction and clinical features in children. J Hepatobiliary Pancreat Sci. 2017;24(8):449–55.
16. Vater A. Dissertatio de scirrhis viserum occasione sections viri typanite defunte. Wittenburgae, 4 Pamphlers. 1723;881:22.
17. Alonso-Lej F. Congenital choledochal cyst, with a report of 2, and an analysis of 94, cases. Int Abstr Surg. 1959;108(1):1–30.
18. Todani T, Watanabe Y, Narusue M, Tabuchi K, Okajima K. Congenital bile duct cysts: classification, operative procedures, and review of thirty-seven cases including cancer arising from choledochal cyst. Am J Surg. 1977;134(2):263–9.
19. Todani T. Congenital choledochal dilatation: classification, clinical features, and long-term results. J Hepato-Biliary-Pancreat Surg. 1997;4(3):276–82. https://doi.org/10.1007/BF02489025.
20. Todani T, Watanabe Y, Toki A, Morotomi Y. Classification of congenital biliary cystic disease: special reference to type Ic and IVA cysts with primary ductal stricture. J Hepato-Biliary-Pancreat Surg. 2003;10(5):340–4. https://doi.org/10.1007/s00534-002-0733-7.
21. Ishibashi H, Shimada M, Kamisawa T, et al. Japanese clinical practice guidelines for congenital biliary dilatation. J Hepatobiliary Pancreat Sci. 2017;24(1):1–16. https://doi.org/10.1002/jhbp.415.
22. Lipsett PA, Pitt HA. Surgical treatment of choledochal cysts. J Hepato-Biliary-Pancreat Surg. 2003;10(5):352–9. https://doi.org/10.1007/s00534-002-0797-4.
23. Baison GN, Bonds MM, Helton WS, Kozarek RA. Choledochal cysts: similarities and differences between Asian and Western countries. World J Gastroenterol. 2019;25(26):3334–43. https://doi.org/10.3748/wjg.v25.i26.3334.
24. Irwin ST, Morison JE. Congenital cyst of the common bile-duct containing stones and undergoing cancerous change. Br J Surg. 1944;32(126):319–21.
25. Voyles CR, Smadja C, Shands WC, Blumgart LH. Carcinoma in choledochal cysts: age-related incidence. Arch Surg. 1983;118(8):986–8.
26. Ng WT. Bile duct carcinogenesis after excision of extrahepatic bile ducts in pancreaticobiliary maljunction. Surgery. 2000;128(3):492–4.
27. Imazu M, Iwai N, Tokiwa K, Shimotake T, Kimura O, Ono S. Factors of biliary carcinogenesis in choledochal cysts. Eur J Pediatr Surg. 2001;11(01):24–7.
28. Ohashi T, Wakai T, Kubota M, et al. Risk of subsequent biliary malignancy in patients undergoing cyst excision for congenital choledochal cysts. J Gastroenterol Hepatol. 2013;28(2):243–7.
29. Todani T. Carcinoma arising from the bile duct in choledochal cyst and anomalous arrangement of the pancreaticobiliary ductal union. Tan to Sui (The Biliary Tract and Pancreas). 1985;6:525–35.

30. McConnell AA. Cyst of the common bile-duct. Br J Surg. 1919;7(28):520–4.
31. Todani T, Watanabe Y, Toki A, Urushihara N. Carcinoma related to choledochal cysts with internal drainage operations. Surg Gynecol Obstet. 1987;164(1):61–4.
32. Tocchi A, Mazzoni G, Liotta G, Lepre L, Cassini D, Miccini M. Late development of bile duct cancer in patients who had biliary-enteric drainage for benign disease: a follow-up study of more than 1,000 patients. Ann Surg. 2001;234(2):210.
33. Visser BC, Suh I, Way LW, Kang SM. Congenital choledochal cysts in adults. Arch Surg. 2004;139(8):855–62.
34. Kasai M, Asakura Y, Taira Y. Surgical treatment of choledochal cyst. Ann Surg. 1970;172(5):844.
35. Ishida M, Tsuchida Y, Saito S, Hori T. Primary excision of choledochal cysts. Surgery. 1970;68(5):884–8.
36. Takeshita N, Ota T, Yamamoto M. Forty-year experience with flow-diversion surgery for patients with congenital choledochal cysts with pancreaticobiliary maljunction at a single institution. Ann Surg. 2011;254(6):1050–3.
37. Ando H, Kaneko K, Ito T, et al. Complete excision of the intrapancreatic portion of choledochal cysts. J Am Coll Surg. 1996;183(4):317–21.
38. Watanabe Y, Toki A, Todani T. Bile duct cancer developed after cyst excision for choledochal cyst. J Hepato-Biliary-Pancreat Surg. 1999;6:207–12. https://doi.org/10.1007/s005340050108.
39. Todani T, Watanabe Y, Toki A, Urushihara N, Sato Y. Reoperation for congenital choledochal cyst. Ann Surg. 1988;207(2):142–7. https://doi.org/10.1097/00000658-198802000-00005.
40. Todani T, Watanabe Y, Fujii T, Toki A, Uemura S, Koike Y. Congenital choledochal cyst with intrahepatic involvement. Arch Surg. 1984;119(9):1038–43.
41. Ando H, Ito T, Kaneko K, Seo T. Congenital stenosis of the intrahepatic bile duct associated with choledochal cysts. J Am Coll Surg. 1995;181(5):426–30.
42. Ando H, Kaneko K, Ito F, Seo T, Ito T. Operative treatment of congenital stenoses of the intrahepatic bile ducts in patients with choledochal cysts. Am J Surg. 1997;173(6):491–4.
43. Pal K, Singh VP, Mitra DK. Partial hepatectomy and total cyst excision is curative for localized type IV-A biliary duct cysts -report of four cases and review of management. Eur J Pediatr Surg. 2009;19(3):148–52. https://doi.org/10.1055/s-0029-1202365.
44. Kawarada Y, Das BC, Tabata M, Isaji S. Surgical treatment of type IV choledochal cysts. J Hepato-Biliary-Pancreat Surg. 2009;16(5):684–7. https://doi.org/10.1007/s00534-009-0052-3.
45. Zheng X, Gu W, Xia H, et al. Surgical treatment of type IV-A choledochal cyst in a single institution: children vs. adults. J Pediatr Surg. 2013;48(10):2061–6. https://doi.org/10.1016/j.jpedsurg.2013.05.022.
46. Dong JH, Yang SZ, Xia HT, et al. Aggressive hepatectomy for the curative treatment of bilobar involvement of type IV-A bile duct cyst. Ann Surg. 2013;258(1):122–8. https://doi.org/10.1097/SLA.0b013e318285769e.
47. He XD, Wang L, Liu W, et al. The risk of carcinogenesis in congenital choledochal cyst patients: an analysis of 214 cases. Ann Hepatol. 2014;13(6):819–26.
48. Brown ZJ, Baghdadi A, Kamel I, Labiner HE, Hewitt DB, Pawlik TM. Diagnosis and management of choledochal cysts. HPB. 2023;25(1):14–25. https://doi.org/10.1016/j.hpb.2022.09.010.
49. Ouaïssi M, Kianmanesh R, Belghiti J, et al. Todani type II congenital bile duct cyst: European multicenter study of the French surgical association and literature review. Ann Surg. 2015;262(1):130–8. https://doi.org/10.1097/SLA.0000000000000761.
50. Ohtsuka T, Inoue K, Ohuchida J, et al. Carcinoma arising in choledochocele. Endoscopy. 2001;33(7):614–9. https://doi.org/10.1055/s-2001-15324.
51. Horaguchi J, Fujita N, Kobayashi G, Noda Y, Ito K, Takasawa O. Clinical study of choledochocele: is it a risk factor for biliary malignancies? J Gastroenterol. 2005;40(4):396–401. https://doi.org/10.1007/s00535-005-1554-7.
52. Lobeck IN, Dupree P, Falcone RA, et al. The presentation and management of choledochocele (type III choledochal cyst): a 40-year systematic review of the literature. J Pediatr Surg. 2017;52(4):644–9. https://doi.org/10.1016/j.jpedsurg.2016.10.008.
53. Law R, Topazian M. Diagnosis and treatment of choledochoceles. Clin Gastroenterol Hepatol. 2014;12(2):196–203. https://doi.org/10.1016/j.cgh.2013.04.037.
54. Ozawa K, Yamada T, Matumoto Y, Tobe R. Carcinoma arising in a choledochocele. Cancer. 1980;45(1):195–7. https://doi.org/10.1002/1097-0142(19800101)45:1<195::AID-CNCR2820450131>3.0.CO;2-S.
55. Desmet VJ. Congenital diseases of intrahepatic bile ducts: variations on the theme “ductal plate malformation”. Hepatology. 1992;16(4):1069–83. https://doi.org/10.1002/hep.1840160434.
56. Dayton MT, Longmire WP, Angeles L, Ronald Tompkins CK. Carob’s disease: a premalignant condition? Am J Surg. 1983;145(1):41–8. https://doi.org/10.1016/0002-9610(83)90164-2.
57. Mabrut JY, Kianmanesh R, Nuzzo G, et al. Surgical management of congenital intrahepatic bile duct dilatation, caroli’s disease and syndrome: long-term results of the french association of surgery multicenter study. Ann Surg. 2013;258(5):713–21. https://doi.org/10.1097/SLA.0000000000000269.
58. Kassahun WT, Kahn T, Wittekind C, et al. Caroli’s disease: liver resection and liver transplantation. Experience in 33 patients. Surgery. 2005;138(5):888–98. https://doi.org/10.1016/j.surg.2005.05.002.
59. Mabrut JY, Partensky C, Jaeck D, et al. Congenital intrahepatic bile duct dilatation is a potentially curable disease: long-term results of a multi-institutional study. Ann Surg. 2007;246(2):236–45. https://doi.org/10.1097/SLA.0b013e3180f61abf.

60. Habib S, Shakil O, Couto OF, et al. Caroli's disease and orthotopic liver transplantation. Liver Transpl. 2006;12(3):416–21. https://doi.org/10.1002/lt.20719.
61. Harring TR, Nguyen NTT, Liu H, Goss JA, O'Mahony CA. Caroli disease patients have excellent survival after liver transplant. J Surg Res. 2012;177(2):365–72. https://doi.org/10.1016/j.jss.2012.04.022.
62. Farello GA, Cerofolini A, Rebonato M, Bergamaschi G, Ferrari C, Chiappetta A. Congenital choledochal cyst: video-guided laparoscopic treatment. Surg Laparosc Endosc. 1995;5(5):354–8.
63. Shen HJ, Xu M, Zhu HY, et al. Laparoscopic versus open surgery in children with choledochal cysts: a meta-analysis. Pediatr Surg Int. 2015;31(6):529–34. https://doi.org/10.1007/s00383-015-3705-0.
64. Liem NT, Pham HD, Dung LA, Son TN, Vu HM. Early and intermediate outcomes of laparoscopic surgery for choledochal cysts with 400 patients. J Laparoendosc Adv Surg Tech A. 2012;22(6):599–603. https://doi.org/10.1089/lap.2012.0018.
65. Sun R, Zhao N, Zhao K, et al. Comparison of efficacy and safety of laparoscopic excision and open operation in children with choledochal cysts: a systematic review and update meta-analysis. PLoS One. 2020;15(9):e0239857.
66. Woo R, Le D, Albanese CT, Kim SS. Robot-assisted laparoscopic resection of a type I choledochal cyst in a child. J Laparoendosc Adv Surg Tech A. 2006;16(2):179–83. https://doi.org/10.1089/lap.2006.16.179.
67. Nazki S, Kanojia RP, Bawa M, et al. Robotic excision of choledochal cyst with hepaticoduodenostomy (HD): report of HD technique, initial experience, and early outcome. Eur J Pediatr Surg. 2021;31(3):286–91. https://doi.org/10.1055/s-0040-1713933.
68. Morikawa T, Ohtsuka H, Takadate T, et al. Laparoscopic and robot-assisted surgery for adult congenital biliary dilatation achieves favorable short-term outcomes without increasing the risk of late complications. Surg Today. 2022;52(7):1039–47. https://doi.org/10.1007/s00595-021-02438-8.
69. Jin Y, Zhang S, Cai D, et al. Robot-assisted resection of choledochal cyst in children. Front Pediatr. 2023;11:1162236. https://doi.org/10.3389/fped.2023.1162236.
70. Nguyen SH, Abella M, Gutierrez JV, et al. Robotic surgery for pediatric choledochal cysts: an American case series and literature review. J Surg Res. 2023;291:473–9. https://doi.org/10.1016/j.jss.2023.06.034.
71. Faust RA. Paradigm shift in pediatric surgery: invasion of the robots. Clin Pediatr (Phila). 2008;47(2):122–7. https://doi.org/10.1177/0009922807307152.
72. Koga H, Murakami H, Ochi T, Miyano G, Lane GJ, Yamataka A. Comparison of robotic versus laparoscopic hepaticojejunostomy for choledochal cyst in children: a first report. Pediatr Surg Int. 2019;35(12):1421–5. https://doi.org/10.1007/s00383-019-04565-3.
73. Xie X, Li K, Wang J, Wang C, Xiang B. Comparison of pediatric choledochal cyst excisions with open procedures, laparoscopic procedures and robot-assisted procedures: a retrospective study. Surg Endosc. 2020;34(7):3223–31. https://doi.org/10.1007/s00464-020-07560-1.
74. Zhang MX, Chi SQ, Cao GQ, Tang JF, Tang ST. Comparison of efficacy and safety of robotic surgery and laparoscopic surgery for choledochal cyst in children: a systematic review and proportional meta-analysis. Surg Endosc. 2023;37(1):31–47. https://doi.org/10.1007/s00464-022-09442-0.
75. Lee H, Kwon W, Han Y, Kim JR, Kim SW, Jang JY. Comparison of surgical outcomes of intracorporeal hepaticojejunostomy in the excision of choledochal cysts using laparoscopic versus robot techniques. Ann Surg Treat Res. 2018;94(4):190–5. https://doi.org/10.4174/astr.2018.94.4.190.
76. Han J, Lee JH, Park Y, et al. Comparison of surgical outcomes of laparoscopic and robotic surgery in adult choledochal cysts. J Laparoendosc Adv Surg Tech A. 2023;34(1):55–60. https://doi.org/10.1089/lap.2023.0376.
77. Ishibashi T, Kasahara K, Yasuda Y, Nagai H, Makino S, Kanazawa K. Malignant change in the biliary tract after excision of choledochal cyst. Br J Surg. 1997;84(12):1687–91. https://doi.org/10.1002/bjs.1800841212.
78. Kobayashi S, Asano T, Yamasaki M, Kenmochi T, Nakagohri T, Ochiai T. Risk of bile duct carcinogenesis after excision of extrahepatic bile ducts in pancreaticobiliary maljunction. Surgery. 1999;126(5):939–44. https://doi.org/10.1016/s0039-6060(99)70036-x.
79. Ikegame K, Takano A, Watanabe H, et al. Biliary cancer developed after the reparative surgery for congenital choledochal cyst: a case report and review of the literature. Int Cancer Conf J. 2017;6(2):43–9. https://doi.org/10.1007/s13691-016-0270-x.
80. Mizuguchi Y, Nakamura Y, Uchida E. Subsequent biliary cancer originating from remnant intrapancreatic bile ducts after cyst excision: a literature review. Surg Today. 2017;47(6):660–7. https://doi.org/10.1007/s00595-016-1366-9.

Pregnancy and Liver Diseases

28

Aiste Gulla, Diana Ramasauskaite,
and Babak Sarani

28.1 Incidence

Worldwide, about 3–5% of pregnant women face liver function abnormalities. Liver diseases in pregnancy are defined as hepatic conditions with a prevalence of less than 1 in 10,000 pregnancies. These conditions pose diagnostic and therapeutic dilemmas because their presentation often mimics common obstetric complications or physiologic changes of pregnancy. They can be broadly classified into genetic and metabolic disorders (e.g., Wilson disease, hereditary hemorrhagic telangiectasia), vascular disorders (e.g., Budd-Chiari syndrome, portal vein thrombosis), autoimmune conditions (e.g., autoimmune hepatitis, primary biliary cholangitis), and neoplastic conditions (e.g., hepatic adenomatosis). Furthermore, there is often significant overlap with pregnancy-specific liver diseases such as acute fatty liver of pregnancy (AFLP) and hemolysis, elevated liver enzymes, and low platelets (HELLP) syndrome, complicating the clinical picture. It can be associated with significant maternal and fetal morbidity and mortality. The International Federation of Gynecology and Obstetrics guideline aims to use the latest evidence to inform practice relevant to a global population [9]. Liver diseases in pregnancy can be divided into two main categories: gestational liver disorders and acute and chronic liver disorders occurring co-incidentally in pregnancy. Both are associated with increased rates of maternal and fetal morbidity and mortality. Gestational liver disorders affect 3% of the pregnant population [10].

28.2 Epidemiology and Prevalence

The epidemiology of these conditions varies. Wilson disease affects approximately 1 in 30,000 live births, frequently presenting in females during their childbearing years. Budd-Chiari syndrome has an incidence of approximately 1 in 100,000 pregnancies; however, the hypercoagulable state of pregnancy increases the risk of development five- to tenfold. Hereditary hemorrhagic telangiectasia (HHT) affects 1 in 5000 births, with hepatic involvement occurring in

A. Gulla (✉)
Department of Surgery, George Washington University, School of Medicine and Health Sciences, Washington, DC, USA

Clinic of Surgery, Gastroenterology and Nephrourology, Institute of Clinical Medicine, Faculty of Medicine, Vilnius, Lithuania
e-mail: a.gulla@gwu.edu

D. Ramasauskaite
Department of Obstetrics and Gynecology, Institute of Clinical Medicine, Faculty of Medicine, Vilnius University, Vilnius, Lithuania
e-mail: diana.ramasauskaite@mf.vu.lt

B. Sarani
Department of Surgery, The George Washington University Hospital, Washington, DC, USA

T. Hackert, A. Gulla (eds.), *Rare Liver and Biliary Tract Diseases*,
https://doi.org/10.1007/978-3-032-15076-9_28

roughly 30% of patients; symptoms often manifest or worsen during pregnancy due to hemodynamic stress. Autoimmune hepatitis affects 1 in 10,000 pregnancies and is notable for a high risk of postpartum flares (30–50%). Primary biliary cholangitis is typically a disease of older women but can occur in childbearing age. Hepatic adenomatosis is extremely rare, yet the risk of adenoma rupture during pregnancy is significant, estimated at 20–40%.

28.3 Pathophysiological Effects of Pregnancy

Pregnancy induces profound physiological changes that can destabilize compensated liver disease. Hemodynamically, cardiac output increases by 40–50%, and blood volume expands, placing stress on vascular malformations and collateral circulation. Hormonal surges in estrogen and progesterone affect hepatic metabolism and vascular tone, potentially promoting the growth of hepatic adenomas. The systemic hypercoagulable state, characterized by increased clotting factors and decreased protein S, heightens the risk for thrombotic events like Budd-Chiari syndrome. Immunologically, the shift toward Th2 dominance (relative immunosuppression) helps prevent fetal rejection but can alter the course of autoimmune diseases. Mechanically, the gravid uterus compresses the inferior vena cava and increases portal pressure, further complicating portal hypertension. Failure to recognize these rare conditions contributes to high maternal mortality rates, ranging from 5% to 30% depending on the specific etiology and severity. Fetal mortality is similarly high, often exceeding 20–40%. Early diagnosis and prompt intervention are paramount to survival. Management should be centralized at specialized hepatology and transplant centers where rapid access to advanced diagnostics, interventional radiology, and liver transplantation is available. A multidisciplinary team approach is essential to navigate the complex interplay between maternal well-being and fetal safety.

28.4 Wilson Disease and Pregnancy

Wilson disease is an autosomal recessive disorder caused by mutations in the ATP7B gene, leading to impaired biliary excretion of copper. This results in the accumulation of copper in the liver, brain, and cornea. Copper toxicity causes direct hepatocyte necrosis and chronic inflammation, eventually leading to cirrhosis. In severe cases, massive release of copper into the bloodstream can cause fulminant Wilson disease, characterized by acute liver failure and Coombs-negative hemolytic anemia. *Pregnancy Considerations and Outcomes*: Pregnancy is generally safe for women with Wilson disease if the condition is well controlled on maintenance therapy. It is imperative that chelation therapy (using agents such as penicillamine, trientine, or zinc) be continued throughout pregnancy. Discontinuation of therapy poses a 10–15% risk of acute liver failure. While there is a theoretical teratogenic risk with penicillamine, the benefits of preventing maternal liver failure far outweigh the risks. Maternal outcomes are favorable with treatment, achieving a 90–95% success rate; conversely, untreated patients face a 30–50% risk of acute liver failure. Fetal outcomes are also good with continued therapy, showing 80–90% live birth rates. *Risk of Acute Liver Failure*: Acute liver failure may occur if the diagnosis is missed or if treatment is interrupted. Clinical presentation includes jaundice, coagulopathy, encephalopathy, and hemolytic anemia. Diagnostic features often include low serum ceruloplasmin, elevated free serum copper, Coombs-negative hemolysis, and an AST/ALT ratio of less than 2 (often with relatively low alkaline phosphatase). The King's College Criteria and the Revised Wilson Index are useful for prognosis; a high score predicts poor survival without transplantation. Without transplantation, maternal mortality in acute failure approaches 70–90%. *Liver Transplantation*: Acute liver failure in Wilson disease is an indication for emergency liver transplantation. The timing of the procedure depends on fetal viability; if the fetus is viable (>28–32 weeks), delivery via cesarean section is typically performed first, followed immediately by transplantation. In pre-viable pregnancies with maternal deterioration, a combined procedure or transplant with the fetus in situ may be considered. Technical considerations include managing portal hypertension and correcting profound coagulopathy. Outcomes for transplantation in this setting are respectable, with 1-year maternal survival rates of 60–75% and fetal survival rates of 50–70% for viable gestations. Pregnancy after transplantation is generally successful (75–80% live birth rate) if conception occurs 1–2 years post-transplant. Post-transplant management involves lifelong immunosuppression. Tacrolimus and azathioprine are generally considered safe during pregnancy. Patients require continued monitoring for copper metabolism issues, although the transplanted liver corrects the metabolic defect. Genetic counseling is essential, as there is a 25% risk of the offspring being affected if the partner is a carrier.

28.5 Budd-Chiari Syndrome and Pregnancy

Budd-Chiari syndrome results from hepatic venous outflow obstruction, leading to sinusoidal congestion, ischemic hepatocyte necrosis, and eventual fibrosis or cirrhosis. Obstruction can occur at the level of the microscopic hepatic veins (primary) or the inferior vena cava (secondary). Underlying causes include hypercoagulable states, myeloproliferative disorders, paroxysmal nocturnal hemoglobinuria, and use of oral contraceptives. A hallmark anatomical feature is hypertrophy of the caudate lobe, which often preserves direct venous drainage into the inferior vena cava. Pregnancy is a major risk factor, increasing the likelihood of Budd-Chiari syndrome by five- to tenfold due to the physiological hypercoagulable state. Approximately 20–30% of cases present during pregnancy, while 40–50% present in the early postpartum period. Common risk factors include inherited thrombophilias such as Factor V Leiden and the prothrombin G20210A mutation, as well as JAK2 mutations. Presentation typically peaks in the third trimester or immediately postpartum. The clinical presentation varies by acuity. Acute cases (3 months) present with established cirrhosis, portal hypertension, and variceal bleeding. The classic triad of hepatomegaly, ascites, and abdominal pain is present in 60–70% of patients. Doppler ultrasound is the first-line diagnostic modality, with a sensitivity of 75–90%. It typically reveals absent or reversed flow in the hepatic veins, IVC thrombosis, and caudate lobe enlargement. CT with contrast shows a characteristic "flip-flop" pattern of central hypodensity with peripheral enhancement but is generally avoided in pregnancy due to radiation unless necessary. MRI is the gold standard for diagnosis in pregnancy, providing detailed visualization of thrombosis and parenchymal changes without ionizing radiation; gadolinium should be avoided.

28.6 Hereditary Hemorrhagic Telangiectasia with Hepatic Arteriovenous Malformations

Hereditary hemorrhagic telangiectasia (HHT) is an autosomal dominant disorder caused by mutations in ENG (HHT1), ACVRL1 (HHT2), or SMAD4. These mutations lead to defective TGF-beta signaling in the vascular endothelium, resulting in arteriovenous malformations (AVMs) that lack capillary beds. In the liver, this manifests as direct shunting between the hepatic artery and hepatic vein, hepatic artery and portal vein, or portal vein and hepatic vein. Hepatic AVMs are present in 30–80% of HHT patients but are symptomatic in only 8–15% prior to pregnancy. Symptoms often emerge or worsen during pregnancy, affecting 30–50% of previously asymptomatic women. The three main clinical patterns are high-output cardiac failure (60%), portal hypertension (30%), and biliary ischemia/cholangiopathy (10%). The 40–50% increase in cardiac output and blood volume during pregnancy significantly exacerbates shunting through AVMs. Additionally, hormonal changes may promote vascular dilation. Consequently, the incidence of high-output heart failure increases tenfold during pregnancy in women with significant hepatic involvement. High-output cardiac failure presents with dyspnea, tachycardia, bounding pulses, and peripheral edema. Echocardiography typically reveals a hyperdynamic circulation. Portal hypertension manifests as ascites, splenomegaly, and variceal bleeding. Biliary ischemia can present with cholestatic jaundice and biliary strictures, mimicking intrahepatic cholestasis of pregnancy. Diagnosis is based on the Curaçao clinical criteria and confirmed by imaging. Doppler ultrasound is the initial imaging of choice, showing enlarged hepatic arteries and hypervascularity. MRI is preferred in pregnancy for detailed assessment of hepatic morphology and AVMs. Genetic testing confirms the diagnosis and informs risk for the offspring (50% risk). Management of high-output heart failure includes diuretics (furosemide is safe) and beta-blockers (labetalol is preferred). ACE inhibitors and ARBs are contraindicated due to teratogenicity. Portal hypertension is managed with beta-blockers and endoscopic band ligation for bleeding varices. Supportive care includes iron supplementation for chronic bleeding. Transcatheter embolization is generally avoided or used only as a temporizing measure due to high recurrence rates (50–70%) and the risk of extensive liver infarction. Hepatic artery ligation is a historical procedure with high mortality and necrosis risk, now rarely performed. Bevacizumab (anti-VEGF) has shown promise in reducing AVMs but is limited in pregnancy due to potential anti-angiogenic effects on the fetus. *Liver Transplantation*: Liver transplantation is the only curative treatment for hepatic AVMs and is indicated for refractory high-output heart failure, progressive portal hypertension, or biliary ischemia. If indicated during pregnancy, delivery of a viable fetus (>28–32 weeks) usually precedes transplant. Maternal survival at 1 year is 70–85%, with fetal survival ranging from 50% to 70%. Technical considerations include managing extensive vascular collaterals and the potential need for cardiopulmonary bypass.

28.7 Autoimmune Hepatitis and Primary Biliary Cholangitis

Autoimmune hepatitis (AIH) is a chronic inflammatory liver disease characterized by T cell–mediated destruction of hepatocytes. It is associated with autoantibodies such as ANA, anti-smooth muscle antibodies (Type 1), and anti-LKM1 (Type 2). The disease primarily affects women and can progress to fibrosis and cirrhosis. Primary biliary cholangitis (PBC) is characterized by the immune-mediated destruction of small intrahepatic bile ducts, leading to cholestasis and cirrhosis. It is strongly associated with anti-mitochondrial antibodies (AMAs). While more common in older women, it can present during childbearing years. Pregnancy often induces a state of relative immunosuppression, which can stabilize or improve AIH in 50–60% of patients. However, 20–30% may experience flares. Postpartum, the reconstitution of the immune system leads to a high risk of AIH flare (30–50%) within the first 6 months. PBC is typically stable during pregnancy, though pruritus may worsen. Outcomes correlate with the degree of liver fibrosis. In non-cirrhotic patients, live birth rates are 80–85%. In patients with compensated cirrhosis, live birth rates drop to 65–75%, with higher rates of preterm birth (40–50%) and IUGR. Pregnancy is contraindicated in decompensated cirrhosis due to high maternal mortality (15–30%) and fetal loss (40–60%). Prednisone and azathioprine are the mainstays of treatment and are considered safe for use during pregnancy. Mycophenolate mofetil is teratogenic and must be switched to azathioprine prior to conception. Tacrolimus is generally safe. Treatment should never be stopped due to the high risk of flare and subsequent acute liver failure. For PBC, ursodeoxycholic acid is safe and should be continued. Liver function tests should be monitored every 4–6 weeks, or more frequently if a flare is suspected. Flares are managed by increasing prednisone doses or adding azathioprine. Severe flares involving coagulopathy or encephalopathy require hospitalization and may necessitate delivery. Patients with cirrhosis should be screened for varices prior to conception. During pregnancy, non-selective beta-blockers are safe. Acute variceal bleeding is managed with endoscopic variceal ligation and octreotide. Vaginal delivery is preferred unless obstetric indications for cesarean section exist; assisted second stage labor helps avoid excessive Valsalva maneuvers. Emergency liver transplantation in pregnancy is indicated for acute liver failure due to severe flare, decompensated cirrhosis with multi-organ failure, or refractory variceal bleeding. Maternal survival is 60–75% at 1 year. The timing strategy involves delivering a viable fetus prior to transplant when possible. Pregnancy after liver transplantation for autoimmune disease is feasible 1–2 years post-transplant if graft function is stable. Medication adjustments (switching MMF to azathioprine) should occur pre-conception. Disease recurrence in the graft is possible (10–30% for AIH, 20–40% for PBC) but does not typically worsen with pregnancy. Live birth rates are 70–75%, with increased risks of preeclampsia (20–30%) and preterm birth.

28.8 Hepatic Adenomatosis

Hepatic adenomatosis is defined by the presence of multiple (>10) hepatic adenomas. These are benign hepatocellular tumors associated with oral contraceptive use and certain metabolic conditions. Subtypes include inflammatory, HNF1-alpha inactivated, and beta-catenin activated adenomas, the latter having higher malignant potential. Adenomas are hormone-sensitive, and the high levels of estrogen and progesterone in pregnancy promote growth. Adenomas often increase in size by 20–50%. The risk of rupture is significant, particularly for lesions >5 cm (10–20% risk) and >10 cm (20–40% risk). Rupture most commonly occurs in the third trimester (50%) or postpartum (30%). Unruptured adenomas are often asymptomatic. Rupture presents dramatically with sudden severe RUQ pain, hemodynamic instability, and signs of hemoperitoneum. Maternal mortality from rupture has historically been 10–20% but has decreased to 2–5% with modern management. Diagnosis relies on imaging. Ultrasound shows hyperechoic masses. MRI (without gadolinium) is useful for characterizing lesions. CT is avoided unless rupture is suspected, in which case it reveals hypervascular lesions with hemorrhage. Biopsy is generally avoided due to bleeding risk. Pregnancy adenomas >5 cm should ideally be resected pre-conception. If discovered during pregnancy, close surveillance with ultrasound every 4–6 weeks is recommended. For large lesions, early delivery at 34–36 weeks may be considered to avoid the peak rupture risk period, followed by postpartum resection. Adenoma rupture is a surgical emergency. Initial management involves aggressive resuscitation and activation of massive transfusion protocols. Surgical options include damage control (packing, Pringle maneuver) for unstable patients or definitive resection (segmentectomy/lobectomy) for stable patients. If the fetus is viable, cesarean section is often performed concurrently or immediately prior to hepatic resection. Selective hepatic artery embolization is an effective alternative to surgery for hemodynamically stable patients or as a bridge to surgery. It controls bleeding with a 70–80% success rate. Radiation exposure is a consideration but is justified by the life-threatening nature of the condition. Maternal mortality with rupture is 2–5% with prompt intervention. Fetal survival after rupture is 60–75%. Postpartum, patients require imaging surveillance and elective resection of remaining large adenomas. Estrogen-containing contraception is contraindicated.

28.9 Portal and Hepatic Artery Thrombosis

The risk of thrombosis is elevated five- to tenfold in pregnancy. Portal vein thrombosis (PVT) occurs in 1 in 50,000–100,000 pregnancies. Hepatic artery thrombosis (HAT) is extremely rare outside of transplantation. Risk factors include thrombophilias, myeloproliferative disorders, and infection. *Pathophysiology*: Acute PVT causes sudden occlusion, leading to intestinal congestion and potential mesenteric ischemia. Chronic PVT leads to collateral formation (cavernoma) and portal hypertension. HAT compromises arterial supply, potentially causing liver infarction and biliary ischemia. Acute PVT presents with sudden abdominal pain, nausea, and fever. Chronic PVT may present with complications of portal hypertension like variceal bleeding. Acute HAT presents with RUQ pain and massive transaminase elevation, potentially progressing to fulminant failure. Doppler ultrasound is the first-line diagnostic tool. MR angiography is preferred in pregnancy for detailed vascular mapping. Labs typically show thrombophilia markers. Immediate anticoagulation with LMWH or unfractionated heparin is required for acute thrombosis. Therapy should continue for at least 6 months or lifelong if underlying disorders persist. Monitoring with anti-Xa levels is recommended for LMWH.

Surgical thrombectomy is indicated for acute PVT with mesenteric ischemia. Percutaneous mechanical thrombectomy via transjugular approach is an option but has variable success rates. TIPS is indicated for chronic PVT with symptomatic portal hypertension or refractory bleeding. It is technically challenging in cavernous transformation but has a success rate of 60–80%. Liver transplantation is indicated for acute liver failure from HAT or massive PVT with hepatic necrosis. Maternal survival is 50–70% in the acute setting. With anticoagulation, maternal mortality for acute PVT is <5%, and live birth rates are 70–80%. Acute HAT carries higher mortality (50–70%) without transplant.

28.10 Clinical Presentation (Summary Table 28.1)

Failure to recognize these rare conditions contributes to high maternal mortality rates, ranging from 5% to 30% depending on the specific etiology and severity. Fetal mortality is similarly high, often exceeding 20–40%. Early diagnosis and prompt intervention are paramount to survival. Management should be centralized at specialized hepatology and transplant centers where rapid access to advanced diagnostics, interventional radiology, and liver transplantation is available. A multidisciplinary team approach is essential to navigate the complex interplay between maternal well-being and fetal safety.

Technically, the gravid uterus limits surgical exposure and alters abdominal anatomy. Fetal considerations, such as continuous monitoring and the avoidance of teratogenic medications or excessive radiation, complicate perioperative care. Hemodynamic management must account for aortocaval compression and expanded blood volume. Coagulation management is difficult due to the baseline hypercoagulability of pregnancy conflicting with disease-related coagulopathy. Anesthetic management requires careful planning for aspiration risk and difficult airways. Finally, decision-making regarding the timing of delivery versus surgery versus combined procedures requires careful coordination between surgical and obstetric teams.

Table 28.1 Comparison of rare liver diseases in pregnancy

Clinical reference guide for obstetric and surgical management

Disease entity	Clinical features	Key laboratory findings	Timing of onset	Maternal mortality	Fetal outcomes	Definitive treatment	Distinguishing features
Acute fatty liver of pregnancy (AFLP)	Nausea/vomiting (75%), jaundice (90%), polydipsia/ polyuria, epigastric pain, encephalopathy	*Swansea criteria*: ↑ AST/ALT (>3×), ↑ Bili, ↑ Uric acid, hypoglycemia, ↑ WBC, coagulopathy (↑ PT/INR)	Third trimester (30–38 weeks)	1–18% (high)	Stillbirth, fetal distress, preterm birth	*Immediate delivery* (within 24 h) ICU support, glucose, coagulopathy correction	Hypoglycemia, elevated uric acid, microvesicular steatosis on biopsy (rarely needed)
HELLP syndrome	RUQ/epigastric pain, hypertension, edema, malaise, nausea	*Hemolysis*: ↑ LDH, Schistocytes *EL*: AST/ALT >70 IU/L *LP*: Platelets <100k	Third trimester (>27 weeks) or postpartum	1–5%	IUGR, placental abruption, perinatal death (7–20%)	Delivery (steroids if <34w), $MgSO_4$, BP control	Strong association with preeclampsia; rapid clinical deterioration
Hepatic rupture/ hematoma	Sudden severe RUQ pain (often radiating to shoulder), hemodynamic shock, abdominal distension	Acute drop in hemoglobin/Hct Labs consistent with HELLP syndrome	Late third trimester or <48 h postpartum	~39% (surgical emergency)	High perinatal mortality (up to 60%)	*Damage control surgery* (packing), hepatic artery embolization, transfusion	Catastrophic hemodynamic collapse in setting of HELLP/ preeclampsia
Budd-Chiari syndrome	Abdominal pain, hepatomegaly, ascites (rapid onset), lower limb edema	Mild-moderate ↑ AST/ ALT Imaging: hepatic vein thrombosis/occlusion (Doppler/MRI)	Any trimester or postpartum	Low (with tx)	Preterm birth, fetal loss (if unmanaged)	LMWH anticoagulation TIPS or thrombolysis (if severe)	Caudate lobe hypertrophy on imaging; absence of flow in hepatic veins
Intrahepatic cholestasis (ICP)	Intense pruritus (palms/soles), worse at night. No primary rash. Dark urine	*Total bile acids >10 μmol/L* (severe >40) Mild ↑ ALT/AST (2–10×)	Late second/ third trimester	~0%	Spontaneous preterm birth, meconium staining, stillbirth (correlated with bile acid levels)	UDCA (10–15 mg/ kg) Delivery at 37–38 weeks (earlier if severe)	Pruritus without skin rash; resolves rapidly postpartum
Hyperemesis Gravidarum	Intractable nausea/ vomiting, >5% weight loss, dehydration, ketosis	Mild ↑ ALT/AST (transient) Ketonuria Hypokalemia	First trimester (4–12 weeks)	~0%	SGA/low birth weight (if severe/ prolonged)	IV fluids, thiamine, antiemetics, nutritional support	Early onset; resolves by 20 weeks; exclusion of other causes

(continued)

Table 28.1 (continued)

Clinical reference guide for obstetric and surgical management

Disease entity	Clinical features	Key laboratory findings	Timing of onset	Maternal mortality	Fetal outcomes	Definitive treatment	Distinguishing features
Wilson disease	Jaundice, hepatic failure (if treatment stopped), neuro/psych symptoms	↓ Ceruloplasmin, ↑ Urinary copper, coombs-neg hemolytic anemia	Pre-existing	Variable (risk of acute failure)	Miscarriage risk (if untreated)	*Continue chelation*: zinc or dose-reduced D-penicillamine/ trientine	Kayser-Fleischer rings; history of copper metabolism disorder
Hereditary hemorrhagic telangiectasia	Dyspnea, high-output heart failure, epistaxis, RUQ pain (biliary ischemia)	↑ ALP/GGT (cholestatic) Imaging: Hepatic AVMs, telangiectasias	Pre-existing (worsens in pregnancy)	1% (risk of hemorrhage)	IUGR (due to vascular shunting)	Supportive (heart failure) Embolization/LT (rare/refractory)	Systemic AVMs, epistaxis history, hyperdynamic circulation
Primary biliary cholangitis (PBC)	Fatigue, pruritus May flare postpartum	Cholestatic (↑ ALP/ GGT) *AMA positive*. ↑ IgM	Pre-existing	Low	Increased risk of preterm birth & adverse outcomes	UDCA (safe) Treat pruritus (cholestyramine/ rifampicin)	Autoimmune markers (AMA); florid duct lesion on histology
Primary sclerosing cholangitis (PSC)	Pruritus, fatigue, fever (cholangitis)	Cholestatic (↑ ALP) MRCP: Multifocal strictures ("beading")	Pre-existing	Low	Preterm birth	UDCA Antibiotics for cholangitis ERCP for dominant strictures	Strong association with IBD (ulcerative colitis); biliary strictures

Abbreviations & Key Definitions: *AFLP* acute fatty liver of pregnancy, *ALT/AST* alanine/aspartate aminotransferase, *ALP* alkaline phosphatase, *AMA* antimitochondrial antibody, *AVM* arteriovenous malformation, *DIC* disseminated intravascular coagulation, *ERCP* endoscopic retrograde cholangiopancreatography, *GGT* gamma-glutamyl transferase, *HELLP* hemolysis, elevated liver enzymes low platelets, *HF* heart failure, *IBD* inflammatory bowel disease, *ICP* intrahepatic cholestasis of pregnancy, *INR* international normalized ratio, *IUGR* intrauterine growth restriction, *LDH* lactate dehydrogenase, *LMWH* low molecular weight heparin, *LT* liver transplantation, $MgSO_4$ magnesium sulfate, *MRCP* magnetic resonance cholangiopancreatography, *PT* prothrombin time, *RUQ* right upper quadrant, *SGA* small for gestational age, *Swansea Criteria* diagnostic tool for AFLP (req. ≥6 criteria), *TIPS* transjugular intrahepatic portosystemic shunt, *UDCA* ursodeoxycholic acid, *WBC* white blood cell count, *MELD* model for end-stage liver disease

28.11 Medical Management Anticoagulation and Pregnancy

Low molecular weight heparin (LMWH) or unfractionated heparin is safe during pregnancy and should be initiated immediately. Lifelong anticoagulation is typically required. Ascites is managed with diuretics (furosemide, spironolactone) and paracentesis as needed. Variceal bleeding requires management with beta-blockers and endoscopic therapy. Transjugular intrahepatic portosystemic shunt (TIPS) is effective for decompressing the liver. It creates a connection between the portal and hepatic veins. While radiation exposure is a concern, TIPS can be performed during pregnancy with shielding and minimal fluoroscopy. Success rates are 70–90%, significantly improving pregnancy outcomes. Surgical shunts (mesocaval, portocaval) are more invasive and rarely performed given the availability of TIPS. Thrombolysis may be considered in acute cases but carries a high bleeding risk. Emergency liver transplantation is indicated for acute liver failure unresponsive to medical therapy or TIPS. Timing involves delivering the fetus first if viable (>28–32 weeks), followed by transplantation. Combined procedures may be necessary for maternal decompensation in previable pregnancies. Technical challenges include the need for IVC reconstruction and management of extensive collaterals. Maternal 1-year survival is 50–70%, which is lower than in nonpregnant recipients, while fetal survival is approximately 40–60%. Outcomes depend heavily on prompt diagnosis and treatment. With appropriate management, maternal mortality is 5–10%, with a live birth rate of 70–80%, though preterm delivery occurs in 40–60% of cases. Without treatment, maternal mortality can reach 30–70%, with fetal loss rates of 50–80%. Subsequent pregnancies are possible with stable disease and anticoagulation but remain high-risk.

28.12 Acute Liver Surgery in Pregnancy

Emergency hepatic surgery is rare, indicated for ruptured adenomas, hepatic rupture in HELLP/AFLP, trauma, or spontaneous hemorrhage. Rapid assessment of maternal stability and fetal viability is crucial. Multidisciplinary coordination involving obstetrics and surgery is required. Resuscitation should follow massive transfusion protocols (1:1:1 ratio) to correct coagulopathy. General anesthesia with rapid sequence induction is standard due to aspiration risk. Positioning should avoid aortocaval compression. Continuous fetal monitoring is indicated for viable pregnancies. Early complications include hemorrhage, biliary leak, and infection. Late complications include incisional hernia and biliary stricture. Maternal mortality for emergency resection ranges from 5% to 15%.

Traumatic hepatic rupture is managed according to standard ATLS principles, with maternal stabilization taking absolute priority under the 'mother first' approach. Initial steps focus on rapid assessment, airway protection, circulatory support, and correction of shock, followed by targeted imaging to define the extent of injury. Definitive management may involve operative or non-operative strategies depending on hemodynamic stability, but the overarching goal remains prompt resuscitation and control of hemorrhage to optimize both maternal and fetal outcomes.

28.13 Liver Transplantation for Rare Diseases in Pregnancy

Liver transplantation is indicated for acute liver failure or decompensated cirrhosis. Maternal life is prioritized ethically. Delivery before transplant preferred for viable fetuses (>28 weeks) if mother is stable enough. For pre-viable fetuses, urgent maternal liver transplantation may be required when the mother's survival depends on immediate intervention. In pregnancies with a viable fetus, transplantation is considered when there is rapid maternal deterioration despite maximal supportive management, with decisions guided by both maternal stability and the potential for safe delivery. The 1-year survival rate for maternal outcomes is 50–75%. Sicker patients and surgical complexity contribute to lower survival compared to non-pregnant recipients. Fetal outcomes survival ranges from 40% to 70%, heavily dependent on gestational age. Prematurity is nearly universal. Maternal life takes priority. Organ allocation does not explicitly prioritize pregnancy, requiring case-by-case consideration.

Pregnancy after liver transplantation is feasible and generally safe 1–2 years post-transplant.

Bibliography

1. Ch'ng CL, Morgan M, Hainsworth I, Kingham JG. Prospective study of liver dysfunction in pregnancy in Southwest Wales. Gut. 2002;51(6):876–80.
2. Knight M, Nelson-Piercy C, Kurinczuk JJ, Spark P, Brocklehurst P, UK Obstetric Surveillance System. A prospective national study of acute fatty liver of pregnancy in the UK. Gut. 2008;57(7):951–6.
3. Westbrook RH, Yeoman AD, Joshi D, et al. Outcomes of pregnancy following liver transplantation: the UK experience. J Hepatol. 2015;63(3):743–50.
4. Reau N, Andreana L, Schilsky ML. Maternal and fetal outcomes in pregnancy complicated by Wilson's disease. Am J Gastroenterol. 2013;108(5):799–806.
5. Aggarwal N, Sawhney H, Vasishta K, Dhiman RK, Chawla Y. Pregnancy and cirrhosis: maternal and fetal outcome. Aust N Z J Obstet Gynaecol. 1999;39(4):503–6.
6. Janssen HL, Garcia-Pagan JC, Elias E, Mentha G, Hadengue A, Valla DC, European Group for the Study of Vascular Disorders of the Liver. Budd-Chiari syndrome: a review by an expert panel. J Hepatol. 2003;38(3):364–71.
7. Bari K, Khan AR. Budd-Chiari syndrome and pregnancy—a review. J Pak Med Assoc. 2021;71(9):2273–7.
8. Faughnan ME, Palda VA, Garcia-Tsao G, et al. International guidelines for the diagnosis and management of hereditary haemorrhagic telangiectasia. J Med Genet. 2011;48(2):73–87.
9. De Gussem EM, Lausman AY, Beder AJ, et al. Outcomes of pregnancy in women with hereditary hemorrhagic telangiectasia. Obstet Gynecol. 2014;123(3):514–20.
10. Garcia-Tsao G, Korzenik JR, Young L, et al. Liver disease in patients with hereditary hemorrhagic telangiectasia. N Engl J Med. 2000;343(13):931–6.
11. Heneghan MA, Norris SM, O'Grady JG, Harrison PM, McFarlane IG. Management and outcome of pregnancy in autoimmune hepatitis. Gut. 2001;48(1):97–102.
12. Werner M, Bjornsson E, Prytz H, et al. Autoimmune hepatitis among fertile women: strategies during pregnancy and breastfeeding? Scand J Gastroenterol. 2007;42(8):986–91.
13. Lindor KD, Bowlus CL, Boyer J, Levy C, Mayo M. Primary biliary cholangitis: 2018 practice guidance from the American Association for the Study of Liver Diseases. Hepatology. 2019;69(1):394–419.
14. Trivedi PJ, Kumagi T, Al-Harthy N, et al. Good maternal and fetal outcomes for pregnant women with primary biliary cirrhosis. Clin Gastroenterol Hepatol. 2014;12(7):1179–85.
15. Bieze M, van den Esschert JW, de Graaf W, et al. Outcomes of liver transplantation for hepatocellular adenoma: a case series with long-term follow-up. Liver Transpl. 2012;18(7):763–72.
16. Toso C, Majno P, Andres A, et al. Management of hepatocellular adenoma: solitary-uncomplicated, multiple and ruptured tumors. World J Gastroenterol. 2005;11(36):5691–5.
17. Chui AK, Rao AR, Yeo W, et al. Spontaneous rupture of hepatocellular adenoma in pregnancy: a case report and review of literature. Int J Hepatol. 2011;2011:908253.
18. Fickert P, Fuchsbichler A, Wagner M, et al. Regurgitation of bile acids from leaky bile ducts causes sclerosing cholangitis in Mdr2 (Abcb4) knockout mice. Gastroenterology. 2004;127(1):261–74.
19. Condat B, Pessione F, Hillaire S, et al. Current outcome of portal vein thrombosis in adults: risk and benefit of anticoagulant therapy. Gastroenterology. 2001;120(2):490–7.
20. Plessier A, Darwish-Murad S, Hernandez-Guerra M, et al. Acute portal vein thrombosis unrelated to cirrhosis: a prospective multicenter follow-up study. Hepatology. 2010;51(1):210–8.
21. Leebeek FW, Kluijtmans LA, Knol HM, et al. Hyperhomocysteinemia as a risk factor for venous thrombosis: relationship with MTHFR polymorphisms. Thromb Haemost. 2001;86(3):809–15.
22. Saab S, Brown RS Jr. Management of thrombocytopenia in patients with chronic liver disease. Dig Dis Sci. 2019;64(10):2757–68.
23. Gäckler A, Rohn B, Lisman T, et al. Evaluation of hemostasis in patients with end-stage liver disease. Semin Thromb Hemost. 2015;41(5):465–73.
24. Saab S, Nguyen A, Bui M, Durazo FA, Han S, Yersiz H, Farmer DG, Ghobrial RM, Goldstein LI, Tong MJ, Busuttil RW. Pregnancy in liver transplant recipients. Liver Transpl. 2007;13(4):457–64.
25. Jabiry-Zieniewicz Z, Kaminski P, Pietrzak B, et al. Outcome of four high-risk pregnancies in liver transplant recipients on tacrolimus immunosuppression. Transplant Proc. 2006;38(1):255–7.

26. Radomski JS, Moritz MJ, Muñoz SJ, et al. National Transplantation Pregnancy Registry: analysis of pregnancy outcomes of female liver transplant recipients. Liver Transpl Surg. 1995;1(5):281–4.
27. Christopher V, Al-Chalabi T, Richardson PD, et al. Pregnancy outcome after liver transplantation: a single-center experience of 71 pregnancies in 45 recipients. Liver Transpl. 2006;12(8):1138–43.
28. Coscia LA, Armenti DP, King RW, Sifontis NM, Constantine MM, Doyle AM, Moritz MJ, Armenti VT. Update on the teratogenicity of maternal mycophenolate mofetil. J Pediatr Genet. 2015;4(2):42–55.
29. Jain A, Venkataramanan R, Fung JJ, et al. Pregnancy after liver transplantation under tacrolimus. Transplantation. 1997;64(4):559–65.
30. European Liver Transplant Registry. www.eltr.org. Accessed 2024.
31. Armenti VT, Radomski JS, Moritz MJ, et al. Report from the National Transplantation Pregnancy Registry (NTPR): outcomes of pregnancy after transplantation. Clin Transpl. 2006:57–70. 2006 edition
32. Glantz A, Marschall HU, Lammert F, Mattsson LA. Intrahepatic cholestasis of pregnancy: a randomized controlled trial comparing dexamethasone and ursodeoxycholic acid. Hepatology. 2005;42(6):1399–405.
33. Sibai BM, Ramadan MK, Usta I, Salama M, Mercer BM, Friedman SA. Maternal morbidity and mortality in 442 pregnancies with hemolysis, elevated liver enzymes, and low platelets (HELLP syndrome). Am J Obstet Gynecol. 1993;169(4):1000–6.
34. Rolfes DB, Ishak KG. Liver disease in pregnancy. Histopathology. 1986;10(6):555–70.
35. Society for Maternal-Fetal Medicine (SMFM), Sibai BM. Evaluation and management of severe preeclampsia before 34 weeks' gestation. Am J Obstet Gynecol. 2011;205(3):191–8.

29 Benign Hepatic Cysts

A. M. Schreuder, A. Furumaya, V. Lam, J. Verheij, F. Struik, J. P. H. Drenth, and J. I. Erdmann

29.1 Introduction

Hepatic cysts are a diverse group of liver lesions with a wide clinical presentation. While most hepatic cysts are asymptomatic and benign, they can occasionally cause symptoms or lead to complications, and it is important to differentiate between benign and (pre-)malignant cysts. Increased use of imaging has lowered the threshold of the detection of hepatic cysts, as they are often reported as an incidental finding on cross-sectional imaging and abdominal ultrasound. The most common benign cystic liver lesions include simple hepatic cysts, polycystic liver disease (PLD), and hepatic mucinous cystic neoplasms (MCNs). Understanding the nature of hepatic cysts, the diagnostic approach, and the appropriate management strategies is essential for optimizing patient outcomes. This chapter focuses on benign hepatic cysts, emphasizing clinical presentation, diagnostic evaluation, and treatment options.

29.2 Types of Benign Hepatic Cysts, Pathophysiology, and Clinical Presentation

Cysts are fluid-filled cavities that can develop through a number of pathophysiological mechanisms, including developmental anomalies, infectious processes, or benign neoplastic transformations.

Most benign hepatic cysts are epithelial-lined and arise from bile ducts. Most patients with liver cysts remain asymptomatic, and most cysts are

A. M. Schreuder · V. Lam · J. I. Erdmann (✉)
Department of Surgery, Amsterdam UMC, Cancer Center Amsterdam/Amsterdam Gastroenterology Endocrinology Metabolism (AGEM), Amsterdam, Netherlands
e-mail: am.schreuder@amsterdamumc.nl; v.lam@amsterdamumc.nl; ji.erdmann@amsterdamumc.nl

A. Furumaya · J. P. H. Drenth
Department of Gastroenterology, Amsterdam UMC, Cancer Center Amsterdam/Amsterdam Gastroenterology Endocrinology Metabolism (AGEM), Amsterdam, Netherlands
e-mail: a.furumaya@amsterdamumc.nl; jph.drenth@amsterdamumc.nl

J. Verheij
Department of Pathology, Amsterdam UMC, Cancer Center Amsterdam/Amsterdam Gastroenterology Endocrinology Metabolism (AGEM), Amsterdam, Netherlands
e-mail: j.verheij@amsterdamumc.nl

F. Struik
Department of Radiology, Amsterdam UMC, Cancer Center Amsterdam/Amsterdam Gastroenterology Endocrinology Metabolism (AGEM), Amsterdam, Netherlands
e-mail: f.struik@amsterdamumc.nl

T. Hackert, A. Gulla (eds.), *Rare Liver and Biliary Tract Diseases*,
https://doi.org/10.1007/978-3-032-15076-9_29

discovered as an incidental finding on imaging for other reasons [1]. Although benign, these cysts can grow over time, occasionally becoming large enough to cause symptoms or compress adjacent structures. Larger cysts or multiple cysts can produce symptoms depending on their size and location. Symptoms may include the following:

- Abdominal pain or discomfort
- Nausea or vomiting
- Early satiety or bloating

In rare cases, patients present with cyst-related complications such as hemorrhage and infection. In general, patients with cyst hemorrhage present with acute abdominal or back pain. Patients with cyst infection often have fever and may also present with pain.

1. Simple Hepatic Cysts

Simple hepatic cysts are the most common type of benign hepatic cyst, found in up to 18% of patients on abdominal computed tomography for unrelated pathology [2]. They are more commonly seen in women and tend to increase in frequency with age. Simple hepatic cysts are thought to arise from bile duct malformations during liver development, which become isolated and accumulate fluid. They are typically filled with clear, serous fluid and are lined by a single layer of cuboidal epithelium.

However, larger cysts may cause symptoms such as abdominal discomfort, early satiety, or bloating. Rarely, complications such as infection, hemorrhage, or rupture can occur, necessitating medical intervention [3]. Treatment is rarely needed, but when symptomatic, aspiration with sclerotherapy or surgical cyst fenestration may be performed, see below under the Sect. 29.5.

2. Polycystic Liver Disease

Polycystic liver disease (PLD) is characterized by the presence of multiple hepatic cysts. In general, PLD should be considered in the presence of more than 10 hepatic cysts [4]. It is commonly associated with autosomal dominant polycystic kidney disease (ADPKD), a genetic disorder that affects both kidneys and the liver. Mutations in the *PKD1* and *PKD2* genes, encoding the polycystin-1 protein in the primary cilium, are responsible for the development of ADPKD [5]. Approximately 80–90% of patients with ADPKD will develop hepatic cysts by the age of 60. In ADPKD, the renal function deteriorates over time, often requiring renal replacement therapy. In polycystic liver disease, liver function is generally spared. Most patients with PLD remain asymptomatic and require no treatment. In some cases, severe symptoms may arise from the volume of the liver and its cysts, leading to abdominal distension and discomfort. In extreme cases, these livers can grow to enormous sizes (up to 20 kg) and can lead to complications such as biliary obstruction or portal hypertension.

In symptomatic patients, management may consist of medication, aspiration with sclerotherapy or surgical cyst fenestration, or liver transplant. If there is one dominant cyst or group of cysts, local treatment can be considered. When the burden of disease is severe, patients may have an indication for liver transplant (see 'treatment strategies'). The optimal treatment modality for polycystic liver disease depends on cyst size and distribution. Since treatment of PLD is complex, it is best performed in expert centers.

3. Mucinous Cystic Neoplasms of the Liver

These cysts were previously classified as "biliary cystadenoma," a term which was abandoned in the 2010 World Health Organization (WHO) classification. These cysts are rare and account for less than 5% of hepatic cysts [6]. Women are disproportionately affected, and mucinous cystic neoplasms of the liver (MCN-L) tend to occur between the ages of 40 and 60. They present as multiloculated cysts lined by a layer of biliary epithelium and are often surrounded by a thick fibrous capsule. The epithelium is cuboidal or columnar, and there is no connection to the bile ducts. What differentiates mucinous cystic neoplasms from other cystic lesions is their mucin production and ovarian-like stroma. Current knowledge suggests an embryological origin of mucinous cystic neoplasms through the inclusion of ectopic gonadal precursor cells in the liver [7].

MCN-L are premalignant, mucinous cystic neoplasms with high-grade dysplasia (previously called mucinous cystadenocarcinoma in situ) or invasive carcinoma arising in a mucinous cystic neoplasm may develop. The lifetime risk of transformation is uncertain but is probably around 2%, making early diagnosis and management critical [8].

It may be difficult to distinguish MCN-L from more commonly occurring simple hepatic cysts on imaging. Symptoms are nonspecific and of little differentiating value. However, several typical characteristics should trigger suspicion. Obstructive jaundice is a telltale sign of malignancy. Simple cysts may lie near the bile ducts and even cause some bile duct dilatation, but never jaundice. Imaging features that suggest an MCN-L instead of a simple cyst are nodules, wall thickening, calcifications, septations, bile duct dilatation, and portal flow anomalies. These characteristics are, however, not very specific [9].

When an MCN-L is suspected, complete resection is advocated, similar to solid (pre-) malignant lesions. It is advised to discuss the risk of malignancy based on history, radiological findings, and histopathological evaluation, and weigh this against the morbidity and potential mortality of a complete resection. For example, performing an extended left hepatectomy for a low-risk lesion may not be justified, but a left lateral minimally invasive resection can be considered even in low-risk cases.

29.3 Differential Diagnosis

Benign hepatic cysts are generally straightforward in their presentation, but distinguishing them from other liver pathologies is critical to avoid misdiagnosis, especially when malignancy or infection is a concern. Imaging features, clinical history, and laboratory tests help guide the differential diagnosis. The following are key differential diagnoses to consider when evaluating cystic lesions in the liver:

1. Malignant Liver Cysts

Mucinous cystic neoplasms with invasive carcinoma: This is the malignant counterpart of MCN-L. It often presents as a multiloculated cyst with irregular or thickened walls. Other suspicious imaging signs are solid components or rapid growth.

Intraductal papillary neoplasms of the bile duct (IPNB): IPNB is a pre-malignant lesion arising from the bile ducts with a significant risk of progressing to cholangiocarcinoma. IPNB often contains both solid and cystic components. A history of chronic inflammation or biliary obstruction is often present. On imaging, the lesions show biliary communication and papillary projections.

Cystic Hepatocellular Carcinoma (HCC): Though rare, HCC can occasionally present as a cystic lesion, especially subsequent to necrosis or internal bleeding. Cystic HCC may be difficult to distinguish from benign cysts on imaging, but viable portions of the tumor generally still demonstrate arterial enhancement and washout, one of the key characteristics of HCC. Elevated alpha-fetoprotein (AFP) levels and a history of cirrhosis or chronic liver disease may help guide the diagnosis.

Metastatic Cysts: Some metastatic cancers, such as ovarian or pancreatic cancers, may form cystic lesions in the liver. Neuroendocrine tumors may also metastasize to the liver and, in rare cases, present as cystic lesions. These lesions often have irregular margins, with arterial enhancement and are associated with a known primary malignancy. Neuroendocrine tumors often have characteristic imaging findings such as rim enhancement or calcifications. A known primary NET (e.g., in the pancreas or gastrointestinal tract) and elevated hormone levels can guide the diagnosis.

Malignant liver lesions with a cystic component generally are rapidly growing malignancies and, therefore, demonstrate typical imaging features such as vascular involvement, solid components, and multifocality. Several typical clinical characteristics should also trigger suspicion of malignancy. Obstructive jaundice is a telltale sign of malignancy. Other, more general clinical signs suggestive of a malignancy include fatigue and weight loss.

2. Infectious Cystic Lesions

Hydatid Cyst (Echinococcal Cyst): Hydatid cysts are caused by infection with the Echinococcus granulosus tapeworm [10]. Humans become accidental intermediate hosts by ingesting food or water contaminated with parasite eggs, leading to the formation of cysts in various organs, including the liver. Echinococcal infections are predominantly found in endemic areas in Central Asia, South America, East Africa, and Eastern Europe. A history of traveling or living in these areas and consumption of meat is crucial for differential diagnosis. On imaging, they appear as in a typical septated cyst with "daughter" cysts (cyst-in-cyst lesions). Serology may be positive, making the diagnosis likely, but it is often deceivingly negative. These cysts require specialized treatment, which consists of antiparasitic medications (e.g., mebendazole or albendazole) and either percutaneous aspiration and injection with hypertonic saline or alcohol or surgical removal of the cyst. Care must be taken to avoid cyst rupture, which can lead to dissemination of the parasite and anaphylactic shock.

Amoebic Liver Abscess: Caused by Entamoeba histolytica, amoebic liver abscesses can present as cystic lesions with fever, abdominal pain, and systemic symptoms. A history of travel to endemic areas or exposure to contaminated water or food is a key clue.

Pyogenic Abscess: Bacterial liver abscesses can mimic cystic lesions but typically present with signs of infection such as fever, leukocytosis, and elevated inflammatory markers. Pyogenic abscesses often have thick, irregular walls on imaging, and treatment involves antibiotics and drainage.

Tuberculous Abscess: In endemic regions, tuberculosis (TB) can cause hepatic abscesses that may mimic cystic lesions. These lesions are often accompanied by systemic symptoms of TB such as night sweats, weight loss, and fever.

3. Vascular Lesions

Hepatic Hemangioma: Although typically solid, hemangiomas can sometimes undergo cystic degeneration or hemorrhage, giving them a cyst-like appearance on imaging. Hemangiomas are benign vascular malformations and often have a characteristic enhancement pattern on contrast-enhanced imaging (early peripheral nodular enhancement with centripetal filling on delayed phases).

Arteriovenous Malformations (AVMs): AVMs are abnormal connections between arteries and veins that can present as complex cystic or vascular lesions. Doppler ultrasound or contrast-enhanced imaging can help differentiate AVMs from simple cysts based on their vascular flow patterns.

4. Congenital and Developmental Biliary Lesions

Ductal plate malformations can occur at various stages of embryogenesis and may lead to a spectrum of fibrocystic diseases, including choledochal malformations, Caroli's disease, cysts, biliary hamartomas, and congenital hepatic fibrosis.

Choledochal malformations: These are congenital dilations of the bile ducts and may be mistaken for hepatic cysts on imaging. Choledochal cysts are often located in the biliary tree and can cause symptoms of jaundice or cholangitis. Magnetic resonance cholangiopancreatography (MRCP) can help visualize the biliary anatomy and differentiate these from intrahepatic cysts and from other causes of biliary dilatation, such as gallstones and biliary malignancy.

Caroli's disease is a rare congenital disorder characterized by segmental dilation of the intrahepatic bile ducts. Caroli's disease can present as multiple cystic structures within the liver, often associated with recurrent cholangitis and liver fibrosis. MRCP is diagnostic and can differentiate between Caroli's disease and simple cystic lesions, showing multiple saccular or fusiform dilations of the intrahepatic bile ducts. These may be diffuse, lobular, or segmental.

Biliary hamartoma (Von Meyenburg Complex): Biliary hamartomas are small, benign malformations of the bile ducts, often appearing as multiple small cystic or solid nodules within the liver. They may communicate with the biliary tree, but generally they do not. They are thought to arise from embryonic bile duct remnants that have failed to involute, leading to clusters of dilated bile duct surrounded by fibrocollagenous stroma. On imaging, these lesions are typically hypointense on T1-weighted magnetic resonance imaging (MRI) and hyperintense on T2-weighted images, but they do not enhance post-contrast. Although they are benign and asymptomatic, they can mimic metastatic disease, making it important to distinguish them based on clinical and imaging features.

5. Other Cystic Liver Lesions

Intrahepatic Pseudocyst: Pseudocysts are non-epithelialized collections of fluid, often following pancreatitis, trauma, or surgery. These may appear cystic on imaging but lack a true cyst wall. A history of pancreatitis or abdominal trauma can help differentiate pseudocysts from true hepatic cysts.

29.4 Diagnostic Workup

The diagnosis of benign hepatic cysts typically starts with imaging studies, as many cysts are discovered incidentally during abdominal imaging for unrelated reasons (Fig. 29.1) [11].

- Ultrasound: Often the first imaging modality used, ultrasound can differentiate between simple and complex cysts. Simple cysts appear as anechoic (dark) structures with smooth walls and no internal echoes.
- Computed Tomography (CT): CT scans provide more detailed anatomical information and can help identify complications such as hemorrhage or infection within a cyst. CT is highly sensitive in identifying calcifications and gas configurations within hepatic cysts. Enhancement after administration of intravenous contrast can guide the differential diagnosis.
- Magnetic Resonance Imaging (MRI): MRI is particularly useful for characterizing complex cystic lesions. Specific MRI sequences, such as T2-weighted images, can highlight cyst fluid characteristics and delineate cyst borders. Furthermore, T1-weighted images can be used to reveal a previous hemorrhage.

The diagnostic evaluation of liver cysts focuses on identifying (pre)malignant liver lesions, for example, mucinous cystic neoplasms, and assessing the correlation between liver cysts and symptoms. In general, simple hepatic cysts and polycystic liver disease are characterized by thin cyst walls filled with fluid and the absence of septations and intracystic debris or gas. Characteristically, the cysts are homogeneous and anechoic (ultrasound), hypoattenuating (CT) and high on T2-weighted imaging (MRI) [4]. Often, simple hepatic cysts and polycystic liver disease can be reliably diagnosed in the presence of these typical imaging features, and the absence of worrisome clinical or imaging features.

In contrast, if clinical features such as fever, weight loss or jaundice, increased liver function tests or complex imaging features are present, such as thick cyst wall, septations, or intracystic debris or gas, this warrants further evaluation. Liver function tests are generally normal in patients with benign hepatic cysts unless there is compression of the bile ducts or portal vein, which is very rare. If present, it is more common in malignant cystic lesions. Tumor markers such as CEA and CA19.9 can be helpful in cases of suspicion of malignancy. The differential diagnosis of cysts with complex features includes mucinous cystic neoplasms, echinococcal cysts, simple hepatic cysts with hemorrhage or infection, primary liver malignancy or metastasis with cystic component or biliary cysts. Biliary cysts are differentiated from hepatic cysts by biliary communication, which is best assessed using MRCP. Mucinous cystic neoplasms are challenging in view of their malignant potential. Therefore, they often lack the typical clinical characteristics associated with malignancy. In

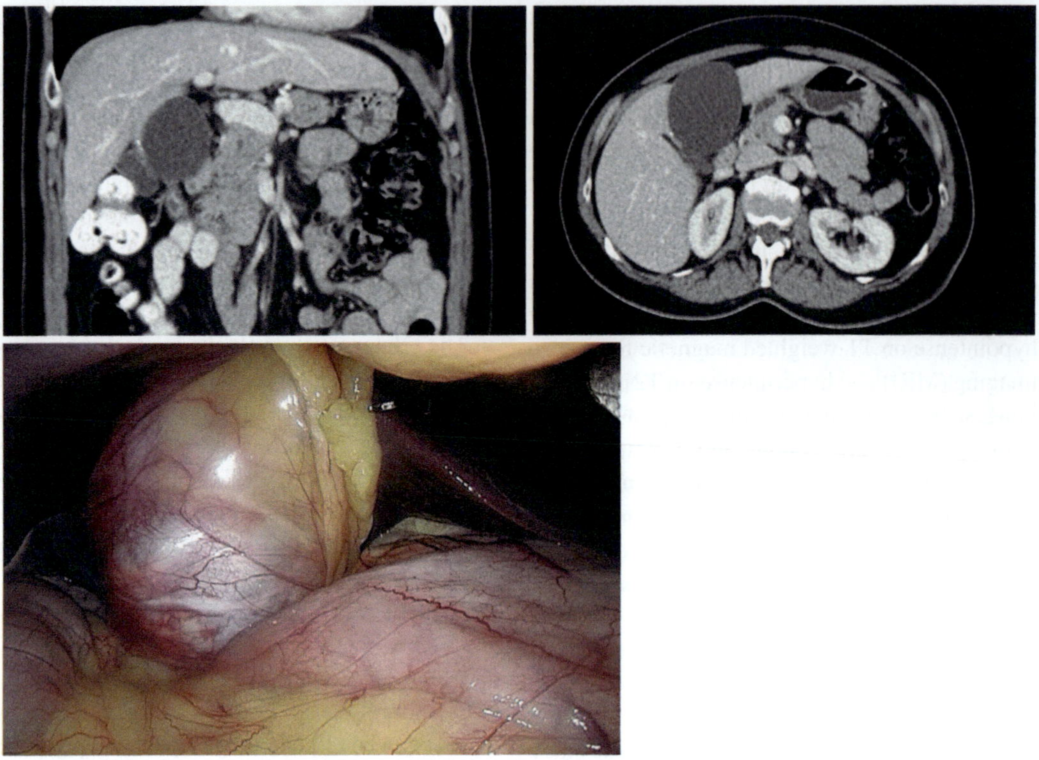

Fig. 29.1 To illustrate a common diagnostic dilemma for "simple cysts," an example of a simple appearing cyst is shown with a macroscopically unremarkable appearance. Pathology proved this lesion to be an MCN-L. The typical location, small calcification and reported recent increase in size raised suspicion and a radical minimally invasive surgical resection was performed. This case demonstrates the difficulty in differentiating MCN-L from simple cysts and shows that a thorough history and critical approach are needed. (Scan and picture used with permission of the patient)

addition, they are challenging to differentiate from simple hepatic cysts with complex features on CT or MRI [9].

In cases where the nature of the hepatic cysts is unclear from imaging studies, aspiration of cyst fluid can be helpful. Cytological analysis may identify malignant or atypical cells to confirm malignancy. In addition, microbiological analysis, such as culture of cyst content, can identify infectious cystic hepatic cysts. Histopathological evaluation should be performed in cases where the nature of the cystic lesion is unclear from imaging studies. Histological evaluation can confirm the benign nature of the cyst and rule out malignancy. Histopathological assessment with estrogen receptor (ER) and progesterone receptor (PR) stainings may help to differentiate mucinous cystic neoplasms from simple hepatic cysts. However, when an echinococcal cyst is suspected, biopsy is contraindicated, and clinicians should also be aware of the risk of sampling error.

29.5 Treatment Strategies

Management of benign hepatic cysts depends on the type of lesion, the presence of symptoms, the risk of complications, and the potential for malignant transformation. Most patients with benign hepatic cysts are asymptomatic and require no intervention. The approach to management can range from observation to minimally invasive procedures or surgery, depending on the specific lesion and patient factors.

29.5.1 Nonsurgical Management

Most patients with simple hepatic cysts and polycystic liver disease can be treated conservatively [4, 12]. If the patient has no symptoms and a liver cyst without any complex features (i.e., simple hepatic cysts or polycystic liver disease) is diagnosed incidentally on imaging (ultrasound, CT or MRI), no further diagnostic evaluation, follow-up or treatment is warranted.

The main reason to follow-up or treat simple hepatic cysts or polycystic liver disease is the presence of severe symptoms caused by the liver cysts. Symptoms may include cysts causing significant mass effect on surrounding structures, such as the stomach (causing abdominal discomfort or early satiety) or bile ducts (causing biliary obstruction). Follow-up mainly consists of clinical follow-up to assess for the development of symptoms such as abdominal discomfort, nausea, or early satiety. Regular imaging follow-up (ultrasound, CT or MRI) is usually not indicated. Laboratory tests are usually not required unless there are concerns about liver function or malignancy.

In case of cyst infection, antibiotic treatment is often required. Cyst hemorrhage usually resolves spontaneously; however, cessation or re-evaluation of anticoagulative therapy is advised. Patients with a higher chance of cyst hemorrhage or cyst rupture (i.e. large cysts or polycystic liver disease) may be advised to avoid activities that could cause trauma to the liver (e.g., contact sports), but clear evidence to support this advice is lacking. Furthermore, female patients with polycystic liver disease are advised to avoid the use of estrogen-containing oral contraceptives [15].

Symptomatic patients with hepatomegaly from polycystic liver disease with multiple small- to medium-size cysts spread throughout the liver (without one or a few dominant liver cysts) may benefit from treatment with somatostatin analogues.

29.5.2 Indications for Intervention

Invasive treatment of simple hepatic cysts and PLD is only indicated in the presence of symptoms. Symptoms may include cysts causing significant mass effect on surrounding structures, such as the stomach (causing abdominal discomfort or early satiety) or bile ducts (causing biliary obstruction). Before resorting to treatment, the likelihood of the cyst causing the symptoms should be established based on the cyst size, number, and location. Large cysts, for example, larger than eight centimeters, are probably more likely to cause symptoms [13, 14]. However, patients with large cysts may also be asymptomatic [13]. Therefore, other conditions such as cholelithiasis and peptic ulcer disease should be considered based on clinical symptoms. A period of observation can be taken to assess if symptoms may spontaneously resolve. Complete resection of all MCN-L is recommended.

Simple hepatic cysts causing mechanical complaints may be treated with aspiration and sclerotherapy or laparoscopic cyst fenestration. MCNs require radical surgical resection. Polycystic liver disease, particularly when associated with ADPKD, can present unique challenges due to the presence of numerous cysts. The optimal treatment modality for polycystic liver disease depends on cyst size and distribution.

29.5.3 Aspiration and Sclerotherapy

Aspiration alone may be used diagnostically in cases with unclear symptom-cause relations; if treatment is warranted, a combination of percutaneous aspiration and sclerotherapy should be performed [16]. Aspiration and sclerotherapy are more effective than aspiration alone, with lower recurrence rates (approximately 10–20% versus up to 80% for aspiration alone). Shortly after percutaneous aspiration and sclerotherapy, cyst sizes might temporarily increase due to an inflammatory reaction, which then subsides over time. Therefore, the effect of treatment can only be established within 3–6 months, and repeated instillation within this period is generally not advised.

The procedure is generally performed by interventional radiologists. During the procedure, ultrasound-guided or CT-guided drainage is followed by the injection of a sclerosing agent, usually ethanol. Alternative sclerosing agents include tetracycline or minocycline. These agents cause fibrosis of the cyst lining and prevent refilling. Connection with the biliary system should be ruled out, as injection of a sclerotic agent into the biliary tree causes severe damage and fibrosis of the bile duct.

Percutaneous aspiration and sclerotherapy initially alleviate symptoms in more than 96% of patients. Major complications are rare (less than 1%) but may include cyst infection, hemorrhage, bile leak, or damage to surrounding structures.

This method is typically reserved for simple hepatic cysts or polycystic liver disease with one or a few large dominant cysts, and it is not recommended for MCN-L with a potential for malignancy. Aspiration and sclerotherapy may be less effective in PLD compared to simple hepatic cysts, due to the presence of multiple hepatic cysts in PLD. In case of recurrence or persistent symptoms more than 6 months after the index treatment, repeat percutaneous aspiration, sclerotherapy, or surgical cyst fenestration can be considered. A step-up approach is recommended, starting with sclerotherapy. If sclerotherapy is repeatedly ineffective in alleviating symptoms, surgery can be considered. Repeated treatment should be guided by symptoms, not the size of the remaining cyst after an intervention.

29.5.4 Surgical Management

Surgical treatment of benign liver cysts may consist of cyst fenestration, partial liver resection, or liver transplantation. In general, minimally invasive methods such as laparoscopic and robotic surgery are preferred over open surgery due to the shorter recovery time and lower risk of complications; however, the size and location of the cyst may warrant open surgery.

Cyst fenestration, also known as cyst deroofing, is a surgical procedure used to treat large, symptomatic hepatic cysts. The goal of this procedure is to remove part of the cyst wall, allowing the remaining cyst to collapse and the fluid to drain into the abdominal cavity, where it is absorbed. Indications include cysts that have recurred after aspiration and sclerotherapy and cysts at risk for complications such as infection, hemorrhage, or rupture.

The procedure is performed laparoscopically or via laparotomy, depending on the size and location of the cyst. The cyst is opened using diathermia or a coagulation/sealing device, and the fluid is drained. The cyst wall is partially excised (deroofed), leaving the remainder to collapse. These cysts do not require complete excision; deroofing and removing as much cystic wall as possible is sufficient. The surgeon must be aware of the anatomical structures that may run through or close to a cyst wall to avoid damaging the bile ducts or vessels to adjacent segments.

Laparoscopic fenestration has a high success rate, and patients typically experience significant symptom relief. Recurrence is common but only requires re-intervention when symptomatic. Therefore, routine follow-up with imaging is not required. A step-up approach, which reserves laparoscopic cyst deroofing for symptomatic recurrence after one or two procedures of percutaneous aspiration and sclerotherapy, may be the best course of treatment [3].

Surgical resection is indicated for cysts that are at risk of malignancy, cysts with complex features, or when less invasive methods fail to control symptoms. The goal of surgery is to completely remove the cyst and any associated pathological tissue.

Indications include MCN-L in young patients with a favorable location for resection (e.g., segmental resection), or an increased risk of malignant transformation into MCN-L with associated invasive carcinoma, cysts with atypical features on imaging (e.g., solid components, irregular walls, or mural nodules), large cysts causing significant symptoms or complications (e.g., biliary obstruction, portal hypertension), and recurrent cysts after prior treatments such as aspiration or fenestration. It is advised to discuss the risk of malignancy based on history, radiological findings, and histopathological evaluation, and weigh this against the morbidity and potential mortality of a complete resection. Performing an extended left hepatectomy for a low-risk lesion may not be justified, but a left lateral minimally invasive resection can be considered even in low-risk cases.

The procedure may be performed minimally invasive or open, depending on the size and location of the lesion. The cyst and part of the surrounding liver tissue are excised, ensuring complete removal of the cyst to prevent recurrence. Especially when there is a high suspicion of malignancy, a margin of healthy liver tissue may be resected to ensure complete removal and reduce the risk of recurrence. Frozen section may help in determining the definitive surgical procedure in cases where there is uncertainty regarding the presence of malignancy.

As with any major liver surgery, risks include bleeding, infection, bile leaks, and liver dysfunction. The risk of recurrence is low if the cyst is completely excised, especially in the case of MCN-L.

Liver Transplantation: In rare, severe cases where polycystic liver disease leads to complications such as portal hypertension, liver failure, or significant impairment of quality of life, and less extensive surgical treatment is deemed insufficient, liver transplantation may be considered.

29.6 Summary/Recommendations

- Benign hepatic cysts include simple hepatic cysts, polycystic liver disease, and mucinous cystic neoplasms. Hepatic cysts have an extensive differential diagnosis, including malignant liver lesions with cystic components, biliary cysts, and echinococcal cysts.
- Simple hepatic cysts are very common and rarely require treatment. When symptomatic, they can be treated in a step-up strategy by percutaneous aspiration and sclerotherapy, or minimally invasive surgical cyst fenestration.
- Polycystic liver disease can be treated by somatostatin analogues, percutaneous aspiration and sclerotherapy, cyst fenestration, surgical resection, or liver transplantation. Treatment should be performed in expert centers.
- Mucinous cystic neoplasms are premalignant and therefore warrant complete surgical resection.

References

1. Charny CK, Jarnagin WR, Schwartz LH, Frommeyer HS, DeMatteo RP, Fong Y, Blumgart LH. Management of 155 patients with benign liver tumours. Br J Surg. 2001;88(6):808–13.
2. Carrim ZI, Murchison JT. The prevalence of simple renal and hepatic cysts detected by spiral computed tomography. Clin Radiol. 2003;58(8):626–9.
3. Furumaya A, van Rosmalen BV, de Graeff JJ, Haring MPD, de Meijer VE, van Gulik TM, et al. Systematic review on percutaneous aspiration and sclerotherapy versus surgery in symptomatic simple hepatic cysts. HPB (Oxford). 2021;23(1):11–24.
4. European Association for the Study of the Liver. Electronic address eee, European Association for the Study of the L. EASL clinical practice guidelines on the management of cystic liver diseases. J Hepatol. 2022;77(4):1083–108.
5. Zhang ZY, Wang ZM, Huang Y. Polycystic liver disease: classification, diagnosis, treatment process, and clinical management. World J Hepatol. 2020;12(3):72–83.
6. Erdogan D, Kloek J, Lamers WH, Offerhaus GJ, Busch OR, Gouma DJ, van Gulik TM. Mucinous cystadenomas in liver: management and origin. Dig Surg. 2010;27(1):19–23.
7. Hutchens JA, Lopez KJ, Ceppa EP. Mucinous cystic neoplasms of the liver: epidemiology, diagnosis, and management. Hepat Med. 2023;15:33–41.
8. Zen Y, Jang KT, Ahn S, Kim DH, Choi DW, Choi SH, et al. Intraductal papillary neoplasms and mucinous cystic neoplasms of the hepatobiliary system: demographic differences between Asian and Western populations, and comparison with pancreatic counterparts. Histopathology. 2014;65(2):164–73.
9. Furumaya A, Schulz HH, Verheij J, Takkenberg RB, Besselink MG, Kazemier G, et al. Diagnosis and

treatment of patients with suspected mucinous cystic neoplasms of the liver: a retrospective cohort study. Langenbeck's Arch Surg. 2024;409(1):66.
10. Brunetti E, Kern P, Vuitton DA. Writing panel for the W-I. Expert consensus for the diagnosis and treatment of cystic and alveolar echinococcosis in humans. Acta Trop. 2010;114(1):1–16.
11. Mavilia MG, Pakala T, Molina M, Wu GY. Differentiating cystic liver lesions: a review of imaging modalities, diagnosis and management. J Clin Transl Hepatol. 2018;6(2):208–16.
12. Frenette C, Mendiratta-Lala M, Salgia R, Wong RJ, Sauer BG, Pillai A. ACG clinical guideline: focal liver lesions. Am J Gastroenterol. 2024;119(7):1235–71.
13. Scheuerlein H, Rauchfuss F, Franke J, Jandt K, Dittmar Y, Trebing G, Settmacher U. Clinical symptoms and sonographic follow-up after surgical treatment of nonparasitic liver cysts. BMC Surg. 2013;13(1):42.
14. van Aerts RMM, van de Laarschot LFM, Banales JM, Drenth JPH. Clinical management of polycystic liver disease. J Hepatol. 2018;68(4):827–37.
15. van Aerts RMM, Bernts LHP, Gevers TJG, Kievit W, Koopmans L, Nieboer TE, et al. Estrogen-containing oral contraceptives are associated with polycystic liver disease severity in premenopausal patients. Clin Pharmacol Ther. 2019;106(6):1338–45.
16. Wijnands TF, Gortjes AP, Gevers TJ, Jenniskens SF, Kool LJ, Potthoff A, et al. Efficacy and safety of aspiration sclerotherapy of simple hepatic cysts: a systematic review. AJR Am J Roentgenol. 2017;208(1):201–7.

Maple Syrup Urine Diseases: Organic Acidemias

30

Kimberly A. Chapman

30.1 Background

Organic acidemias or acidurias (OAs) are disorders that spill organic acids in the urine and blood. They come in two types, cerebral and systemic. The cerebral OA (usually represented by Glutaric Acidemia type 1 or GA1) can have detectable organic acids in blood and urine, but major symptoms are neurological. The systemic OAs are represented by propionic acidemia (PA), methylmalonic aciduria (MMA), and isovaleric acidemia (IVA), and typically have metabolic acidosis as a component and systemic issues. Most patients with systemic OAs are at risk for developing secondary urea cycle dysfunction, resulting in hyperammonemia.

In general, both types are identifiable by newborn screening (NBS) and are on the NBS in all states in the United States (US). The symptoms can vary from a few, if any, to life-threatening and life-limiting. The systemic OAs can present prior to NBS, resulting in the classic neonatal presentation of vomiting, lethargy, decreased intake, and, if not treated, coma and death. This combination of symptoms is also seen in metabolic decompensations of the more severe patients.

K. A. Chapman (✉)
Prenatal Pediatrics Institute, Rare Disease Institute-Genetics and Metabolism, Cardiogenetics Program, Children's National Hospital, Washington, DC, USA
e-mail: kchapman@childrensnational.org

The systemic organic acidemias are mostly caused by dysfunction of enzymes that metabolize proteins, especially the branched chains.

30.2 Incidence

The estimated prevalence for GA1 in the general population ranges from 1 in 30,000 to 1 in 110,000 [7, 8, 12]. Certain ethnic groups have higher prevalence rates due to founder variants.

Isolated MMA has an estimated prevalence of 1 in 159,614 in the general population of the United States [4, 11]. MMA with homocystinuria (MMA + HCU) has a higher prevalence in some populations within the United States.

For PA, the estimated prevalence in the United States is between 1 in 105,000 and 1 in 130,000 [3, 5], but the incidence according to newborn screening data is 1 in 242,741 [4].

IVA has a prevalence of 1 in 250,000 individuals in the United States, with some estimates suggesting a prevalence of 1 in 100,000 [9, 10].

30.3 Clinical Presentation

Both types of OAs are detectable through newborn screening (NBS), which is conducted in all states across the United States. The symptoms of these conditions can range from mild to life-threatening and life-limiting.

T. Hackert, A. Gulla (eds.), *Rare Liver and Biliary Tract Diseases*,
https://doi.org/10.1007/978-3-032-15076-9_30

GA1 (OMIM #231670) is an example of a cerebral OA and is typically detected through NBS. All patients with GA1 are at increased risk of striatal injury, which can lead to movement disorders, particularly between the ages of 3 months and 6 years. These issues often arise during periods of illness, fever, or surgery, although some patients may develop brain abnormalities more gradually.

Patients with GA1 frequently exhibit macrocephaly and are at higher risk for tearing of cerebral venous sinuses, which can result in subdural hemorrhages. Recent studies have also highlighted an increased risk of renal dysfunction with age in these patients.

GA1 is caused by dysfunction of glutaryl-CoA dehydrogenase, an enzyme involved in the catabolic pathways for lysine and tryptophan. Diagnostic markers include elevated levels of glutarylcarnitine (C5DC) on acylcarnitine profile, and increased levels of 3-hydroxyglutaric acid and glutaconic acid in urine organic acid tests. Additionally, urine acylglycine testing may reveal elevated glutaric acid and 3-methylglutaconic acid. A subset of patients may have nearly normal levels on these screens while they are in good health.

Systemic OAs may present with classic neonatal symptoms before NBS results are available, including vomiting, lethargy, decreased intake, and, if not treated, potentially leading to coma and death. Metabolic decompensations can occur at any age and are often triggered by illness, fever, or psychological or physical stress.

Milder presentations may include hyperglycemia and ketones, which can resemble diabetes, as well as cardiomyopathies and renal dysfunction, particularly during illness.

IVA (OMIM #243500) is a systemic OA that can range from severe, requiring aggressive treatment and presenting with hyperammonemia, to very mild or asymptomatic forms. The severity of the condition can sometimes be correlated with specific genotypes, but decompensation can lead to hyperammonemia and life-threatening complications, making it essential to ensure adequate calories during medical procedures.

IVA results from a dysfunction of the isovaleryl-CoA dehydrogenase, an enzyme responsible for converting isovaleryl-CoA to 3-methylcrotonyl-CoA in the leucine catabolic pathway. Patients typically show elevated isovalerylcarnitine on acylcarnitine profile, isovalerylglycine, and 3-hydroxyisovaleric acid in their urine, as detected by urine organic acids tests.

Without proper supplementation, individuals with IVA can become carnitine deficient, which increases their risk for cardiomyopathies, myopathies, and cardiac arrhythmias. In severe cases, a leucine-restricted diet may be necessary. Treatment often includes supplemental levocarnitine and glycine.

PA (OMIM #606054) is a systemic OA that can range from mild to severe, with the latter frequently presenting with metabolic acidosis and hyperammonemia. Approximately 30% of patients may exhibit symptoms before NBS results are available.

PA is caused by a dysfunction of the propionyl-CoA carboxylase enzyme, which converts propionyl-CoA to methylmalonyl-CoA in the catabolic pathways for valine, isoleucine, odd-chain fatty acids, methionine, and threonine. Patients with PA typically show elevated propionylcarnitine (C3) on acylcarnitine profiles and have increased levels of 2-methylcitrate and 3-hydroxypropionate in their urine, as detected by urine organic acids tests.

Over their lifetime, patients with PA can develop metabolic encephalopathy, which can cause damage to the basal ganglia, leading to movement disorders. They are also at risk for cardiomyopathies, long QTc intervals, renal dysfunction, and optic atrophy, which may present or worsen during metabolic decompensations.

MMA can occur in isolated forms (OMIM #251000, #251100, #251110) or in combination with homocystinuria (MMA + HCU). Both forms can be identified by the NBS, though the combined form may sometimes be missed. MMA + HCU is typically due to a cobalamin (vitamin B12) processing disorder, such as cobalamin C deficiency (OMIM #277400) or cobalamin D deficiency (OMIM #277410). While isolated MMA may respond to hydroxocobalamin, MMA + HCU requires hydroxocobalamin, which is a form of vitamin B12.

Both isolated MMA and MMA + HCU can present with metabolic decompensation, including metabolic acidosis and hyperammonemia, leading to symptoms such as vomiting, lethargy, coma, and death. Isolated MMA is more likely to present with these severe symptoms.

Isolated MMA is caused by dysfunction of the methylmalonyl-CoA mutase complex, which includes methylmalonyl-CoA mutase, cobalamin A, and cobalamin B. In MMA + HCU, cobalamin processing defects prevent the proper loading of cobalamin into the methylmalonyl-CoA mutase complex, affecting the same catabolic pathway as PA. Appropriate cobalamin processing is also necessary for methionine synthetase function, and so MMA + HCU also impacts the methionine cycle, resulting in elevated total homocysteine.

Patients with both isolated MMA and combined MMA + HCU show elevated propionylcarnitine (C3) and methylmalonylcarnitine (C4DC) on acylcarnitine profiles. They also have increased methylmalonic acid in urine and blood, along with elevated 2-methylcitrate and 3-hydroxypropionate in urine, as detected by urine organic acid tests. In combined MMA + HCU, these markers may be lower, but total homocysteine levels are elevated (increasing risk for thrombosis). Individuals with vitamin B12 deficiency can also present with similar markers.

Patients with MMA may develop metabolic encephalopathy, which can cause basal ganglia damage and movement disorders. They are also at higher risk for renal dysfunction, with a significant percentage (20–80%, depending on genotype) eventually requiring therapy for renal failure.

Patients with MMA + HCU are also at increased risk for retinal disease leading to vision loss, peripheral neuropathy, venous thrombosis, and hemolytic-uremic syndrome, especially without therapy.

30.4 Workup Investigations

OAs are typically identified by newborn screening in the United States; however, this testing can occasionally miss cases, especially milder ones. Most adults have not been screened for these disorders, as newborn screening programs for these conditions began in the early 2000s, so if diagnosed, most likely symptomatic or family screening. Below are lists of common and less common presentations of these disorders.

Red flags for possible OA if not known (a.k.a. When to Call a Metabolic Specialist for Workup Help)

Unusual presentations (without other explanations)

- Requires insulin when ill for ketones and hyperglycemia, but not while healthy
- Hyperammonemia (must check ammonia) (without liver failure)
- Recurrent confusion or coma with illness (frequently hyperammonemia)
- Sudden development of cardiomyopathy
- Electrolyte wasting without explanation
- Urine ketones, which are hard to clear

There are a number of systems impacted in the OAs. Below is system-based approach to screening and risk for these disorders.

Cardiac Systemic OAs, particularly PA and MMA, are at increased risk for long QTc syndrome and associated arrhythmias, with risk increasing with age. It is recommended to conduct an annual EKG [1, 6] or to perform one prior to any medical procedure if not done annually. Additionally, PA and MMA patients are at higher risk for cardiomyopathy, so an annual echocardiogram is also recommended [1, 6].

Currently, there are no specific cardiac recommendations for IVA or GA1.

Renal Both the systemic and cerebral OAs carry a risk of renal dysfunction. Annual laboratory tests to evaluate renal function are recommended [2, 6]. For patients on low-protein diets, measuring cystatin C may provide a better assessment than blood urea nitrogen (BUN) and creatinine (Cr) [2, 6].

Thrombosis In MMA + HCU, inadequately treated patients have elevated total homocysteine levels. Levels greater than 120 μmol/L are associated with an increased risk of spontaneous thrombosis. Administering at least 1 mg of hydroxocobalamin (not cyanocobalamin) intramuscularly or intravenously can usually reduce these levels to a safer range.

30.5 Treatment

For all organic acidemias, the primary goals are to:

1. *Manage Untolerated Amino Acids and Metabolites*: Control the levels of amino acids and other metabolites that the patient cannot tolerate through diet, typically.
2. *Prevent or Reverse Catabolism*: Avoid or counteract the breakdown of body tissues to prevent the release of untolerated substrates.
3. *Scavenge Toxins*: Use medications to remove accumulated toxic substances. For example, levocarnitine is commonly used, and occasionally nitrogen scavengers are employed.
4. *Replace Deficient Substances*: Provide supplements for substances that the body is unable to produce, such as citrate for PA and MMA.
5. *Enhance Enzyme Function*: Improve the activity of dysfunctional enzymes by using specific supplements. For example, biotin for PA, cobalamin for MMA, and thiamine for IVA.

30.6 Surgical Planning/Management

For patients with organic acidemias:

1. *Intravenous Fluids*: Avoid using lactated Ringer's solution, as lactate is not metabolized as readily in patients with organic acidemias.
2. *Nutritional Support*: To prevent catabolism during surgery, provide calories, such as through 10% dextrose and electrolytes, unless the patient is on a ketogenic diet. Ensure the patient can tolerate feeds, whether oral or G-tube.
3. *Blood Glucose Management*: Be prepared to administer insulin if the patient is hyperglycemic.
4. *Anesthesia Considerations*:
   (a) *Propofol*: Patients with propionic and methylmalonic acidemia may or may not tolerate extended use of propofol due to the risk of lactic acidosis; therefore, it should be limited to short procedures.
   (b) *Volatile Anesthetics*: Titrate slowly to avoid rapid changes in mitochondrial function, especially in patients with systemic organic acidemias.
   (c) *Local Anesthetics*: Generally, well tolerated in patients with organic acidemias.
5. *Renal or Liver Medication Dosing*: Organic acidemias can impact both the kidneys and liver (particularly in GA1 and MMA). Screening for organ dysfunction before surgery and dosing medications appropriately is necessary.
6. *Cardiac Complications*: Patients with Propionic acidemia are at risk for cardiomyopathy and arrhythmias, including long QTc syndrome. A thorough history and physical examination can assist in assessing this risk.
7. *Organ Transplant*: Patients with methylmalonic acidemia and propionic acidemia may undergo liver or liver/kidney transplant to alleviate some symptoms of their disease. Both types of transplants carry an increased risk for intraoperative and immediate perioperative lactic acidosis. To manage this, maintain calorie intake through fluids, and use acetate, bicarbonate, or citrate, along with insulin, to stabilize the patient. Typically, lactic acidosis resolves within 48–72 h postoperatively, assuming no other sources are present, such as GI bleeds, hypoxia/ischemia, and brain bleeds, which can also elevate lactate levels unrelated to the underlying metabolic disorder.

Careful management in these areas is crucial to mitigate risks and optimize outcomes for patients with organic acidemias undergoing surgery.

30.7 Follow-Up and Recommendations

1. *Pre-procedure Planning*: Contact the metabolic provider before the procedure to assist with planning and ensure appropriate management.
2. *Prevent Catabolism*: Avoid fasting, if possible. If fasting is necessary, start dextrose-containing fluids, aiming for approximately 6–10 mg/kg/min glucose infusion rate (GIR). Typically, a 10% dextrose solution with electrolytes at 1.5 times the maintenance rate is sufficient.
3. *Caloric Fluids Management*: Do not reduce or stop calorie-containing fluids until the patient can tolerate feeds. When transitioning from dextrose fluids, gradually wean by first reducing to maintenance level, then to half of the maintenance rate, with no less than 30-min intervals between reductions.
4. *Insulin Management*: Intrinsic insulin release may not be sufficient to maintain glucose within the target range. Monitor glucose levels closely and add additional insulin if needed, but do not decrease dextrose delivery.
5. *Initiate Feeds*: Start oral or tube feeds as soon as possible to provide necessary nutrition and prevent catabolism. If delayed more than 24 h, then plan parental nutrition with protein, dextrose, and intralipids.
6. *Levocarnitine*: If the patient is on levocarnitine, switch from oral to intravenous at a 1:1 ratio relative to the home dose.
7. *Home Medications*: Continue or restart as soon as possible. Convert those that can be to intravenous if necessary.

Careful adherence to these recommendations will help manage metabolic needs and optimize patient outcomes.

References

1. Baumgartner MR, Hörster F, Dionisi-Vici C, Haliloglu G, Karall D, Chapman KA, Huemer M, Hochuli M, Assoun M, Ballhausen D, Burlina A, Fowler B, Grünert SC, Grünewald S, Honzik T, Merinero B, Pérez-Cerdá C, Scholl-Bürgi S, Skovby F, Wijburg F, MacDonald A, Martinelli D, Sass JO, Valayannopoulos V, Chakrapani A. Proposed guidelines for the diagnosis and management of methylmalonic and propionic acidemia. Orphanet J Rare Dis. 2014;9:130. https://doi.org/10.1186/s13023-014-0130-8. PMID: 25205257; PMCID: PMC4180313.
2. Boy N, Mühlhausen C, Maier EM, Ballhausen D, Baumgartner MR, Beblo S, Burgard P, Chapman KA, Dobbelaere D, Heringer-Seifert J, Fleissner S, Grohmann-Held K, Hahn G, Harting I, Hoffmann GF, Jochum F, Karall D, Konstantopoulous V, Krawinkel MB, Lindner M, Märtner EMC, Nuoffer JM, Okun JG, Plecko B, Posset R, Sahm K, Scholl-Bürgi S, Thimm E, Walter M, Williams M, Vom Dahl S, Ziagaki A, Zschocke J, Kölker S. Recommendations for diagnosing and managing individuals with glutaric aciduria type 1: third revision. J Inherit Metab Dis. 2023;46(3):482–519. https://doi.org/10.1002/jimd.12566. Epub 2022 Nov 17. PMID: 36221165.
3. Chace DH, DiPerna JC, Kalas TA, Johnson RW, Naylor EW. Rapid diagnosis of methylmalonic and propionic acidemias: quantitative tandem mass spectrometric analysis of propionylcarnitine in filter-paper blood specimens obtained from newborns. Clin Chem. 2001;47(11):2040–4. PMID: 11673377.
4. Chapman KA, Gramer G, Viall S, Summar ML. Incidence of maple syrup urine disease, propionic acidemia, and methylmalonic aciduria from newborn screening data. Mol Genet Metab Rep. 2018;15:106–9. https://doi.org/10.1016/j.ymgmr.2018.03.011. PMID: 30023298; PMCID: PMC6047110.
5. Couce ML, Castiñeiras DE, Bóveda MD, Baña A, Cocho JA, Iglesias AJ, Colón C, Alonso-Fernández JR, Fraga JM. Evaluation and long-term follow-up of infants with inborn errors of metabolism identified in an expanded screening programme. Mol Genet Metab. 2011;104(4):470–5. https://doi.org/10.1016/j.ymgme.2011.09.021. Epub 2011 Sept 22. PMID: 22000754.
6. Forny P, Hörster F, Ballhausen D, Chakrapani A, Chapman KA, Dionisi-Vici C, Dixon M, Grünert SC, Grunewald S, Haliloglu G, Hochuli M, Honzik T, Karall D, Martinelli D, Molema F, Sass JO, Scholl-Bürgi S, Tal G, Williams M, Huemer M, Baumgartner MR. Guidelines for the diagnosis and management of methylmalonic acidaemia and propionic acidaemia: first revision. J Inherit Metab Dis. 2021;44(3):566–92. https://doi.org/10.1002/jimd.12370. Epub 2021 Mar 9. Erratum in: J Inherit Metab Dis. 2022;45(4):862. doi: 10.1002/jimd.12535. PMID: 33595124; PMCID: PMC8252715.

7. Kyllerman M, Steen G. Glutaric aciduria. A "common" metabolic disorder? Arch Fr Pediatr. 1980;37(4):279. PMID: 7406647.
8. Lindner M, Kölker S, Schulze A, Christensen E, Greenberg CR, Hoffmann GF. Neonatal screening for glutaryl-CoA dehydrogenase deficiency. J Inherit Metab Dis. 2004;27(6):851–9. https://doi.org/10.1023/B:BOLI.0000045769.96657.af. PMID: 15505392.
9. Moorthie S, Cameron L, Sagoo GS, Bonham JR, Burton H. Systematic review and meta-analysis to estimate the birth prevalence of five inherited metabolic diseases. J Inherit Metab Dis. 2014;37(6):889–98. https://doi.org/10.1007/s10545-014-9729-0. Epub 2014 Jul 15. PMID: 25022222.
10. Mütze U, Henze L, Gleich F, Lindner M, Grünert SC, Spiekerkoetter U, Santer R, Blessing H, Thimm E, Ensenauer R, Weigel J, Beblo S, Arélin M, Hennermann JB, Marquardt T, Marquardt I, Freisinger P, Krämer J, Dieckmann A, Weinhold N, Keller M, Walter M, Schiergens KA, Maier EM, Hoffmann GF, Garbade SF, Kölker S. Newborn screening and disease variants predict neurological outcome in isovaleric aciduria. J Inherit Metab Dis. 2021;44(4):857–70. https://doi.org/10.1002/jimd.12364. Epub 2021 Feb 7. PMID: 33496032.
11. Therrell BL Jr, Lloyd-Puryear MA, Camp KM, Mann MY. Inborn errors of metabolism identified via newborn screening: ten-year incidence data and costs of nutritional interventions for research agenda planning. Mol Genet Metab. 2014;113(1–2):14–26. https://doi.org/10.1016/j.ymgme.2014.07.009. Epub 2014 Jul 16. PMID: 25085281; PMCID: PMC4177968.
12. Tsai FC, Lee HJ, Wang AG, Hsieh SC, Lu YH, Lee MC, Pai JS, Chu TH, Yang CF, Hsu TR, Lai CJ, Tsai MT, Ho PH, Lin MC, Cheng LY, Chuang YC, Niu DM. Experiences during newborn screening for glutaric aciduria type 1: diagnosis, treatment, genotype, phenotype, and outcomes. J Chin Med Assoc. 2017;80(4):253–61. https://doi.org/10.1016/j.jcma.2016.07.006. Epub 2017 Mar 13. PMID: 28302372.

31 Primary Sclerosing Cholangitis

Miah Lingelbach, Tobias Keck, and Aiste Gulla

31.1 Introduction

Primary sclerosing cholangitis (PSC) is a chronic, progressive cholangiopathy characterized by ongoing inflammation and fibrosis of both the intrahepatic and extrahepatic bile ducts, ultimately leading to cholestasis and parenchymal scarring. The disease is marked by the development of periductal concentric fibrosis, producing the classic "onion-skin" [1] pattern of biliary injury. Because PSC can mimic a range of secondary causes of biliary stricturing, it remains a diagnosis of exclusion, established only after alternative etiologies of biliary sclerosis have been ruled out—most commonly through cholangiographic imaging. As fibrosis advances, persistent biliary obstruction and inflammation drive the progression to hepatic fibrosis, secondary biliary cirrhosis, and eventual liver failure. At this stage, liver transplantation becomes the only definitive therapeutic option, underscoring the significant morbidity associated with this disease.

M. Lingelbach
A.T. Still University – School of Osteopathic Medicine: Renton, Renton, WA, USA
e-mail: miah.lingelbach@atsu.edu

T. Keck
Department of Surgery, University of Lübeck, Lübeck, Germany

A. Gulla (✉)
Department of Surgery, George Washington University, School of Medicine and Health Sciences, Washington, DC, USA

Clinic of Surgery, Gastroenterology and Nephrourology, Institute of Clinical Medicine, Faculty of Medicine, Vilnius, Lithuania
e-mail: aiste.kielaite-gulla@mf.vu.lt

31.2 Incidence and Origin

With the progression of minimally invasive imaging modalities and the progression of liver transplantation centers, global meta-analyses of primary sclerosing cholangitis (PSC) incidence have been performed. In these studies, there was a bimodal age distribution noted in the cohort of patients with PSC, peaking at 12–17 years old and again at 37–42 years old [2]. One meta-analysis found that the mean incidence of PSC was 0.60 per 100,000 PY [2]. Incidence rates within the US population studies vary with gender, as PSC occurs twice as frequently in men as in women, with an incidence rating of 1.25 compared to 0.54 per 100,000 PY, respectively [2]. Similarly to the US meta-analysis results, the male predominance of PSC is seen in the UK, as males make up 60–63.5% of reported cases [2].

A single cause of PSC is unknown, though many mechanisms are suspected to be contributing factors. Recent studies have suggested an inflammatory reaction origin induced by chronic or recurrent entry of bacteria into the portal circulation. With increasing recognition of the gut-liver axis, many have begun using this theory in conjunction with differences in gut microbiomes as a possible explanation for the origin of PSC [3]. Immune activation has been suspected, as elevated anti-smooth muscle

T. Hackert, A. Gulla (eds.), *Rare Liver and Biliary Tract Diseases*,
https://doi.org/10.1007/978-3-032-15076-9_31

antibodies and antinuclear antibodies are seen in 75% of patients with PSC [4]. Genetic factors are also strong contributors, as first-degree relatives of patients with PSC have an increased risk of PSC and ulcerative colitis [5]. Other studies and speculations suggest ischemic duct damage or environmental exposures as contributing factors, though they have yet to be confirmed.

31.2.1 SC–Irritable Bowel Disease Concurrence (PSC-IBD)

The prevalence of irritable bowel disease (IBD) in PSC has a large variance, ranging from 46.5% to 98.7%, with ulcerative colitis (UC) making up >75% of cases [6]. The mean concurrence of PSC-IBD is 50%, again with UC compromising 76% of those cases and Crohn's disease representing 17% of the cases [2]. Diagnosis of concurrent PSC and IBD is made in patients who have diagnostic features of ulcerative colitis or Crohn's disease in addition to diagnostic features of PSC, which will be explored later in this section.

31.2.2 PSC-Autoimmune Hepatitis (PSC-AIH)

PSC-AIH is a subphenotype of PSC rather than a separate clinical disease. PSC-AIH represents 6–14% of patients with PSC [4]. Studies have shown that most of these cases occur in patients without concurrent IBD and should therefore be explored more thoroughly in patients who do not have IBD at the time of diagnosis [4]. PSC-AIH is typically seen in children and young adults, within the early bimodal peak of incidence at ages 12–17 [4]. Diagnosis is made when patients have diagnostic features of PSC with biochemical or histological features on liver biopsy of AIH.

31.3 Clinical Presentation

Roughly 50% of patients with primary sclerosing cholangitis are asymptomatic in early disease progression and are incidentally diagnosed when abnormal liver function tests are examined for other reasons [1, 7]. 22% of patients develop symptoms within 5 years of diagnosis [7]. When patients become symptomatic, 20% endorse RUQ abdominal pain, and 10% endorse episodic pruritus and fatigue [1]. When PSC is suspected, liver function tests will present with a cholestatic pattern, with elevated alkaline phosphatase (ALP) being the dominant finding [1, 7]. With intrahepatic cholestasis, elevation of liver function tests can be seen at two to three times the upper limit [1].

As the disease progresses, symptoms of advanced liver disease and liver failure become apparent, including jaundice, ascites, GI bleeding, and hepatic encephalopathy. At this point, physical examination would reveal hepatomegaly in 44% of patients and splenomegaly in 39% of patients. Excoriations from debilitating pruritus may be present [1]. Elevated serum bilirubin level is a poor prognostic factor, suggesting advanced disease and/or cirrhosis [1].

31.4 Differential Diagnosis and Workup

31.4.1 Imaging

The various causes of cholestatic liver function tests are seemingly endless, including anatomic, autoimmune, infectious, ischemic, malignant, and even drug-induced causes (Table 31.1). Patients with persistent cholestatic liver tests should undergo RUQ ultrasound to exclude biliary obstruction due to various etiologies, which could be a cause of secondary sclerosing cholangitis [1]. Once excluded and if cholestatic liver tests persist, patients should undergo cholangiography obtained using magnetic resonance cholangiopancreatography (MRCP), endoscopic retrograde cholangiopancreatography (ERCP), or percutaneous transhepatic cholangiography (PTC) [7]. MRCP is the preferred first-line test for cholangiography as it is less invasive with greater diagnostic accuracy compared to ERCP (Fig. 31.1) [7]. PTC is used as a last resort in diagnosing PSC for patients who are not able to undergo MRCP or ERCP [7].

Table 31.1 Differential diagnosis of cholestatic liver function tests [1–4, 8]

Infectious	HIV syndrome Parasitic cholangiopathy: hydatid cyst, echinococcosis, ascariasis, schistosomiasis Chronic bacterial cholangitis
Ischemic	Critically ill patients Hereditary hemorrhagic telangiectasis Hepatic artery thrombosis
Malignant	Cholangiocarcinoma Diffuse intrahepatic metastasis Langerhans cell histiocytosis Lymphoma
Autoimmune	Eosinophilic cholangitis Hepatic inflammatory pseudotumor IgG4 associated cholangitis Mast cell cholangiopathy Sarcoidosis
Anatomic	Choledocholithiasis Intrahepatic lithiasis Cystic fibrosis liver disease Surgical biliary trauma Anastomotic bile duct strictures Portal hypertensive biliopathy Recurrent pancreatitis Sickle cell cholangiopathy Choledochal cyst
Drug-induced	Immunotherapy from checkpoint inhibitors: pembrolizumab, nivolumab, atezolizumab

Diagnosis of PSC generally can be made with demonstration of characteristic focal and/or multiple areas of stricturing and dilation of intrahepatic and/or extra-hepatic bile ducts without evidence of other disease processes [1]. It is important to note, in patients with high pretest probability of PSC, there is still a 30% probability of PSC even if MRCP is negative [7].

Common bile duct and hepatic duct strictures seen on MRI with >75% reduction in duct lumen are called high-grade strictures [7]. A common bile duct stricture with a diameter of ≤1.5 mm or a hepatic duct stricture ≤1 mm on ERCP can be defined as a dominant stricture [7]. High-grade strictures or dominant strictures are most likely the clinically relevant stricture that may be responsible for symptomatic PSC. Strictures that do not meet these specific criteria but demonstrate symptoms of obstructive cholestasis are termed relevant strictures [7]. As the disease and fibrosis progress and the strictures worsen, the bile ducts become obliterated. With this, focal signal abnormalities of liver parenchyma on T2w and diffusion-weighted images on MRCP suggest intrahepatic cholestasis and inflammation [7].

Diagnostic criteria of PSC diagnosis require three items: increased serum alkaline phosphatase level persisting for >6 months, cholangiographic findings of bile duct strictures on MRCP or ERCP, and the exclusion of secondary sclerosing cholangitis causes [7].

31.4.2 Liver Biopsy

Liver biopsy should be considered if small-duct PSC or PSC-AIH are of concern. If prior imaging (MRI/MRCP) is non-diagnostic with continuous cholestatic liver function tests, then there may be concern for small-duct PSC. If elevation of transaminases is the predominant finding or is greater than five times the upper limit of normal, this could signify PSC-AIH [7].

Diagnostic findings in a liver biopsy in PSC will show periductal fibrosis and fibro-obliterative duct lesions, bile duct loss or ductular proliferation, a biliary pattern of interface activity, and chronic cholestatic changes in periportal hepatocytes [7]. The presence of these findings and a non-diagnostic MRCP is diagnostic for small-duct PSC. If liver biopsy shows histologic features of AIH, such as lymphoplasmacytic interface hepatitis in the setting of diagnostic MRCP findings of PSC, then this suggests PSC-AIH [7].

31.4.3 Measurements of Liver Fibrosis and Cirrhosis

Liver stiffness measurement (LSM) in patients with PSC by vibration-controlled transient elastography (VCTE) or magnetic resonance elastography (MRE) is used for the estimation of liver fibrosis and correlates with long-term patient outcomes [8]. LSM by VCTE or MRE is currently the preferred method for estimation of fibrosis stage in PSC [7, 8]. LSM was independently

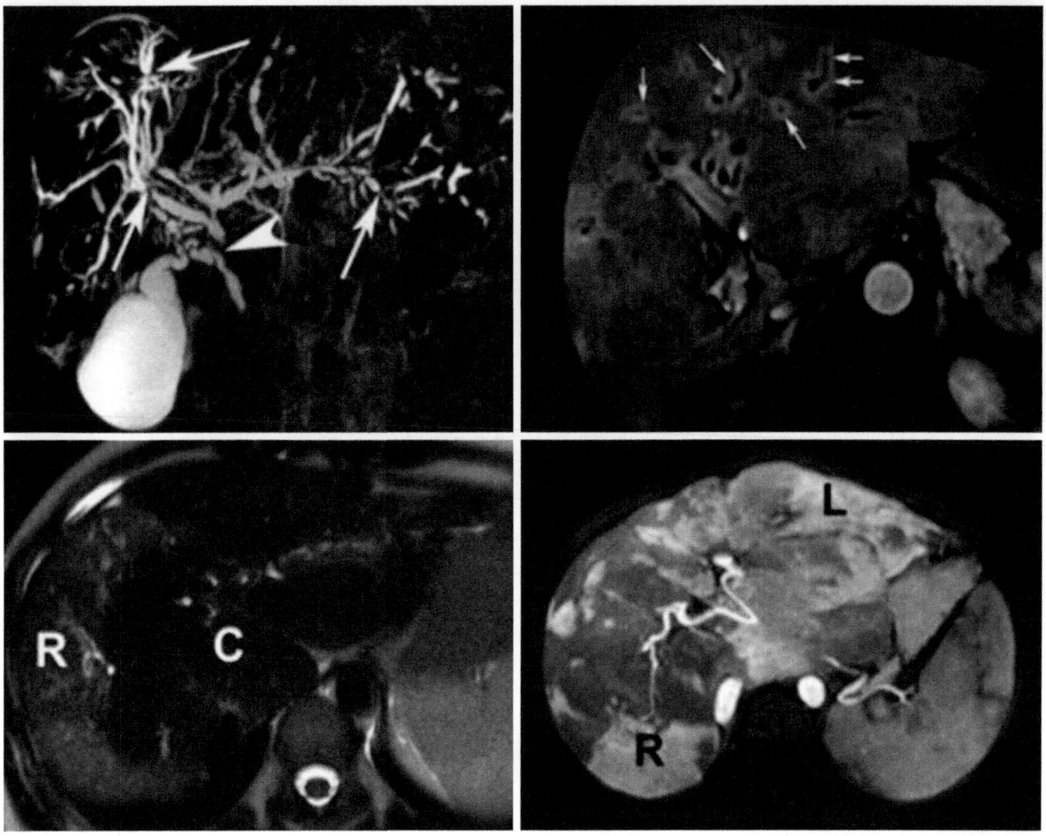

Fig. 31.1 MRI findings of PSC. MRCP (top left) demonstrates multiple severe strictures of intrahepatic ducts (arrows) and a high-grade stricture of the main biliary duct (arrowhead). T2w MRI (bottom left) demonstrates dysmorphology with marked enlargement of the caudate lobe and atrophy with high signal intensity of the right liver lobe. Contrast-enhanced MRI (top right) demonstrates biliary wall thickening with marked mural contrast enhancement (arrows). Contrast-enhanced MRI (bottom right) demonstrated marked contrast enhancement heterogeneity with high signal intensity of the right and left liver lobes in comparison with the caudate lobe [7]

linked to the stage of histological fibrosis, with cutoff values of 9.6 kPa for extensive fibrosis and 14.4 kPa for cirrhosis, and a diagnostic accuracy higher than 0.80 [8]. An association between clinical outcomes and both LSM values (especially >9.9 kPa) and prediction of changes over time has been demonstrated in several retrospective studies [8].

The enhanced liver fibrosis (ELF) test is a proprietary algorithm that considers hyaluronic acid level, amino-terminal propeptide of type III collagen level, and TIMP-1 [9]. The ELF test has recently been studied in the setting of liver fibrosis due to PSC while studying the clinical endpoints of disease progression. ELF test levels were higher in patients reaching the combined endpoint of liver transplantation or death compared to controls. The ELF test, expressed as mild, moderate, and severe fibrosis, was associated with the risk of reaching the clinical endpoint [10, 9]. ELF test independently predicted clinical outcome, and enabled good discrimination between PSC patients with and without the clinical endpoint [10, 9].

It is with the VCTE and ELF testing that we can then stage PSC, defined as the histologic progression from initial disease onset to fulminant cirrhosis (Table 31.2). Histological signs of cirrhosis are a clinically significant endpoint of staging. Cirrhosis in PSC patients is significant for LSM >14.4 kPa by VCTE or ELF score >9.8 [11]. A large prospective study found that

Table 31.2 Risks of adverse disease events after diagnosis

Low-risk of events includes patients who:	Intermediate-risk of events includes patients who:	Significant-risk of events includes patients who: (if any of the following are present)
Have small duct PSC and no evidence of cirrhosis Classic PSC and are asymptomatic with (all of the following present): Bilirubin, albumin, platelets and PT all within normal limits Serum ALP < 1.5 times upper limit of normal LSM by VCTE <6.5 kPa or ELF test <7.7 Limited biliary changes on MRCP [8]	Classic PSC with criteria in between low-risk and significant-risk such as VCTE <9.9 kPa but >6.5 kPa or minimal biochemical liver test abnormalities [8]	Are symptomatic ALP > 1.5 times upper limit of normal Abnormal levels of Bilirubin, albumin, platelets or PT LSM by VCTE >9.9 kPa or ELF test >10.6 Extensive biliary changes seen on MRCP [8].

13.1 kPa was the optimal cutoff to differentiate low and high-risk groups of patients in terms of transplant-free survival and liver complications after a median follow-up of 3 years [8].

31.5 Treatment and Surgical Planning

31.5.1 Medical Management

There are two major treatment goals for PSC: slowing or reversing the disease process and managing the progressive disease complications. There is no proven pharmacological or medical treatment that slows or reverses PSC progression.

Ursodeoxycholic acid (UDCA) has been widely studied as a supportive therapy for PSC patients. Treatment guidelines for PSC are conflicting. The American College of Gastroenterology and the American Association for the Study of Liver Diseases do not support the use, though the European Association for the Study of the Liver approves doses of 15–20 mg/kg daily [1]. UDCA can be considered and continued if well tolerated by the patient and if there is a meaningful reduction or normalization in ALP and/or if clinical symptoms improve within 6–12 months of treatment [1, 7]. Otherwise, UDCA should be discontinued as it has not shown any significant improvement in disease outcomes.

All patients with PSC should be considered for participation in clinical trials, as a variety of regimens are being studied in patients with PSC, but have had varying outcomes. Clinical trials could include treatments with glucocorticoids, cyclosporine, methotrexate, vancomycin, azathioprine, and 6-mercaptopurine, tacrolimus, D-penicillamine, or etanercept.

31.5.2 Endoscopic Dilation of Biliary Strictures

A subset of patients with PSC who have a single or focal dominant, high-grade, or relevant extrahepatic stricture are amendable by endoscopy. In this subset of patients, an ERCP with balloon dilation and/or stenting is recommended to alleviate symptoms such as pruritus and/or cholangitis [11]. During this time, these strictures should be evaluated for possible malignancy during ERCP with brushings for cytology, biopsies, and fluorescence in situ hybridization (FISH) [11].

The decision to perform balloon dilation and stenting of a single, dominant stricture in a noncirrhotic patient should be based on individual patient considerations, including the perceived adequacy and durability of response. When performed, balloon dilation of a biliary stricture should not exceed the diameter of the bile ducts immediately surrounding the stricture [12]. If a plastic biliary stent is placed, it should be removed within 4 weeks to minimize the risk of adverse events [12].

31.5.3 Extra-Hepatic Biliary Resection

Since the early 1980s, studies of biliary-enteric drainage have reported various outcomes for several years after the procedure [13]. While this may provide some symptomatic relief to the patient, it does not alter the disease course, in which continued fibrosis and scarring will occur [13]. The act of surgery on the biliary tree alone carries a risk of postoperative scarring in the porta hepatis, which could potentially complicate future liver transplantation, the only proven treatment method to alter disease course in cirrhotic patients.

A subset of patients with isolated focal extra-hepatic strictures without cirrhosis, as determined by the LSM, VCTE, or FibroScan, may consider extra-hepatic biliary resection (EHBR). Between 1981 and 2006, 126 patients with PSC underwent surgical treatment, 73 of whom were treated with extra-hepatic biliary resection (EHBR) with hepatic duct bifurcation [12]. After 3 years, 57.1% of patients had no PSC-related readmissions, and 16.2% had more than 3 PSC-related hospital admissions [12]. The 5- and 10-year survival rates were 76.4% and 52.7%, respectively [12]. In patients undergoing EHBR, noncirrhotic patients had significantly better long-term outcomes (60.2%) versus cirrhotic patients (12.0%) [12]. This analysis suggests that EHBR for noncirrhotic patients is associated with low perioperative morbidity, few readmissions, and 10-year survival of 60.2% [12].

Surgical therapy via liver transplantation is the only proven methodology for altering the PSC disease course and is the treatment of choice for patients with advanced liver disease due to PSC.

31.6 Surgical Risk Stratification and Planning

There are many risk stratification and prognosis predictors tools currently being developed in the PSC literature. To date, the PSC Risk Estimate Tool (PREsTO), Amsterdam-Oxford model, and Mayo Risk Score are the most widely used models [7, 4]. Risk stratification and fibrosis scoring with VCTE or ELF testing should be completed during diagnosis of PSC and regularly repeated during follow-up [7, 4] (Fig. 31.2).

PSC Risk Estimate Tool (PREsTo) focuses on hepatic decompensation and has a high predictive ability, with a C-statistic of 0.90 [11]. PREsTo consists of nine variables: bilirubin, albumin,

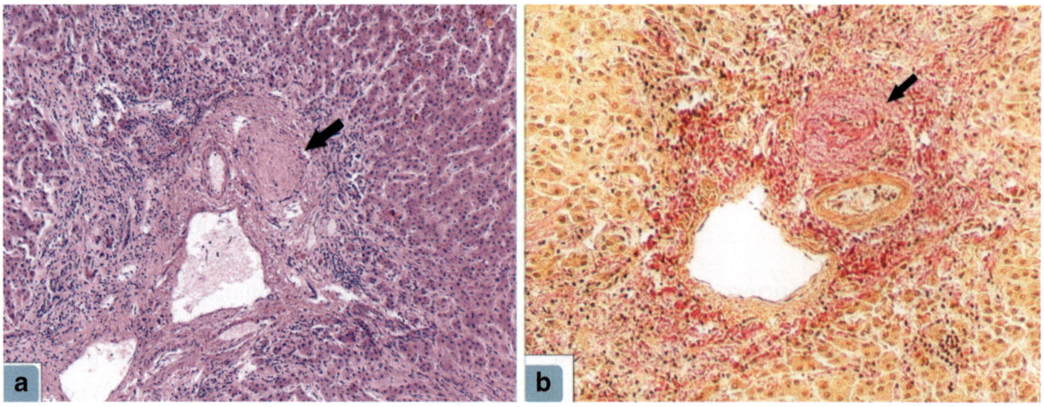

Fig. 31.2 A portal tract showing a bile duct scar (arrow) in a liver biopsy from a primary sclerosing cholangitis patient (**a**). Van Gieson stain confirms that the bile duct has been replaced by fibrous tissue (arrow) (**b**) (**a**: hematoxylin-eosin; original magnification 10×; **b**: Van Gieson stain; original magnification 20×) [4]

Table 31.3 Comparing risk stratification scores for disease progression in PSC [7, 4, 14]

Test	Variables included	C-statistic and confidence interval
PSC Risk Estimate Tool (PREsTo)	Serum bilirubin Serum albumin Serum ALP times the upper limit of normal Platelets AST Hemoglobin Serum sodium Patient age # of years since PSC diagnosis	C statistic 0.90, 95% CI 0.84–0.95
MELD 3.0 Score	Serum bilirubin Serum albumin Serum creatinine INR Serum sodium Patient sex at birth	C statistic 0.869, 95% CI 0.57–0.84
Mayo PSC Risk Score	Serum bilirubin Serum albumin AST Patient age Prior history of variceal bleeding	C statistic 0.85, 95% CI 0.77–0.92

serum alkaline phosphatase (SAP) times the upper limit of normal, platelets, AST, hemoglobin, sodium, patient age, and the number of years since PSC was diagnosed [14]. Statistical validation confirms PREsTo accurately predicts clinical decompensation and performed well compared to the MELD 3.0 score [15] and Mayo PSC risk score [14] (Table 31.3). PREsTo continued to be accurate in the early stages of the disease among individuals with a bilirubin <2.0 mg/dL [14]. This is important as elevated bilirubin levels are a poor prognostic factor, so assessing risk prior to elevation in bilirubin levels may allow for improved disease observation [14].

The median time to death or liver transplantation has been reported to be as low as 9 years from referral centers, but more recent population studies have shown it to be 21 years or longer [4]. As an increasing proportion of patients can receive liver transplantations with the growth of transplant centers and transplant technology, deaths from end-stage liver disease have decreased [7].

Liver transplantation is the definitive treatment for patients with decompensated cirrhosis. Typical transplant indications for PSC patients are life-threatening complications of cirrhosis and portal hypertension, intractable pruritus, recurrent bacterial cholangitis, and/or early-stage cholangiocarcinoma (CCA) [4]. Patients with PSC with cirrhosis and at least two admissions to the hospital within a 1-year period for acute cholangitis with a documented bloodstream infection or evidence of sepsis, including hemodynamic instability requiring vasopressors, qualify for MELD, PREsTo, and Mayo Risk Score exceptions [4]. MELD, PREsTo, and Mayo Risk Score exceptions indicate a higher need for liver transplantation. In addition, patients with PSC with CCA diagnosed by the presence of malignant-appearing stricture and cytology/biopsy, a CA-19-9 >100 U/mL in the absence of cholangitis aneuploidy, or a hilar mass < 3 cm in radial diameter can also qualify for MELD, PREsTo, and Mayo Risk Score exception points [7]. 40% of patients will eventually require OLT. The 1- and 5-year survival rates were 85% and 72%, with disease recurrence in 25% of cases [4].

After liver transplantation, there is a risk of recurrent PSC in the non-native or transplanted liver. Recurrent PSC (rPSC) in the transplanted liver progresses similarly to that of the native liver [16]. rPSC occurs in 10%–37% of transplanted patients [16]. The diagnostic criteria of rPSC include a confirmed diagnosis of PSC before transplant, a cholestatic pattern of liver enzyme elevations, cholangiography via MRCP demonstrating multifocal non-anastomotic biliary strictures, and an absence of chronic ductopenic rejection, hepatic ischemia, or donor–recipient blood type incompatibility, which all occur at least 90 days after LT [7, 16]. The rate of retransplantation for rPSC overall has been reported to be 12.4% at 10-year post-liver transplant date [16].

31.7 Follow-Up/ Recommendations

Close follow-up every 6–12 months is recommended, depending on patient stability and disease progression, to monitor for signs and symptoms of a clinical endpoint like fibrosis or liver failure, or cancer development, at which time the patient will need surgical intervention. Patients with small-duct PSC should be screened for the development of progressive disease or dominant stricture formation by MRI/MRCP every 3–5 years [7].

The risk of colorectal carcinoma in patients with PSC is 5–12 times greater than in the general population, and even still 4–5 times greater than in patients with IBD alone [7]. In patients without known concurrent IBD, diagnostic colonoscopy with histological sampling should be performed at the time of diagnosis to screen for asymptomatic IBD. If no IBD is detected at initial colonoscopy, it should be repeated every 5 years or sooner if symptoms of IBD develop [7]. In patients with known concurrent PSC-IBD, colonoscopy screenings should begin at age 15 and be repeated every 1–2 years [7].

The risk of cholangiocarcinoma (CCA) in patients with PSC is 160–400 times greater than the general population [7]. CCA can occur at any time during PSC disease progression. As CCA develops, patients can often see a rapid worsening of symptoms, cholestasis, or weight loss, while other patients remain entirely asymptomatic [7]. In these asymptomatic patients or patients with non-specific symptoms due to liver failure, an elevated tumor marker of CA 19-9 may be the only indication of CCA [7]. The combination of MRI/MRCP in addition to serum CA 19-9 levels with a cutoff of 20 U/mL reaches a sensitivity of 100% but has a low specificity of 38% [7]. Thus, CCA and other gallbladder cancer screening should be performed annually with MRI/MRCP with or without serum CA 19-9. Screening should not be performed in patients under the age of 18 or in patients with small-duct PSC [7].

Patients should also be monitored for steatorrhea in the setting of subsequent chronic pancreatitis or concurrent IBD. This malabsorptive state can cause complications arising from vitamin deficiencies, most commonly fat-soluble vitamin deficiencies. As such, metabolic bone disease has been seen in many patients with PSC. It is because of this, the AASLD 2022 guidelines recommended bone density scans at the time of diagnosis and every 2–3 years thereafter [7].

31.8 Conclusion

PSC is a progressive disorder of fibrosis and inflammation of the intra- and extra-hepatic biliary tract, eventually progressing to cholestasis and hepatic parenchymal fibrosis. This is a diagnosis of exclusion when all secondary causes of biliary sclerosis have been ruled out, primarily by imaging. Disease progression leads to ultimate liver cirrhosis and failure, requiring liver transplantation.

References

1. Rawla P, Samant H. Primary sclerosing cholangitis. StatPearls; 2023.
2. Mehta TI, Weissman S, Fung BM, Sotiriadis J, Lindor KD, Tabibian JH. Global incidence, prevalence and features of primary sclerosing cholangitits: a systematic review and meta-analysis. Liver Int. 2021;41:2418–26.
3. Dyson JK, Beuers U, Jones DEJ, Lohse AW, Hudson M. Primary sclerosing cholangitis. Lancet. 2018;391(10139):2547–59. https://doi.org/10.1016/S0140-6736(18)30300-3. Epub 2018 Feb 13. PMID: 29452711.
4. Sarcognato S, Sacchi D, Grillo F, et al. Autoimmune biliary diseases: primary biliary cholangitis and primary sclerosing cholangitis. Pathologica. 2021;113:170–84.
5. Bergquist A, Montgomery SM, Bahmanyar S, Olsson R, Danielsson A, Lindgren S, Prytz H, Hultcrantz R, Lööf LA, Sandberg-Gertzén H, Almer S, Askling J, Ehlin A, Ekbom A. Increased risk of primary sclerosing cholangitis and ulcerative colitis in first-degree relatives of patients with primary sclerosing cholangitis. Clin Gastroenterol Hepatol. 2008;6(8):939–43. https://doi.org/10.1016/j.cgh.2008.03.016. PMID: 18674735.

6. de Vries AB, Janse M, Blokzijl H, Weersma RK. Distinctive inflammatory bowel disease phenotype in primary sclerosing cholangitis. World J Gastroenterol. 2015;21(6):1956–71.
7. Bowlus CL, Arrivé L, Bergquist A, Deneau M, Forman L, Ilyas SI, et al. American Association for the Study of Liver Diseases practice guidance on primary sclerosing cholangitis and cholangiocarcinoma. Hepatology. 2023;77:659–702.
8. European Association for the Study of the Liver. EASL Clinical Practice Guidelines on sclerosing cholangitis. J Hepatol. 2022;77(3):761–806.
9. Parkes J, Guha IN, Roderick P, Harris S, Cross R, Manos MM, Irving W, Zaitoun A, Wheatley M, Ryder S, Rosenberg W. Enhanced liver fibrosis (ELF) test accurately identifies liver fibrosis in patients with chronic hepatitis C. J Viral Hepat. 2011;18(1):23–31.
10. de Vries EMG, Färkkilä M, Milkiewicz P, Hov JR, Eksteen B, Thorburn D, Chazouillères O, Pares A, Nygård S, Gilja OH, Wunsch E, Invernizzi P, Carbone M, Bernuzzi F, Boberg KM, Røsjø H, Rosenberg W, Beuers UH, Ponsioen CY, Karlsen TH, Vesterhus M. Enhanced liver fibrosis test predicts transplant-free survival in primary sclerosing cholangitis, a multi-centre study. Liver Int. 2017;37(10):1554–61.
11. Ponsioen CY, Assis DN, Boberg KM, Bowlus CL, Deneau M, Thorburn D, Aabakken L, Färkkilä M, Petersen B, Rupp C, Hübscher SG, PSC Study Group. Defining primary sclerosing cholangitis: results from an international primary sclerosing cholangitis study group consensus process. Gastroenterology. 2021;161(6):1764–1775.e5.
12. Pawlik TM, Olbrecht VA, Pitt HA, Gleisner AL, Choti MA, Schulick RD, Cameron JL. Primary sclerosing cholangitis: role of extrahepatic biliary resection. J Am Coll Surg. 2008;206(5):822–30; discussion 830–2.
13. Cameron JL, Pitt HA, Zinner MJ, Herlong HF, Kaufman SL, Boitnott JK, Coleman J. Resection of hepatic duct bifurcation and transhepatic stenting for sclerosing cholangitis. Ann Surg. 1988;207(5):614–22.
14. Eaton JE, Vesterhus M, McCauley BM, Atkinson EJ, Schlicht EM, Juran BD, Gossard AA, LaRusso NF, Gores GJ, Karlsen TH, Lazaridis KN. Primary sclerosing cholangitis risk estimate tool (PREsTo) predicts outcomes of the disease: a derivation and validation study using machine learning. Hepatology. 2020;71(1):214–24.
15. Mazumder NR, Fontana RJ. MELD 3.0 in advanced chronic liver disease. Annu Rev Med. 2024;75:233–45.
16. Visseren T, Erler NS, Polak WG, Adam R, Karam V, Vondran FWR, Ericzon BG, Thorburn D, IJzermans JNM, Paul A, van der Heide F, Taimr P, Nemec P, Pirenne J, Romagnoli R, Metselaar HJ, Darwish Murad S, European Liver and Intestine Transplantation Association (ELITA). Recurrence of primary sclerosing cholangitis after liver transplantation – analysing the European Liver Transplant Registry and beyond. Transpl Int. 2021;34(8):1455–67.

32 Hepatic Inflammatory Pseudotumor

Takeshi Takamoto and Daisuke Ban

32.1 Introduction

An inflammatory pseudotumor (IPT) is literally an inflammatory lesion that appears like a tumor but does not contain neoplastic cells. IPT is composed primarily of inflammatory cell infiltrates and fibrosis. Therefore, the diagnosis of "inflammatory pseudotumor" is ambiguous and sometimes used to describe any non-neoplastic solid mass accompanied by inflammation, especially in the clinical setting and medical imaging diagnosis. Histopathologically, IPT can be obviously distinguished from abscess scars or granulations. However, the confusion and broad interpretation of "inflammatory pseudotumor" are due to the difficulty in diagnosis. The definite diagnosis of IPT requires the excision of an entire tumor followed by a complete histopathological examination because of the potential sampling error in a needle or incisional biopsy. It may lead to underdiagnosis by examining necrotic tissue or inflammation associated with a neoplasm. Therefore, clinical articles on IPT with insufficient pathological examinations should be interpreted carefully.

IPT involves nearly all body sites, with the most common being the lung [1]. Most IPTs present as a single mass, except for a few case reports of multiple IPTs [2–4]. Histologically, IPTs have polymorphous inflammatory cell infiltration, variable amounts of fibrosis, necrosis, granulomatous reaction, and myofibroblastic spindle cells. Hepatic IPT (HIPT) was first described in 1953 by Pack and Baker et al. [5]. In addition to the liver, IPTs have been documented in the ovary, lung, spleen, lymph nodes, central nervous system, salivary glands, breast, skin, soft tissues, and the orbit since the late 1930s [6]. The term "inflammatory pseudotumor" was first used by Umiker and Iverson in 1954 because the clinical features and imaging findings mimic those of malignant tumors [7]. There is a variety of synonyms for this entity, including plasma cell granuloma, post-inflammatory tumor, xanthomatous pseudotumor, and inflammatory fibrosarcoma [8, 9]. This entity has been described by several names and histological presentations and is known as a "great mimicker," masquerading as malignant neoplasms [10]. Recent pathological findings revealed that the inflammatory myofibroblastic tumor and the inflammatory pseudotumor-like follicular dendritic cell tumor

T. Takamoto
Hepato-Biliary-Pancreatic Surgery Division, Artificial Organ and Transplantation Division, University of Tokyo, Tokyo, Japan
e-mail: takamotot-sur@h.u-tokyo.ac.jp

D. Ban (✉)
Department of Hepatobiliary and Pancreatic Surgery, Graduate School of Medicine, Institute of Science Tokyo, Tokyo, Japan

Hepato-Biliary-Pancreatic Surgery Division, Artificial Organ and Transplantation Division, University of Tokyo, Tokyo, Japan
e-mail: ban.d.11a0@m.isct.ac.jp

T. Hackert, A. Gulla (eds.), *Rare Liver and Biliary Tract Diseases*,
https://doi.org/10.1007/978-3-032-15076-9_32

can be clearly distinguished and excluded from IPT. The IPT has become a less heterogeneous and more uncommon entity.

32.2 Epidemiology

More than 200 cases of HIPT have been reported in PubMed by 2020, while most were from case reports. According to case reports, HIPT has been described in patients of all ages, from infants to octogenarians, and more than 70% are male [11–15]. Published data suggest that HIPT is being recognized with increased frequency, predominantly in Asian countries [16]. The incidence of HIPT has been reported to be around 0.5–0.7% in retrospective studies reviewing the institutional history of all liver resections [17]. A survey by Torzilli et al. evaluated the outcomes of 403 consecutive patients who underwent liver resection for a focal liver lesion. Patients with HIPT accounted for 20% of patients whose preoperative diagnosis proved to be incorrect, and 33% of cases were incorrectly assigned to a surgical procedure [17].

32.3 Clinical Features

Ninety percent of patients with HIPT had some symptoms [12]. The most common presenting symptoms were fever, abdominal pain, and fatigue/weight loss. Other symptoms included gastrointestinal upset, jaundice, weakness, and myalgia [18]. In the blood tests, less than half of the patients with HIPT had elevated levels of common inflammatory markers, including C-reactive protein (CRP) [19], white blood cell count, and erythrocyte sedimentation rate. Liver function tests may show abnormal values, including elevated alkaline phosphatase and γ-glutamyl transferase levels [20]. Cases of biliary obstruction or portal hypertension have also been reported. In general, tumor markers were negative; however, mild elevations in carbohydrate antigen 19-9 (CA19-9) and alpha-fetoprotein (AFP) have been reported in some patients [21, 22].

32.4 Differential Diagnosis

The major considerations as differential diagnoses are pyogenic abscess, metastases, and peripheral cholangiocarcinoma. Patients with typical pyogenic abscesses may present with symptoms related to infection, such as leukocytosis or fever. Liquefied abscesses have typical central fluid-containing areas that differ from the solid nature of IPTs. In general, peripheral cholangiocarcinomas have the imaging features of a heterogeneous mass with delayed enhancement and cannot be completely excluded from the differential diagnosis by imaging alone. Kitajima et al. [18] postulated diffusion-weighted imaging (DWI) with a low b value to differentiate IPT from cholangiocarcinoma because IPT demonstrates a higher signal than cholangiocarcinoma. Some atypical IPTs may present with arterial enhancement and are difficult to distinguish from hepatocellular

Table 32.1 Updated classification of hepatic inflammatory pseudotumor based on IgG4

	Lymphoplasmacytic type	Fibrohistiocytic type
Age	>50 years	>30 years
Sex, male	>80%	>60%
Serology	Serum IgG4 elevation (80%)	None
Location in liver	Periductal masses in perihilar or intrahepatic large portal tracts	Intraparenchymal nodular lesions (80%) or perihilar nodules (20%)
Histopathological findings	Plasma cell-rich inflammation Storiform fibrosis Obliterative phlebitis	Xanthogranulomatous change Suppurative inflammation Microabscess
Extrahepatic lesions	Autoimmune pancreatitis Retroperitoneal fibrosis Sclerosing sialodacryoadenitis Other IgG4-related diseases	None

carcinoma (HCC). Because the imaging features of IPTs overlap with those of other primary hepatic malignancies, imaging diagnosis should be performed only after excluding these malignancies [23, 24] (Table 32.1).

32.5 Histopathology and Etiology

HIPT consists of fibrous stroma and infiltration of chronic inflammatory cells with a predominance of plasma cells or histiocytes. The pathologic diagnosis of IPL is relatively straightforward, with lesions consisting of densely hyalinized collagenous tissue with an inflammatory infiltrate of predominantly plasma cells [25].

There is still no consensus on the classification of HIPT. However, a histological classification was proposed by Someren in 1978, who classified HIPT into three groups, namely (1) xanthogranuloma-type pseudotumors, (2) plasma cell granuloma-type pseudotumors, and (3) sclerosing pseudotumors [26]. After that, Makhlouf et al. (insert citation number here or at the end of the sentence) identified five main histologic subgroups: a plasma-cell-rich subgroup with aggregates or sheets of lymphocytes, a mixed inflammatory cell subgroup, a granulomatous subgroup, a granulomatous subgroup with eosinophils, and a predominantly purulent subgroup. The smooth muscle actin (SMA) and vimentin are usually positive in the spindle cells, whereas cytokeratin, desmin, CD34, S100 protein, and anaplastic lymphoma kinase (ALK) are negative [27]. In 2001, Hamano et al. reported elevated serum IgG4 levels in patients with autoimmune pancreatitis, suggesting a close relationship between IgG4-related immune reactions and inflammatory pseudotumor [28]. Autoimmune pancreatitis shows tumorous swelling of the pancreatic parenchyma, which is sometimes called an inflammatory pseudotumor. This finding was extrapolated in HIPT, and IgG4-related immune reactions were highlighted as playing an essential role in HIPT. Zen et al. have reported severe lymphoplasmacytic infiltration by IgG4-positive plasma cells, causing obliterative phlebitis and irregular fibrosis in a part of sclerosing cholangitis [29]. In 2007, a new pathological classification of IPT was proposed with respect to IgG4-related disease: fibrohistiocytic and lymphoplasmacytic types, as summarized in Table 32.1 [30, 31]. Features of fibrohistiocytic IPT include xanthogranulomatous inflammation, neutrophilic infiltration, and multinucleated giant cells that form lesions primarily in the peripheral hepatic parenchyma. In contrast, lymphoplasmacytic IPT is characterized by the presence of eosinophil-dominant infiltration and diffuse lymphoplasmacytic infiltration surrounding the hepatic hilum, as well as obliterative phlebitis and cholangitis with periductal fibrosis. IgG4-positive plasma cells were significantly more dominant in the lymphoplasmacytic than in the fibrohistiocytic type. The lymphoplasmacytic type could belong to the so-called IgG4-related diseases. In contrast, the fibrohistiocytic type might still be a heterogeneous group of disorders. This type appears to be pathologically different from IgG4-related disease, although cases with relatively abundant IgG4-positive plasma cells should be distinguished from IgG4-related disease with secondary histopathologic modifications. Several case reports have presented patients who developed HIPT and autoimmune pancreatitis (AIP) simultaneously, which showed peripheral eosinophilia [32] or abundant IgG4-positive plasma cells [33, 34]. The IgG4-related disease is highlighted as a possible cause of HIPT.

Epstein-Barr virus (EBV) may play a role in nearly half of IPT involving the liver and spleen [35]. Most of the reported cases of follicular dendritic cell (FDC) tumors in the liver and spleen are infected with EBV and demonstrate an IPT-like morphology. A tumor with those features has been termed an inflammatory pseudotumor-like follicular dendritic cell (IPTFDC) tumor [36, 37]. A proportion of HIPTs are thought to be secondary to infection [36]. Balabaud et al. summarized histologic subgroups of IPT: a plasma cell-rich subgroup with aggregates of or diffuse lymphocytes, a mixed inflammatory cell subgroup, a granulomatous subgroup, a granulomatous subgroup with eosinophils, and a predominantly purulent subgroup [38].

Other probable etiologies include infections such as *Actinomyces*, *Bacteroides*, *Escherichia coli*, *Klebsiella*, *Enterococcus*, Gram-positive cocci, and beta-hemolytic streptococci. These seeding gut infectious bacteria may gain entry to the liver through the portal circulation and subsequently provoke an inflammatory response. These seeding gut infectious bacteria may gain entry to the liver through the portal circulation and subsequently provoke an inflammatory response, which sometimes decreases or completely resolves upon administration of antibiotics. However, benign liver tumors complicated by bacterial cholangitis or posthepatic abscess granulation nodules should be excluded from IPT. Some cases of HIPT are associated with autoimmunity, trauma, and surgical-related infections [10].

32.6 Radiological Features

HIPT appears as a single or multifocal mass in medical diagnostic modalities. However, the imaging findings are nonspecific. HIPT displays a variety of enhancement patterns due to pathological changes in the course of disease progression. The main components reflected in imaging findings are fibrous component proliferation and inflammatory cell infiltration. In addition, fatty deposits, necrosis, and hemorrhage are considered to be the main components reflected in the imaging findings, but the heterogeneous mixture of these components in various proportions results in diverse imaging findings.

Generally, CT appearances of IPT were low attenuation relative to the surrounding liver in plain CT, with irregular delayed enhancement in contrast-enhanced CT [39–41]. Contrast-enhanced CT imaging also shows various enhancement patterns, including heterogeneous enhancement, homogeneous enhancement, enhancement of septa, peripheral enhancement with delayed central filling, and no enhancement or central necrosis (Fig. 32.1).

Nam et al. reported that the proportion of the components varies depending on the inflammatory phase of IPT, resulting in changes in imaging findings [42]. The early staining is less pronounced in areas with proliferated fibrous components, and the proliferated fibrous components delay the wash-out of the contrast agent. Several authors described peripheral enhancement in the early phases of dynamic CT [43]; however, it is not a specific finding for IPT. Enhancement patterns in contrast CT are variable, between none at all to heterogeneous or homogenous enhancement [1] (Fig. 32.2). IPT sometimes mimics hypovascular tumors due to the abundant fibrosis and shows a delayed enhancement on dynamic CT, showing similar appearances of metastatic liver tumors and intrahepatic cholangiocarcinoma [41]. Some atypical IPTs may present with arterial enhancement and are difficult to distinguish from hepatocellular carcinomas (HCCs) (Figs. 32.3 and 32.4). Koea et al. described dynamic CT findings of IPT as follows [44]: the enhancement pattern of hepatocellular carcinoma is different from that of IPL in that it is hyperdense in the arterial phase, and hypodense, with only the capsule enhancing, on delayed-phase CT scans. In addition, the portal vein occlusion often seen with hepatocellular carcinoma is from venous invasion with an intraluminal tumor present and vessel expansion. The venous occlusion seen in association with IPL is from gross thickening of the wall of the vein and obliteration of the lumen.

Magnetic resonance imaging (MRI) of HIPT reveals varying images, appearing hypointense on T1-weighted images and hyperintense on T2 [45]. Gd-enhancement MRI showed poorly defined peripheral rim-like enhancement at the arterial phase [14]. HIPT should be considered when focal liver lesions present with a “targetoid-like” aspect on T1–T2W images, with hypointensity on the HBP and ADC values higher than those of the surrounding parenchyma.

On ultrasound images, HIPTs appear as hypoechoic or hyperechoic lesions with increased through-transmission and septation [42, 46]. However, the ultrasound imaging features were also nonspecific. IPTs may show hyper-echoic, hypoechoic, or mixed-echoic findings with an

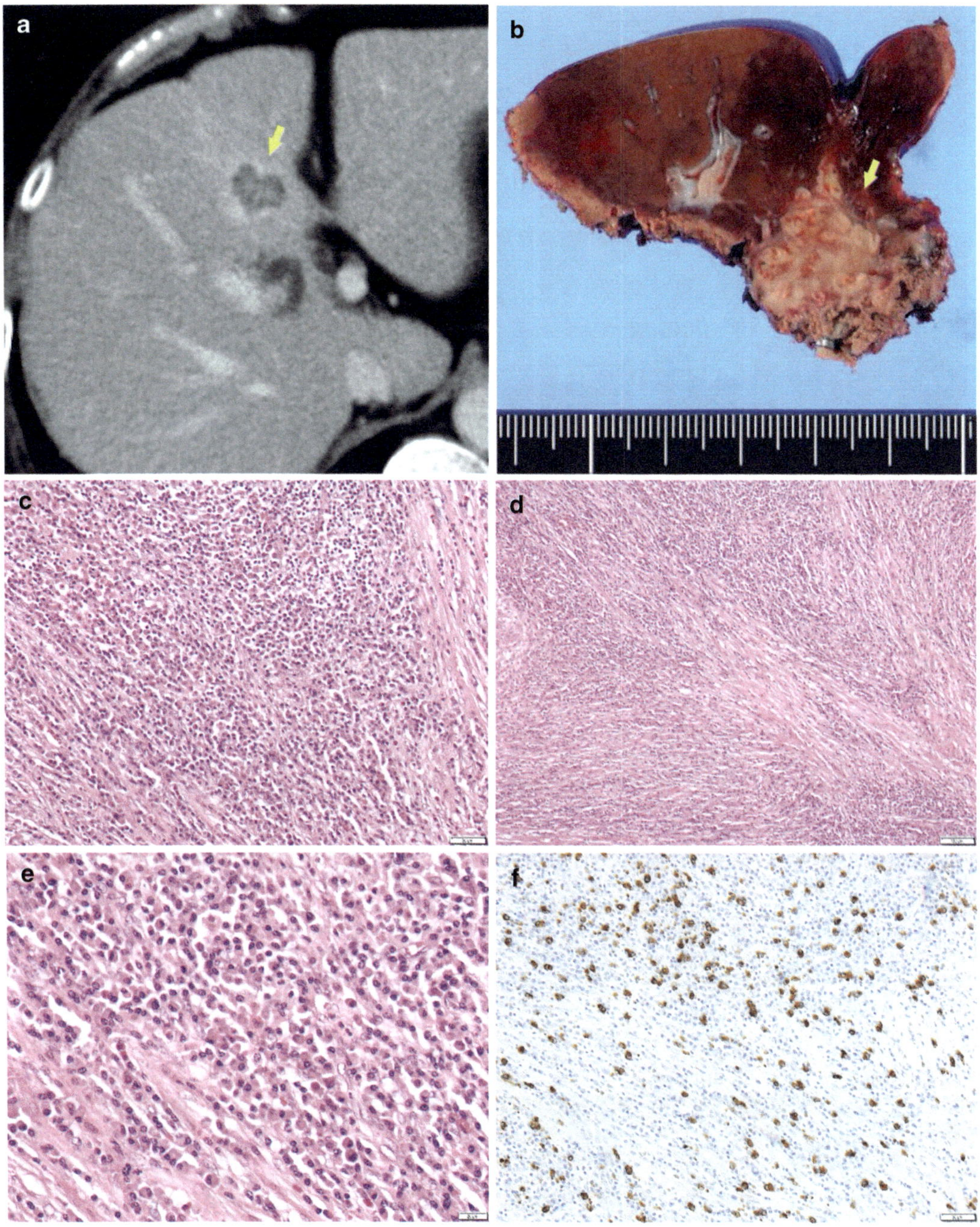

Fig. 32.1 A 72-year-old woman with a liver tumor in S4 underwent laparoscopic limited liver resection (**a**; yellow arrow). The tumor was 15 mm in diameter and irregularly shaped. It expanded along the peripheral small portal tracts and bile ducts with inflammation (**b**). The Hematoxylin-Eosin staining shows inflammatory infiltration and fibrosis (**c**, **d**). The infiltrating cells are lymphocytes and plasma cells (**e**). Many plasma cells are IgG4 positive (**f**)

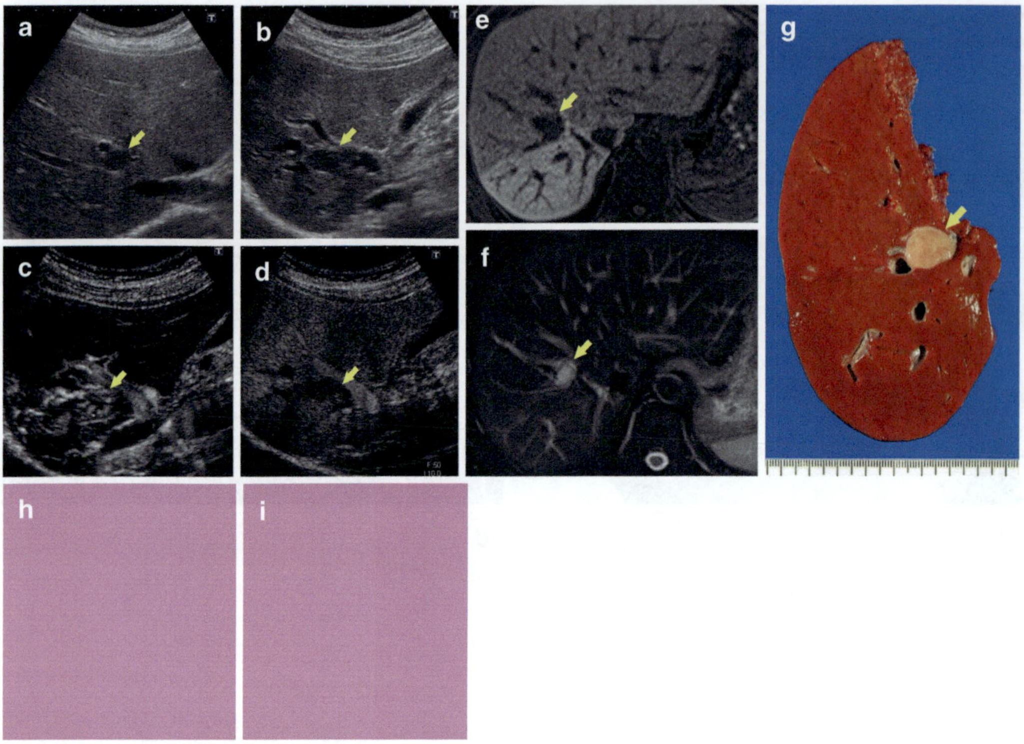

Fig. 32.2 A 46-year-old man with no symptoms presented with liver dysfunction on his annual check-up blood tests. He had a medical history of leukemia and underwent bone marrow transplantation 7 years ago. Transabdominal ultrasonography (B-mode) showed a hypoechoic lesion (yellow arrow) of 1.5 cm in diameter in the right hepatic hilum (**a**). And the tumor obstructs the right hepatic bile duct, causing the dilatation of the anterior and posterior bile ducts (**b**). Contrast-enhanced ultrasonography (CEUS) using perfluorobutane microbubbles (Sonazoid®, Daiichi-Sankyo Co., Ltd., Tokyo, Japan) shows diffuse enhancement in the tumor in the early vascular phase (**c**). The tumor appeared as a complete defect (**d**) in the post-vascular phase. On MRI, the tumor showed a T1 hypointense (**e**) and T2 hyperintense lesion (**f**). In the gadolinium ethoxybenzyl diethylenetriamine pentaacetic acid (Gd-EOB-DTPA) MRI, the tumor was detected as a hypointensity lesion both in the early phase and hepatobiliary phase. Under the diagnosis of intrahepatic cholangiocarcinoma, the patient underwent right hepatectomy and extra bile duct resection. The tumor was well-circumscribed, solid, and yellowish white in color (**g**). No evidence of necrosis or hemorrhage was present (**h**, **i**)

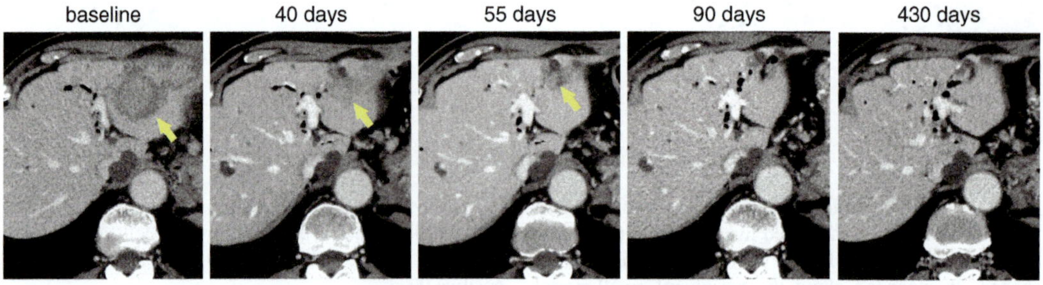

Fig. 32.3 A 79-year-old man presented with a fever and upper abdominal pain. He underwent pancreaticoduodenectomy for invasive ductal carcinoma of the pancreatic head 1 year ago. He had emphysema and a history of hepatitis B virus infection. The contrast-enhanced CT image shows a heterogeneous lesion (yellow arrow) with a low-density rim, 3.5 cm in diameter, in the left lateral section of the liver. Liver metastasis was initially suspected as a recurrence of pancreatic cancer, and an ultrasound-guided transabdominal needle biopsy was performed. Histopathologic examination revealed many foamy cells and multinucleated giant cells without evidence of malignancy. Antibiotics were administered, and follow-up with contrast CT was continued. After 40 days, the tumor shrank significantly, and 90 days after the initial episode, the tumor almost disappeared

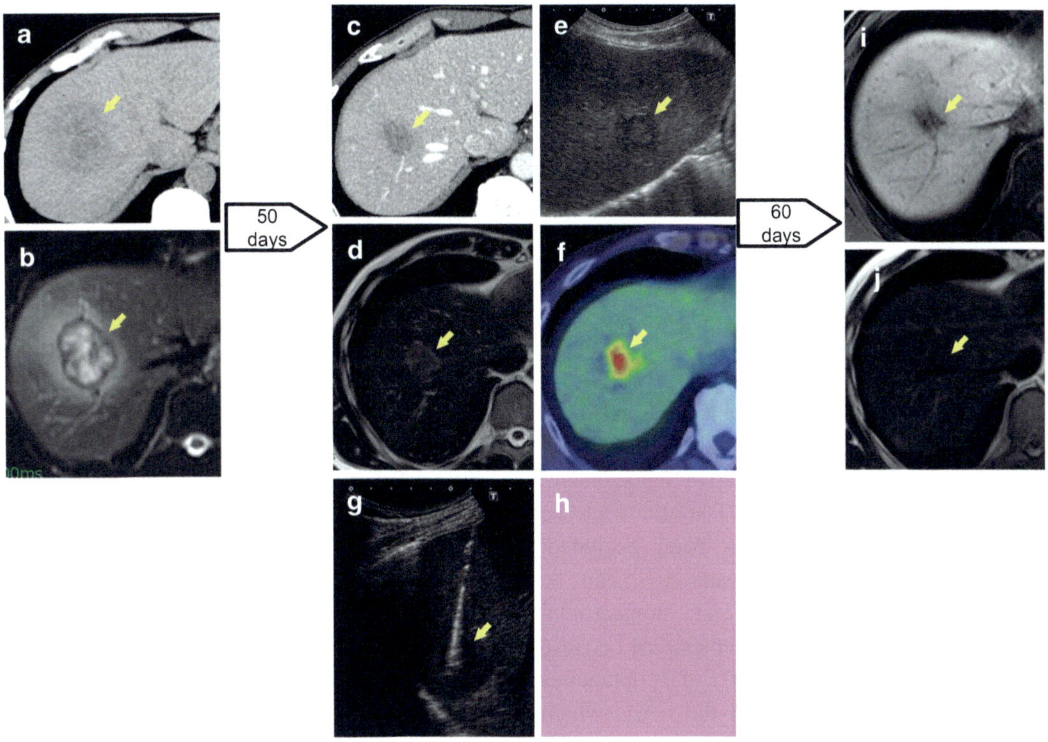

Fig. 32.4 A 64-year-old man presented with body weight loss and general fatigue. He had diabetes mellitus. His past medical history included a duodenal ulcer and an acute myocardial infarction. Unenhanced CT revealed a solid low-density area (yellow arrow) in the liver in segment 8 (**a**). MRI found a liver tumor with a hypointense peripheral rim and a central T2 hyperintense lesion (**b**). Then, the patient was transferred to our hospital for further treatment of suspected primary liver cancer. Additional imaging examinations were performed. Transabdominal ultrasonography (B-mode) showed a heterogeneous liver tumor in segment 8 with a hypoechoic rim and a blurred border (**e**). The ^{18}F-FDG PET-CT showed strong uptake with an SUV-max of 7.73. No other abnormal uptake was observed (**f**). However, the tumor decreased in size, and the tumor component changed on contrast CT (**c**) and MRI (**d**) compared to those obtained 50 days before in the previous hospital. An ultrasound-guided needle biopsy was performed (**g**), and the histopathologic findings showed only inflammatory cells and no evidence of malignancy (**h**). A close follow-up plan was taken, and the patients underwent Gd-EOB-DTPA MRI examination again with an interval of 60 days. The second Gd-EOB-DTPA MRI showed evident tumor shrinkage (**i**), and the tumor exhibited low signal intensity on T2WI, implying fibrosis (**j**)

obscure margin, and the inside of the nodules is heterogenous on fundamental ultrasonography [47]. Some nodules can show internal blood flow on color Doppler flow imaging. Larger nodules were prone to have an irregular shape, unclear margin, and heterogeneous echo [44]. Kong et al. postulated that some contrast-enhanced ultrasonography (CEUS) imaging characteristics could be a clue for diagnosing HIPT whenever the following are present: mild hyper-enhanced or iso-enhanced, quick wash-out, unclear border after contrast administration, and a small internal non-enhanced area in the nodule [44]. The heterogeneous enhancement of IPT by the US using ultrasound contrast agent (CEUS) is also observed, related to different pathologic components within the nodules [44]. Several perfusion patterns in CEUS were reported, showing the dominance of diffuse enhancement or non-enhancement patterns [44]. The enhancement time of IPT was relatively short in duration. Most of the nodules became iso and hypo-enhanced quickly after reaching peak level, which differs from HCC.

Fluorine-18-fluorodeoxyglucose (18F-FDG) uptake in IPTs varied from low to high in positron emission tomography [48, 49]. The uptake of FDG is supposed to depend on tumor cellularity, the biological behaviors of the tumor cells, the composition and the proportion of inflammatory cells, and the extent of activation of the inflammatory cells.

32.7 Treatments

Knowledge of HIPT can prevent incorrect diagnosis and unnecessary surgery, since HIPTs have a good prognosis with conservative management. If the pathologic features of IPT are known to be present, and malignancy has been excluded, patients with peripheral hepatic IPT can be treated with observation and nonsteroidal anti-inflammatory/steroid therapies [25] because there have been several reports of spontaneous regression of IPT throughout the body, which may reflect its inflammatory nature [12, 41]. Dynamic CT and Gd-enhanced MRI could provide clues to the diagnosis in patients with a liver mass and normal levels of serum tumor markers, such as AFP, CA19-9, and carcinoembryonic antigen (CEA), especially in those with clinical or laboratory findings of inflammation. Close follow-up with these imaging modalities is practically essential in diagnosing HIPT. Lesion disappearance or involution in a dehydrated pattern resembling coagulative necrosis on MRI can be observed in HIPT [50]. In addition, active histological diagnosis, including percutaneous fine needle biopsy, is warranted for patients with suspected HIPT. However, the persistence of the nodules was observed for a few years [50]. If the mass grows or other abnormal findings are found, more aggressive treatment, including surgical resection, should be taken into account [51].

References

1. Goldsmith PJ, Loganathan A, Jacob M, Ahmad N, Toogood GJ, Lodge JPA, et al. Inflammatory pseudotumours of the liver: a spectrum of presentation and management options. Eur J Surg Oncol. 2009;35(12):1295–8.
2. Patankar T, Prasad S, Shenoy A, Rathod K. Pulmonary inflammatory pseudotumour in children. Australas Radiol. 2000;44(3):318–20.
3. Yang X, Zhu J, Biskup E, Cai F, Li A. Inflammatory pseudotumors of the liver: experience of 114 cases. Tumour Biol. 2015;36(7):5143–8.
4. Ishii-Kitano N, Enomoto H, Nishimura T, Aizawa N, Shibata Y, Higashiura A, et al. Multiple inflammatory pseudotumors of the liver demonstrating spontaneous regression: a case report. Life. 2022;12(1):124.
5. Pack GT, Baker HW. Total right hepatic lobectomy; report of a case. Ann Surg. 1953;138(2):253–8.
6. Coffin CM, Humphrey PA, Dehner LP. Extrapulmonary inflammatory myofibroblastic tumor: a clinical and pathological survey. Semin Diagn Pathol. 1998;15(2):85–101.
7. Umiker WO, Iverson L. Postinflammatory tumors of the lung; report of four cases simulating xanthoma, fibroma, or plasma cell tumor. J Thorac Surg. 1954;28(1):55–63.
8. Pettinato G, Manivel JC, De Rosa N, Dehner LP. Inflammatory myofibroblastic tumor (plasma cell granuloma). Clinicopathologic study of 20 cases with immunohistochemical and ultrastructural observations. Am J Clin Pathol. 1990;94(5):538–46.
9. Narla LD, Newman B, Spottswood SS, Narla S, Kolli R. Inflammatory pseudotumor. Radiographics. 2003;23(3):719–29.
10. Patnana M, Sevrukov AB, Elsayes KM, Viswanathan C, Lubner M, Menias CO. Inflammatory pseudotumor: the great mimicker. AJR Am J Roentgenol. 2012;198(3):W217–27.
11. Shek TW, Ng IO, Chan KW. Inflammatory pseudotumor of the liver. Report of four cases and review of the literature. Am J Surg Pathol. 1993;17(3):231–8.
12. Tang L, Lai EC, Cong WM, Li AJ, Fu SY, Pan ZY, et al. Inflammatory myofibroblastic tumor of the liver: a cohort study. World J Surg. 2010;34(2):309–13.
13. Nagarajan S, Jayabose S, McBride W, Prasadh I, Tanjavur V, Marvin MR, et al. Inflammatory myofibroblastic tumor of the liver in children. J Pediatr Gastroenterol Nutr. 2013;57(3):277–80.

14. Park JY, Choi MS, Lim YS, Park JW, Kim SU, Min YW, et al. Clinical features, image findings, and prognosis of inflammatory pseudotumor of the liver: a multicenter experience of 45 cases. Gut Liver. 2014;8(1):58–63.
15. Al-Hussaini H, Azouz H, Abu-Zaid A. Hepatic inflammatory pseudotumor presenting in an 8-year-old boy: a case report and review of literature. World J Gastroenterol. 2015;21(28):8730–8.
16. Lévy S, Sauvanet A, Diebold M-D, Marcus C, Da Costa N, Thiéfin G. Spontaneous regression of an inflammatory pseudotumor of the liver presenting as an obstructing malignant biliary tumor. Gastrointest Endosc. 2001;53(3):371–4.
17. Torzilli G, Inoue K, Midorikawa Y, Hui A-M, Takayama T, Makuuchi M. Inflammatory pseudotumors of the liver: prevalence and clinical impact in surgical patients. Hepato-Gastroenterology. 2001;48(40):1118–23.
18. Kitajima K, Shiba H, Nojiri T, Uwagawa T, Ishida Y, Ichiba N, et al. Intrahepatic cholangiocarcinoma mimicking hepatic inflammatory pseudotumor. J Gastrointest Surg. 2007;11(3):398–402.
19. Yin L, Zhu B, Lu X-y, Lau WY, Zhang YJ. Misdiagnosing hepatic inflammatory pseudotumor as hepatocellular carcinoma: a case report. JGH Open. 2017;1(2):76–8.
20. Horiuchi R, Uchida T, Kojima T, Shikata T. Inflammatory pseudotumor of the liver. Clinicopathologic study and review of the literature. Cancer. 1990;65(7):1583–90.
21. Ogawa T, Yokoi H, Kawarada Y. A case of inflammatory pseudotumor of the liver causing elevated serum CA19-9 levels. Am J Gastroenterol. 1998;93(12):2551–5.
22. Shirai Y, Shiba H, Fujiwara Y, Eto K, Misawa T, Yanaga K. Hepatic inflammatory pseudotumor with elevated serum CA19-9 level mimicking liver metastasis from rectal cancer: report of a case. Int Surg. 2013;98(4):324–9.
23. Ahn KS, Kang KJ, Kim YH, Lim TJ, Jung HR, Kang YN, et al. Inflammatory pseudotumors mimicking intrahepatic cholangiocarcinoma of the liver; IgG4-positivity and its clinical significance. J Hepatobiliary Pancreat Sci. 2012;19(4):405–12.
24. Wu CH, Chiu NC, Yeh YC, Kuo Y, Yu SS, Weng CY, et al. Uncommon liver tumors: case report and literature review. Medicine (Baltimore). 2016;95(39):e4952.
25. Koea JB, Broadhurst GW, Rodgers MS, McCall JL. Inflammatory pseudotumor of the liver: demographics, diagnosis, and the case for nonoperative management. J Am Coll Surg. 2003;196(2):226–35.
26. Someren A. "Inflammatory pseudotumor" of liver with occlusive phlebitis: report of a case in a child and review of the literature. Am J Clin Pathol. 1978;69(2):176–81.
27. Makhlouf H, Fanburg-Smith J, Wang G, Mujahid M, Vesoulis Z, Goodman Z, editors. Inflammatory pseudotumor (IPF) of liver: an entity distinct from inflammatory myofibroblastic tumor (IMFT): a clinicopathologic, immunohistochemical, and molecular genetic study of 145 cases. Laboratory investigation. New York: Nature Publishing Group; 2011.
28. Hamano H, Kawa S, Horiuchi A, Unno H, Furuya N, Akamatsu T, et al. High serum IgG4 concentrations in patients with sclerosing pancreatitis. N Engl J Med. 2001;344(10):732–8.
29. Zen Y, Harada K, Sasaki M, Sato Y, Tsuneyama K, Haratake J, et al. IgG4-related sclerosing cholangitis with and without hepatic inflammatory pseudotumor, and sclerosing pancreatitis-associated sclerosing cholangitis: do they belong to a spectrum of sclerosing pancreatitis? Am J Surg Pathol. 2004;28(9):1193–203.
30. Zen Y, Fujii T, Sato Y, Masuda S, Nakanuma Y. Pathological classification of hepatic inflammatory pseudotumor with respect to IgG4-related disease. Mod Pathol. 2007;20(8):884–94.
31. Torbenson M, Zen Y, Yeh M. Tumors of the liver, AFIP Atlas of tumor pathology series 4. Washington, DC: American Registry of Pathology; 2018. p. 336–40.
32. Sasahira N, Kawabe T, Nakamura A, Shimura K, Shimura H, Itobayashi E, et al. Inflammatory pseudotumor of the liver and peripheral eosinophilia in autoimmune pancreatitis. World J Gastroenterol. 2005;11(6):922–5.
33. Kanno A, Satoh K, Kimura K, Masamune A, Asakura T, Unno M, et al. Autoimmune pancreatitis with hepatic inflammatory pseudotumor. Pancreas. 2005;31(4):420–3.
34. Klöppel G, Sipos B, Zamboni G, Kojima M, Morohoshi T. Autoimmune pancreatitis: histo- and immunopathological features. J Gastroenterol. 2007;42(Suppl 18):28–31.
35. Arber DA, Kamel OW, van de Rijn M, Davis RE, Medeiros LJ, Jaffe ES, et al. Frequent presence of the Epstein-Barr virus in inflammatory pseudotumor. Hum Pathol. 1995;26(10):1093–8.
36. You Y, Shao H, Bui K, Bui M, Klapman J, Cui Q, et al. Epstein-Barr virus positive inflammatory pseudotumor of the liver: report of a challenging case and review of the literature. Ann Clin Lab Sci. 2014;44(4):489–98.
37. Li XQ, Cheuk W, Lam PW, Wang Z, Loong F, Yeong ML, et al. Inflammatory pseudotumor-like follicular dendritic cell tumor of liver and spleen: granulomatous and eosinophil-rich variants mimicking inflammatory or infective lesions. Am J Surg Pathol. 2014;38(5):646–53.
38. Balabaud C, Bioulac-Sage P, Goodman ZD, Makhlouf HR. Inflammatory pseudotumor of the liver: a rare but distinct tumor-like lesion. Gastroenterol Hepatol (N Y). 2012;8(9):633–4.
39. Materne R, Van Beers BE, Gigot J-F, Horsmans Y, Lacrosse M, Pringot J. Inflammatory pseudotumor of the liver: MRI with mangafodipir trisodium. J Comput Assist Tomogr. 1998;22(1):82–4.
40. Sakai T, Shiraki K, Yamamoto N, Kawakita T, Ohmori S, Itoh I, et al. Diagnosis of inflammatory pseudotumor of the liver. Int J Mol Med. 2002;10(3):281–5.

41. Yamaguchi J, Sakamoto Y, Sano T, Shimada K, Kosuge T. Spontaneous regression of inflammatory pseudotumor of the liver: report of three cases. Surg Today. 2007;37(6):525–9.
42. Nam KJ, Kang HK, Lim JH. Inflammatory pseudotumor of the liver: CT and sonographic findings. AJR Am J Roentgenol. 1996;167(2):485–7.
43. Seki S, Kitada T, Sakaguchi H, Iwai S, Hirohashi K, Higaki I, et al. A clinicopathological study of inflammatory pseudotumors of the liver with special reference to vessels. Hepato-Gastroenterology. 2004;51(58):1140–3.
44. Kong WT, Wang WP, Shen HY, Xue HY, Liu CR, Huang DQ, et al. Hepatic inflammatory pseudotumor mimicking malignancy: the value of differential diagnosis on contrast enhanced ultrasound. Med Ultrason. 2021;23(1):15–21.
45. Yan FH, Zhou KR, Jiang YP, Shi WB. Inflammatory pseudotumor of the liver: 13 cases of MRI findings. World J Gastroenterol. 2001;7(3):422–4.
46. Celik H, Özdemir H, Yücel C, Gultekin S, Oktar SO, Arac M. Characterization of hyperechoic focal liver lesions: quantitative evaluation with pulse inversion harmonic imaging in the late phase of levovist. J Ultrasound Med. 2005;24(1):39–47.
47. Saito M, Seo Y, Yano Y, Miki A, Morinaga Y, Itoh T, et al. Sonazoid-enhanced ultrasonography and Ga-EOB-DTPA-enhanced MRI of hepatic inflammatory pseudotumor: a case report. Intern Med. 2012;51(7):723–6.
48. Kawamura E, Habu D, Tsushima H, Torii K, Kawabe J, Ohsawa M, et al. A case of hepatic inflammatory pseudotumor identified by FDG-PET. Ann Nucl Med. 2006;20(4):321–3.
49. Dong A, Wang Y, Dong H, Gong J, Cheng C, Zuo C, et al. Inflammatory myofibroblastic tumor: FDG PET/CT findings with pathologic correlation. Clin Nucl Med. 2014;39(2):113–21.
50. Calistri L, Maraghelli D, Nardi C, Vidali S, Rastrelli V, Crocetti L, et al. Magnetic resonance imaging of inflammatory pseudotumor of the liver: a 2021 systematic literature update and series presentation. Abdom Radiol (NY). 2022;47(8):2795–810.
51. Oh K, Hwang S, Ahn CS, Kim KH, Moon DB, Ha TY, et al. Clinicopathological features and postresection outcomes of inflammatory pseudotumor of the liver. Ann Hepatobiliary Pancreat Surg. 2021;25(1):34–8.

GPSR Compliance

The European Union's (EU) General Product Safety Regulation (GPSR) is a set of rules that requires consumer products to be safe and our obligations to ensure this.

If you have any concerns about our products, you can contact us on ProductSafety@springernature.com

In case Publisher is established outside the EU, the EU authorized representative is:

Springer Nature Customer Service Center GmbH
Europaplatz 3
69115 Heidelberg, Germany

Batch number: 10732799

Printed by Printforce, the Netherlands